FUNDAMENTALS AND FRONTIERS OF MEDICAL EDUCATION AND DECISION-MAKING, VOLUME 2

This volume examines education and decision-making in the health professions across diverse implementation contexts, exploring the negotiation between biomedical Western medicine and local traditions, practices, or constraints. Theoretical approaches such as collective competence, socioecology, and heterarchy provide lenses to understand how systems adapt and evolve. The result is a comparative exploration of how medical education reflects broader social, cultural, and political forces.

Combining both theory and case studies, the volume identifies factors that have contributed to the success and failure of medical innovations around the world. Drawing on cases from Canada, Nepal, Ukraine, sub-Saharan Africa, India, Brazil, Guatemala, and East Asia, the chapters explore how history, culture, and crises shape the development and delivery of medical education. Multiple chapters examine the continuing influence of colonial legacies, whether through the marginalization of Indigenous peoples in Canada and Guatemala, the influence of caste hierarchies in India, or structural inequalities in sub-Saharan Africa. Others focus on curricular innovations, from the integration of medical humanities in Nepal to ethics training in Canadian neonatal care, and from traditional medicine in Brazil and East Asia to adaptive learning in contexts of war and displacement.

It is essential reading for academics, clinicians, and administrators in medical education as well as students in psychological and cognitive sciences.

Jordan Richard Schoenherr is an Adjunct Research Professor in the Department of Psychology, and a member of the Institute for Data Science at Carleton University, Canada, Adjunct Fellow, School of Systems & Computing, University of New South Wales, Australia, Co-Editor-in-Chief, IEEE Transactions on Technology and Society.

FUNDAMENTALS AND FRONTIERS OF MEDICAL EDUCATION AND DECISION-MAKING, VOLUME 2

Innovation, Implementation, and Translational Research

Edited by Jordan Richard Schoenherr

Routledge
Taylor & Francis Group
NEW YORK AND LONDON

Designed cover image: Donguibogam by the royal physician Heo Jun. (1613) National Museum of Korea, National Institutes of Health, and Alex Hu (@alexandwich) via Unsplash

First published 2027
by Routledge
605 Third Avenue, New York, NY 10158

and by Routledge
4 Park Square, Milton Park, Abingdon, Oxon, OX14 4RN

Routledge is an imprint of the Taylor & Francis Group, an informa business

ISBN: 9781032806877 (hbk)
ISBN: 9781032806853 (pbk)
ISBN: 9781003498155 (ebk)

DOI: 10.4324/9781003498155

Typeset in Times New Roman
by Newgen Publishing UK

For my sister and brother

CONTENTS

SECTION 2
Implementation Case Studies: Institutional and Nations Perspectives 189

ABOUT THE EDITOR

Jordan Richard Schoenherr, PhD, is Adjunct Research Professor in the Department of Psychology and a member of the Institute for Data Science at Carleton University and a research fellow in the School of Systems & Computing at University of New South Wales. He is currently the Co-Editor-in-Chief of *IEEE Transactions on Technology and Society*. Dr. Schoenherr's research and writing focuses on the cognitive psychology of decision-making, learning, and metacognition, history and logic of psychometrics, and the sociotechnical system. Prior to the receipt of his PhD, he began his postdoctoral research in medical education at the University of Ottawa Skills and Simulation Centre. In addition to his academic duties, he has worked for, and consulted with, Health Canada (Office of the Chief Scientist) and the Public Health Agency of Canada (Ombudsman Integrity and Resolution Office) on health and science policy, scientific communication, and ethical decision-making. He is the author of the *Ethics of Artificial Intelligence from Popular Science to Cognitive Science, Fundamentals and Frontiers in Medical Education and Decision-Making*, and numerous chapters, proceedings, and peer-reviewed articles that examine applications of decision-making to health, ethics, and cybersecurity.

CONTRIBUTORS

Akinyele O. Adisa, BDS, FMCDS, is Reader in the Oral Pathology Department, Faculty of Dentistry, University of Ibadan, and Oral Pathologist consulting at the University College Hospital, Ibadan, Nigeria. He is also Associate Research Fellow of the Frankfurt Orofacial Regenerative Medicine Laboratory, Frankfurt, Germany. He was a visiting researcher to the Oral Pathology Department of the School of Dentistry, Sheffield, UK, in 2016. He is a sub-editor for the *African Journal of Medicine and Medical Sciences* and serves as a reviewer for several local and international journals.

Rachel Aparecida Ferreira Fernandes, MD, graduated from the Federal University of Minas Gerais, Brazil (UFMG), specializing in Pediatrics and Hematology, with credentials recognized by the Ministry of Education. She holds a master's and a PhD in Hematology and Medical Education from UFMG. Currently, she serves as Associate Professor in the Department of Pediatrics at the Faculty of Medicine, UFMG, and coordinates the outpatient rotation for Hematology residents at the Hospital das Clínicas, UFMG. She led the Department of Pediatrics during the implementation of the new medical curriculum in Brazil. In the field of medical education, her research focuses on clinical reasoning, formative assessment, and feedback literacy. In the field of Hematology, her research focuses on childhood leukemia, nutritional anemias, and Gaucher disease.

Catherine B. Chan is a settler researcher of Irish, English, French, and German ancestry. She is forever grateful to women from the Tk'emlúps First Nation for delivering her great-grandmother, Rose Schubert who was the first White baby born in the southern interior of British Columbia. Rose's parents and siblings traversed the prairies to seek Cariboo Gold. Their party relied on meat supplied by

First Nations hunters and nearly starved because the people of the North Thompson River had been wiped out by a smallpox epidemic. Catherine is married to Patrick Chan, whose Cree grandmother Caroline McNabb was born into the George Gordon First Nation in Treaty 4 Territory (present-day Saskatchewan) in 1910. She is privileged to author this work with colleagues of diverse lived experiences.

Thierry Daboval is a dedicated, fully trained Royal College of Physicians and Surgeons of Canada (RCPSC) neonatologist and pediatrician. He also holds Full Professor academic rank. Dr. Daboval earned his MD from the University of Sherbrooke in 1992, followed by specializations in pediatrics at the University of Montreal, Ste-Justine, and the RCPSC. In 2013, he completed a Master of Science in Clinical Sciences from the University of Quebec. Dr. Daboval has served in various academic and leadership positions since 1998, initially at the University of Sherbrooke and later at the University of Ottawa, where he became Full Professor in 2021. He has also been Chief of Staff at Montfort Academic Hospital and previously served as Site Chief at the Children's Hospital of Eastern Ontario (CHEO), contributing significantly to neonatal care and medical education. His research interests include ethics and communication in neonatology. Dr. Daboval's work in shared decision-making processes has been recognized and incorporated into the Canadian Pediatric Society's guidelines for counseling mothers at risk of preterm delivery and been recognized as one of the ethical models in neonatology, communicative ethics, and the ethics of choice architecture.

José Eduardo Baroneza, MD, PhD, from University of São Paulo (USP), graduated in Biomedical Sciences from State University of Londrina (UEL), specializing in Modern Education from Pontifical Catholic University of Rio Grande do Sul (PUC). He is Professor and researcher of Embryology and Medical Education at the University of Brasília (UnB) Faculty of Medicine. Currently, he is the Director of the Midwest region of the Brazilian Association of Medical Education (ABEM) and the assistant coordinator of the professional master's program in biology teaching (PROFBIO). He led the Medicine course at the University of Brasilia and is one of the members of the Center for Didactic Support and Teaching Experience at the same institution.

Emanuela Ferretti, MD, MSc, FRCPC, is Professor of Pediatrics at the University of Ottawa and neonatologist at the Children's Hospital of Eastern Ontario (CHEO) and the Ottawa Hospital (General Campus). Affiliated member of the CHEORI, her research interest has pertained to multicenter CIHR-funded study on necrotizing enterocolitis (NEC) which includes the study of a non-invasive biological marker to help predict NEC in premature infants, the impact of human milk micro-vesicles – exosomes and drugs – on the development of the human premature intestine. She has co-led Medical Education Research and implemented an international innovative Neonatal Ethics Teaching Program focused on parent–physician communication skills for postgraduate trainees. Lastly, her experiences as team leader of the local Perinatal Palliative Care Committee and expert content advisor for international Neonatal Societies led to develop a Regional Perinatal Pain guideline and the buildout of a QI project on the use of opioids in post-op neonates at CHEO.

Jenna Ganske is a Métis master's student born and raised on Region 3 Territory. She grew up in a Western upbringing and has been learning more about herself and her heritage over the past few years. Her ancestors originated from the Red River Settlement outside of Selkirk, Manitoba, where they eventually migrated to the outskirts of Edmonton, Alberta. Jenna's Métis grandmother once spoke French and had lost her language due to attending a convent in Edmonton at a young age. To honor her grandmother, Jenna took French classes throughout her academics. Once Jenna reached university, she decided to take on Indigenous health studies that have served as a catalyst for her involvement as a health researcher and in her own personal discovery as a Métis woman. Jenna continues to practice her heritage at home and has become an advocate striving for Indigenous health equity.

Rajesh Nath Gongal, FRCS, FRCP, MSc (Palliative Care), is Professor of Surgery at Patan Academy of Health Sciences (PAHS). He served as Medical Director of Patan Hospital in 2007 and worked to upgrade Patan Hospital to an Academy after which he became the Founding Dean of School of Medicine of PAHS. He then went on to serve as Rector and recently completed his tenure as the Vice-Chancellor of PAHS. He played a pivotal role in integrating palliative care and medical humanities in the undergraduate medical and nursing curriculum of PAHS. He is also the Founding Chairperson of Hospice Nepal, the first palliative care center to be established in Nepal in 2000. He completed fellowship and MSc in palliative care from Belfast, Northern Ireland. He is also the Founding President of Nepal Ambulance Service (NAS), a not-for-profit organization which for the first time in Nepal used a toll-free three-digit number to reach a call center which then mobilizes ambulances with EMTs. In the 10 years of its service, it has transferred more than 100,000 patients and played a vital role during the 2015 earthquake and the Covid pandemic. He is also the Founding Chair of Primary Trauma Care Nepal, which started training courses in Trauma for the first time in Nepal since 2003 and continues to train many physicians across the country in trauma care.

Leah Gramlich is a settler doctor of Scottish and German ancestry whose grandparents emigrated to Alberta in the early 1900s. She was born in Inuvik where her father was working as a doctor. She is grounded in family with six siblings and more than 100 first cousins on each side of her family. She values the relationship with the land that is exemplified by First Nations peoples. She recognizes and wants to use her role as a physician, a health leader, and an educator to contribute to truth and reconciliation, acknowledging the colonial past and present of her ancestors. She has learned from her experiences with Indigenous patients to bring a broad view that includes the mouse view, the deer view, and the eagle view to the fore, which allows her to contribute to creating harmony in care for Indigenous peoples.

Nazik Hammad, MD, FRCPC, MSc, MEHP, FACP, is Sudanese Canadian Professor of medical oncology at Saint Michael Hospital, Department of Medicine, University of Toronto. She was the Chair of the Education and Training Committee for the African Organization for Research and Training in Cancer (AORTIC), Director of Global Health, Faculty of Health Sciences, Queen's University, and Visiting Professor at the University of Nairobi, Kenya. She has facilitated several research initiatives and training workshops on curriculum development and capacity building in Oncology in sub-Saharan Africa.

Jehu Erapu Iputo, MBBS, PhD, is currently Head of Department of Physiology at the Faculty of Health Sciences, Busitema University. A medical graduate of the Makerere University Medical School, he was formerly Head of the Departments of Physiology and Medical Education at the Walter Sisulu University, Mthatha, South Africa. He has been a member of several WHO and other international expert committees and training workshops on curriculum development, health systems research and development, and quality assurance in medical education. He was also a member of the Sub-Saharan Medical Schools Survey Implementation Committee and an adviser to the Coordinating Center of the Medical Education Partnership Initiative of the US Government. He is a member of the Executive Committee of the Association of Medical Schools in Africa.

Khalid Khan is an economist and Assistant Professor at the Indian Institute of Dalit Studies (IIDS), New Delhi, with a research focus on education, inequality, labor markets, and identity-based discrimination. He holds a PhD and MPhil in Economics from Jawaharlal Nehru University, New Delhi, and an MSc in Economics from the University of Burdwan. With over a decade of academic and research experience, Dr. Khan has worked with leading institutions including the Institute of Economic Growth and India Development Foundation. Dr. Khan has authored and contributed to numerous project reports, working papers, and book chapters on social exclusion, educational access, and employment disparities across caste, religion, and gender. Dr. Khan's work significantly contributes to the discourse on inclusive development and equitable access to education and employment in India.

Inna Ivanivna Kucherenko, PhD, is the Head of the Department of Educational and Methodological Work, Licensing and Accreditation, Bogomolets National Medical University, one of Ukraine's leading medical institutions. A distinguished academic and administrator, she plays a key role in shaping the university's educational standards, ensuring compliance with national accreditation requirements, and guiding curriculum development in alignment with international best practices.

Taiwo A. Lawal, MBBS, MSc, MD, FWACS, FACS, is Senior Lecturer/Honorary Consultant Pediatric Surgeon at the University of Ibadan/University College Hospital, Ibadan, Nigeria. He served as the Sub-Dean (Undergraduate) in charge of the training of medical students in the Faculty of Clinical Sciences between 2014 and 2018. He has been the Sub-Dean Postgraduate since August 2020. He also heads the Clinical Skills Sub-Unit of the College of Medicine Education Unit where he superintends over simulation training for undergraduate students at the College of Medicine, University of Ibadan. He is a reviewer for several international journals.

Rick Lightning is a Cree elder from Maskwacîs. He is a third-generation residential school survivor. He works toward reconciliation with partners who share a similar vision and stick with you, rather than allies. He encourages ceremonial-based thinking based on spirituality rather than ritual-based thinking.

Lisa M. Littlechild is an Ermineskin Cree Nation member, one of the four reserves in Maskwacîs. She is a mother of seven, of whom one was a type 1 diabetic. Her son was from the Louis Bull tribe. Lisa's views on treatment and equality are a voice that hopes to stop or slow down systemic racism.

Funmilayo E. Olopade, MBBS, PhD, is Senior Lecturer in the Department of Anatomy, University of Ibadan, Nigeria. She is a medical graduate who teaches Neuroscience, Gross Anatomy and Embryology to second- and third-year medical and dental students. She is currently the Head of the sub-committee on curriculum of the College of Medicine Education Unit (CMEU), and the departmental coordinator for postgraduate studies. She has been a member of several international expert committees on curriculum development and capacity building in medical education.

Emiola Oluwabunmi Olapade-Olaopa, MBBS, MD, FRCS, FWACS, FAS, FNAMed, FAMedS, is Professor of Surgery at the University of Ibadan, and Honorary Consultant Urologist to the University College Hospital, Ibadan. He is the Immediate-Past Provost of the College of Medicine, University of Ibadan, and has been Adviser on health-professionals training and health systems development to several African countries, WHO, and the Governments of the United States and Finland. He was a member of the Sub-Saharan Medical Schools Survey Implementation Committee. He is currently the President of the Association of Medical Schools in Africa, and the International Relations Director (Africa and the Middle East) of the Societe Internationale d'Urologie. He has been elected to the Fellowship of the Nigerian Academies of Science, Medicine and Medicine Specialities.

Alessandra Ramos Venosa, MD, PhD, graduated from the University of São Paulo (USP) with a specialization in Otorhinolaryngology and obtained her PhD in Neurotology from the same institution. She is currently Associate Professor at the Faculty of Medicine of the University of Brasília (FMUnB) and served as Head of the surgery department at the Faculty of Medicine of UnB during the implementation of the new Brazilian Curricular Guidelines, with active contribution to this process. She has coordinated the Medical Program and the Faculty Development Center at the Faculty of Medicine of UnB. She also works at the University Hospital of Brasília, where she is Head of the Neurotology outpatient clinic and is responsible for the residency rotation in this area.

Ajovi B. Scott-Emuakpor, MD, PhD, FAAP, FWACP, FAMedS, is Professor and Emeritus Division Chief, Pediatric and Adolescent Hematology and Oncology in the Department of Pediatrics/Human Development at Michigan State University in East Lansing, Michigan. He was Director of Michigan State University's Pediatric Residency Program and Director of Clinical Genetics at Michigan State University. He was also Chairman of Department of Pediatrics at Ingham Regional Medical Center in Lansing, Michigan. In Nigeria, he was Director of the Institute of Child Health, Director of Clinical Services and Training of the University of Benin Teaching Hospital, and Acting Chief Medical Director of University of Benin Teaching Hospital, Benin City, Nigeria. He is Fellow Emeritus of the Academy of Medicine Specialities of Nigeria.

Madhusudan Subedi is a Nepali sociologist and medical anthropologist and currently Professor at the Patan Academy of Health Sciences, Nepal. His teaching repertoire encompasses subjects such as Sociology of Health, Sociology of Ageing and Disability, Social Determinants of Health, Health Humanities, Health Equity and Social Justice, and Qualitative Research. He has authored and co-authored four books, 12 chapters, and over 100 academic articles. Beyond academia, he has provided consultancy services to various international and national organizations, including CARE, DFID, EU, Plan International, ILO, UNICEF, UNFPA, and WHO. He is also a life member of several professional societies, such as the Nepal Red Cross Society and Nepal Ethnographic Museum. Professor Subedi is the pioneering faculty member who established humanities in medicine and nursing in Nepal, laying the foundation for a more holistic approach to healthcare education. As a dedicated advocate, he has championed the integration of humanities into medical and nursing trainings, emphasizing the importance of compassion and ethical reasoning in patient care. Professor Subedi's commitment to integrating sociological and anthropological perspectives into medicine, public health, and nursing sciences has significantly influenced health education and policy in Nepal, particularly in promoting community-based approaches and addressing social determinants of health.

Jessica Thorlakson is a settler librarian of Métis and European ancestry, born and raised in Amiskwaciwâskahikan. Their Métis family came from Manitoba to Alberta in 1903, initially settling in Lac St. Anne and eventually moving around Alberta and British Columbia; her grandfather's family hid him in the woods around Kamloops to evade residential schools. Jessica's paternal ancestors were Scandinavian settlers. They came from Iceland to Manitoba in the 1800s and settled in the Okanagan by 1880 on the traditional and unceded territory of the Syilx Okanagan People. She recognizes the privilege of being able to reconnect with her Indigeneity and acknowledges the colonial past and present of her white-settler ancestors.

SECTION 1

Implementation and Innovation Issues

1

INNOVATION AND IMPLEMENTATION IN THE HEALTH PROFESSIONS

Translating Research in Education and Healthcare Delivery

Jordan Richard Schoenherr

Healthcare is inseparable from society. Promoting, maintaining, and improving the health and welfare of patients is critical to sustaining communities. Healthcare professionals (HCPs) must not only possess an understanding of disease prevalence, incidence, diagnostic criteria, and treatment practices, they must also understand the attitudes, beliefs, resources, and historical context of the community and its health seekers (Schoenherr & McConnell, 2024a). These demands necessitate the development of education and training programs that enable HCPs to develop the competencies and skills required to ensure patient safety, promote effective stewardship of healthcare resources and patient information, advocate for healthcare issues and patient groups, and support continuous innovation.

Education and training programs must equip HCPs with the necessary tools to effectively respond to dynamic environments that present new cognitive, social, and cultural challenges. The heterogeneous practice settings – rural private practice, urban teaching hospitals, or combat zones – often require distinct approaches to the healthcare delivery. Training and education programs must also account for the demands on HCPs and learners' time, evolving demographic profiles of both learners and patient communities, the dynamics of healthcare organizations, regional, national, political priorities of elected representatives, and international healthcare policies and standards, as well as new and technological ecosystems.

In health professions education, educators, program developers, and technicians should not assume that practices which are effective in one context will work in another. Academic research or program evaluations might also have limited generalizability, as results might only be applicable to specific learners, educators, or institutional, regional, or national settings (Henrich et al., 2010; Messick, 1995; for reviews, see Schoenherr & Hamstra, 2016, 2024). Successful program

DOI: 10.4324/9781003498155-1

implementation requires an effective innovation system: the design, creation, and refinement of practices, products, and professional roles used to educate professionals and deliver care. This system must operate within the social networks of healthcare, integrating stakeholders from academia, government, and industry (Breschi & Malerba, 2013; Carlsson, 2006; Hekkert et al., 2007; Lundvall, 2007).

Educators and program developers face many unique challenges. Despite extensive research in the learning sciences,[1] HCPs must identify critical features of the educational activities and assessment instruments, how they are aligned, and can be aligned with educational outcomes. Moreover, they must determine how available human, financial, and material resources can be adapted to the immediate and future needs of learners and institutions (Hamstra et al., 2014; O'Doherty et al., 2018; Schoenherr & Hamstra, 2024).

Existing institutions (e.g., universities, hospitals, local medical services), technologies (e.g., learning management systems (LMSs), image processing, mannequin simulators), social networks (e.g., interregional and international collaborations, private and public sector interaction), and professional organizations (e.g., accreditation bodies, professional societies) influence the ease with which innovators can access, adapt, and utilize resources. As organizations thrive on stability, educational systems should be designed to be principled, efficient, reliable, and continuously monitored and regulated by institutional and professional bodies, such as through program reviews (Wiemers et al., 2018; Karavas-Doukas, 2014). Healthcare organizations must also address societal demands, government regulations, and regional competition. While novel innovations in assessment, pedagogy, and healthcare technologies can help meet these needs, HCPs must remain vigilant, as disruptive innovations can introduce unforeseen challenges that require stakeholders to adapt, modify, or even reject these innovations (Coad et al., 2022; Khessina et al., 2018; Simpson et al., 2006; cf. Rosenbusch et al., 2011).

Volumes have been devoted to understanding the factors, stages, stakeholders, and levels that define innovation processes (Edquist, 2010; Fleuren et al., 2004; Garud et al., 2013; House, 1979; Piening & Salge, 2015; Salerno, et al., 2015; Slappendel, 1996) including those specific to education (Berman & McLaughlin, 1976; Cai, 2017; Cohen & Ball, 2007; Looney, 2009; Sein-Echaluce et al., 2017; Serdyukov, 2017). This chapter provides a brief review of essential concepts of knowledge translation, innovation, and implementation in health professions education to support subsequent chapters in this volume. It assumes that effective innovation requires consideration of the sociotechnical ecology of the implementation context – how learning technologies, educators, learners, and their communities interact leading to the success or failure of innovations.

Section 1 situates innovation in health professions education within the broader sociotechnical ecology of healthcare delivery, tracing how paradigms emerge, stabilize, and are challenged, with CBME as the primary example. Section 2 describes approaches to the study of innovation adoption. Rather than focus on the individual and interpersonal processes that lead to innovation, models of innovation processes are considered from the social network perspective. Finally, Section 3 reviews the broad themes and problems of innovation discussed in the remaining chapters of this volume, including implementation and de-implementation challenges, the integration of pluralistic healthcare practices, the impact of spatial factors on healthcare education and delivery, and the immediate and long-term effects of societal conflict.

1.1 Innovation in the Health Professions

Many principles, practices, and products are labeled 'innovations' with little qualification. In the health professions, any novel educational intervention, assessment instrument, supporting technology, and program evaluation tool can be dubbed an innovation, often based on the evaluations of the innovators themselves.[2] However, for something to be genuinely innovative, it must not only address a well-defined problem, it must also lead to measurable improvements in practice and outcomes. Moreover, innovation requires widespread adoption across key stakeholders, including health seekers, learners, educators, practitioners, administrators, or broader community members. The extent and nature of this adoption – whether at an individual, institutional, or systemic level – should be considered when evaluating the true impact of an innovation.[3]

In this context, it is crucial to distinguish between incremental improvements, transformative innovations, and mere novelties (fads). A truly innovative product, process, or intervention must offer novel solutions that are sustainable, scalable, and adaptable across various healthcare settings. The process of adoption itself is influenced by many factors, including organizational culture, resource availability, and the alignment of the innovation with the needs and values of both healthcare providers, patients, communities, and existing healthcare systems.

Even if adopted, an innovation might primarily be selected due to its perceived *prestige* (i.e., symbolic value) rather than the demonstrable *functional utility* it introduces into a program (Schoenherr, 2017). For instance, the widespread adoption of 'high fidelity' simulation-based healthcare training has been characterized by a belief that they offer educational experiences that promote skill transfer from simulated environments to real-world clinical settings (Cook et al., 2012; Hamstra, et al., 2014; Norman et al., 2012: Schoenherr & Hamstra, 2017). Even when reputable institutions adopt these technologies, or professional organizations advocate for their use, it is not necessarily the case that they represent the most effective educational or care practices available to HCPs. More systematic evaluation criteria are required to ensure that the affordances of these technologies satisfy the desired outcomes of educators and institutions.

Adopters and Adaptation. Adaptation is a critical feature of the innovation process, requiring that products or processes are aligned with the unique features of an institutional environment. For instance, the presence of high-fidelity environments and simulation mannequins alone does not guarantee that a learner will develop competencies. Without skilled educators designing relevant scenarios with clear learning outcomes and directing learners attention to critical affordances, these tools might fail to achieve their potential. The critical determinants of success of an innovation processes are ultimately the agency and autonomy of educators, technicians, program developers, and learners as they integrate and normalize an educational intervention or assessment instrument within an healthcare or educational organization (May & Finch, 2009; May et al., 2022).

When searching for innovations, people often seek out 'leaders' in a field or 'champions' within an organization who can define problems, propose solutions, and validate their efficacy. In the United States, the Flexner Report (Flexner, 1910)[4] is often regarded as a radical shift in medical education in the United States. Flexner's report advocated for the reconceptualization of medical schools as public trusts, closely associated with academic institutions, grounded in scientific knowledge, and inclusive of both male and female clinicians. While the report is largely seen as transformative, it effectively consolidated healthcare authority and established a consensus among elite medical professionals rather than presenting a truly novel educational paradigm change (Figure 1.3). Retrospectively, its implementation also created significant trade-offs such as disadvantaging groups of practitioners, e.g., African American clinicians (Campbell et al., 2020; Miller & Weiss, 2012). The process of adopting and adapting innovations in the health professions is not only a matter of introducing new tools or practices but also requires critical evaluation of their impact on all stakeholders, ensuring that the benefits of innovation are distributed equitably.

By focusing on leaders who translate ideas and practices from one domain to another, the collaborative contributions of other stakeholders and adopters are often underappreciated (Douthwaite et al., 2001; Fullan, 1972; Mignon, 2017; Owusu-Agyeman, 2021).[5] This restricted focus on leadership can overshadow the cumulative contributions of many individuals who have shaped innovations in health professions education. Historically, many innovations that have laid the foundation of biomedicine are not the product of any single innovator, leader, or cultural group, but rather the outcome of multiple thinkers, healers, and educators across diverse traditions (e.g., Islamic and African medicine; Kananoja, 2021; Nasser et al., 2009; Syed, 2002; van Middendorp et al., 2010).

Innovation processes require situating the development of an instrument, procedure, or program within a larger, interconnected system that combines people, technology, and organizational structures, often referred to as a sociotechnical systems (Schoenherr & Michael, 2026).[6] At each level of this system, problems are identified, framed, and prioritized, while solutions are proposed, implemented, and iteratively refined by a variety of stakeholders. These interactions are often dynamic and non-linear, with each stakeholder contributing unique expertise and feedback, leading to the continuous adjustment of the innovation to more effectively adapt to implementation context. For instance, healthcare innovations ideally go through multiple iterative cycles of feedback from clinicians, patients, administrators, and policymakers, each refining the solution from their perspective.

Healthcare integrates physical, biological, psychological, and sociocultural domains, making it a highly dynamic field for innovation. As a result, healthcare innovations often emerge from the interaction of these domains, where clinical, cultural, and technological factors converge to address complex challenges (Clarke et al., 2003). The occurrence of diseases has historically prompted urgent needs for innovation – whether by advancing educational activities to train clinicians or addressing the broader societal challenges these diseases present to healthcare systems (Porter, 2005). For instance, pandemics such as the Black Plague, smallpox, and Spanish Flu not only led to significant changes in public health practices but also acted as catalysts for the formalization of medical education, the establishment of hospitals, and the early adoption of distance education (McIsaac, 2001; McNeill, 1976; Speilman & Sunavala-Dossabhoy, 2021).

The COVID-19 pandemic provides a more recent demonstration: during a time when healthcare resources were stretched beyond capacity, and the demand for qualified HCPs was at an all-time high, public health restrictions prompted rapid changes in how healthcare education was delivered (Gordon et al., 2020; Gaur et al., 2020; Papapanou et al., 2022). The adoption of remote learning techniques, particularly the use of LMSs, became essential in meeting the immediate need for continued education. However, as a qualitative review of nine medical schools found, while LMSs allowed for the swift transition to online course delivery, the rapid adoption of novel software posed significant challenges for both students and educators. These challenges included issues with technical proficiency, engagement, academic misconduct, and accessibility, reflecting the sociocultural and technological gaps that interfered with effective use of these tools (Binks et al., 2021; Schoenherr, in preparation a).

The apparent costs and benefits of innovations cannot be taken at face value. Ongoing program evaluation is crucial to ensure that the evolving needs of practitioners and institutions are being met, as well as to anticipate and address potential challenges. Effective evaluation processes consider the contextual factors influencing innovation, including institutional resources, cultural dynamics, and stakeholder engagement. For instance, the same telemedicine initiative might have varying levels of success depending on technological infrastructure, patient demographics, and healthcare policies in different settings (urban versus rural or low-income versus high-income communities). Assessing the efficacy of innovations across diverse institutional and cultural contexts is essential for developing realistic implementation models. These models enable more effective planning and predictive forecasting, helping to identify potential barriers and anticipate challenges before they emerge.

By engaging in comprehensive evaluations, educators and program evaluators can refine implementation strategies that allow for the sustainable adoption of innovations. Reviewing various dissemination approaches – such as knowledge translation frameworks, collaborative partnerships, and implementation science models – can provide valuable insights into how best to evaluate the impact of innovations on healthcare delivery and education (Damschreoder et al., 2009; Walsh & Rundall, 2001).

1.1.1 Innovation and Human-Centered Design

The human-centered design approach provides a critical starting point for healthcare and educational innovations, focusing on the social, psychological, and affective/emotional processes of all stakeholders involved (Buchanan, 2004; Hanington, 2010; Michael et al., 2024; Schoenherr & McConnell, 2024; Schoenherr et al., 2023). By focusing on the social and psychological processes of learners, educators, health seekers, and administrators, program designers can better align innovations with the needs and preferences of individuals, increasing the likelihood of successful adoption and responsivity to stakeholders.

Beyond institutional, social, and cultural differences, human, financial, and material resources all present challenges in program delivery (Bero et al., 1998; Davis & Taylor-Vaisey, 1997; Kitson et al., 1998; Schoenherr & Hamstra, 2024; Titler, 2008). The trade-offs created during organizational change must also be addressed as technologies need to be modified or replaced, workforces need to be hired, retrained, or retired, and learners need to be familiarized with new paradigms and modalities of learning. Careful consideration is always necessary to determine when and where an innovation should be adopted to overcome knowledge and resource gaps to ensure program sustainability.

Paradigms and Redomaining: Adapting Innovations. Innovation in healthcare education can emerge from a variety of sources, both inside and outside communities of research, education, and practice. Innovators in medical education are individuals or groups who recognize deficiencies and efficiencies and how existing resources can be used, or configured, to improve care, learning outcomes, efficient administration of resources.[7] They must perceive the novel affordances of technologies[8] and learning environments, as well as the traits, motivations, and preferences of educators, learners, and their broader sociocultural context.[9]

Innovations can also be adopted from outside of a community through a process of *redomaining* (e.g., Arthur, 2009; Mulgan, 2012).[10] Redomaining occurs when an innovation is created for one purpose by one group of people and is adopted and adapted for another purpose by another group of people. The process is comparable to analogical reasoning, where features and relationships from an old domain are mapped onto a new domain (Gentner & Maravilla, 2017; Holyoak, 2012).[11] For instance, aspirin was originally developed as an analgesic but was later used to help in the management of cardiovascular disease. In healthcare education, simulation-based educational practices have drawn extensively from aviation, where principles like high-stakes decision-making and crisis management are integral. Similarly, the concept of the therapeutic alliance, which originated in clinical psychology, has been generalized to broader healthcare practices, emphasizing the importance of a collaborative relationship between patients and healthcare providers.

BOX 1.1 SELECTIVE MILESTONES IN MEDICAL EDUCATION

The First Medical School, Degrees, and Licensure

Creation of the first medical schools represents a critical milestone toward a formal means of standardized learning and assessment. While degrees do not guarantee competencies, the formalization and standardization of medical knowledge and practice provide a means to confer status (and prestige) onto learners. Examples are available in Europe and Asia (Schoenherr & Beaudoin, 2027). The first formal degree was awarded by the Schola Medica Salernitana in Salerno, the school was widely viewed as a focal point for medical treatment, being dubbed *Hippocratica Civitas* (Town of Hippocrates). The degree would come to consist of three years of logic, five years of medical studies, and a one-year apprenticeship (De Divitiis et al., 2004).

Advancements in Anatomical Instruction

The creation of anatomy books provided a point of reference for all learners, providing them with insight into the anatomical structure that defined humans (Figure 1.1). Most of these early volumes suffered from inaccuracies due to being based on idealized accounts and incompatible animal models due to prohibition against dissection. As general models, these references are imperfect. Along with medical texts, they nevertheless prove invaluable for developing a shared understanding of anatomical features that is more durable and accessible than verbal instruction.

Bedside Teaching

Teaching a learner in the presence of a patient, or bedside teaching, provides a critical counterpoint to theoretical studies, captured by William Osler's 'Medicine is learned by the bedside and not in the classroom' and the 'see one' do one, 'teach one' approach often attributed to him. Exposure to idiosyncratic features of cases, observations of interpersonal processes between healers and health seekers, and the ability to interact with clinical educators provide unique educational opportunities.

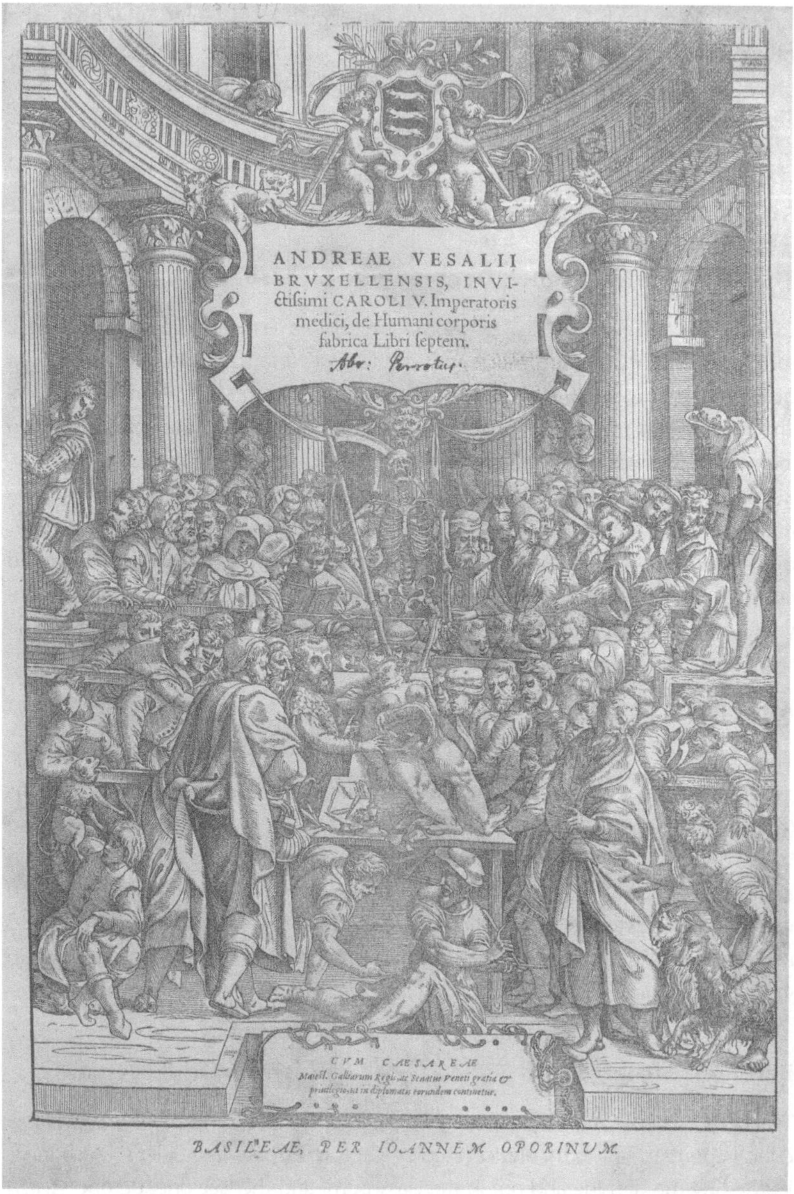

FIGURE 1.1 Credit: De humani corporis fabrica libri septem / [Andreas Vesalius]. Public Domain Mark.

Source: Wellcome Collection.

The inner cover images of Vesalius' *De Humani Corporis Fabrica Libri Septem* depicting a dissection of a human body (cadaver) with the Grim Reaper depicted as a skeleton with a scythe above the corpse surrounded by observers.

Professional Organizations and Accreditation Bodies

A clear means to ensure consistency is to establish centralized organizations to identify norms and conventions that all practitioners in a field should adhere to specific standards or practices. Using such standards, professional organizations examine whether an institution satisfies these standards. While introducing additional administrative layers, relying on consensus processes, and constraining who can be a clinician introduces its own issues, the benefits of ensuring consistent, quality education generally create an acceptable trade-off.

The Flexner Report

In the United States, medical schools proliferated along with concerns over the variable quality in education. Informed by German style of medical education based on science, Flexner was requested by the Carnegie Foundation to review medical schools in Canada and the United States. The review and subsequent publication of these schools in the Flexner Report (Flexner, 1910) resulted in radical changes, reducing the total number of institutions that could provide medical education.

Dissection and Simulation Studies

Concerns with patient safety coupled with developments in technology led to the creation of simulation-based training. Precursors can be observed in the use of cadavers; however, these practices were initially quite controversial due to views about the integrity of the human body. Modern simulations vary in size and realism, ranging from large-scale mock-ups of operating rooms and examination rooms, to the use of cadavers, human standardized patients (SPs), simulation mannequins, and virtual reality. Unlike bedside teaching, simulation allows for a systematic presentation and assessment of learners' competencies.

Competency-Based Medical Education (CBME)

The recognition of the limits of the apprenticeship model coupled with concerns over the bases for assessment of HCP, resulted in a shift toward a competency-based paradigm that emphasized specific competencies, milestones, and entrustable professional activities (EPAs). Due to their generality, definition and operationalization of competencies largely remains at the discretion of a medical field, institution, department, or practitioner.

Understanding how paradigms are created, stabilized, and changed is crucial to evaluating the innovation process in health professions education.

The development of tasks and assessment instruments in this field can be described in terms of three stages: a Pre-Paradigmatic Stage, a Paradigmatic Stage, and a Post-Paradigmatic Stage (Schoenherr & Hamstra, 2016; for alternative models, see Hughes, 1987, Rogers, 1962/2003).

In the early stages of inventions, designers, researchers, and practitioners debate the essential concepts and problems that are important, the appropriate technologies used for research, representation, and instruction, and the quantity and diversity of evidence that can be used to make coherent arguments, e.g., outcome measures, diagnostic criteria and categories, instruments, procedures, behavioral markers, educational milestones, performance levels. Due to the lack of consensus between experts, this represents a *Pre-Paradigmatic Stage*. For instance, apprenticeships are highly variable, based on the learners and instructors when no formal norms and conventions are available, gaps can also exist *between* expert diagnosis and their confidence in novel diagnosis and associated treatment recommendations (Millington et al., 2018), or educators might disagree about what kinds of skills defined clinical practice or how best to assess them. Historically, healthcare education and practice in the United States has experienced similar pre-paradigmatic tensions, as seen in the debates on the standardization of medical training and professionalization of the field (Coburn, 1988; Coburn et al., 1983; Friedson, 1985; Rosen, 1983/2016; Sinclair, 1997; Starr, 1982; Strauss et al., 1963; Turner, 1995).[12]

Over time a consensus concerning problems and diagnostic categories, the diagnostic criteria, instruments, treatments, learning and patient outcomes, and roles and responsibilities emerges within a community of experts, referred to as the *Paradigmatic Stage*. This stage represents a normal period of science and practice, wherein researchers, practitioners, and educators use past innovations without questioning the basis for their use, e.g., the apprenticeship model or CBME (Batt et al., 2020; ten Cate, 2017).[13] Increased patient safety, decreased hospital stays, improved reliability of assessment and learning outcomes, and higher graduation rates provide evidence for the utility of the core features of a paradigm.[14] These practices become the standard of care and create a core curriculum that is integrated into the organizational structure, institutional procedures, and professional practices. To maintain these outcomes, practitioners can monitor and self-regulate each other's behavior. Over time, the number of practitioners becomes sufficiently large that formal regulatory structures emerge. The accreditation process follows this paradigmatic logic: institutions must adopt the paradigm and are evaluated relative to it. However, paradigms are also limited in terms of the methods and topics learners can acquire in a reasonable amount of time, leading to the emergence of multiple subspecialities (e.g., medicine and public health; Ruis & Golden, 2008).

Finally, once people outside the original domain are exposed to an existing innovation within another community, they can adopt it. This reflects the *Post-Paradigmatic Stage* in the innovation process. Redomaining can either occur with or without adaptation within the novel implementation context. For instance, rather than directly examining an innovation's utility, educational interventions and assessment instruments are often adopted because they have been *validated* by other practitioners (Schoenherr & Hamstra, 2017). The real and perceived success or failure of redomaining will ultimately depend on how the innovation is aligned, implemented, and evaluated within an organization or community. Without understanding the strengths and weaknesses of an invention and evaluating the outcomes within a program, it cannot safely be defined as an innovation. Similarly, whatever formal regulatory organizations and structures might exist, they might not have the capacity or capabilities to evaluate the success of redomained innovations.

Innovation and Institutionalization of CBME. The processes of standardization, professionalization, and accreditation have been some of the most influential drivers of change within health professions education. As power becomes centralized in hospitals, academic institutions, and professional societies (e.g., AMA; Rosen, 1983/2016; Starr, 1982), innovations can spread rapidly through these networks. The Flexner Report serves as a key example of how paradigm consensus among a majority, or an influential subset, of practitioners can shape educational reform. In contemporary healthcare professions education, CBME stands as the most widespread attempt to achieve standardization (e.g., ACGME; RCPSC; World Federal for Medical Education (WFME), 2020; World Health Organization (WHO), 2022). In contrast to the apprenticeship model, which it was developed to replace, the CBME paradigm assumes that certain competencies (e.g., medical expertise, communication, collaboration) can be systematically acquired and assessed through appropriate educational interventions and assessment instruments.

Developing criteria to evaluate the efficacy of a CBME-based approach is not a straightforward task. Educators and developers must not only assess the extent to which these methods are supported by evidence (i.e., *construct validity*; Kane, 1992; Messick, 1995) but also consider their feasibility within the local institutional and broader sociocultural context (i.e., *implementation validity*; Schoenherr & Hamstra, 2024). For instance, the implementation of 'global' biomedicine in hospitals is determined by the constraints of local resources, values, and traditions (Hoke et al., 2022). While educators might be aware of the standards and methods that have proven effective elsewhere, HCPs and administrators might lack the necessary resources, experience, or training to effectively replicate and integrate these methods into an institution's curriculum. As the behavioral and social sciences have demonstrated, concepts and methods cannot always be transferred without adaptation and validation from their place of origin.[15]

1.1.2 Defining and Designing Competency in the Health Professions

Effective education in health professions requires an understanding of the dynamic relationships between learners and educators. The apprenticeship model – along with its faults – embodies these concerns. By relying on supervisors' and mentors' judgments often based on tradition rather than evidence (Asch & Weinstein, 2014), we cannot guarantee that learners will have the same quality and quantity of experiences. Rather than relying on expert intuition, learning objectives must be based on the learner's current state of knowledge, the appropriate stage of professional practice (milestones), and the associated affective, cognitive, and behavioral processes that define competencies (Schoenherr & McConnell, 2024b).

Educators and curriculum designers must create and select specific pedagogical techniques, course content, and assessment instruments to operationalize general competencies. For instance, van der Aa et al. (2020) present a generic competency-based framework that outlines key competencies such as 'patient-centered care', 'teamwork', 'system-based practice', and 'personal and professional development'. Their framework is offered as a guidance document, rather than prescriptive standards, which aligns it with other competency-based frameworks (Schoenherr & McConnell, 2024b). To operationalize competency in accordance with the CBME, educators must conduct extensive research in controlled experiments and *in situ* studies. These studies must also be translated cautiously across research paradigms and disciplines to ensure that findings are both valid and relevant to different educational contexts (Schoenherr, 2025).

1.1.2.1 The Problems of Competency-Based Medical Education

CBME is often presented as a novel and disruptive educational paradigm (e.g., Ferguson et al., 2017; Holmboe et al., 2017; Nousiainen et al., 2017; Park et al., 2016). Unlike traditional models that rely on fixed timeframes and hierarchical teacher–learner relationships, CBME promotes non-hierarchical learning environments characterized by diverse instructional strategies, multi-modal assessment, real-world problem-solving, and team-based training that vary based on the task, context, and learner competencies (Carraccio et al., 2002; Frank et al., 2010; Gruppen et all., 2012; McGaghie et al., 1978).

Despite claims that CBME has become the dominant educational paradigm, its implementation often appears more aspirational than actualized, lacking several features of an established paradigm (Schoenherr & McConnell, 2024). The slow refinement and adoption and uneven implementation of CBME practices can be attributed to a set of interrelated issues. First, competencies are not naturally occurring constructs that can be objectively identified. Rather, they are socially negotiated definitions created through consensus among groups of practitioners, national regulators, and international accreditation organizations. To address the needs of a national or international community of practitioners, competencies are typically formulated in broad terms. Such generality introduces more degrees of freedom for interpretation, selection of interventions and assessment, and variability in the implementation of CBME programs. For instance, McGaghie et al. (1978) notes that '[t]he intended output of a competency-based programme is a health professional who can practise medicine at a defined level of proficiency, in accord with local conditions, to meet *local needs*' (p. 18; italics added). Similarly, in their principles-based standards, the World Federation for Medical Education (WFME, 2020) they note that

> [p]rinciples-based standards are not prescriptive and detailed, but are stated at a broad level of generality. They address the components of the educational programme, such as student support, or a curriculum model, or an assessment system. But they do not say how support should be offered, nor what curriculum model should be adopted, nor what assessment methods should be used. They ask that the medical school states its mission and values, but they do not say what that mission or those values should be. Those are contextual decisions for local agencies and schools.
>
> *(p. 6)*

If educators and practitioners are left to interpret the gaps between principles and practice, it remains unclear whether a competency-based approach is more structured and systematic than apprenticeship models. Rather, the adoption of naïve empiricism wherein educators uncritically rely on flexible, incommensurable criteria might lead to confirmation bias and rationalization, encouraging educators to seek out evidence that supports the techniques that they have learned and developed.[16]

Second, to meaningfully assess competencies, CBME requires a level of specificity in assessment that is not currently feasible. Other than general roles and skills (e.g., 'communicator', 'collaborator', 'advocate'), each speciality in the health professions requires its own set of competencies, associated milestones and entrustable professional activities (EPAs), and the affective, cognitive, and behavioral performance standards that define competent performance.

While health professions education researchers have increased the development of assessment instruments as evidenced by academic publications, they do not constitute a coherent CBME paradigm. Comparisons of educational interventions and instruments are rarely conducted, and the level of testing and documentation required can contribute to assessment fatigue among both learners and faculty.

Moreover, CBME's emphasis on quantitative assessment risks obscuring wholistic features of practice, gloss over important differences in learner performance by focusing on standard competencies, and lead to homogeneity in practice that is not necessarily desirable (Hodges, 2013; cf. Schoenherr & Hamstra, 2016). Indeed, such homogeneity can be anathema to innovation.

Third, although the adaptation of a general competency-based approach is widely recognized as desirable, the extent to which HCPs have been drawn from a representative international population remains questionable. The World Health Organization's recent efforts to acknowledge the significance of indigenous medicine (WHO, 2002, 2013, 2019) and its development of global competency-based frameworks (WHO, 2022, 2023) represent an important symbolic and structural starting point. However, in attempting to accommodate regional variability, such frameworks risk being too general or inconsistently applied to support effective assessment and evaluation across diverse implementation contexts.

Nevertheless, it remains unclear how specific educational traditions influence the practices of traditional healers, or how HCPs with limited time or resources can acquire and retain meaningful knowledge of such a pluralistic global system. Addressing this challenge requires systematic and principled translation of research from cross-cultural learning sciences into practical guidance for health professions education (Betancourt et al., 2003).

1.1.3 Health Professions Education as Translational Research

Research in health professions education is applied. Rather than attempting to develop general models of learning, research is directed toward specific outcomes: to develop, maintain, and assess the competencies of HCPs and to promote accurate and efficient delivery of care.[17] To support these goals, health professions education draws on the results of basic research from the learning sciences while acknowledging the demands of knowledge translation (Schoenherr & McConnell, 2024; Swanwick et al., 2018; Thomas et al., 2021). Clinicians have long recognized the need to translate scientific principles and experimental results into practice (e.g., Ibn Sina's rules for experimental pharmacology; see Box 1.1; for the history of animal models, see Altman, 1998; Ericsson et al., 2013). Here, the basic pathways that define the translational research process are described (Box 1.2).

BOX 1.2 SCIENTIFIC AND KNOWLEDGE TRANSLATION IN THE MUSLIM WORLD

The biomedical tradition has been influenced by many indigenous traditions rather than being solely 'Western' in its origins. Ibn Sina contributed greatly to the scientific medicine. Ibn Sina's *On Knowledge of the Potency of Drugs through Experimentation* (tajribah) illustrates both scientific principles and knowledge translation principles (translation except from Nasser et al., 2009, pp. 79–80):

2. The experiment must be done on a single, not a composite, condition. In the latter case, if the condition consists of two opposite diseases and the drug is tried and found beneficial in both, we cannot infer the real cause of the cure…
3. The drug must be tested on two contrary conditions. If it is effective on both, we cannot judge which condition benefited directly from the drug. It is possible that the drug acted directly against one disease, and acted against the symptom of the other…
6. The effect of the drug should be the same in all cases or, at least, in most. If that is not the case, the effect is then accidental, because things that occur naturally are always or mostly consistent.
7. Experiments should be carried out on the human body. If the experiment is carried out on the bodies of [other animals] it is possible that it might fail [because] … the quality of the medicine might … affect the human body differently from the animal body.

1.1.3.1 Translation Research Process

Knowledge translation and translational research have been described by many models.[18] An educational framework developed by Ellis and Fouts (1993, 1994) classified research supporting educational interventions into three progressive levels: (1) basic research, (2) small-scale classroom comparative studies, and (3) large-scale school- or district-wide comparative studies. More generally, translational research is often described through three broad, bi-directional pathways, commonly labeled T1, T2, and T3. These phases reflect the flow of knowledge across research stages that can inform practice (Dougherty & Conway, 2008; Rubio et al., 2010; cf., see El Khoury et al., 2007; Schully et al., 2010; Westfall et al., 2007). Each pathway is bi-directional, with concepts, evidence, and methods flowing from one area to another (Figure 1.2).

The **first translational pathway (T1)** focuses on improving outcomes for learners (and patients). This research starts with methods, findings, and data from the learning sciences and adapts it to the context of learners, e.g., classroom, simulation environment, e-learning. For instance, studies of attentional blindness where individuals miss relevant features in a display (Simons & Chabris, 1999) can be observed in lapses in radiologists' diagnostics detection (Drew et al., 2013). Similarly, controlled experiments that examine how prior knowledge affects learners' accuracy in assessing their own performance (e.g., overconfidence bias; Schoenherr & Lacroix, 2020) can be found in learners' and experts' acquisition of specific skills in the health professions (e.g., point-of-care ultrasound (POCUS); Millington et al., 2018; Schoenherr et al., 2024). Conversely, studies conducted within medical education settings can reciprocally inform the learning sciences.

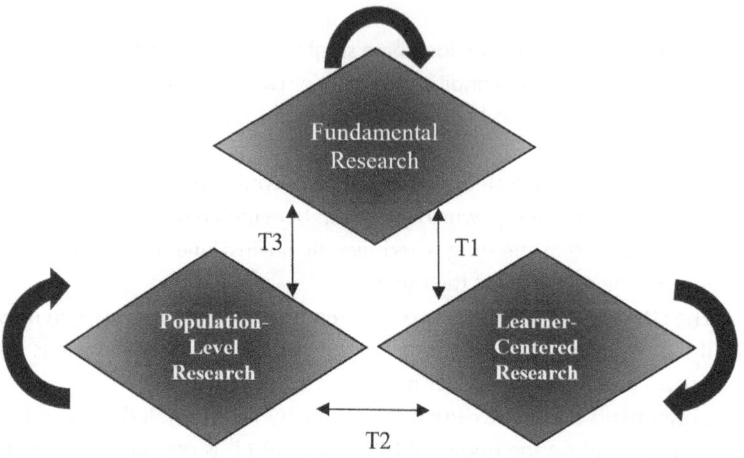

FIGURE 1.2 Translational research approaches. The results of fundamental research are used to inform learner-centred research. Results from patient-centred research can be used at the population-level.

A diagram showing three kinds of research. The interactions between Fundamental Research and Learned-Centered Research (Pathway 1), Learned-Centered Research and Population-Level Research (Pathway 2), and Fundamental Research and Population-Level Research (Pathway 3) are defined by internal feedback and bidirectional interactions.

For instance, Schoenherr et al. (2018) observed domain-specific overconfidence bias: clinicians with less experience in cardiac ultrasound tended to be overconfident, whereas those with extensive experience were underconfident. In that expertise can take years to develop, such studies provides more evidence for the validity of theories of metacognition.

The **second translational pathway (T2)** focuses on improving learner outcomes at a programmatic, institutional, regional, national, or professional level. This approach attempts to identify factors that account for individual, institutional, or cultural differences that occur at scale. For instance, innovations like problem-based learning (PBL) might work for specific groups of learners in one institution or sociocultural context. However, outcomes can be suboptimal at another institution due to challenges such as implementation fidelity, variations in educational culture, differences among raters, or divergent institutional paradigms (OSCE; Gupta et al., 2010; Schoonheim-Klein et al., 2007; Troncon, 2004; Wilby et al., 2016; cf. Kelly et al., 2014).

The **third translational pathway (T3)** considers how the outcomes of current educational practices within a national or professional community can provide insight into the learning sciences as well as how evidence from the learning sciences can be used to directly inform the development of large-scale educational initiatives such as CBME. Accreditation, program evaluation, and assessing alignment with clinical competencies can likely best be defined by this research pathway. Analogous to how epidemiological studies can suggest research questions for the basic sciences, the findings from program evaluation examining milestones across educational institutions can focus educators' efforts onto specific gaps in curriculum development, educational interventions, and corresponding assessment instruments (Edgars et al., 2018; Lewis et al., 2021; Natesan et al., 2018). Similarly, the successes or failures of artificial intelligence implementations in healthcare delivery or education can suggest specific inquiries into the utility of models and their recommendations, and the trust they engender in patients, learners, and healthcare professionals (Schoenherr, 2027a). Critically, practice-based research networks (PBRNs) play a critical role in facilitating this translational research, enabling collaboration across institutions to improve the relevance and applicability of educational innovations in real-world practice (Westfall et al., 2007).

Researchers and practitioners engaged in each type of translational research face distinct challenges, requiring different competency profiles. T1 researchers must understand learning sciences paradigms and how abstract principles and processes can be applied and scaled to various learning environments, such as classrooms, laboratories, or clinical settings. T2 researchers must be familiar with curriculum design, institutional structures, and the operational demands of healthcare systems, alongside best practices informed by learner-centered research. Finally, T3 researchers must be able to isolate and control relevant variables within large datasets, analyze their covariance, interactions, and dependencies, and align these findings with professional, institutional, and national policies and guidelines. Additionally, T3 research will also benefit from advances in big data analytics, requiring HCPs to develop new competencies in data science and informatics (Bilgic et al., 2024) as well as understand larger features of the sociocultural and political–economic context of healthcare delivery. Institutions must ensure that they develop curricula to foster these competency profiles and that HCPs have the requisite skills needed to work at these interfaces.

1.1.4 Evidence and Validity

Translational research allows individuals to adapt existing instruments and methods, evidence, and theories to new settings, thereby reducing the costs associated with paradigm development. The shift to CBME raises important questions about what counts as evidence for the efficacy of an educational intervention or the adequacy of an assessment instrument. Many pedagogical methods simply are not evaluated beyond arguments from authority: clinicians should be able to determine what constitutes the knowledge, skills, methods, and materials required to educate learners. As a form of translational research, health professions education must identify appropriate assessment dimensions, clarify the types of evidence that can support claims about a program's effectiveness or an assessment's validity, and critically evaluate the strength and scope of the available literature.

1.1.4.1 Evaluation Dimensions

By adopting a paradigm-based view of innovation, program developers can identify the key features and dimensions necessary for evaluating the efficacy of educational innovations. Four evaluation dimensions have been proposed to describe translational research processes (Dougherty & Conway, 2008): (1) research, (2) implementation and system design, (3) measurement and accountability, and (4) scaling and spread of interventions. These dimensions are interconnected and together define a comprehensive evaluation paradigm. As the chapters in this volume demonstrate, these dimensions can be examined explicitly or implicitly when considering the implementation validity of educational innovations (for checklists, see Lis et al., 2022; Appendix A).

Following the identification of a potentially innovative educational intervention, assessment instrument, or program evaluation strategy within the literature, programs and institutions should consider the processes of *implementation and redesign*. Following an initial examination of the readiness of an organization for the implementation of changes, organizational change must be evaluated in the short- and medium-term to determine its success (Al-Haddad & Kotnour, 2015; Ján & Veronika, 2017; Shea et al., 2014). Human, material, and financial resources must be considered to assess the validity of implementation (Schoenherr & Hamstra, 2024). When an innovation replaces existing methods of healthcare delivery, this must also address issues related to *de*-implementation, i.e., how physical and social organizational structures will change to accommodate a novel innovation (Norton & Chambers, 2020). This requires change management strategies (Van Rossum et al., 2016).

Effective evaluation requires both *measurement and accountability*. Stakeholders have a responsibility to ensure that a high standard of care is provided to patients, along with the efficient use of available resources. Outcome measures must be carefully selected and applied over appropriate time scales to assess the efficacy of a treatment or procedure. This included patient-centered information (e.g., objective outcomes such as complication rates, patient self-report measures) as well as professional (e.g., stress, burnout, workplace satisfaction) and organizational measures (e.g., costs, aggregated patient outcomes, efficient use of resources).

In CBME, administrators and educators must ensure that they provide learners with meaningful learning opportunities, assess learners in a fair and valid manner, and evaluate programs based on rigorous standards. These outcome measures should be selected to allow for interdepartmental, interinstitutional, interregional, and international comparisons. Provided that these measures offer a valid means to evaluate innovations in terms of competencies (constructs) and organizational factors, they can be used to create a comprehensive program evaluation framework.[19]

Innovations are defined by large-scale adoption. Estimating the *scaling and spread of interventions* require that we consider how scientific and procedural knowledge spread through processes such as social learning within healthcare and research social networks (Cain & Mittman, 2002; Jippes et al., 2013; Ratna et al., 2008; Zheng et al., 2010). For instance, during the implementation process, surgical interventions might be adapted to an institutional context, with specific features changed to meet the demands of local communities of practitioners, e.g., due to available of materials and equipment. Identifying how a procedure was adapted can guide the development of future procedures and increase the likelihood that they will be adopted by practitioners. Consequently, effective implementation strategies require concerted research by interprofessional and interdisciplinary groups with diverse sets of skills and expertise to understand the impact on learners, leadership, organizations, and communities of health seekers. Coordination of multi-departmental and multi-site implementation studies will demonstrate the generalizability of the outcomes of an intervention.

1.1.4.2 The Quality of Evidence

CBME requires an evidence-based approach to selecting and evaluating innovations. When HCPs use evidence-based decision-making during program development, they must not accept the findings of studies at face value. Journal peer-review processes are overburdened, the quality of publications is often difficult to judge, site-specific factors can skew or obscure results, and biases can affect the acceptance of evidence, both individually and within teams (Allcott, 2015; Barnow, 1980; Heckman, 1990; Schiekirka et al., 2014; Woodman & Wayne, 1985).[20] Perhaps the most problematic issues for translational research in the health professions are *publication bias* and *survivorship bias*. At the same time, 'research' is often provided in conference proceedings, talks, blogs, or reports from manufacturers, collectively referred to as the *grey literature*. These formats are typically defined by limited details on the methods, evidence, or peer review. These biases must be acknowledged and accounted for during translational research.

1.1.4.3 Publication Biases

Individuals and organizations might discount negative results, believe there is little chance such findings will be published, or avoid drawing attention to the unreliability of a method leading to publication and reporting biases (Begg & Berlin, 1988; Dickersin, 1990; Every-Palmer & Howick, 2014; McGauran et al., 2010; Moscati et al., 1994; Murad et al., 2018; Van Aert et al., 2019). For instance, special interests can influence the selective publication of findings that support the efficacy of an innovation, the selective reporting of data, or the questionable use of references to support claims[21] (De Vries & Lemmens, 2006; Fooks et al., 2019; Smith, 2005; Spielmans & Parry, 2010). Systematic reviews and meta-analyses in both education and medicine are not immune to these biases and are similarly affected (Cook & Therrien, 2017; Gage et al., 2017; Ioannidis, 2016;

Page et al., 2021; Ropovik et al., 2021).[22] At the same time, there is also an apparent ambivalence toward adopting measures that might address biases. For instance, Wager and Williams (2013) found that under one-third of journals (28%) required trial registration and that journal editors were did not see a clear benefit to adopting such measures.

Adoption decisions are often made because an innovation has proven successful in a different institutional context. However, a focus on successful innovation neglects important lessons that can be learned from failure and the vulnerabilities of an innovation, referred to as *survivorship bias* (Lockwood, 2021; Wald, 1943). Like feedback in medical simulations, program evaluation provides invaluable information about why an innovation failed. Patterns of failure can be as informative as those of success. Failure conditions must be identified and compared across institutional contexts. Given that educational interventions are often assessed in isolation, we must also acknowledge that this might be nothing more than *placebo effect*.[23] For instance, De Giovanni et al. (2006) found that a 'high fidelity' simulator produced learning outcomes that were no better than a 'low fidelity' simulator (for an early review, see Norman et al., 2012). Thus, direct comparison of education interventions and programs must be conducted.

Compounding this, most studies examine interventions in Western, educated industrialized, rich, and democratic countries (WEIRD problem; Henrich et al., 2010). Such observations suggest that even when evidence appears to support the adoption of an intervention or assessment method, these outcomes might not translate into a new program, organization, or sociocultural context. For instance, cross-cultural evidence suggests that techniques such as PBL and self-directed learning (SDL) have proven less effective in promoting learning, with adoption being consistent with local educational paradigms but inconsistent with the original techniques (Chan et al., 2024; Frambach et al., 2012 Premkumar et al., 2018: for a brief discussion in this volume, see Schoenherr & Beaudoin, 2027). Accounting for the implementation context by understanding economic and sociocultural differences along with engaging stakeholders is critical for ensuring robust educational innovations.

1.1.4.4 The Grey Literature and Training

Models of translational research must also acknowledge research published and presented in the *grey literature*, the set of methods and results described in publications that are outside of formal academic channels, often with little to no peer review (Adams et al., 2016; Adams et al., 2017; Haddaway et al., 2015; Mahood et al., 2014; Rothstein & Hopewell, 2009). Although the findings and conclusions of such research can be difficult to verify, they nevertheless have come to influence health professions education. For instance, manufacturer representatives ('reps') and industry-funded training opportunities play an undeniable role in the delivery of education related to specific technologies, e.g., surgery (Johnson & Hutchison, 2018; O'Connor et al., 2016). Unlike educators, who focus on a theory or practice, reps instead focus on a specific product and the promotion of its adoption. Claims made by reps must be assessed with more caution as other studies, as research suggests that many are unsupported (Grundy et al., 2020). Even if there is no intent to misrepresent results, people often only consider confirmatory evidence. However, while research might not be published because of dubious quality, publication biases might also result in the rejection of valid studies, with protocols for meta-analyses requiring the collection of such research to compensate. Educators and program developers must carefully weigh the costs and benefits of accepting or rejecting the results of such studies and be transparent about the decision processes that informed these judgments.

1.2 Innovation, Implementation, and Evidence

Provided that valid sources of evidence can be obtained, educators and program developers can begin to evaluate the success of innovations. The innovativeness of a new principle, pedagogy, practice, or product is ultimately dependent on the extent to which it is adopted by a group of individuals, how technology is transferred from one group or problem to another, and whether it acts as a catalyst for growth, cooperation, and competition in technological systems and innovation ecosystems (Cobben et al., 2022; Geels, 2004; Hughes, 1987). A review of general models demonstrates how innovation and implementation can be quantitatively assessed within communities of practice.

1.2.1 Human Factors in Innovation

Innovations are created, adapted, and accepted by people. Models of innovation have considered the general factors that affect adoption as well as the agency of adopters (May et al., 2022; May et al., 2009). At the individual and interpersonal levels, innovation can be best understood as a creative problem-solving process. Problem-solving requires perceiving a problem and recognizing how learners and educators approach a task. If available methods are deemed insufficient, creativity requires divergent thinking. Rather than becoming fixated on common task features and attempting previous solutions, people perceive alternative uses and make distant connections. Mapping of features from known domains to new domains can facilitate the transfer of methods and technology through a process of analogical reasoning, i.e., redomaining. Multicultural or multisector experiences can be especially beneficial, as innovators can draw ideas from different social networks (Cheng & Leung, 2013; Kadam et al., 2020; Leung et al., 2008; Wang et al., 2019).

Working in diverse teams can also be beneficial (Kurtzberg & Amabile, 2001; Kurtzberg, 2005; cf. Mannix & Neale, 2005; Polzer et al., 2002). No matter how creative a single individual might be, they benefit from working with others who have different experiences, perceive different patterns, challenge their approach and have novel linguistic and cultural concepts. Members of a team must nevertheless have an accurate understanding of the competencies of others that they work with, i.e., collective competence. Educators must also be receptive to the ideas of others outside their immediate social network, whether in formal academic publications, professional conferences, or industry.

1.2.2 Innovation in Social Networks

Innovation in education combines both social processes (e.g., pedagogical techniques, assessment methods) and technological artifacts (e.g., instruments, learning technologies, integrated learner records). Understanding why educators and learners adopt specific innovations requires viewing this process within a social network. Here, four broad approaches to the innovation process are reviewed: diffusion models, induced innovation, the evolutionary approach, and path-dependent models (Ruttan, 1997, 2000).

1.2.2.1 Diffusion Models

Diffusion processes reflect the patterns of adoption of an idea, practice, or technology by agents (e.g., individuals, groups, computers), using one or more communication channels (e.g., interpersonal interaction, textbooks, websites) within a defined social network over time (Katz et al., 1963; Kadushin, 2012; Rogers, 1962/2003; Sultan et al., 1990; Swanson, 1994; Valente, 2010). In an analogous manner to epidemiological research, diffusion models require a study of the prevalence and incidence of innovation adoption over time and the factors that affect the rate.

Rogers (1962/2003) provides a basic model of five characteristics that determine whether an idea, product, or practice is adopted by individuals within a social network: their relative advantage, compatibility, trialability, complexity, and the observability of its characteristics (cf. Rogers et al., 2014). Together, these processes contextualize changes in medical teaching paradigms. For instance, decreases in bedside teaching offered in the curriculum from 75% to 8–19%[24] have been attributed to changes in diagnostic paradigms, i.e., reliance on imaging and laboratory testing, increasing demands on clinicians' time, and the comparative advantage of other pedagogical methods, e.g., simulation-based training (Chapman et al., 2014; Verghese et al., 2015; Williams et al., 2008).

Beyond the transfer of information, social factors also affect the diffusion process, including normative social pressure (Coleman et al., 1966; Davis et al., 1989; DiMaggio & Powell, 1983) and competition between agents or groups of agents (e.g., Burt, 1987; Hannan & McDowell, 1987). While diffusion can occur

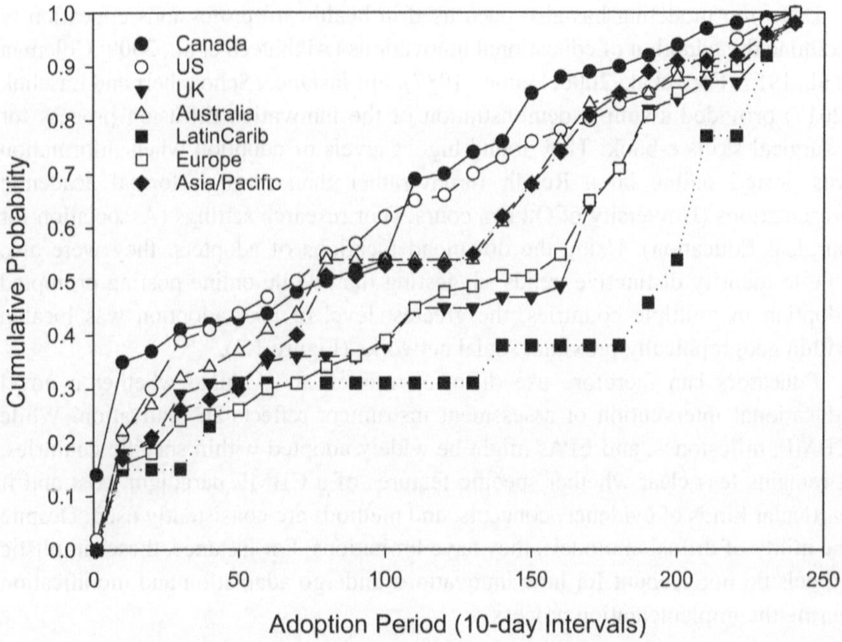

FIGURE 1.3 Diffusion of surgical skills eBook as measured by iTunes download rate within five countries. Adapted from Schoenherr et al. (2015).

A figure depicting cumulative proportion adopted (y-axis) based on the days since release (x-axis). Canada and US curves demonstrate consistent levels of adoption across the time span (0–250 days since release). Australia, the UK, and Latin America demonstrate lower and less consistent adoption, with all demonstrating increased adoption around 125 days after initial release.

passively or through word-of-mouth, advertising and marketing often frame the comparative advantages of an innovation (Van den Bulte & Lilien, 2001). For instance, clinicians presenting instructional methods and purported innovations at conferences can lead to greater adoption (Figure 1.3).

Diffusion models have been widely applied in public health research (Haider & Kreps, 2004; Lee, 2004; Luke & Harris, 2007; Rogers, 2004), examining the spread of health information and practices in areas such as HIV/AIDS, dietary behaviors, diabetes care, alcohol consumption, and vaccinations (e.g., Becker, 1970; Bertrand, 2004; Green et al., 2009; Lien & Jiang, 2017; Polgar, 1962; Schoenherr, 2022; Valente & Fosados, 2006; Valente & Pitts, 2017). For instance, a study using a regional sample from the United States differing in cultural conformity biases (cultural tightness[25]; Gelfand et al., 2006, 2011) found that states with higher cultural tightness exhibited lower vaccination rates (Schoenherr, 2022b). Thus, diffusion models provide a valuable tool for demonstrating how innovation adoption occurs within defined populations.

Diffusion modeling has also been used in healthcare professions education to examine the adoption of educational innovations (Alkhateeb et al., 2009; Coleman et al., 1957; Ford et al., 2006; Homer, 1987). For instance, Schoenherr and Laschuk (2017) provided a simple demonstration of the innovation diffusion process for a surgical skills e-book. They found higher levels of adoption when information was posted online on a Reddit forum rather than through formal academic presentations (University of Ottawa courses) or research settings (Association for Surgical Education). Using the download locations of adopters, they were also able to identify distinctive trends suggesting that, while online posting prompted adoption in multiple countries, the greatest level of user adoption was located within geographically proximal social networks (Figure 1.3).

Educators can therefore use diffusion models to evaluate whether a novel educational intervention or assessment instrument reflects an innovation. While CBME, milestones, and EPAs might be widely adopted within specific countries, it remains less clear whether specific features of a CBME paradigm exist and if particular kinds of evidence, concepts, and methods are consistently used. Despite the utility of diffusion models, they have limitations. For instance, these simplistic models do not account for how innovations undergo adaptation and modification during the implementation process.

1.2.2.2 Induced Innovation

Innovations are not always the result of intrinsic motivation on the part of their creators. *Induced innovation* arises as a response to external changes such as the relative availability or accessibility of resources, perceived costs and benefits (or return-on-investment), advances in technology, sociopolitical events, or conflict and competition between organizations or states (Hicks, 1932; Kennedy, 1964; Ruttan, 2000; von Weizsäcker, 1962/2010). In such cases, educators and program developers are responding to externalities within a sociotechnical system that would otherwise be in equilibrium.

Induced innovations are a ubiquitous feature of education. For instance, when a LMS is no longer supported by its developers, an institution must adopt a new system; if the availability of cadavers is limited, a department will need to adopt simulation alternatives; or if a region is repeatedly attacked, educators and administrators must find ways to continue delivering healthcare and educating clinicians with reduced resources. The impact of the Flexner Report can be understood in these terms, as many colleges were closed, resulting in a decline in the number of clinicians (Figure 1.4). Similarly, the introduction of CBME by national accreditation organizations (e.g., ACGME, RCPSC) and recommendations by the WHO (2022, 2023) reflect induced innovations as institutions respond to external professional standards and strive to maintain 'best practices'. Whether the adoption of these principles will affect the practices of institutions and educators remains an empirical question.[26]

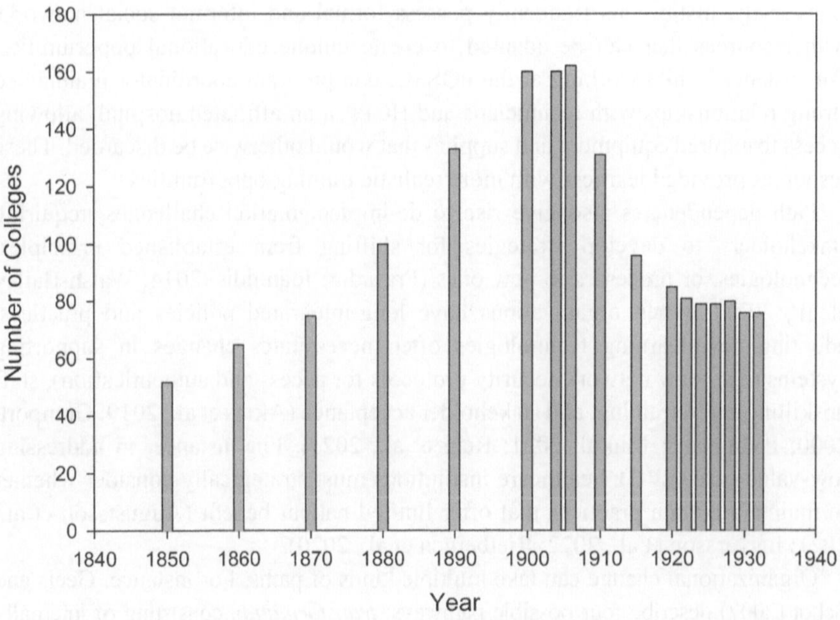

FIGURE 1.4 The rise and decline of US medical colleges. Squares represent the number of medical schools. Triangles represent the number of medical school graduates. Vertical reference line indicates the publication of Flexner Report (1910). Discontinuities reflect an absence of records.

A figure depicting the effect of the Flexner Report over a period of a century (1840–1940). The number of colleges demonstrates an increase until 1905. A sharp decrease is observed during 1910. The number of graduates demonstrates a corresponding decrease until shortly after 1920 when a monotonic increase is observed.

1.2.2.3 Path-Dependent Models

Innovation rarely begins with a blank canvas. Path-dependent models assume that organizations are constrained by prior decisions and existing infrastructure, social organizations, supply chains, governmental regulations, policies, and technology (Arthur, 1994; David, 1985). These models emphasize the embeddedness of organizations within regional, national, and international innovation systems (Gallaud & Torre, 2005; Grillitsch & Trippl, 2015; Isaken & Trippl, 2016; Ross, 2007; Rycroft & Kash, 2002; Salge, 2012; Thrane et al., 2010; Wilsford, 1994). In higher education, curriculum and program development are constrained by accreditation processes, policies (e.g., intellectual property, conflicts of interest), available personnel, and educational technologies. Innovators often face limited degrees of freedom due to existing organizational structures, technologies, and the collective knowledge and skills of educators, administrators, and technicians within the social networks of universities, hospitals, and vendors. Consequently, many alternatives are unavailable or require significant time and resources to implement.

Conversely, institutions frequently possess formal and informal social networks with resources that can be adapted to create unique educational opportunities. For instance, while working at the uOSSC, one program coordinator maintained strong relationships with technicians and HCPs at an affiliated hospital, allowing access to expired equipment and supplies that would otherwise be discarded. These resources provided learners with more realistic training opportunities.

Path dependencies also give rise to de-implementation challenges, requiring stakeholders to develop strategies for shifting from established principles, technologies, or processes to new ones (Prasad & Ioannidis, 2014; Walsh-Bailey et al., 2021). When organizations have long-integrated policies and practices, adopting new learning technologies often necessitates changes in supporting systems (e.g., new network security protocols for access and authentication), staff upskilling and retraining, and stakeholder acceptance (Akins et al., 2019; Gumport, 2000; Padmaja & Mukul, 2021; Reig et al., 2021). For instance, in addressing low-value care (LVC), healthcare institutions must strategically consider whether to maintain certain practices that offer limited patient benefit (Augustsson et al., 2021; Ingvarsson et al., 2022; Rietbergen et al., 2020).

Organizational change can take multiple kinds of paths. For instance, Geels and Schot (2007) describe four possible pathways: *transformation* consisting of internally motivated change either within an institution or society, *reconfiguration* consisting of cumulative component changes due to functional or economic factors, *technological substitution* consisting of competition due to novel innovations from old and new developers and manufacturers, or *de- or re-alignment* consisting of stakeholders and/or paradigms losing credibility or collapse of a system or introduction of multiple innovations. While these are ideal types, identifying the features of the current and future innovation systems will increase the likelihood of successful implementation. Additionally, recognizing the interaction between these pathways and the broader sociotechnical context is critical for understanding the complexities of organizational change, as shifts do not always follow a single, linear pathway (Geels, 2011).

The qualification that CBME has not been fully implemented in practice can partially be understood as a problem of de-implementation (Schoenherr & McConnell, 2024). Changing the dominant paradigm to a competency-based model requires time: to retrain and develop educators and support staff, develop valid assessment methods, reallocate funds to facilities, change evaluation methods, and more. Instead, the adaptation of old methods *framed* as CBME approaches might be far more widespread than systematic approaches that conform to the principles of CBME shaped by learning science and learning engineering. This appears to be a transition process defined by de- and re-alignment.

1.2.2.4 Evolutionary Approach

Parallels with biological evolution have also inspired models of how ideas are generated, modified, and replicated within communities (Dennett, 1996; Jablonka

& Lamb, 2014). Like diffusion models, evolutionary models of innovation can be agnostic regarding the extent to which deliberation about the utility of a product or process occurs. In this model, innovations are variants that are adopted deliberately or incidentally, which are more or less adapted to varied degrees to the needs of adopters and their environments. Innovation is thus represented as a semi-stochastic process, with each innovation conferring a comparative survival advantage to an individual, institution, or society that adopts it. This approach highlights path dependency, uncertainty, multiple stable states, and the heterogeneity of contributing stakeholders unevenly distributed in an ecosystem (Castellacci, 2008; Cooke et al., 2024; Nill & Kemp, 2009; Saviotti, 2013).

The benefits of an evolutionary approach are especially apparent in healthcare, where innovations support, enhance, or undermine the health and well-being of members of society (Consoli & Mina, 2009; Mokyr, 2010). Educational practices can be understood similarly. Rather than fully understanding the benefits of a pedagogical approach or assessment instrument, administrators and educators might engage in a process of comparatively 'blind imitation', adopting educational models that produce satisfactory outcomes, such as improvements in performance, increases in learner confidence, or alignment with accreditation body requirements. For instance, research into learning styles that assesses whether there is an ideal mode of instruction for certain learners has revealed only limited support with one study finding that learning styles accounted for only 3% of the variance in academic performance (Kirschner, 2017; Komarraju et al., 2011; Newton & Salvi, 2020; cf. Litzinger et al., 2007).[27]

Even with care, stakeholders can spend years and considerable funding developing innovations that ultimately fail to be adopted due to changes in society, instruction, or technology. If designers and educators do not understand innovation as an ecosystem shaped by sociopolitical climate, and material and human resources, even the best ideas can fail to take hold if they are not intentionally aligned with the needs, values, and beliefs of prospective adopters.

Trends and fads in education are frequent and often costly for institutions and learners who unwittingly adopt them. Summarizing this issue, Cohen and Ball (2007) note that 'many innovations consist more of ideas and hopes than of the carefully designed details of daily operations that often are required to make appreciable change' (p. 19). The rapid adoption and abandonment of innovations is so common that it has been termed the 'pendulum syndrome' (Maddux, 1986). Moreover, even when research is available, educators' teaching practices are not always significantly influenced by it (Gall et al., 2003; Grossen, 1998). Similar concerns have been raised about the adoption of technologies such as AI within the healthcare professions (Maddux & Cummings, 2004; Manlhiot, 2018; Oosterhoff & Doornberg, 2020; Sanami et al., 2017). Without understanding the basis for the validity of an educational intervention or assessment instrument, adoption can lead to unnecessary problems for learners, educators, and institutions.

The widespread adoption of high-fidelity simulation likely provides the best example of blind copying. Many studies and commentaries have noted that the concept of fidelity is often left unqualified, that outcomes are often not aligned with specific learning objectives, and that fidelity is neither necessary nor sufficient to promote the acquisition of competencies (Schoenherr & Hamstra, 2016, 2017). Many chapters in this volume identify such issues. In many cases, the evidence-based approach used in biomedicine often neglects sociocultural aspects of the delivery of care. Similarly, we cannot expect that educational paradigms developed in one context can be effortlessly adopted by stakeholders in other settings.

1.3 Implementation and the Sociocultural Context of Education

Innovations must be positioned within the curriculum, a community of practitioners, and the broader sociocultural context of healthcare delivery. In this final section, I review three major themes related to disruptive innovations in health professions education and healthcare delivery that are discussed in this volume. First, technologies and technological systems offer new solutions while creating new challenges. As technologies become available from outside a social network or are adopted by administrators, educators can – or must – adapt their practices. By examining education as a sociotechnical system that combines learners and educators mediated by technology, we can identify gaps, vulnerabilities, and opportunities to supplement or replace human instruction in situations where there is a limited number of available educators. Second, educational paradigms and programs are ultimately rooted within specific sociocultural contexts. The compatibility of educational innovations with the properties of social organizations and institutions will be a significant determinant of their success. Third, the foundations of education are also affected by short- and long-term disruptive events such as natural disasters, armed conflicts, colonialism, and climate change. Understanding how healers and HCPs have adapted to ongoing crises, managed and substituted limited resources to facilitate learning, and created stable learning environments provides critical lessons for creating robust educational programs.

1.3.1 Technology Change and Sociotechnical Systems of Education

Technology is inseparable from education and educators. Whether through multiple-choice questions, plastic anatomical models, e-learning platforms, mobile apps, patient simulators, or AI-based training systems, technologies can support learning objectives if deliberately integrated into instructional design, pedagogy, and the curriculum (Guze, 2015; Han et al., 2013; Moran et al., 2018; Ruiz et al., 2006; Vozenilek et al., 2004). Without competent educators and program developers to create, calibrate, modify, and evaluate them, no technology can guarantee learning outcomes. Worse still, technologies can obscure invalid educational practices beneath a patina of legitimacy.

Technologies are also inseparable from learners and the cognitive and affective processes involved in learning. Learning technologies are ultimately based on design principles derived from the learning sciences (Thai et al., 2022; Schoenherr & McConnell, 2024). Human-centered design requires that the capabilities, capacities, biases, values, and motivations of learners be placed at the center of the design process (Schoenherr, 2021, 2022; Schoenherr et al., 2024; for a general review, see Schoenherr et al., 2023). Designers must direct the attention of educators and learners to the affordances of a technology that increases the likelihood of achieving learning outcomes.

Designers and program developers must also ensure that educators, learners, and administrators understand how these technologies are created, how they operate, and the consequences of incorporating them into decision-making processes. This understanding is necessary to ensure users can critically assess, question, and challenge the operations and outputs of these systems (i.e., transparency, explainability, and contestability; Alfrink et al., 2023; Gorry et al., 1973; Ploug & Holm, 2020; Schoenherr, 2021; Thomson & Schoenherr, 2020).[28] For instance, there is widespread recognition that many AI-based technologies are susceptible to sex, gender, and ethnic biases (Cau et al., 2024; Cirillo et al., 2020; Huang et al., 2022; Noseworthy et al., 2020; Seyyed-Kalantari et al., 2021). Failing to understand the limitations of these technologies can place patients at risk and compromise the integrity of learning and assessment, reinforcing institutionalized forms of discrimination.

When working together, learners, educators, and technicians create sociotechnical systems based on the nature and extent of their interaction with technology (Adams Ivanov, 2015; Navarro-Bringas et al., 2020). In health professions education, educators' time is often limited, leaving learners with few opportunities to receive one-on-one instruction. Learning technologies can provide learners with novel training opportunities: rather than placing patient safety at risk, VR or mannequin-based simulations can be used to practice basic skills. If educators are in limited supply or inaccessible to a community of learners, online courses can integrate instruction and assessment to engage them. Similarly, adaptive instructional systems (AIS) can adjust to learner competencies, providing a personalized learning experience (Anderson et al., 1985; Graesser et al., 2012; Lee & Park, 2008; Park & Lee, 2013). Advances in educational technologies can also facilitate program evaluation, with approaches such as learning analytics offering a systematic means to evaluate and represent outcomes (Bilgic et al., 2024).

When new technologies are introduced into healthcare delivery, curricula must be adapted to reflect the new skills and competencies required to use them effectively (e.g., Jimenez et al., 2020; Johnson, 2019). Disruptive technologies such as AI, chatbots, data analytics, and telemedicine require a shift in how HCPs are trained (Schoenherr, 2027a). These technologies also introduce their own unique ethical concerns (Schoenherr, 2021, 2022; Schoenherr et al., 2024; Schoenherr & DeFalco, 2021). Simply possessing competence in one domain does not guarantee success in another. For instance, following the introduction of robotic surgery, over 10,000 adverse incidents were reported between 2000 and 2013. The magnitude of these patient safety events represented a serious challenge, prompting calls for the integration of standardized training within medical curricula (Ahmed et al., 2015). Similarly, Schoenherr et al. (2018) found that general prior experience with ultrasound was not associated with performance when learning cardiac POCUS. These findings reinforce the broader observation that expertise is highly domain-specific (Monterio et al., 2024; Norman et al., 2018).

1.3.2 Culture, Social Structures, and Institutionalized Discrimination

Learning occurs in diverse sociocultural environments. Beyond the cognitive and technological dimensions of learning and decision-making, sociocultural differences influence learning across the lifespan (Heffernan et al., 2010; Hofstede, 1986; Schulman, 1987). Cultural factors include linguistic conventions and social categories, the roles of peers and parents in the learning environment, the history, status, and identities of learning communities, the prioritization of holistic versus analytic thought, and how responsibility is distributed among individuals (Henrich, 2020; Nisbett, 2010). The threads of sociocultural values, social structures, and discrimination are recurrent factors that create, maintain, and receive the benefits of innovations.

1.3.2.1 Social Organization

Accreditation bodies, hospitals, educational institutions, pharmacies, and other professional organizations define interconnected social networks that have evolved to meet the demands of their respective societies (Starr, 1982). Within these systems, roles and identities are central to determining the flow of information, who is permitted to practice healthcare, and the relative accessibility of healthcare services and resources (Cockerham, 2017). Medical pluralism occurs when there are two or more practices and healthcare paradigms within one society. These paradigms are embodied within distinct social networks affected by different attitudes, beliefs, norms, and conventions. So-called cultural bound syndromes exemplify the intersubjective nature of health and illness, underscoring the need to understand how patients, kin networks, and healers engage in collective sensemaking to diagnose, monitor, and treat illness (Simons & Hughes, 2012).

Many healthcare traditions focus on the individual as a whole or within the context of their peer and kin networks, rather than viewing illness exclusively biological and physical models, as is typical in biomedicine. Despite biomedicine's overt dominance in global health systems, health seekers continue to explore alternative approaches, often relying on trial-and-error, adopting folk beliefs, or gravitating toward health traditions rooted in other cultures. Notably, the implementation of biomedicine itself has varied across sociocultural context (e.g., Finkler, 2019; Lock, 2003).

In this volume, Schoenherr (2027b) reviews the sociocognitive and historical development of healthcare beliefs and services in Mayan communities. These communities, along with their regional counterparts, developed coherent systems of health beliefs and healing practices long before the introduction of biomedicine. In these communities, the adoption of biomedical models has introduced significant barriers: dependency on limited medical resources, reduced accessibility for rural communities, and substantial discrepancies in language and belief systems between HCPs and health seekers. Understandably, traditional healthcare practices continue to play a vital role in many regions, particularly in light of the shortcomings of biomedical systems (WHO, 2002, 2013, 2019).

To be effective, HCPs must be aware of these sociocultural dynamics and how they influence whether patients adopt or reject clinical advice. Cultural competence is therefore essential to successful implementation of educational interventions as well as an ethical imperative for the health professions.

As innovations emerge to diagnose and treat illness, organizing healthcare practitioners, identifying essential knowledge, and delivering education continue to emerge, program developers should recognize that evolutionary processes – both biological and cultural – will ultimately jointly determine which innovations persist. In this volume, Schoenherr and Beaudoin (2027) provide an overview of cultural evolution in health professions education using East Asia as a case study. Rather than assuming a hierarchical dominance of medical professions, they review six nations whose histories and cultures have intersected through both cooperation and conflict, i.e., China, Japan, Korea (North and South), Taiwan, and Vietnam. These complex dynamics continue to influence contemporary health professions education in the region and have impacted global health practices directly and indirectly.

Enduring ancient (Imperial China) and brief contemporary empires (Imperial Japan) have profoundly shaped this region of the continent, developing their own indigenous healthcare practices and institutions. Collectively, Traditional East Asian Medicine (TEAM) represents a healthcare system that exemplifies the dynamics of medical pluralism, both competing with and complementing Western biomedical traditions.

Ancient indigenous systems, combined with exposure to Western educational traditions, have led to the development of accreditation systems across the region. However, these systems differ substantially in their form, structure, and implementation. In their study Schoenherr and Beaudoin find that countries have adopted various models, e.g., some maintain parallel accredited education systems for TEAM, others have integrated TEAM with biomedicine, while in Vietnam, formal accreditation remains absent. These systems represent heterarchical (non-vertically organized) rather than true hierarchical structures and are often incommensurable in terms of standards, practices, and institutional goals.

BOX 1.3 A SIMPLE SOCIAL COGNITIVE MODEL OF INSTITUTIONAL DISCRIMINATION

By restricting who is and who is not a healthcare professional (HCP), institutions can support discriminatory practices. A social cognitive approach, that defines the basic social cognitive processes that create institutionalized discrimination can be used to provide specific recommendation on where and how to intervene at an individual, group, institutional, and societal level.

First, studies have repeatedly demonstrated that people are more inclined to prefer people who are like themselves (Froelich et al., 2021; Gibbons & Olk, 2003; McPherson et al., 2001; cf. Collisson et al., 2014) and group members even if the basis for a 'group' is minimal, i.e., an arbitrary label (Spears & Otten, 2012). Any similarity such as appearance, affective responsiveness, language, manner of speech, belief system can prime people to think about another as a group member. In interviews, interviewers are much more likely to prefer applicants that are like themselves (Roth et al., 2020) thereby reinforcing existing values, competencies, and demographic characteristics of groups.

Second, human cognition tends to rely on social categories (stereotypes) for faster, efficient processing. These stereotypes are associated with beliefs about the warmth (cooperativeness) and competence (ability) of people or occupational categories. For instance, studies demonstrated that doctors and nurses are associated with high levels of warmth and competence whereas homeless and drug addicts are outgroups assigned low competence and warmth (Fiske et al., 2002). Other studies have suggested that groups of 'others' are devalued relative to in-group members (Cikara et al., 2010). People that feel discriminated against can also engage in self-defeating behaviors (Smith, 2004; Spencer et al., 1999; Steele & Aronson, 1995).

Third, public representations of social categories can lead to associations between kinds of persons and roles. If a 'kind' of person has occupied a leadership or subordinate position, this creates a stereotype of the kind of person that can or should occupy this position. Recent developments in artificial intelligence such as generative AI reinforce these concerns. For instance, the relatively homogenous images produced by generative AI provide a glimpse into the unrepresentative way in which HCPs are presented (Figure 1.5)[29] while similar results have been obtained with early candidate selection algorithms (Köchling & Wehner, 2020). These biases are a result of existing over- or underrepresentation of ethnic, gender, and religious categories. Similarly, biases can also be reinforced through scientification and medicalization: when respected groups 'validate' differences through test-taking, diagnoses while others are discounted or dismissed, e.g., 'traditional medicine'.

Fourth, intragroup and intergroup interactions are guided by different norms and conventions, also defined by differences in power and expected communication practices. For instance, the doctor–patient interactions are typically hierarchical, with the patient 'complying' with a doctor's recommendations (see also, 'sick role'; Schoenherr & LeBouar, 2024). Power can also adversely affect information processing, ignoring alternative perspectives and options (Guinote & Vescio, 2010), leading to confirmation biases.

Finally, informal and formal social mechanisms of group regulation will lead to the reinforcement of existing norms and conventions. Studies have demonstrated that negative feedback is directed toward deviants in group settings, leading to conformity, ostracism, or organizational exit. Other subtle forms of behavior (i.e., incivility) can be harder to address. The individuals who remain in a group are relatively homogenous.

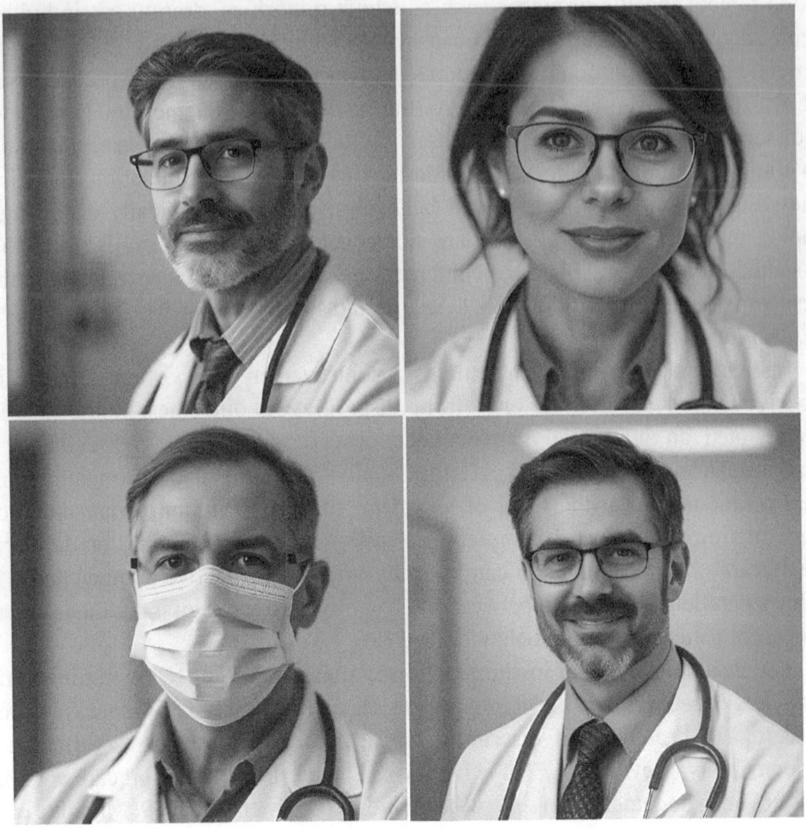

FIGURE 1.5 Randomly generated images created with AI (prompt: "an image of a doctor"). Images generated with DeepAI.

Four randomly generated AI-generated images. The four images depict healthcare professionals. Stereotypical feature of HCPs, they are all depicted with a blue, collared shirt, a white lab coat, and a stethoscope around the necks, all have very light skin colour, 3/4 wear glasses, 3/4 are men, and 2/4 wear a tie. One is depicted wearing a face mask.

Heterarchical structures are undoubtedly a prevalent feature in healthcare, reflecting the diversity of healthcare ecosystems. HCPs must also recognize that many innovations that transform healthcare often originate outside their existing social networks. Learners' use of novel technologies can create new educational opportunities, while health seekers increasingly rely on 'folk medical technologies' (Schoenherr, 2022a, 2022b) that bypass traditional models of expertise in healthcare delivery.

1.3.2.2 Institutional Discrimination

Inequalities have been a persistent feature of both healthcare delivery and health professions education. Rather than being idiosyncratic or isolated, discrimination often targets specific groups – such as ethnic minorities, drug users, individuals with alcohol dependency, or those with mental health conditions – and is embedded in institutional procedures and practices (Lim et al., 2022; Nong et al., 2020; Shavers et al., 2012). As the Institute of Medicine (2003) observed, '[d]iscrimination … results from biases, prejudices, stereotyping, and uncertainty in clinical communication and decision-making' (p. 4). Discrimination stems from individual cognitive, affective, and behavioral responses, typically occurring as rapid, automatic judgments that are not considered deliberately. Beyond these instances of ephemeral biases, the interaction of multiple social agents within their respective roles can result in more systemic and systematic barriers, or *institutional discrimination.*

Institutional discrimination remains a controversial topic, often because it is poorly defined or inferred only from disparities in outcomes. Some scholars have noted an inferential gap between observed disparities and evidence of discrimination (Epstein, 2005). Definitionally, institutional discrimination must be operationalized at the level of a system. In that institutions represent social networks directed toward completing a task – seeking, receiving, or delivering healthcare – the phenomenon can be analyzed using collective competence. This allows parallels to be drawn between the cognitive processes of individuals and the emergent patterns of group behavior (see Box 1.3).

The insidious aspect of institutional discrimination is that HCPs, administrative staff, health seekers, and the community might not be aware of how specific actions lead to larger patterns of discrimination, a process referred to as diffusion of responsibility (Beyer et al., 2017; Darley & Latane, 1968). In healthcare contexts, this has been documented in several case studies (Christensen, 2019; Marcotte et al., 2020; McIntosh, 2019). As healthcare systems increasingly integrate technology into clinical workflows and decision-making, such discriminatory practices can become further obscured behind technological veil, complicating efforts to detect and address the underlying basis of the problem.

In addition to the discussions of discrimination and inequalities in healthcare access presented in other chapters of this volume (e.g., Chan et al., 2027;

Venosa et al., 2027; Schoenherr, 2027; Schoenherr et al., 2027), Khan (2027) examines the unique challenges of developing the health workforce in India. While India is often described in terms of a caste-based social system, such characterizations can obscure the dynamic and complex social processes that exist within any society (Dugar et al., 2012; Pew Research, 2021; Rao & Rao, 1980; Ray et al., 2020). Rather than focusing on individual institutions, Khan considers the broader medical education system in India by analyzing the representation of different social groups. Khan highlights how entrenched social institutions and inequalities external to the healthcare system directly affect the composition of the workforce. By examining who enters the healthcare professions, the demographics of those who succeed, and the communities that ultimately gain or lack access to care, health educators and program developers can identify structural barriers and make informed, targeted changes to address gaps in curriculum and recruitment. These insights can support more equitable workforce development strategies that better reflect and serve the needs of diverse communities.

1.3.2.3 Culturally Sensitive and Relevant Pedagogy

To ensure a culturally competent and diverse health professions workforce, education must recognize that effective health communication with patients and instruction with learners requires an understanding of cultural processes, making their inclusion in the curriculum essential. Approaches such as *culturally appropriate* and *compatible pedagogy* were developed to align teaching practices with the cultural practices of specific learner communities, with the objective of facilitating the acquisition of knowledge valued by the dominant majority group (Au & Jordan, 1981; Cazden & Leggett, 1981; Erickson & Mohatt, 1982; Jordan, 1985; Mohatt & Erickson, 1981; Vogt et al., 1987). From this perspective, instructional and assessment methods that are culturally congruent increase the likelihood that learners will retain and apply knowledge effectively.

Critiques of this model have suggested that it homogenizes knowledge and functions as an assimilative strategy. For instance, Ladson-Billings (1995) suggests that such approaches reinforce inequity/inequality. She instead advocated for *culturally relevant pedagogy* which emphasizes distinctions such as the relationship between self and others (e.g., teaching that fosters community and belief in student competence), social relationships (e.g., building connectivity with students and developing a learning community), and the conceptualization of knowledge (e.g., critical reflection on content and multifaceted assessment). By adopting this educational paradigm, Ladson-Billings argues that learners can maintain their sense of community and heritage including language and practice (cf. Paris, 2012). Integrating this approach into health professions education will require further refinement of competency profiles for HCPs and how curricula are adapted and delivered.

In this volume, multiple chapters examine the importance of understanding and incorporating indigenous and folk approaches to healthcare delivery and education.[30] Health beliefs are products of cultural evolution, stemming from the need to sustain health and promote well-being through interaction with the physical and social environment. Over time, the exchange of principles, practices, and people between groups can act as a catalyst for significant innovation. Concurrently, inequalities can arise, leading to social stratification and discrepancies regarding who structures learning environments, what information is presented, and how learners are assessed. Moreover, intergroup exchanges are not always consensual, with the process of colonization creating significant challenges to the development of trust and recognition of the value of traditional approaches. Perceptions of health seekers' concerns, diagnostic methods, communities, and therapeutic techniques should be accommodated in policies and practices (Chan et al., 2027; Venosa et al., 2027). Regardless of their own attitudes and beliefs toward so-called complementary and alternative medicines, HCPs can benefit from the ability to identify, articulate, and respond to the concerns of community members (Schoenherr & Le-Bouar, 2024).

The availability of multiple approaches to health professions education and healthcare delivery creates novel challenges for healthcare practitioners, providers, and health seekers. As Schoenherr and Beaudoin (2027) review in this volume, TEAM exists alongside biomedicine, with some countries exhibiting comparatively limited regulations (Vietnam), strict separations between the two (Korea), or permitting some form of blending or syncretism (e.g., China, Japan). While regional and national accreditation bodies serve as initial regulatory loci, international efforts are also necessary (e.g., WHO, 2022, 2023). Focusing on another continent, Olapade-Olaopa et al. (2026) provide an extensive overview of the medical education landscape in Africa. They highlight ongoing challenges such as inadequate funding, staff shortages, and a failure to fully address community needs, which have spurred collaborative efforts to build capacity. However, political instability and conflict remain creating persistent threats to establishing stable evaluation and educational paradigms.

Recognizing that patients and practitioners are embedded within broader traditions underscores the importance of exposing HCPs to the humanities, positioning healthcare delivery within its wider social and historical contexts (Wald et al., 2019). Through engagement with the arts, literature, philosophy, and history, HCPs can deepen their understanding of their relationships with health seekers, communities, and diverse groups. In this volume, Gongal and Subedi (2027) describe their experience developing and delivering a humanities curriculum in Nepal, which adopts a community-based approach centered on cultivating empathy. Beyond general topics such as the doctor–patient relationship, learners engage with critical issues including social justice, disabilities, aging, and death through a variety of media. While not explicitly focused on culture, this approach complements the work of Daboval et al. (2027), who develop communication learning objectives and educational activities aimed at equipping neonatologists with the skills necessary to navigate ethically sensitive situations. Rather than emphasizing patient 'compliance' with healthcare recommendations, their approach prioritizes the therapeutic alliance, recognizing the clinician's role in fostering a safe environment that encourages open sharing of information, perspectives, treatment options, and difficult prognoses regarding a child's health. Central to these concerns is an awareness that barriers such as language proficiency, differing values and norms, and health literacy can significantly impact communication (Fune et al., 2021; Schoenherr & Le-Bouar, 2024). Failure to effectively address these challenges can lead to psychological or physical withdrawal from the interaction (Ferretti et al., 2023).

1.3.3 Conflict and Colonialism

Beyond comparatively passive processes such as technology diffusion, migration, and global trade, external natural and anthropogenic threats are also catalysts for innovation. The heterogeneous healthcare ecosystems that define much of the world have been undeniably affected for good and ill by intergroup conflict and colonialism. As groups seek to defend themselves or compete with others, healthcare practices must adapt to impositions such as scarce resources, power asymmetries, time constraints.

1.3.3.1 Armed Conflict

Armed conflict poses some of the greatest challenges to healthcare delivery and health professions education. At the very time when healthcare is most needed, human, financial, and material resources are often depleted or decimated – sometime intentionally (Schoenherr, in preparation a). Battlefield conditions further reduce survival rates for medical procedures. For instance, clinicians have a 15% failure rate for battlefield cricothyrotomy, but this rate more than doubles when performed by medics (Mabry & Frankfurt, 2012).

Managing the available resources and finding additional ones becomes critical during conflict. Adaptation requires that civilian and military leaders, hospital and university administrators, and HCPs collaborate to develop flexible strategies and use whatever resources are at hand in innovative and efficient ways. They must also create or adapt new technologies and treatments to meet the unique challenges posed by conflict. For instance, the clinical diagnoses of 'battle hypnosis' and 'shell shock' (now recognized as PTSD) emerged from a growing understanding of the psychological effects of war on soldiers (Crocq & Crocq, 2000; Saigh & Bremner, 1999). Importantly, many healthcare innovations developed during armed conflicts have since been translated into civilian medical applications (Givens et al., 2017).

Wars have driven the introduction and rapid advancement of numerous healthcare innovations, including emergency medicine, surgery, splints, prosthetics, antiseptics, blood transfusion, rehabilitation, and vaccination (Adrienne, 2022; Gabriel, 2013; Helling, 2022). The large-scale armed conflicts of the twentieth century created unprecedented tests of social organizations and healthcare systems. Unlike peacetime, where there are a relatively small number of patients, the massive volume of cases during war provides HCPs with increased experience, insights, and opportunities for medical experimentation. For instance, the incidence of compromised airways and the need for blood transfusions in non-conflict settings is comparatively low (<0.5% and <3.0%, respectively), while these rates more than double during armed conflicts (Como et al., 2004; Mabry & Frankfurt, 2012). Such observations highlight the critical importance of public health approaches, as well as the logistics involved in transporting and treating the wounded to facilitate recovery and return to duty, as well as the increased importance and prominence of physicians and surgeons (Van Way, 2016).

Conflicts vary widely in scale and duration. Short, small-scale conflicts are less likely to severely disrupt well-established healthcare systems unless adversaries deliberately target infrastructure or civilian populations. In contrast, persistent or large-scale conflicts demand significant innovation and adaptation, as their heavy physical and psychological toll taxes soldiers, citizens, and HCPs. Challenges such as mental trauma, physical injuries, infectious diseases, population displacement, food insecurity, reproductive health issues, and sexual violence can become greatly magnified. Moreover, in total war scenarios where healers, HCPs, and medical infrastructure are intentionally targeted, healthcare delivery must account for the risks of verbal threats and physical attacks (Garry & Checchi, 2020; Haar et al., 2021).[31]

Many communities, countries, and regions around the globe have been faced with these challenges, e.g., sub-Saharan Africa, Kashmir, Palestine, Ukraine (Agbo et al., 2024; Chol et al., 2018). These challenges range from broad issues like rebuilding infrastructure and restoring the healthcare workforce (Martineau et al., 2017) to more fundamental concerns, such as addressing power imbalances and rebuilding trust in national institutions, including healthcare systems, after civil war (Gele et al., 2017; Leather et al., 2006). For instance, in a study of Kashmir – a region disputed by India, Pakistan, and China – Varma (2020) highlights that suspicion toward government-provided healthcare leads health seekers to avoid these resources. Even in the absence of formal conflict, state-based healthcare can be misused by government representatives, fostering distrust. In Iran, ambulances have reportedly been used for non-medical purposes such as transporting military forces and arresting protestors (Ghasemiardekani et al., 2023). Similar distrust exists in other countries affected by civil war (e.g., Guatemala), in 'borderland' regions (e.g., US–Mexico border; Goldberg, 2016; McKeirnan-González, 2012), and within countries impacted by colonialism (e.g., Africa, Canada, the United States; Chan et al., 2026; Wells & Gowda, 2020). Below, I briefly consider two recent armed conflicts.

1.3.3.2 Israel–Palestine

The Israel–Palestine conflict presents another complex case study of two nations struggling to coexist.[32] In contrast to Israel,[33] Palestinian medical education faces significant physical, financial, and psychological barriers stemming from its subordinate relationship with Israel. Until the 1990s, Palestinian medical students had to seek education and training abroad due to a lack of local facilities. The first medical education institution in Palestine opened in 1994. Prior to the outset of the recent conflict, there were seven medical schools in the region (Abu Alamrain et al., 2026). One learner described the healthcare system as

> a disjointed sector comprised of the Palestinian Ministry of Health (MoH), non-governmental organizations (NGOs), United Nations Relief and Work Agency (UNRWA), and private services… As a result of [this] fragmented healthcare system with a scattered population, creating a well-organized and connected medical education system posed a significant challenge.
>
> *(Shellah, 2022)*

Beyond the challenges posed by social organizations, the requirement to obtain permits and pass security checkpoints significantly reduced the time available for study and clinical practice, while also increasing stress on learners. These barriers negatively impact the motivation of both students and educators, leading to variable educational outcomes. Differences in training quality were evident depending on where students receive their education. For instance, one informant described their pediatric training:

> For Pediatrics, we felt a huge difference [in our training] in other hospitals compared to Al-Makassed, where they have formal bedside teaching. We only had one doctor in Hebron responsible for us, no lectures, no exams, no teaching. There wasn't a system.
>
> *(p. 7; informant cited in Shahawy & Diamond, 2018)*

More recently, the Hamas-led attack of 7 October 2023 and the Israeli military operations that followed have devastated Gaza's healthcare system and medical-education infrastructure (Abu Alamrain et al., 2026; OHCHR, 2024a). Israeli forces raided hospitals and detained medical personnel, including hospital directors (OHCHR, 2024b). Israeli authorities attributed these operations to the military use of hospitals by Palestinian armed groups, whereas OHCHR reported that Israel had not provided sufficient information to substantiate these allegations and that publicly available information contradicted some of them (OHCHR, 2024a). Detentions and the killing of health workers further depleted Gaza's already limited healthcare workforce (OHCHR, 2024a, 2024b). Many medical students continued training through online courses, transfer to universities abroad, and remote teaching programs despite displacement, resource scarcity, power outages, and internet restrictions. To recover and establish an effective system, medical education requires expansion of online programs, a wider range of training pathways, safe learning environments, and mental health support (Abu Alamrain et al., 2026). Reconstruction of healthcare education and delivery in Gaza will require international collaboration, substantial resources, and sustained institutional and sociopolitical support (Abu Alamrain et al., 2026; Alkhaldi & Alrubaie, 2024; Shellah et al., 2025).

1.3.3.3 Ukraine

The end of the Cold War brought with it the promise that old enmities might give way to greater collaboration. However, following the earlier annexation of the Crimea in 2014, Russia invaded Ukraine in 2022. The survival of Ukraine as an autonomous state seemed unlikely. More than two years later, the adaptation of the Ukrainian healthcare system to delivering healthcare to its citizens and soldiers while continuing educational programs stands as a testament to the ability of HCPs to adapt to the demands of armed conflict (Schoenherr, in preparation b).

In this volume, Ivanivna and Schoenherr (2027) provide an overview of the Ukrainian healthcare system leading up to the 2022 invasion. Until recent years, Ukraine operated under the Semashko Model, a centralized, hierarchical healthcare system imposed during the Soviet era. Within this system, HCPs and staff were state employees. Recent reforms have aimed to decentralize regulatory authority to regional centers to better address the unique needs of local populations, while simultaneously developing national educational frameworks to maintain consistency. At the same time, Ukraine has worked to align its healthcare standards with those of European and international bodies.

Like many other countries, this progressively decentralizing system was faced extreme challenges during the COVID-19 pandemic. As Ukraine continued its efforts to align itself with global health practices and those of Europe in particular, attacks on civilian targets such as hospitals which further threatened the well-being of Ukrainian society. Nearly 2,000 attacks resulted in over 11,000 civilian deaths and 24,000 injuries, with 86% of these attacks targeting healthcare facilities. As Ivanivna and Schoenherr (2027) demonstrate in their qualitative account, Ukrainian HCPs were forced to reallocate resources, revise and emphasize new curricular priorities (e.g., battlefield trauma), and adapt program delivery methods (Schoenherr, in preparation b). Despite the ongoing conflict, national-level formal assessments (KROK) remained mandatory, though passing criteria were temporarily relaxed to accommodate the realities of conducting exams amid attacks. Alongside establishing a new equilibrium for delivering healthcare education during armed conflict, they highlight the need to develop post-conflict strategies for recovery and rebuilding.

1.3.3.4 Health and Imperial Legacies, Colonialism, and Their Borders

Conflicts have a long-lasting impact, often leading to disrupting and restructuring societies. The most obvious and widespread outcomes are those of imperialism and colonialism, especially those of European powers who redefined and imposed national boundaries and group identities while intentionally and unintentionally threatening and altering the health and lifeways of indigenous populations in Africa, the Americas, and Asia (Lehning, 2013; Ziltener & Künzler, 2013). Colonialism was not confined to European powers. In East Asia, a modernizing Japan sought to replicate the perceived success of Europe in the pacific, with equally disastrous consequences for countries it occupied and sought to control (Booth & Deng, 2017; Myers & Peattie, 2020; Schoenherr & Beaudoin, 2027).

As a polarizing issue, colonialism remains a comparatively neglected topic in health professions education. Given its continued legacy affects relationships in the communities that hospitals and teaching institutions serve in developed and less developed countries alike, this is an indefensible oversight (Bleakley et al., 2008; Daffé, et al. 2021; Eichbaum et al., 2021; Naidu, 2021; Perkins et al., 2023; Steinke & Hövelmann, 2020; Supe, 2016; Whitehead, 2016). If disadvantaged communities are distrustful of HCPs due to historical trauma resulting from colonial practices (Gone et al., 2019; Mohatt et al., 2014; Nutton & Fast, 2015), this distrust can result in failures to seek treatment, discounting medical support and rejecting advice, or engaging in psychological reactance toward dominant health practices (Canales et al., 2011). Similarly, the development of international healthcare education standards must carefully accommodate local cultural, social, and historical conditions to avoid perpetuating colonial legacies and to better serve diverse populations (Adams et al., 2016; Bleakey et al., 2008; Gosselin et al., 2016; Karle et al., 2008; Wu et al., 2022).

Indigenous health has increasingly become a primary concern within global health discourse (Ferdinand et al., 2022; Gracey & King, 2009; King et al., 2009; Peiris et al., 2008; Montenegro & Stephens, 2006; Reid et al., 2019; Schuch et al., 2021; Valeggia & Snodgrass, 2015; Willis et al., 2006). Numerous countries have documented substantial disparities in health outcomes between indigenous and non-indigenous populations (Adelson, 2005; Ahmed et al., 2023; Frohlich et al., 2006). These disparities extend beyond differing mental models that influence the effectiveness of public health communication and healthcare delivery (Schoenherr & Le-Bouar, 2024), encompassing broader social and structural inequalities that exacerbate the prevalence and incidence of disease within indigenous communities (Bailey et al., 2017; Diderichsen et al., 2012; Gee & Ford, 2011; Homan, 2019; Marrone, 2007). Addressing these complex challenges requires not only rigorous study of the specific needs of underserved indigenous communities (Harfield et al., 2020) but also the development of authentic partnerships with indigenous and minoritized groups to foster trust, co-design, and culturally respectful healthcare initiatives (Allen et al., 2020).

Geopolitical borders also exert significant influence on health outcomes and healthcare accessibility (Bell et al., 2015; Macias & Morales, 2001; Wismar et al., 2011). Many modern borders are colonial artifacts that divide continents without regard for preexisting indigenous territories, disrupting traditional social, economic, and health networks. These imposed boundaries can create substantial barriers to healthcare coverage both within and across borders (Cohen, 1993; Douoguih, 2008; Simionato et al., 2018; Ssengooba et al., 2021; cf. border closures during COVID-19 in Africa, Emeto et al., 2021). In cases where government services have proven insufficient or collapsed, community members and private healthcare providers often fill the void that remains. However, questions regarding the adequacy, accessibility, and equity of these services remain (e.g., Somalia, Gele et al., 2017). These are also evidenced in larger discussions of the roles and responsibilities of private versus public healthcare in fragile and resource-limited settings continue to be critical (Hanson et al., 2008).

Border and transborder regions have their own unique characteristics and challenges due to a confluence of resources, culture, laws and regulations, nationalisms, and security concerns (Arreola & Curtis, 1994; Diener & Hagen, 2010; Zartman, 2010). For instance, within 100 km of the US–Mexico border, populations in the *colonias*[34] suffer from numerous health issues due to lack of infrastructure, sanitation, essential services, and minimal sociopolitical representation and integration with the dominant culture (Collins-Dogrul, 2006; Schoenherr & Grubesic, in preparation; Weinberg et al., 2003). These deficiencies pose serious challenges to the coordination and interoperability of healthcare systems across national boundaries (Carrillo et al., 2017; Cruz, 2014; Donelson & Esparza, 2016). The existential threats faced by countries such as Ukraine and Taiwan that have geopolitical borders both inside and outside 'the West' provide a larger-scale demonstration of how borders affect support.

In this volume, Chan et al. (2027) provide an illustrative example of how indigenous healthcare and induced innovation intersect. As Canada continues its transition into a post-colonial era, there is growing recognition that the lifeways of First Nations populations were forcibly disrupted through land and resource appropriation, the introduction of novel diseases, exploitation, conflict, and the imposition of (re)education and relocation policies. These actions have had long-lasting impacts on health and well-being (Wilk et al., 2017). Unfortunately, such conditions are not exclusively observed in North America (MacDonald, 2007; Woolford, 2015).[35] Redressing these inequities stands as an important means to address institutionalized racism that often subordinates – or neglects – the traditional wisdom and practices of a group and their current needs of indigenous communities. As they note, addressing discrimination and colonialism requires support for all stakeholders, including communities, institutions, and leadership that must engage with the subject matter in an authentic manner that support reconciliation.

HCPs must understand how prospective patients select from among healthcare options in pluralistic systems to best provide information, diagnostic, and treatment recommendations. Due to the legacy of colonization, the Americas provide numerous examples of pluralistic healthcare systems. In this volume, Schoenherr (2027) reviews the Mayan indigenous healthcare systems that exist alongside BWM practices, highlighting a pluralistic landscape supported by both formal and informal training pathways for a diverse array of healers. In another chapter, Venosa et al. (2027) trace the development of medical education in Brazil from the colonial era to the present. As a large, culturally and ethnically diverse nation with the second highest number of medical schools globally, Brazil offers a valuable case study into the historical and ongoing challenges of establishing medical education institutions and designing curricula within pluralistic and evolving healthcare contexts.

Considering medical education on a larger scale, Olapade-Olaopa et al. (2026) review medical education in sub-Saharan Africa, a region that has undergone colonization, interregional and international warfare, and some of the earliest, richest human cultural traditions. As sub-Saharan Africa transitioned into a post-colonial era, medical education has proven inadequate in meeting the demand for HCPs and health seekers. Governmental and nongovernmental (private and faith-based organizations) increased the establishment of medical schools, leading to an increase from 51 in 1980 to 250 by 2010. Qualifying such a promising increase, they note that multinational collaboration was necessary to address shortfalls in human and financial resources, funding and exacerbated by migration of skilled workers. Limited infrastructure, geopolitical and security issues, and emergent disease remain persistent challenges. By presenting these detailed case studies, we hope to bring into focus the larger issues which HCPs must address when developing education programs and delivering care.

1.4 Summary: Contextualizing Healthcare Education and Practice

Health professions education is defined by the patterns of interactions between learners, educators, administrators, institutions, technologies, and the communities that they serve. To achieve critical milestones, competency-based approaches to education require accurate models of the learners' knowledge, learning processes, perceptions of the environment, professional identity development, and impact of situational variables on their delivery of care and learning outcomes. Despite the lengthy history of research in the learning sciences, there are countless avenues for research that remain unexplored. The specialized nature of the health professions education requires research studies dedicated to evidence-based innovation and implementation frameworks.

Even when innovations have evidence that they have been successfully implemented within an institutional setting (implementation validity) and develop the necessary competencies in a principled manner (construct validity) that allow learners to complete EPAs, these favorable results might not translate to other hospitals, universities, or countries. Dynamic interactions between practitioners, learners, administrators, local resources, policies and guidelines developed by governmental and professional bodies create healthcare ecosystems that provide their own equilibria that cannot be ignored.

Many translational pathways exist that educators, curriculum designers, and HCPs can use to improve their teaching, research, practice, and advocacy. The adoption of CBME often emphasizes the use of findings from basic research, largely because health professions education is often based on the intuitions of clinical educators, often relying on the 'face validity' of instructional methods. While experimental control is necessary to draw generalizable conclusions, other translational pathways can illustrate the importance of acknowledging the unique features of a specific community, healthcare ecosystem, and cultural tradition that have evolved over time in which clinicians learn and practice.

Educators must also be cognizant that if they adopt an evidence-based approach to instructional design that they have carefully considered the strengths and weaknesses of the *studies* used to provide that evidence. Many innovations in health professions education are supported by limited evidence, with evidence often provided by studies in the 'grey literature', conducted by manufacturers or publications that have limited peer review. These findings should not be discounted, but they must be contextualized to understand their validity in making inferences in program design.

When viewed as a system, educational paradigms are clearly embedded within an institutional and sociocultural context. Educators in the health professions are keenly aware that successful educational intervention at an institution are often based on the presence of a particular educator (i.e., leader or champion) or team. Should that educator leave or the composition of that team change, changes in the quality and validity of the program will follow. Whether delivering care or providing instruction, program developers, educators, and learners must acknowledge that their success is predicated on the collective competence of all stakeholders.

A systems-based approach underscores the cumulative contributions of stakeholders. How they perceive, challenge, and contribute to educational interventions are delivered and how they understand performance assessment will be a critical determinant of the successful implementation of a program. The development of culturally sensitive curricula necessitates considering how cultural identity, local resources, and precedent influence the delivery of educational activities and use of assessment methodologies. If the curriculum fails to address key factors that are relevant to a population of learners or communities of health seekers, it will fall short of developing the critical competencies necessary of HCPs.

Notes

1 Learning science includes cognitive and educational psychology, anthropology, computer science, and engineering (Darling-Hammond et al., 2020; Meltzoff et al., 2009; for applications in medical education, see Schoenherr & McConnell, 2024).

2 Face validity represents a pseudo-scientific practice of assuming that experts' judgments within a domain are sufficient to deem a feature of a research paradigm (theory, evidence, or instrument) 'valid' without formally considering the quantity and diversity of evidence or attempting to disconfirm, or seek alternatives to, the practice.

3 Here, the term 'health seeker' refers to those individuals who desire health, while not necessarily being 'patients' of healthcare professionals. 'Community members' refers to anyone in the community who might not necessarily seek health. As advocates, healthcare professionals must ensure that they speak persuasively to a broad audience to promote healthcare services.

4 Commissioned by the American Medical Association and Carnegie Foundation.

5 As I note in the preface, I frequently found that the contributions of 'technicians' – a broad collection of individuals with varied skill sets – were often ignored.

6 Formally referred to as a sociotechnical system.

7 For instance, Kwang and Rodrigues (2002) found that education adapters were more conscientious than innovators. Innovators were more open and extraverted than adapters.

8 Referred to as the functional affordances in human-centered design (Gibson, 1977; Norman, 1999, 2013). These results were replicated and extended by Marcati et al. (2008) who found that both general innovation and domain-specific innovation was positively associated with openness and extraversion and negatively associated with conscientiousness and agreeableness.

9 In health professions education, simulator-based education has been framed in similar terms (for a review, see Schoenherr & Hamstra, 2017). *If* learners see how rubber tubing represents arteries or polygons on a screen represent a bowel, *then* they can improve their laparoscopic performance without needing a cadaver or a patient. *If* an educator uses an assessment instrument properly, *then* they can examine how learners' performance changes before and after an educational intervention. Without perceiving these affordances, the engineering 'fidelity' of a model will not be related to increases in learners' competencies. Learning is ultimately a result of sharing the same mental representations of a problem space and jointly attending to the important features (Schoenherr et al., 2025).

10 When considering a technology, this is also referred to as *technology transfer* (Eveland, 1986). When considering concepts a concept, this is also referred to as *knowledge translation* or *knowledge transfer*.

11 The appropriateness of the analogy (structural similarity) will determine its success.

12 For a discussion in psychological science, see Schoenherr (2017).

13 It arguably covertly remains the dominant paradigm.

14 In science studies, this is referred to as generativity.

15 This general criticism has been extensively considered in the behavioral, social, and learning sciences (the WEIRD problem; Henrich et al., 2010).

16 Confirmation bias occurs when an individual seeks our confirmatory evidence without considering evidence that might disconfirm their beliefs, hypothesis, or formal theories.

17 Whether intentional or not, Cooke et al.'s account of Messick's framework excludes 'generalizability' as a form of evidence suggesting that generalizable – either between institutions or contributing to research on learning sciences is not relevant.

18 While this section focuses on educational research, it is equally applicable to biopsychosocial research conducted in the health sciences.

19 A program evaluation space (PES) is defined by two dimensions: the amount of evidence obtained from studies examining the cognitive, affective, and social factors that impact performance in a task, and the amount of evidence that organizations

have adequate human, financial, and material resources and that the intervention or assessment instrument plays a unique, integral role in the curriculum and institution program. Innovations with high levels of both construct and implementation validity are ecologically optimized (Schoenherr & Hamstra, 2024).

20 Confirmation bias, availability heuristic, self-censorship, and groupthink can affect how individuals gather, assess, and integrate evidence individually and within a team setting.

21 In my experience, these legitimate issues must be distinguished from alternative, non-dominant interpretations of the literature. When reading articles that accused researchers (as a community) of erroneous citations, the accusers often fail to qualify why they believe those articles had committed this error. Some of these discrepancies might instead be attributed to novel interpretations of evidence that are coupled with limited (or inadequate) justification.

22 Methods are available to reduce publication biases, e.g., contacting researchers within a given field to obtain unpublished datasets, compare standard-effect sizes.

23 Rejecting the null hypothesis.

24 For estimates, see Collins et al. (1978), Reichsman et al. (1964), Tremonti and Biddle (1982), Shankel and Mazzaferri (1986), and Williams et al. (2008).

25 Cultural tightness–looseness (CTL) describes the extent to which a group values conformity versus tolerance of deviation, influencing conformity bias, a major factor in whether individuals imitate others' behaviors.

26 For instance, in a multi-year study, Schoenherr and Williams-Jones (2016) demonstrated that the development of national scientific integrity policy induced the creation of academic institutional policies.

27 The 'Whole Language' reading method provides another instance (e.g., Bowers, 2020: Ehri et al., 2001).

28 For a brief review of earlier debates in cognitive science, see Schoenherr (2020).

29 Of those images generated, the majority had agents with lighter skin and were typically male, wearing the stethoscope around their neck. Other generative AI models (e.g., Canva and Imagen3 (Google Gemini)) produced more ethnically diverse images.

30 Here, indigenous refers to beliefs that are associated with evolving traditions, often associated with a group's beliefs about a collective past whereas 'folk' represents popular beliefs that are present within a community, neither explicitly nor implicitly anchored to the history of that group.

31 For a review of the quality of this literature, see Bou-Karroum et al. (2020).

32 There is not sufficient space here to discuss the ethical, social, and cultural factors that have contributed to this division.

33 For example, see Reis et al. (2009), Reis e al. (2016).

34 Unregulated informal low-income housing communities located around the border.

35 For a discussion in Latin America, see Gago et al. (2024), Schoenherr (2027); for a brief discussion of colonial medicine in East Asia, see Schoenherr and Beaudoin (2027).

Appendix A

Implementation Evaluation Checklist

Implementation checklist provides evaluators with critical questions that must be addressed when determining the alignment of an innovation in an organizational setting. Unlike other evaluation grids (e.g., Lis et al., 2022), this grid assumes that sustainability is an emergent property that results from multiple sources of stability.

Features	Questions
Sociocultural Factors	
Stakeholder engagement	• Is the activity being co-designed with multiple stakeholders? • Who are the stakeholders? What proportion from each group has been engaged? • Are there any conflicts between stakeholders? • How will conflicts be addressed and resolved?
Dominant cultural values	• Do cultural norms support the adoption of new approaches? • What is the typical response to new innovations? • Are there any cultural values that can come into conflict? • What is the environmental impact of the activity?
Novelty	• What are the comparable innovations? • How novel (similar) is the innovation relative to others? • Is novelty (over/under) valued? • Does the activity depend on other technologies and resources?
Politics	• Is there a stable political climate (municipally, regionally, nationally)? • How is the governance structure of healthcare organizations related to government? • What are the typical results of changes in leadership and governance?
Regulation	• Is the activity subject to regulatory oversight? • What laws and guidelines are applicable to the activity? • Have regulators been formally engaged?
Organizational Factors	
Human resources	• How many FTEs can an organization commit to an activity? • What is the level of turnover? Are any retention initiatives? • What strategies have been developed to ensure corporate memory is retained?
Material	• What material resources are required? • Have these resources been available historically? Will they be available for the foreseeable future? • What alternative sources have been identified?
Curriculum	• What are the specific milestones of a program? • How frequently is the curriculum reviewed? • What evaluation criteria have been adopted? • Stakeholders had input and provided feedback? • How external parties been engaged in program review to reduce bias? • How integrated is the innovation in the curriculum?
Financial	• How much does the activity cost now? In the future? • How is ROI being evaluated? • Are funding sources stable?

(*Continued*)

Features	*Questions*
Organizational policies	• How does the activity align with organizational policies? • Do new policies need to be developed? • What are the implications for academic integrity? • Are there any real, perceived, or potential conflicts of interests?
Team/Group Factors	
Competencies and contributions	• What are the skills and competencies that are necessary for effective innovation development? • How will competency be assessed? • How will differences in competency be addressed? • Which stakeholders will contribute to the development of the innovation? • How will contributions be assessed and credit be assigned?
Cohesion	• How cohesive is the innovation team? • What activities or strategies can be developed to enhance cohesion? • How will intraprofessional and interprofessional communication be facilitated?
Leadership and organizational mandate	• What leadership framework(s) are being used? • What mandate has been provided to the team? • What organizational guidelines and policies facilitate/interfere with the innovation process? • Who will advocate for the innovation and its implementation internally and externally?
Diversity	• Are team members a representative sample of the stakeholders? • How might skills compliment or conflict? • How will conflicts and consensus be resolved? • Are there any biases that might result in a failure to address stakeholder needs?
Innovation Factors	
Validity	• How is the utility of an innovation being assessed? • What quantity and diversity of evidence currently exist to support the innovation? • What prospective studies need to be conducted? • Have external (peer) reviewers been engaged? • How will outcomes be assessed?
Complexity	• How dependent is the innovation on other technologies? • How much and what kind of training is required? • How much knowledge translation is required? • Are the operations of the innovation explainable to all relevant stakeholders?
Role of innovation	• Does the innovation play a unique role in the curriculum? • What competencies, milestones, and EPAs does the innovation support? • Does the innovation suggest new competencies, milestones, and EPAs?

Bibliography

Abu Alamrain, A., Irfan, B., Irfan, K., Ibsais, A., Leister, M., Raheel, M., ... & Zughbur, M. (2026). Medical education in Gaza: Navigating disruption during the 2023–2025 Israeli military assault and beyond. *Medicine, Conflict and Survival*, 1–29.

Adams, J., Hillier-Brown, F. C., Moore, H. J., Lake, A. A., Araujo-Soares, V., White, M., & Summerbell, C. (2016). Searching and synthesising 'grey literature' and 'grey information' in public health: Critical reflections on three case studies. *Systematic Reviews*, *5*, 1–11.

Adams, L. V., Wagner, C. M., Nutt, C. T., & Binagwaho, A. (2016). The future of global health education: Training for equity in global health. *BMC Medical Education*, *16*, 1–7.

Adams, R. H., & Ivanov, I. I. (2015). Using socio-technical system methodology to analyze emerging information technology implementation in the higher education settings. *International Journal of e-Education, e-Business, e-Management and e-Learning*, *5*(1), 31.

Adams, R. J., Smart, P., & Huff, A. S. (2017). Shades of grey: Guidelines for working with the grey literature in systematic reviews for management and organizational studies. *International Journal of Management Reviews*, *19*(4), 432–454.

Adelson, N. (2005). The embodiment of inequity: Health disparities in Aboriginal Canada. *Canadian Journal of Public Health*, *96*(Suppl 2), S45–S61.

Adrienne, C. (2022). *Healing a Divided Nation: How the American Civil War Revolutionized Western Medicine*. Simon and Schuster.

Agbo, K. C., Haruna, U. A., Oladunni, A. A., & Lucero-Prisno III, D. E. (2024). Addressing gaps in protection of health workers and infrastructures in fragile and conflict-affected states in Africa. *Discover Health Systems*, *3*(1), 36.

Ahmed, K.Y., Allan, J., Dalton, H., Sleigh, A., Seubsman, S., & Ross, A.G. (2023). Reviewing publicly available reports on child health disparities in Indigenous and remote communities of Australia. *International Journal of Environmental Research and Public Health*, *20*(11), 5959.

Ahmed, K., Khan, R., Mottrie, A., Lovegrove, C., Abaza, R., Ahlawat, R., ... & Dasgupta, P. (2015). Development of a standardised training curriculum for robotic surgery: A consensus statement from an international multidisciplinary group of experts. *BJU International*, *116*, 93–101.

Akins, E. E., Giddens, E., Glassmeyer, D., Gruss, A., Kalamas Hedden, M., Slinger-Friedman, V., & Weand, M. (2019). Sustainability education and organizational change: A critical case study of barriers and change drivers at a higher education institution. *Sustainability*, *11*(2), 501.

Alberani, V., Pietrangeli, P. D. C., & Mazza, A. M. (1990). The use of grey literature in health sciences: A preliminary survey. *Bulletin of the Medical Library Association*, *78*(4), 358–363.

Alfrink, K., Keller, I., Kortuem, G., & Doorn, N. (2023). Contestable AI by design: Towards a framework. *Minds and Machines*, *33*(4), 613–639.

Al-Haddad, S., & Kotnour, T. (2015). Integrating the organizational change literature: A model for successful change. *Journal of Organizational Change Management*, *28*(2), 234–262.

Alkhaldi, M., & Alrubaie, M. (2024). Roadmap for rebuilding the health system and scenarios of crisis path in Gaza. *The International Journal of Health Planning and Management*, *40*, 241–253.

Alkhateeb, F. M., Khanfar, N. M., & Loudon, D. (2009). Physicians' adoption of pharmaceutical e-detailing: Application of Rogers' innovation-diffusion model. *Services Marketing Quarterly*, *31*(1), 116–132.

Allcott, H. (2015). Site selection bias in program evaluation. *The Quarterly Journal of Economics*, *130*(3), 1117–1165.

Allen, L., Hatala, A., Ijaz, S., Courchene, E. D., & Bushie, E. B. (2020). Indigenous-led health care partnerships in Canada. *CMAJ*, *192*(9), E208–E216.

Alser, O., & Alser, M. (2023). Urgent call for protecting health-care workers in Palestine. *The Lancet*, *402*(10414), 1746–1747.

Altman, L. K. (1998). *Who Goes First?: The Story of Self-Experimentation in Medicine*. Univ of California Press.

Anderson, J. R., Boyle, C. F., & Reiser, B. J. (1985). Intelligent tutoring systems. *Science*, *228*(4698), 456–462.

Arnold, D. (2005). Europe, technology, and colonialism in the 20th century. *History and Technology*, *21*(1), 85–106.

Aronson, B., & Laughter, J. (2016). The theory and practice of culturally relevant education: A synthesis of research across content areas. *Review of Educational Research*, *86*(1), 163–206.

Arreola, D. D. & Curtis, J. R. (1994). *The Mexican Border Cities: Landscape Anatomy and Place Personality*. University of Arizona Press.

Arthur, W. B. (1994). *Increasing Returns and Path Dependence in the Economy*. University of Michigan Press.

Arthur, W. B. (2009). *The Nature of Technology: What It Is and How It Evolves*. Penguin UK.

Asch, D. A., & Weinstein, D. F. (2014). Innovation in medical education. *New England Journal of Medicine*, *371*(9), 794–795.

Atkinson, R. C. (2014). Adaptive instructional systems: Some attempts to optimize the learning process. In *Cognition and Instruction* (pp. 81–108). Psychology Press.

Au, K., & Jordan, C. (1981). Teaching reading to Hawaiian children: Finding a culturally appropriate solution. *Culture and the Bilingual Classroom: Studies in Classroom Ethnography*, 139–152.

Augustsson, H., Ingvarsson, S., Nilsen, P., von Thiele Schwarz, U., Muli, I., Dervish, J., & Hasson, H. (2021). Determinants for the use and de-implementation of low-value care in health care: A scoping review. *Implementation Science Communications*, *2*, 1–17.

Bailey, Z. D., Krieger, N., Agénor, M., Graves, J., Linos, N., & Bassett, M. T. (2017). Structural racism and health inequities in the USA: Evidence and interventions. *The Lancet*, *389*(10077), 1453–1463.

Barnow, S. N. (1980). Issues in the analysis of selectivity bias. *Evaluation Studies*, *5*, 43–59.

Batt, A. M., Tavares, W., & Williams, B. (2020). The development of competency frameworks in healthcare professions: A scoping review. *Advances in Health Sciences Education*, *25*, 913–987.

Becker, M. H. (1970). Factors affecting diffusion of innovations among health professionals. *American Journal of Public Health and the Nations Health*, *60*(2), 294–304.

Begg, C. B., & Berlin, J. A. (1988). Publication bias: A problem in interpreting medical data. *Journal of the Royal Statistical Society Series A: Statistics in Society*, *151*(3), 419–445.

Bell, D., Holliday, R., Ormond, M., & Mainil, T. (2015). Transnational healthcare, cross-border perspectives. *Social Science & Medicine*, *124*, 284–289.

Berman, P., & McLaughlin, M. W. (1976). Implementation of educational innovation. In *The Educational Forum* (Vol. *40*, No. 3, pp. 345–370). Taylor & Francis Group.

Bero, L. A., Grilli, R., Grimshaw, J. M., Harvey, E., Oxman, A. D., & Thomson, M. A. (1998). Closing the gap between research and practice: An overview of systematic reviews of interventions to promote the implementation of research findings. *BMJ*, *317*(7156), 465–468.

Bertrand, J. T. (2004). Diffusion of innovations and HIV/AIDS. *Journal of Health Communication*, *9*(S1), 113–121.

Betancourt, J. R., Green, A. R., Carrillo, J. E., & Ananeh-Firempong 2nd, O. (2003). Defining cultural competence: A practical framework for addressing racial/ethnic disparities in health and health care. *Public Health Reports*, *118*(4), 293.

Beyer, F., Sidarus, N., Bonicalzi, S., & Haggard, P. (2017). Beyond self-serving bias: Diffusion of responsibility reduces sense of agency and outcome monitoring. *Social Cognitive and Affective Neuroscience*, *12*(1), 138–145.

Bilgic, E., Chen, D. M., & Chan, T. (2024). Implementation of learning analytics in medical education: Practical considerations. In J. R. Schoenherr, & M. M. McConnell (Eds.), *Fundamentals and Frontiers of Medical Education and Decision-Making: Psychological Theory and Educational Practice* (pp. 108–136). Routledge.

Binks, A. P., LeClair, R. J., Willey, J. M., Brenner, J. M., Pickering, J. D., Moore, J. S., ... & Schwartzstein, R. M. (2021). Changing medical education, overnight: The curricular response to COVID-19 of nine medical schools. *Teaching and Learning in Medicine*, *33*(3), 334–342.

Bleakley, A., Brice, J., & Bligh, J. (2008). Thinking the post-colonial in medical education. *Medical Education*, *42*(3), 266–270.

Bogale, B., Scambler, S., Mohd Khairuddin, A. N., & Gallagher, J. E. (2024). Health system strengthening in fragile and conflict-affected states: A review of systematic reviews. *PloS One*, *19*(6), e0305234.

Booth, A., & Deng, K. (2017). Japanese colonialism in comparative perspective. *Journal of World History*, 61–98.

Bou-Karroum, L., El-Harakeh, A., Kassamany, I., Ismail, H., El Arnaout, N., Charide, R., ... & Akl, E. A. (2020). Health care workers in conflict and post-conflict settings: Systematic mapping of the evidence. *PloS One*, *15*(5), e0233757.

Bowers, J. S. (2020). Reconsidering the evidence that systematic phonics is more effective than alternative methods of reading instruction. *Educational Psychology Review*, *32*(3), 681–705.

Brannick, M. T., Erol-Korkmaz, H. T., & Prewett, M. (2011). A systematic review of the reliability of objective structured clinical examination scores. *Medical Education*, *45*(12), 1181–1189.

Breschi, S., & Malerba, F. (2013). CHAPTER SIX sectoral innovation systems: Technological regimes, schumpeterian dynamics, and dpatial boundaries. In *Systems of Innovation* (pp. 130–156). Routledge.

Buchanan, R. (2004). Human-centered design: Changing perspectives on design education in the East and West. *Design Issues*, *20*(1), 30–39.

Burt, R. S. (1987). Social contagion and innovation: Cohesion versus structural equivalence. *American Journal of Sociology*, *92*(6), 1287–1335.

Cai, Y. (2017). From an analytical framework for understanding the innovation process in higher education to an emerging research field of innovations in higher education. *The Review of Higher Education*, *40*(4), 585–616.

Cain, M., & Mittman, R. (2002). *Diffusion of Innovation in Health Care*. California HealthCare Foundation.

Campbell, K. M., Corral, I., Linares, J. L. I., & Tumin, D. (2020). Projected estimates of African American medical graduates of closed historically Black medical schools. *JAMA Network Open*, *3*(8), e2015220–e2015220.

Canales, M. K., Weiner, D., Samos, M., Wampler, N. S., Cunha, A., & Geer, B. (2011). Multi-generational perspectives on health, cancer, and biomedicine: Northeastern Native American perspectives shaped by mistrust. *Journal of Health Care for the Poor and Underserved*, *22*(3), 894–911.

Carlsson, B. (2006). Internationalization of innovation systems: A survey of the literature. *Research Policy*, *35*(1), 56–67.

Carraccio, C., Wolfsthal, S. D., Englander, R., Ferentz, K., & Martin, C. (2002). Shifting paradigms: From Flexner to competencies. *Academic Medicine*, *77*, 361–367.

Carrillo, G., Uribe, F., Lucio, R., Ramirez Lopez, A., & Korc, M. (2017). The United States–Mexico border environmental public health: The challenges of working with two systems. *Revista Panamericana de Salud Publica*, *41*, e98.

Castellacci, F. (2008). Innovation and the competitiveness of industries: Comparing the mainstream and the evolutionary approaches. *Technological Forecasting and Social Change*, *75*(7), 984–1006.

Cau, R., Pisu, F., Suri, J. S., & Saba, L. (2024). Addressing hidden risks: Systematic review of artificial intelligence biases across racial and ethnic groups in cardiovascular diseases. *European Journal of Radiology*, 111867.

Cazden, C. B., & Leggett, E. L. (1981). Culturally responsive education: Recommendations for achieving Lau remedies. In H. T. Trueba, G. P. Guthrie, & K. H. Au (Eds.), *Culture and the Bilingual Classroom: Studies in Classroom Ethnography* (pp. 69–86). Newbury House Publishers.

Chan, C. B., Gramlich, L., Littlechild, L. M., Lightning, R., Ganske, J., & Thorlakson, J. (2027). Innovations in health professions education in Canada to address the Truth and Reconciliation Commission of Canada's Calls to Action and the health inequities experienced by Indigenous peoples. In J. R. Schoenherr (Ed.), *Fundamentals and Frontiers of Medical Education and Decision-Making: Innovation, Implementation, and Translational Research* (pp. 284–309). Routledge.

Chan, S. C. C., Gondhalekar, A. R., Choa, G., & Rashid, M. A. (2024). Adoption of problem-based learning in medical schools in non-western countries: A systematic review. *Teaching and Learning in Medicine*, *36*(2), 111–122.

Chapman, R., Wynter, L., Burgess, A., & Mellis, C. (2014). Can we improve the delivery of bedside teaching? *The Clinical Teacher*, *11*(6), 467–471.

Cheng, C. Y., & Leung, A. K. Y. (2013). Revisiting the multicultural experience–creativity link: The effects of perceived cultural distance and comparison mind-set. *Social Psychological and Personality Science*, *4*(4), 475–482.

Chol, C., Negin, J., Garcia-Basteiro, A., Gebrehiwot, T. G., Debru, B., Chimpolo, M., ... & Abimbola, S. (2018). Health system reforms in five sub-Saharan African countries that experienced major armed conflicts (wars) during 1990–2015: A literature review. *Global Health Action*, *11*(1), 1517931.

Christensen, S. S. (2019). Escape from the diffusion of responsibility: A review and guide for nurses. *Journal of Nursing Management*, *27*(2), 264–270.

Cikara, M., Farnsworth, R. A., Harris, L. T., & Fiske, S. T. (2010). On the wrong side of the trolley track: Neural correlates of relative social valuation. *Social Cognitive and Affective Neuroscience*, *5*(4), 404–413.

Cirillo, D., Catuara-Solarz, S., Morey, C., Guney, E., Subirats, L., Mellino, S., ... & Mavridis, N. (2020). Sex and gender differences and biases in artificial intelligence for biomedicine and healthcare. *NPJ Digital Medicine*, *3*(1), 81.

Clarke, A. E., Shim, J. K., Mamo, L., Fosket, J. R., & Fishman, J. R. (2003). Biomedicalization: Technoscientific transformations of health, illness, and US biomedicine. *American Sociological Review*, *68*(2), 161–194.

Coad, A., Nightingale, P., Stilgoe, J., & Vezzani, A. (2022). The dark side of innovation. In *The Dark Side of Innovation* (pp. 1–11). Routledge.

Cobben, D., Ooms, W., Roijakkers, N., & Radziwon, A. (2022). Ecosystem types: A systematic review on boundaries and goals. *Journal of Business Research*, *142*, 138–164.

Coburn, D. (1988). Canadian medicine: Dominance or proletarianization? *The Milbank Quarterly*, *66*(2), 92–116.

Coburn, D., Torrance, G. M., & Kaufert, J. M. (1983). Medical dominance in Canada in historical perspective: The rise and fall of medicine? *International Journal of Health Services*, *13*(3), 407–432.

Cockerham, W. C. (2017). *Medical Sociology*. Routledge.

Cohen, D. K., & Ball, D. L. (2007). Educational innovation and the problem of scale. Scale up in education: *Ideas in Principle*, *1*, 19–36.

Cohen, L. (1993). Quebec, Ontario battle over cross-border health care charges. *CMAJ: Canadian Medical Association Journal*, *148*(7), 1206.

Coleman, J., Katz, E., & Menzel, H. (1957). The diffusion of an innovation among physicians. *Sociometry*, *20*(4), 253–270.

Coleman, J. S., Katz, E., & Menzel, H. (1966). *Medical Innovation: A Diffusion Study*. Bobbs-Merrill.

Collins-Dogrul, J. (2006). Managing US–Mexico "border health": An organizational field approach. *Social Science & Medicine*, *63*(12), 3199–3211.

Collins, G. F., Cassie, J. M., & Daggett, C. J. (1978). The role of the attending physician in clinical training. *Academic Medicine*, *53*(5), 429–431.

Collisson, B., & Howell, J. L. (2014). The liking-similarity effect: Perceptions of similarity as a function of liking. *The Journal of Social Psychology*, *154*(5), 384–400.

Como, J. J., Dutton, R. P., Scalea, T. M., Edelman, B. B., & Hess, J. R. (2004). Blood transfusion rates in the care of acute trauma. *Transfusion*, *44*(6), 809–813.

Consoli, D., & Mina, A. (2009). An evolutionary perspective on health innovation systems. *Journal of Evolutionary Economics*, *19*, 297–319.

Cook, B. G., & Therrien, W. J. (2017). Null effects and publication bias in special education research. *Behavioral Disorders*, *42*(4), 149–158.

Cook, D. A., Brydges, R., Hamstra, S. J., Zendejas, B., Szostek, J. H., Wang, A. T., ... & Hatala, R. (2012). Comparative effectiveness of technology-enhanced simulation versus other instructional methods: A systematic review and meta-analysis. *Simulation in Healthcare*, *7*(5), 308–320.

Cooke, P., Heidenreich, M., & Braczyk, H. J. (2024). Introduction: Regional innovation systems–An evolutionary approach. In P. Cooke, M. Heidenreich, & H.-J. Braczyk (Eds.), *Regional Innovation Systems* (pp. 1–18). Routledge.

Crocq, M. A., & Crocq, L. (2000). From shell shock and war neurosis to posttraumatic stress disorder: A history of psychotraumatology. *Dialogues in Clinical Neuroscience*, *2*(1), 47–55.

Cruz, P. L. (2014). Cross-border governance on the US–Mexico border: Institutional challenges and developments in health collaboration. *Regions and Cohesion*, *4*(1), 53–71.

Daboval, T., Ferretti, E., & Barkova, A. (2027). Communication in ethically sensitive situations: Implementing a training program in neonatology. In J. R. Schoenherr (Ed.), *Fundamentals and Frontiers of Medical Education and Decision-Making: Innovation, Implementation, and Translational Research* (pp. 191–214). Routledge.

Daffé, Z. N., Guillaume, Y., & Ivers, L. C. (2021). Anti-racism and anti-colonialism praxis in global health—Reflection and action for practitioners in US academic medical centers. *The American Journal of Tropical Medicine and Hygiene, 105*(3), 557.

Damschroder, L. J., Aron, D. C., Keith, R. E., Kirsh, S. R., Alexander, J. A., & Lowery, J. C. (2009). Fostering implementation of health services research findings into practice: A consolidated framework for advancing implementation science. *Implementation Science, 4*(1), 50.

Darley, J. M., & Latané, B. (1968). Bystander intervention in emergencies: diffusion of responsibility. *Journal of Personality and Social Psychology, 8*(4p1), 377.

Darling-Hammond, L., Flook, L., Cook-Harvey, C., Barron, B., & Osher, D. (2020). Implications for educational practice of the science of learning and development. *Applied Developmental Science, 24*(2), 97–140.

David, P. A. (1985). Clio and the economics of QWERTY. *American Economic Review, 75*(2), 332–337.

Davis, D. A., & Taylor-Vaisey, A. (1997). Translating guidelines into practice: a systematic review of theoretic concepts, practical experience and research evidence in the adoption of clinical practice guidelines. *CMAJ, 157*(4), 408–416.

Davis, F. D., Bagozzi, R. P., & Warshaw, P. R. (1989). User acceptance of computer technology: A comparison of two theoretical models. *Management Science, 35*(8), 982–1003.

De Divitiis, E., Cappabianca, P., & De Divitiis, O. (2004). The "schola medica salernitana": The forerunner of the modern university medical schools. *Neurosurgery, 55*(4), 722–745.

De Giovanni, D., Roberts, T., & Norman, G. (2009). Relative effectiveness of high-versus low-fidelity simulation in learning heart sounds. *Medical Education, 43*(7), 661–668.

De Vries, R. & Lemmens, T. (2006). The social and cultural shaping of medical evidence: Case studies from pharmaceutical research and obstetric science. *Social Science & Medicine, 62*, 2694–2706.

Dennett, D. C. (1996). *Darwin's Dangerous Idea: Evolution and the Meaning of Life*. Simon and Schuster.

Dickersin, K. (1990). The existence of publication bias and risk factors for its occurrence. *Journal of the American Medical Association, 263*(10), 1385–1389.

Diderichsen, F., Andersen, I., Manuel, C., Working Group of the Danish Review on Social Determinants of Health, Andersen, A. M. N., Bach, E., ... & Søgaard, J. (2012). Health Inequality-determinants and policies. *Scandinavian Journal of Public Health, 40*(8_ suppl), 12–105.

Diehl, M. (1990). The minimal group paradigm: Theoretical explanations and empirical findings. *European Review of Social Psychology, 1*(1), 263–292.

Diener, A. C., & Hagen, J. (Eds.). (2010). *Borderlines and Borderlands: Political Oddities at the Edge of the Nation-State*. Rowman & Littlefield.

DiMaggio, P. J., & Powell, W. W. (1983). The iron cage revisited: Institutional isomorphism and collective rationality in organizational fields. *American Sociological Review, 48*(2), 147–160.

Donelson, A. J., & Esparza, A. X. (Eds.). (2016). *The Colonias Reader: Economy, Housing and Public Health in US-Mexico Border Colonias*. University of Arizona Press.

Dougherty, D., & Conway, P. H. (2008). The "3T's" road map to transform US health care: The "how" of high-quality care. *JAMA, 299*(19), 2319–2321.

Douoguih, M. (2008). Accessing maternal health services in eastern Burma. *Plos Medicine, 5*(12), e250.

Douthwaite, B., Keatinge, J. D. H., & Park, J. R. (2001). Why promising technologies fail: The neglected role of user innovation during adoption. *Research Policy*, *30*(5), 819–836.

Drew, T., Võ, M. L. H., & Wolfe, J. M. (2013). The invisible gorilla strikes again: Sustained inattentional blindness in expert observers. *Psychological Science*, *24*(9), 1848–1853.

Dugar, S., Bhattacharya, H., & Reiley, D. (2012). Can't buy me love? A field experiment exploring the trade-off between income and caste-status in an Indian matrimonial market. *Economic Inquiry*, *50*(2), 534–550.

Edgar, L., Roberts, S., & Holmboe, E. (2018). Milestones 2.0: A step forward. *Journal of Graduate Medical Education*, *10*(3), 367–369.

Edquist, C. (2010). Systems of innovation perspectives and challenges. *African Journal of Science, Technology, Innovation and Development*, *2*(3), 14–45.

Ehri, L. C., Nunes, S. R., Stahl, S. A., & Willows, D. M. (2001). Systematic phonics instruction helps students learn to read: Evidence from the National Reading Panel's meta-analysis. *Review of Educational Research*, *71*(3), 393–447.

Eichbaum, Q. G., Adams, L. V., Evert, J., Ho, M. J., Semali, I. A., & van Schalkwyk, S. C. (2021). Decolonizing global health education: Rethinking institutional partnerships and approaches. *Academic Medicine*, *96*(3), 329–335.

Ekholm, E., & Chow, J. (2018). Addressing publication bias in educational psychology. *Translational Issues in Psychological Science*, *4*(4), 425–439.

El Khoury, J., Toft, M., Hickman, S. E., Means, T. K., Terada, K., Geula, C., & Luster, A. D. (2007). Ccr2 deficiency impairs microglial accumulation and accelerates progression of Alzheimer-like disease. *Nature Medicine*, *13*(4), 432–438.

Ellis, A., & Fouts, J. (1993). *Research on Educational Innovations*. Eye on Education.

Ellis, A., & Fouts, J. (1994). *Research on School Restructuring*. Eye on Education.

Emeto, T. I., Alele, F. O., & Ilesanmi, O. S. (2021). Evaluation of the effect of border closure on COVID-19 incidence rates across nine African countries: An interrupted time series study. *Transactions of The Royal Society of Tropical Medicine and Hygiene*, *115*(10), 1174–1183.

Epstein, R. A. (2005). Disparities and discrimination in health care coverage: A critique of the Institute of Medicine study. *Perspectives in Biology and Medicine*, *48*(1), 26–S41.

Erickson, F., & Mohatt, G. (1982). Cultural organization of participation structures in two classrooms of Indian students. *Doing the Ethnography of Schooling*, *132*, 174.

Ericsson, A. C., Crim, M. J., & Franklin, C. L. (2013). A brief history of animal modeling. *Missouri Medicine*, *110*(3), 201.

Eveland, J.D., 1986. Diffusion, technology transfer, and implementation. *Knowledge*, *8*, 303–322.

Every-Palmer, S., & Howick, J. (2014). How evidence-based medicine is failing due to biased trials and selective publication. *Journal of Evaluation in Clinical Practice*, *20*(6), 908–914.

Ferdinand, A. S., Paradies, Y., & Kelaher, M. (2022). A comprehensive review of optimal approaches to co-design in health with first nations Australians. *International Journal of Environmental Research and Public Health*, *19*(24), 16733.

Ferguson, P. C., Caverzagie, K. J., Nousiainen, M. T., Snell, L., & ICBME collaborators. (2017). Changing the culture of medical training: An important step toward the implementation of competency-based medical education. *Medical Teacher*, *39*, 599–602.

Ferretti, E., Schoenherr, J. R., Mattiola, A., & Daboval, T. (2023). Vulnerabilities in clinician–parent exchanges and the cascade of communication traps: A review. *Archives of Disease in Childhood*, *108*(2), 86–90.

Finkler, K. (2019). *Physicians at Work, Patients in Pain: Biomedical Practice and Patient Response in Mexico*. Routledge.

Fiske, S. T., Cuddy, A. J. C., Glick, P., & Xu, J. (2002). A model of (often mixed) stereotype content: Competence and warmth respectively follow from perceived status and competition. *Journal of Personality and Social Psychology*, *82*(6), 878–902.

Fiske, S. T., Cuddy, A. J., Glick, P., & Xu, J. (2018). A model of (often mixed) stereotype content: Competence and warmth respectively follow from perceived status and competition. In *Social Cognition* (pp. 162–214). Routledge.

Fleuren, M., Wiefferink, K., & Paulussen, T. (2004). Determinants of innovation within health care organizations: literature review and Delphi study. *International Journal for Quality in Health Care*, *16*(2), 107–123.

Fleuriet, K. J., & Castañeda, H. (2017). A risky place? Media and the health landscape in the (In) secure US-Mexico borderlands. *North American Dialogue*, *20*(2), 32–46.

Flexner, A. (1910). *Medical Education in the United States and Canada: A Report to the Carnegie Foundation for the Advancement of Teaching*. Carnegie Foundation for the Advancement of Teaching.

Fooks, G. J., Williams, S., Box, G., & Sacks, G. (2019). Corporations' use and misuse of evidence to influence health policy: A case study of sugar-sweetened beverage taxation. *Globalization and Health*, *15*(1), 56.

Ford, E. W., Menachemi, N., & Phillips, M. T. (2006). Predicting the adoption of electronic health records by physicians: When will health care be paperless? *Journal of the American Medical Informatics Association*, *13*(1), 106–112.

Frambach, J. M., Driessen, E. W., Chan, L. C., & van der Vleuten, C. P. (2012). Rethinking the globalisation of problem-based learning: How culture challenges self-directed learning. *Medical Education*, *46*(8), 738–747.

Frank, J. R., Snell, L. S., Cate, O. T., Holmboe, E. S., Carraccio, C., Swing, S. R., ... & Harris, K. A. (2010). Competency-based medical education: Theory to practice. *Medical Teacher*, *32*, 638–645.

Freidson, E. (1985). The reorganization of the medical profession. *Medical Care Review*, *42*(1), 11–35.

Froehlich, L., Dorrough, A. R., Glöckner, A., & Stürmer, S. (2021). Similarity predicts cross-national social preferences. *Social Psychological and Personality Science*, *12*(8), 1486–1498.

Frohlich, K. L., & Potvin, L. (2008). Transcending the known in public health practice: The inequality paradox. *American Journal of Public Health*, *98*(2), 216–221.

Fullan, M. (1972). Overview of the innovative process and the user. *Interchange*, *3*, 1–46.

Fune, J., Chinchilla, J. P., Hoppe, A., Mbanugo, C., Zuellig, R., Abboud, A. T., ... & Monica van de Ridder, J. M. (2021). Lost in translation: An OSCE-based workshop for helping learners navigate a limited English proficiency patient encounter. *MedEdPORTAL*, *17*, 11118.

Gabriel, R. A. (2013). *Between Flesh and Steel: A History of Military Medicine from the Middle Ages to the War in Afghanistan*. Potomac Books, Inc.

Gage, N. A., Cook, B. G., & Reichow, B. (2017). Publication bias in special education meta-analyses. *Exceptional Children*, *83*(4), 428–445.

Gall, M.D., Gall, J.P., & Borg, W.R. (2003). *Educational Research: An Introduction*. Allyn and Bacon.

Gallaud, D., & Torre, A. (2005). Geographical proximity and the diffusion of knowledge: the case of SME's in biotechnology. In G. Fuchs & P. Shapira (Eds.), *Rethinking Regional Innovation and Change: Path Dependency or Regional Breakthrough?* (pp. 127–146). Springer New York.

Garry, S., & Checchi, F. (2020). Armed conflict and public health: Into the 21st century. *Journal of Public Health*, *42*(3), e287–e298.

Garud, R., Tuertscher, P., & Van de Ven, A. H. (2013). Perspectives on innovation processes. *Academy of Management Annals*, *7*(1), 775–819.

Gaur, U., Majumder, M. A. A., Sa, B., Sarkar, S., Williams, A., & Singh, K. (2020). Challenges and opportunities of preclinical medical education: COVID-19 crisis and beyond. *SN Comprehensive Clinical Medicine*, *2*(11), 1992–1997.

Gee, G. C., & Ford, C. L. (2011). Structural racism and health inequities: Old issues, New Directions. *Du Bois Review: Social Science Research on Race*, *8*(1), 115–132.

Geels, F. W. (2004). From sectoral systems of innovation to socio-technical systems: Insights about dynamics and change from sociology and institutional theory. *Research Policy*, *33*(6–7), 897–920.

Geels, F. W. (2011). The multi-level perspective on sustainability transitions: Responses to seven criticisms. *Environmental Innovation and Societal Transitions*, *1*(1), 24–40.

Geels, F. W., & Schot, J. (2007). Typology of sociotechnical transition pathways. *Research Policy*, *36*(3), 399–417.

Gele, A. A., Ahmed, M. Y., Kour, P., Moallim, S. A., Salad, A. M., & Kumar, B. (2017). Beneficiaries of conflict: A qualitative study of people's trust in the private health care system in Mogadishu, Somalia. *Risk Management and Healthcare Policy*, 127–135.

Gelfand, M. J., et al. (2006). Cultural tightness-looseness: A multilevel review. *Journal of Applied Psychology*, *91*(6).

Gelfand, M. J., Raver, J. L., Nishii, L., Leslie, L. M., Lun, J., Lim, B. C., ... & Yamaguchi, S. (2011). Differences between tight and loose cultures: A 33-nation study. *Science*, *332*(6033), 1100–1104.

Gentner, D., & Maravilla, F. (2017). Analogical reasoning. In L. J. Ball & V. A. Thompson (Eds.), *International Handbook of Thinking and Reasoning* (pp. 186–203). Routledge.

Ghasemiardekani, M., Dadpour, R., Irannezhad, E., & Bidarmaghz, A. (2023). Endangering trust in health services: Using ambulances to arrest protesters in Iran. *Medicine, Conflict and Survival*, *39*(4), 345–351.

Gibbons, D., & Olk, P. M. (2003). Individual and structural origins of friendship and social position among professionals. *Journal of Personality and Social Psychology*, *84*(2), 340.

Gibson, J. J. (1977). The theory of affordances. In R. E. Shaw & J. Bransford (Eds.), *Perceiving, Acting, and Knowing: Toward an Ecological Psychology* (pp. 67–82). Lawrence Erlbaum Associates.

Givens, M., Muck, A. E., & Goolsby, C. (2017). Battlefield to bedside: Translating wartime innovations to civilian Emergency Medicine. *The American Journal of Emergency Medicine*, *35*(11), 1746–1749.

Goldberg, M. A. (2016). *Conquering Sickness: Race, Health, and Colonization in the Texas Borderlands*. University of Nebraska Press.

Gone, J. P., Hartmann, W. E., Pomerville, A., Wendt, D. C., Klem, S. H., & Burrage, R. L. (2019). The impact of historical trauma on health outcomes for Indigenous populations in the USA and Canada: A systematic review. *American Psychologist*, *74*(1), 20–35.

Gongal, R., & Subedi, M. (2027). Developing and implementing a medical humanities curriculum in the undergraduate medical curriculum in Nepal. In J. R. Schoenherr (Ed.), *Fundamentals and Frontiers of Medical Education and Decision-Making: Innovation, Implementation, and Translational Research* (pp. 215–246). Routledge.

Gordon, M., Patricio, M., Horne, L., Muston, A., Alston, S. R., Pammi, M., ... & Daniel, M. (2020). Developments in medical education in response to the COVID-19 pandemic: A rapid BEME systematic review: BEME Guide No. 63. *Medical Teacher, 42*(11), 1202–1215.

Gorry, G. A., Kassirer, J. P., Essig, A., & Schwartz, W. B. (1973). Decision analysis as the basis for computer-aided management of acute renal failure. *The American Journal of Medicine*, *55*(4), 473–484.

Gosselin, K., Norris, J. L., & Ho, M. J. (2016). Beyond homogenization discourse: Reconsidering the cultural consequences of globalized medical education. *Medical Teacher*, *38*(7), 691–699.

Gracey, M., & King, M. (2009). Indigenous health part 1: Determinants and disease patterns. *The Lancet*, *374*(9683), 65–75.

Graesser, A. C., Conley, M. W., & Olney, A. (2012). Intelligent tutoring systems. In K. R. Harris, S. Graham, T. Urdan, A. G. Bus, S. Major, & H. L. Swanson (Eds.), *APA Educational Psychology Handbook* (pp. 451–473). American Psychological Association.

Green, L. W., Ottoson, J. M., Garcia, C., & Hiatt, R. A. (2009). Diffusion theory and knowledge dissemination, utilization, and integration in public health. *Annual Review of Public Health*, *30*, 151–174.

Greenhalgh, T., Robert, G., Macfarlane, F., Bate, P., & Kyriakidou, O. (2004). Diffusion of innovations in service organizations: Systematic review and recommendations. *The Milbank Quarterly*, *82*(4), 581–629.

Grillitsch, M., & Trippl, M. (2016). Innovation policies and new regional growth paths: A place-based system failure framework. *Papers in Innovation Studies*, *26*, 1–23.

Grossen, B. (1998). What does it mean to be a research-based profession? In W. Evers (Ed.), *What's Gone Wrong in America's Classrooms?* (pp. 24–44). Hoover Institution Press.

Grundy Q., Millington A., Cussen C., Held F., & Dale C. M. (2020). Promotion or education: A content analysis of industry-authored oral health educational materials targeted at acute care nurses. *BMJ Open*, *10*(11), e04054.

Gruppen, L. D., Mangrulkar, R. S., & Kolars, J. C. (2012). The promise of competency-based education in the health professions for improving global health. *Human Resources for Health*, *10*, 1–7.

Guinote, A. E., & Vescio, T. K. (2010). *The Social Psychology of Power*. The Guilford Press.

Guma, P. M., & Mokgoatšana, S. (2020). *The* historical relationship between African indigenous healing practices and Western-orientated biomedicine in South Africa: A challenge to collaboration. *HTS Teologiese Studies/Theological Studies*, *76*(4), a6104.

Gumport, P. J. (2000). Academic restructuring: Organizational change and institutional imperatives. *Higher Education*, *39*(1), 67–91.

Gunawardena, C. N., & McIsaac, M. S. (2013). Distance education. In J. Michael Spector, M. David Merrill, Jeroen van Merriënboer, & Marcy P. Driscoll (Eds.), *Handbook of Research on Educational Communications and Technology* (pp. 361–401). Routledge.

Gupta, P., Dewan, P., & Singh, T. (2010). Objective structured clinical examination (OSCE) revisited. *Indian Pediatrics*, *47*(11), 911–920.

Guze, P. A. (2015). Using technology to meet the challenges of medical education. *Transactions of the American Clinical and Climatological Association*, *126*, 260.

Haar, R. J., Read, R., Fast, L., Blanchet, K., Rinaldi, S., Taithe, B., ... & Rubenstein, L. S. (2021). Violence against healthcare in conflict: A systematic review of the literature and agenda for future research. *Conflict and Health*, *15*(1), 37.

Haddaway, N. R., Collins, A. M., Coughlin, D., & Kirk, S. (2015). The role of Google Scholar in evidence reviews and its applicability to grey literature searching. *PloS One*, *10*(9), e0138237.

Haider, M., & Kreps, G. L. (2004). Forty years of diffusion of innovations: utility and value in public health. *Journal of Health Communication*, *9*(S1), 3–11.

Hamstra, S. J., Brydges, R., Hatala, R., Zendejas, B., & Cook, D. A. (2014). Reconsidering fidelity in simulation-based training. *Academic Medicine*, *89*(3), 387–392.

Han, H., Resch, D. S., & Kovach, R. A. (2013). Educational technology in medical education. *Teaching and Learning in Medicine*, *25*(sup1), S39–S43.

Hannan, T. H., & McDowell, J. M. (1984). The determinants of technology adoption: The case of the banking firm. *RAND Journal of Economics*, *15*(3), 328–335.

Hanington, B. M. (2010). Relevant and rigorous: Human-centered research and design education. *Design Issues*, *26*(3), 18–26.

Hanson, K., Gilson, L., Goodman, C., Mills, A., Smith, R., Feachem, R., ... & Kinlaw, H. (2008). Is private health care the answer to the health problems of the world's poor? *PLoS Medicine*, *5*(11), e233.

Harfield, S. G., Davy, C., McArthur, A., Munn, Z., Brown, A., & Brown, N. (2018). Characteristics of Indigenous primary health care service delivery models: a systematic scoping review. *Globalization and Health*, *14*(1), 12.

Heckman, J. (1990). Varieties of selection bias. *The American Economic Review*, *80*(2), 313–318.

Hedin, R. J., Umberham, B. A., Detweiler, B. N., Kollmorgen, L., & Vassar, M. (2016). Publication bias and nonreporting found in majority of systematic reviews and meta-analyses in anesthesiology journals. *Anesthesia & Analgesia*, *123*(4), 1018–1025.

Heffernan, T., Morrison, M., Basu, P., & Sweeney, A. (2010). Cultural differences, learning styles and transnational education. *Journal of Higher Education Policy and Management*, *32*(1), 27–39.

Hekkert, M. P., Suurs, R. A., Negro, S. O., Kuhlmann, S., & Smits, R. E. (2007). Functions of innovation systems: A new approach for analysing technological change. *Technological Forecasting and Social Change*, *74*(4), 413–432.

Helling, T. (2022). *The Great War and the Birth of Modern Medicine: A History*. Simon and Schuster.

Henrich, J. (2020). *The WEIRDest People in the World: How the West Became Psychologically Peculiar and Particularly Prosperous*. Penguin.

Henrich, J., Heine, S. J., & Norenzayan, A. (2010). The weirdest people in the world? *Behavioral and Brain Sciences*, *33*(2-3), 61–83.

Hicks, J. R. (1932). *Theory of Wages*. Macmillan.

Hodges, B. (2013). Assessment in the post-psychometric era: Learning to love the subjective and collective. *Medical Teacher*, *35*, 564–568.

Hofstede, G. (1986). Cultural differences in teaching and learning. *International Journal of Intercultural Relations*, *10*(3), 301–320.

Hoke, M. K., Stumo, S. R., Leatherman, T. L., Hannig, A., Mattingly, C., Janzen, J. M., ... & Wendland, C. (2022). *The Work of Hospitals: Global Medicine in Local Cultures*. Rutgers University Press.

Holmboe, E. S., Sherbino, J., Englander, R., Snell, L., Frank, J. R., & Icbme Collaborators. (2017). A call to action: the controversy of and rationale for competency-based medical education. *Medical Teacher*, *39*(6), 574–581.

Holyoak, K. J. (2012). Analogy and relational reasoning. In K. J. Holyoak & R. G. Morrison (Eds.), the *Oxford Handbook of Thinking and Reasoning* (pp. 234–259). Oxford University Press.

Homan, P. (2019). Structural sexism and health in the United States: A new perspective on health inequality and the gender system. *American Sociological Review*, *84*(3), 486–516.
Homer, J. B. (1987). A diffusion model with application to evolving medical technologies. *Technological Forecasting and Social Change*, *31*(3), 197–218.
Hopewell, S., Clarke, M., & Mallett, S. (2005). Grey literature and systematic reviews. In *Publication Bias in Meta-Analysis: Prevention, Assessment and Adjustments.* (pp. 49–72). John Wiley.
House, E. R. (1979). *Three Perspectives on Innovation, the Technological, the Political and the Cultural.* US Department of Education, Office of Educational Research and Improvement.
Huang, J., Galal, G., Etemadi, M., & Vaidyanathan, M. (2022). Evaluation and mitigation of racial bias in clinical machine learning models: Scoping review. *JMIR Medical Informatics*, *10*(5), e36388.
Hughes, T. P. (1987). *The Evolution of Large Technological Systems. The Social Construction of Technological Systems: New Directions in the Sociology and History of Technology.* MIT Press.
Ingvarsson, S., Hasson, H., von Thiele Schwarz, U., Nilsen, P., Powell, B. J., Lindberg, C., & Augustsson, H. (2022). Strategies for de-implementation of low-value care—A scoping review. *Implementation Science*, *17*(1), 1–15.
Institute of Medicine. (2003). *Unequal Treatment: Confronting Racial and Ethnic Disparities in Health Care*. National Academies Press.
Ioannidis, J. P. (2016). The mass production of redundant, misleading, and conflicted systematic reviews and meta-analyses. *The Milbank Quarterly*, *94*(3), 485–514.
Isaksen, A., & Trippl, M. (2016). Path development in different regional innovation systems: A conceptual analysis. In M. D. Parrilli, R. D. Fitjar, & A. Rodríguez-Pose (Eds.), *Innovation Drivers and Regional Innovation Strategies* (pp. 66–84). Routledge.
Ismaeel, R., Pusic, L. J., Gottlieb, M., Chan, T. M., Oyedokun, T. O., & Thoma, B. (2023). Bias in observed assessments in medical education: A scoping review. *Academic Medicine*, 99, 1438–1450.
Ivanivna, K. I., & Schoenherr, J. R. (2027). Medical education despite war: Innovation in the health professions during armed conflict. In J. R. Schoenherr (Ed.), *Fundamentals and Frontiers of Medical Education and Decision-Making: Innovation, Implementation, and Translational Research* (pp. 247–283). Routledge.
Jablonka, E., & Lamb, M. J. (2014). *Evolution in Four Dimensions: Genetic, Epigenetic, Behavioral, and Symbolic Variation in the History of Life, Revised Edition*. MIT Press.
Jain, A., Brooks, J. R., Alford, C. C., Chang, C. S., Mueller, N. M., Umscheid, C. A., & Bierman, A. S. (2023). Awareness of racial and ethnic bias and potential solutions to address bias with use of health care algorithms. *JAMA Health Forum*, *4*(6), e231197–e231197.
Ján, D., & Veronika, T. (2017). Examination of factors affecting the implementation of organizational changes. *Journal of Competitiveness*, *9*(4).
Jimenez, G., Spinazze, P., Matchar, D., Huat, G. K. C., van der Kleij, R. M., Chavannes, N. H., & Car, J. (2020). Digital health competencies for primary healthcare professionals: a scoping review. *International Journal of Medical Informatics*, *143*, 104260.
Jippes, E., Steinert, Y., Pols, J., Achterkamp, M. C., van Engelen, J. M., & Brand, P. L. (2013). How do social networks and faculty development courses affect clinical supervisors' adoption of a medical education innovation? An exploratory study. *Academic Medicine*, *88*(3), 398–404.
Johnson J., & Hutchison K. (2018). They know how to work it, that's their focus in life: The complex role of industry representatives in surgical innovation. *Journal of Empirical Research on Human Research Ethics*, *13*, 461–474.

Johnson, K. F. (2019). Preparing 21st century counselors and healthcare professionals: Examining technology competency and interprofessional education comfort. *Journal of Counselor Preparation and Supervision, 12*(4), 7.

Jordan, C. (1985). Translating culture: From ethnographic information to educational program. *Anthropology & Education Quarterly, 16*(2), 105–123.

Kadam, R., Rao, S. A., Kareem Abdul, W., & Jabeen, S. S. (2020). Diversity climate perceptions and its impact on multicultural team innovation and performance. *Measuring Business Excellence, 24*(3), 301–318.

Kadushin, C. (2012). *Understanding Social Networks: Theories, Concepts, and Findings*. Oxford University Press.

Kananoja, K. (2021). *Healing Knowledge in Atlantic Africa: Medical Encounters, 1500–1850*. Cambridge University Press.

Kane, M. T. (1992). An argument-based approach to validity. *Psychological Bulletin, 112*(3), 527.

Karavas-Doukas, K. (2014). Evaluating the implementation of educational innovations: lessons from the past. In P. Rea-Dickins & K. Germaine (Eds.), *Managing Evaluation and Innovation in Language Teaching* (pp. 25–50). Routledge.

Karle, H., Christensen, L., Gordon, D., & Nystrup, J. (2008). Neo-colonialism versus sound globalisation policy in medical education. *Medical Education, 42*(10), 956–958.

Katz, E., Levin, M. L., & Hamilton, H. (1963). Traditions of research on the diffusion of innovation. *American Sociological Review, 28*(2), 237–252.

Kelly, M. E., Dowell, J., Husbands, A., Newell, J., O'Flynn, S., Kropmans, T., ... & Murphy, A. W. (2014). The fairness, predictive validity and acceptability of multiple mini interview in an internationally diverse student population-A mixed methods study. *BMC Medical Education, 14*, 1–13.

Kennedy, C. (1964). Induced bias in innovation and the theory of distribution. *Economic Journal, 74*, 803–819.

Khan, K. (2027). Inequality and social mobility in the medical professions in India: Career availability and vulnerabilities. In J. R. Schoenherr (Ed.), *Fundamentals and Frontiers of Medical Education and Decision-Making: Innovation, Implementation, and Translational Research* (pp. 336–358). Routledge.

Khessina, O. M., Goncalo, J. A., & Krause, V. (2018). It's time to sober up: The direct costs, side effects and long-term consequences of creativity and innovation. *Research in Organizational Behavior, 38*, 107–135.

King, M., Smith, A., & Gracey, M. (2009). Indigenous health part 2: The underlying causes of the health gap. *The Lancet, 374*(9683), 76–85.

Kirschner, P. A. (2017). Stop propagating the learning styles myth. *Computers & Education, 106*, 166–171.

Kirmayer, L. J., Gone, J. P., & Moses, J. (2014). Rethinking historical trauma. *Transcultural Psychiatry*, 51(3), 299–319.

Kitson, A., Harvey, G., & McCormack, B. (1998). Enabling the implementation of evidence based practice: A conceptual framework. *BMJ Quality & Safety, 7*(3), 149–158.

Köchling, A., & Wehner, M. C. (2020). Discriminated by an algorithm: A systematic review of discrimination and fairness by algorithmic decision-making in the context of HR recruitment and HR development. *Business Research, 13*(3), 795–848.

Komarraju, M., Karau, S. J., Schmeck, R. R., & Avdic, A. (2011). The Big Five personality traits, learning styles, and academic achievement. *Personality and Individual Differences, 51*(4), 472–477.

Kurtzberg, T. R. (2005). Feeling creative, being creative: An empirical study of diversity and creativity in teams. *Creativity Research Journal, 17*(1), 51–65.

Kurtzberg, T. R., & Amabile, T. M. (2001). From Guilford to creative synergy: Opening the black box of team-level creativity. *Creativity Research Journal*, 13(3–4), 285–294.

Kwang, N. A., & Rodrigues, D. (2002). A Big-Five Personality profile of the adaptor and innovator. *The Journal of Creative Behavior, 36*(4), 254–268.

Ladson-Billings, G. (1995). Toward a theory of culturally relevant pedagogy. *American Educational Research Journal, 32*(3), 465–491.

Leather, A., Ismail, E. A., Ali, R., Abdi, Y. A., Abby, M. H., Gulaid, S. A., ... & Parry, E. (2006). Working together to rebuild health care in post-conflict Somaliland. *The Lancet, 368*(9541), 1119–1125.

Lee, J., & Park, O. C. (2008). Adaptive instructional systems. In J. M. Spector, M. D. Merrill, J. van Merrienboer, & M. P. Driscoll (Eds.), *Handbook of Research on Educational Communications and Technology* (pp. 469–484). Routledge.

Lee, T. T. (2004). Nurses' adoption of technology: Application of Rogers' innovation-diffusion model. *Applied Nursing Research, 17*(4), 231–238.

Lehning, J. R. (2013). *European Colonialism Since 1700*. Cambridge University Press.

Leung, A. K. Y., Maddux, W. W., Galinsky, A. D., & Chiu, C. Y. (2008). Multicultural experience enhances creativity: The when and how. *American Psychologist, 63*(3), 169.

Lewis, K. O., Hathaway, S. B., Bratcher, D., Blowey, D., & Knapp, J. F. (2021). Current milestones assessment practices, needs, and challenges of program directors: A collective case study in a pediatric hospital setting. *Cureus, 13*(4).

Lien, A. S. Y., & Jiang, Y. D. (2017). Integration of diffusion of innovation theory into diabetes care. *Journal of Diabetes Investigation, 8*(3), 259.

Lim, S., Boutain, D. M., Kim, E., Evans-Agnew, R. A., Parker, S., & Maldonado Nofziger, R. (2022). Institutional procedural discrimination, institutional racism, and other institutional discrimination: A nursing research example. *Nursing Inquiry, 29*(1), e12474.

Lingard, L. (2012). Rethinking competence in the context of teamwork: A case for collective competence. *Medical Education*, 46(1), 54–63

Lis, J., Chuang, J., & Schoenherr, J. R. (2022). Implementation tools. In J. Goodell & J. Kolodner (Eds.), *Learning Engineering Toolkit* (pp. 347–360). Routledge.

Litzinger, T. A., Lee, S. H., Wise, J. C., & Felder, R. M. (2007). A psychometric study of the index of learning styles. *Journal of Engineering Education, 96*(4), 309–319.

Lock, M. (2003). Globalization and cultures of biomedicine: Japan and North America. In H. Selin (Ed.), *Medicine Across Cultures: History and Practice of Medicine in Non-Western Cultures* (pp. 155–173). Springer Netherlands.

Lockwood, D. (2021). *Fooled by the Winners: How Survivor Bias Deceives Us*. Greenleaf Book Group.

Looney, J. W. (2009). *Assessment and Innovation in Education*. OECD Working Papers.

Luke, D. A., & Harris, J. K. (2007). Network analysis in public health: History, methods, and applications. *Annual Review of Public Health, 28*, 69–83.

Lundvall, B. Å. (2007). National innovation systems—analytical concept and development tool. *Industry and Innovation, 14*(1), 95–119.

Mabry, R. L., & Frankfurt, A. (2012). An analysis of battlefield cricothyrotomy in Iraq and Afghanistan. *Journal of Special Operations Medicine, 12*(1), 17–23.

MacDonald, D. (2007). First Nations, residential schools, and the Americanization of the Holocaust: Rewriting Indigenous history in the United States and Canada. *Canadian Journal of Political Science/Revue canadienne de science politique, 40*(4), 995–1015.

Macias, E. P., & Morales, L. S. (2001). Crossing the border for health care. *Journal of Health Care for the Poor and Underserved*, *12*(1), 77–87.

Maddux, C. D. (1986). The educational computing backlash: Can the swing of the pendulum be halted? *Computers in the Schools*, *3*(2), 27–30.

Maddux, C., & Cummings, R. (2004). Fad, fashion, and the weak role of theory and research in information technology in education. *Journal of Technology and Teacher Education*, *12*(4), 511–533.

Mahood, Q., Van Eerd, D., & Irvin, E. (2014). Searching for grey literature for systematic reviews: challenges and benefits. *Research Synthesis Methods*, *5*(3), 221–234.

Maity, R., Kumar, H., Dhali, A., Biswas, J., & Kumar, B. (2024). The ongoing Israel-Hamas conflict: A humanitarian health crisis. *Annals of Medicine and Surgery*, 20, 4313–4315.

Mallidou, A. A., Atherton, P., Chan, L., Frisch, N., Glegg, S., & Scarrow, G. (2018). Core knowledge translation competencies: A scoping review. *BMC Health Services Research*, *18*(1), 502.

Manlhiot, C. (2018). Machine learning for predictive analytics in medicine: Real opportunity or overblown hype?. *European Heart Journal-Cardiovascular Imaging*, *19*(7), 727–728.

Mannix, E., & Neale, M. A. (2005). What differences make a difference? The promise and reality of diverse teams in organizations. *Psychological Science in the Public Interest*, *6*(2), 31–55.

Marcati, A., Guido, G., & Peluso, A. M. (2008). The role of SME entrepreneurs' innovativeness and personality in the adoption of innovations. *Research Policy*, *37*(9), 1579–1590.

Marcotte, L. M., Krimmel-Morrison, J., & Liao, J. M. (2020). How to keep diffusion of responsibility from undermining value-based care. *AMA Journal of Ethics*, *22*(9), 802–807.

Maretzki, T. W. (1989). Cultural variation in biomedicine: The kur in West Germany. *Medical Anthropology Quarterly*, *3*(1), 22–35.

Marrone, S. (2007). Understanding barriers to health care: A review of disparities in health care services among indigenous populations. *International Journal of Circumpolar Health*, *66*(3), 188–198.

Martineau, T., McPake, B., Theobald, S., Raven, J., Ensor, T., Fustukian, S., ... & Witter, S. (2017). Leaving no one behind: Lessons on rebuilding health systems in conflict-and crisis-affected states. *BMJ Global Health*, *2*(2), e000327.

May, C & Finch, T. (2009). Implementing, embedding, and integrating practices: An outline of normalization process theory. *Sociology*, *43*,:535–554.

May, C. R., Albers, B., Bracher, M., Finch, T. L., Gilbert, A., Girling, M., ... & Rapley, T. (2022). Translational framework for implementation evaluation and research: A normalisation process theory coding manual for qualitative research and instrument development. *Implementation Science*, *17*(1), 19.

McGaghie, W. C., Miller, G. E., Sajid, A. W., & Telder, T. V. (1978). *Competency-Based Curriculum Development in Medical Education. An Introduction*. Public Health Papers.

McGauran, N., Wieseler, B., Kreis, J., Schüler, Y. B., Kölsch, H., & Kaiser, T. (2010). Reporting bias in medical research–A narrative review. *Trials*, *11*, 1–15.

Mcintosh, E. (2019). The implications of diffusion of responsibility on patient safety during anaesthesia, 'So that others may learn and even more may live'–Martin Bromiley. *Journal of Perioperative Practice*, *29*(10), 341–345.

McIsaac, M. S. (2001). Distance education. In *Encyclopedia of Education* (2nd ed.). Macmillan.

Mckiernan-González, J. (2012). *Fevered Measures: Public Health and Race at the Texas-Mexico Border, 1848–1942*. Duke University Press.

McNeill, W. H. (1976). *Plagues and Peoples*. Anchor Books.

McPherson, M., Smith-Lovin, L., & Cook, J. M. (2001). Birds of a feather: Homophily in social networks. *Annual Review of Sociology*, *27*(1), 415–444.

Meltzoff, A. N., Kuhl, P. K., Movellan, J., & Sejnowski, T. J. (2009). Foundations for a new science of learning. *Science*, *325*(5938), 284–288.

Messick, S. (1995). Standards of validity and the validity of standards in performance asessment. *Educational Measurement: Issues and Practice*, *14*(4), 5–8.

Michael, K., Schoenherr, J. R., & Vogel, K. M. (2024). Failures in the loop: Human leadership in AI-based decision-making. *IEEE Transactions on Technology and Society*, *5*(1), 2–13.

Mignon, I. (2017). Intermediary–user collaboration during the innovation implementation process. *Technology Analysis & Strategic Management*, *29*(7), 735–749.

Miller, L. E., & Weiss, R. M. (2012). Revisiting black medical school extinctions in the Flexner era. *Journal of the History of Medicine and Allied Sciences*, *67*(2), 217–243.

Millington, S. J., Arntfield, R. T., Guo, R. J., Koenig, S., Kory, P., Noble, V., ... & Schoenherr, J. R. (2018). Expert agreement in the interpretation of lung ultrasound studies performed on mechanically ventilated patients. *Journal of Ultrasound in Medicine*, *37*(11), 2659–2665.

Mintzberg, H. (1983). *Structure in Fives: Designing Effective Organizations*. Prentice-Hall.

Mohatt, G., & Erickson, F. (1981). Cultural differences in teaching styles in an Odawa school: A sociolinguistic approach. In H. Trueba, G. Guthrie, & K. Au (Eds.), *Culture and the Bilingual Classroom* (pp. 105–119). Newbury House.

Mohatt, N. V., Thompson, A. B., Thai, N. D., & Tebes, J. K. (2014). Historical trauma as public narrative: A conceptual review of how history impacts present-day health. *Social Science & Medicine*, *106*, 128–136.

Mokyr, J. (2010). Induced technical innovation and medical history: An evolutionary approach. In A. Grübler, N. Nakicenovic, & W. D. Nordhaus (Eds.), *Technological Change and the Environment* (pp. 40–60). Routledge.

Monteiro, S., Cavanagh, A., Biswabandan, B., & Sibbald, M. (2024). Separating the noise from the signal: The role of familiarity and pattern recognition in the development of clinical expertise. (pp. 169–185). Routledge. In J. R. Schoenherr & M. M. McConnell (Eds.), *Fundamentals and Frontiers of Medical Education and Decision-Making: Educational Theory and Psychological Practice*.

Montenegro, R. A., & Stephens, C. (2006). Indigenous health in Latin America and the Caribbean. *The Lancet*, *367*(9525), 1859–1869.

Moran, J., Briscoe, G., & Peglow, S. (2018). Current technology in advancing medical education: Perspectives for learning and providing care. *Academic Psychiatry*, *42*, 796–799.

Moscati, R., Jehle, D., Ellis, D., Fiorello, A., & Landi, M. (1994). Positive-outcome bias: Comparison of emergency medicine and general medicine literatures. *Academic Emergency Medicine*, *1*(3), 267–271.

Mulgan, G. (2012). Social innovation theories: Can theory catch up with practice? In H.-W. Franz, J. Hochgerner, & J. Howaldt (Eds.), *Challenge Social Innovation: Potentials for Business, Social Entrepreneurship, Welfare and Civil Society* (pp. 19–42). Springer Berlin Heidelberg.

Murad, M. H., Chu, H., Lin, L., & Wang, Z. (2018). The effect of publication bias magnitude and direction on the certainty in evidence. *BMJ Evidence-Based Medicine*, *23*(3), 84–86

Myers, R. H., & Peattie, M. R. (Eds.). (2020). *The Japanese Colonial Empire, 1895-1945*. Princeton University Press.

Naidu, T. (2021). Modern medicine is a colonial artifact: Introducing decoloniality to medical education research. *Academic Medicine, 96*(11S), S9–S12.

Nasser, M., Tibi, A., & Savage-Smith, E. (2009). Ibn Sina's Canon of Medicine: 11th century rules for assessing the effects of drugs. *Journal of the Royal Society of Medicine, 102*(2), 78–80.

Natesan, P., Batley, N. J., Bakhti, R., & El-Doueihi, P. Z. (2018). Challenges in measuring ACGME competencies: Considerations for milestones. *International Journal of Emergency Medicine, 11*, 1–6.

Navarro-Bringas, E., Bowles, G., & Walker, G. H. (2020). Embracing complexity: A sociotechnical systems approach for the design and evaluation of higher education learning environments. *TheoreTical issues in ergonomics science, 21*(5), 595–613.

Newton, P. M., & Salvi, A. (2020). How common is belief in the learning styles neuromyth, and does it matter? A pragmatic systematic review. *Frontiers in Education, 5*.

Nill, J., & Kemp, R. (2009). Evolutionary approaches for sustainable innovation policies: From niche to paradigm? *Research Policy, 38*(4), 668–680.

Nisbett, R. (2010). *The Geography of Thought: How Asians and Westerners Think Differently*. Simon and Schuster.

Nong, P., Raj, M., Creary, M., Kardia, S. L., & Platt, J. E. (2020). Patient-reported experiences of discrimination in the US health care system. *JAMA Network Open, 3*(12), e2029650.

Norman, D. A. (1999). Affordance, conventions, and design. *Interactions, 6*, 38–43.

Norman, D. A. (2013). *The Design of Everyday Things: Revised and Expanded Edition*. Basic Books.

Norman, G. R., Dore, K., & Grierson, L. (2012). The minimal relationship between simulation fidelity and transfer of learning. *Medical Education, 46*(7), 636–647.

Norman, G. R., Grierson, L. E. M., Sherbino, J., Hamstra, S. J., Schmidt, H. G., & Mamede, S. (2018). Expertise in medicine and surgery. In K. A. Ericsson, R. R. Hoffman, A. Kozbelt, & A. M. Williams (Eds.), *The Cambridge Handbook of Expertise and Expert Performance* (2nd ed., pp. 331–355). Cambridge University Press.

Norton, W. E., & Chambers, D. A. (2020). Unpacking the complexities of de-implementing inappropriate health interventions. *Implementation Science, 15*(1), 2.

Noseworthy, P. A., Attia, Z. I., Brewer, L. C., Hayes, S. N., Yao, X., Kapa, S., ... & Lopez-Jimenez, F. (2020). Assessing and mitigating bias in medical artificial intelligence: the effects of race and ethnicity on a deep learning model for ECG analysis. *Circulation: Arrhythmia and Electrophysiology, 13*(3), e007988.

Nousiainen, M. T., Caverzagie, K. J., Ferguson, P. C., Frank, J. R., & ICBME Collaborators. (2017). Implementing competency-based medical education: What changes in curricular structure and processes are needed? *Medical Teacher, 39*(6), 594–598.

Nutton, J., & Fast, E. (2015). Historical trauma, substance use, and indigenous peoples: seven generations of harm from a "big event". *Substance Use & Misuse, 50*(7), 839–847.

O'Connor, B., Pollner, F., & Fugh-Berman, A. (2016). Salespeople in the surgical suite: Relationships between surgeons and medical device representatives. *PloS One, 11*(8), e0158510.

O'Doherty, D., Dromey, M., Lougheed, J., Hannigan, A., Last, J., & McGrath, D. (2018). Barriers and solutions to online learning in medical education–an integrative review. *BMC Medical Education, 18*, 1–11.

Olapade-Olaopa, E. O., Adisa, A. O., Olopade, F. E., Lawal, T. A., Hammad, N., Iputo, J. E., & Scott-Emuakpor, A. B. (2027). Medical education in sub-Saharan Africa. In J. R. Schoenherr (Ed.), *Fundamentals and Frontiers of Medical Education and Decision-Making: Innovation, Implementation, and Translational Research* (pp. 412–461). Routledge.

Olson, C. A. (2013). Using the grey literature to enhance research and practice in continuing education for health professionals. *Journal of Continuing Education in the Health Professions*, *33*(1), 1–3.

Oosterhoff, J. H., & Doornberg, J. N. (2020). Artificial intelligence in orthopaedics: false hope or not? A narrative review along the line of Gartner's hype cycle. *EFORT Open Reviews*, *5*(10), 593–603.

Owusu-Agyeman, Y. (2021). Transformational leadership and innovation in higher education: A participative process approach. *International Journal of Leadership in Education*, *24*(5), 694–716.

Padmaja, V., & Mukul, K. (2021). Upskilling and reskilling in the digital age: the way forward for higher educational institutions. In S. L. Gupta, N. Kishor, N. Mishra, S. Mathur, & U. Gupta (Eds.), *Transforming Higher Education through Digitalization* (pp. 253–275). CRC Press.

Paez, A. (2017). Gray literature: An important resource in systematic reviews. *Journal of Evidence-Based Medicine*, *10*(3), 233–240.

Page, M. J., Sterne, J. A., Higgins, J. P., & Egger, M. (2021). Investigating and dealing with publication bias and other reporting biases in meta-analyses of health research: A review. *Research Synthesis Methods*, *12*(2), 248–259.

Papapanou, M., Routsi, E., Tsamakis, K., Fotis, L., Marinos, G., Lidoriki, I., ... & Schizas, D. (2022). Medical education challenges and innovations during COVID-19 pandemic. *Postgraduate Medical Journal*, *98*(1159), 321–327.

Paris, D. (2012). Culturally sustaining pedagogy: A needed change in stance, terminology, and practice. *Educational Researcher*, *41*(3), 93–97.

Park, O. C., & Lee, J. (2013). Adaptive instructional systems. In J. M. Spector, M. D. Merrill, J. Elen, & M. J. Bishop (Eds.), *Handbook of Research on Educational Communications and Technology* (pp. 647–680). Routledge.

Park, Y. S., Hodges, B. D., & Tekian, A. (2016). Evaluating the paradigm shift from time-based toward competency-based medical education: implications for curriculum and assessment. *Assessing Competence in Professional Performance Across Disciplines and Professions*, 411–425.

Peiris, D., Brown, A., & Cass, A. (2008). Addressing inequities in access to quality health care for indigenous people. *Canadian Medical Association Journal*, *179*(10), 985–986.

Perkins, S., Nishimura, H., Olatunde, P. F., & Kalbarczyk, A. (2023). Educational approaches to teach students to address colonialism in global health: A scoping review. *BMJ Global Health*, *8*(4), e011610.

Pew Research (2021). *Attitudes about Caste*. Retrieved January 15, 2022, from www.pewresearch.org/religion/2021/06/29/attitudes-about-caste/

Piening, E. P., & Salge, T. O. (2015). Understanding the antecedents, contingencies, and performance implications of process innovation: A dynamic capabilities perspective. *Journal of Product Innovation Management*, *32*(1), 80–97.

Ploug, T., & Holm, S. (2020). The four dimensions of contestable AI diagnostics-A patient-centric approach to explainable AI. *Artificial Intelligence in Medicine*, *107*, 101901.

Polgar, S. (1962). Health and human behavior: Areas of interest common to the social and medical sciences. *Current Anthropology*, *3*(2), 159–205.

Polzer, J. T., Milton, L. P., & Swarm Jr, W. B. (2002). Capitalizing on diversity: Interpersonal congruence in small work groups. *Administrative Science Quarterly*, *47*(2), 296–324.

Porter, D. (2005). *Health, Civilization and the State: A History of Public Health from Ancient to Modern Times*. Routledge.

Prasad, V., & Ioannidis, J. P. (2014). Evidence-based de-implementation for contradicted, unproven, and aspiring healthcare practices. *Implementation Science*, *9*, 1–5.

Premkumar, K., Vinod, E., Sathishkumar, S., Pulimood, A. B., Umaefulam, V., Prasanna Samuel, P., & John, T. A. (2018). Self-directed learning readiness of Indian medical students: A mixed method study. *BMC medical Education*, *18*, 1–10.

Rao, V. P., & Rao, V. N. (1980). Endogamy and exogamy: Particularistic and universalistic attitudes of college students in India. *Journal of Comparative Family Studies*, *11*(4), 485–499.

Ratna, N. N., Dray, A., Perez, P., Grafton, R. Q., Newth, D., & Kompas, T. (2008). Diffusion and social networks: Revisiting medical innovation with agents. *Complex Decision Making: Theory and Practice*, 247–265.

Ray, T., Chaudhuri, A. R., & Sahai, K. (2020). Whose education matters? An analysis of inter caste marriages in India. *Journal of Economic Behavior & Organization*, *176*, 619–633.

Reichsman, F., Browning, F. E., & Hinshaw, J. R. (1964). Observations of undergraduate clinical teaching in action. *Academic Medicine*, *39*(2), 147–163.

Reid, P., Cormack, D., & Paine, S. J. (2019). Colonial histories, racism and health—The experience of Māori and Indigenous peoples. *Public Health*, *172*, 119–124.

Reis, S., Borkan, J. M., & Weingarten, M. (2009). The current state of basic medical education in Israel: Implications for a new medical school. *Medical Teacher*, *31*(11), 984–989.

Reis, S., Urkin, J., Nave, R., Ber, R., Ziv, A., Karnieli-Miller, O., ... & Mevorach, D. (2016). Medical education in Israel 2016: Five medical schools in a period of transition. *Israel Journal of Health Policy Research*, *5*, 1–14.

Rieg, N. A., Gatersleben, B., & Christie, I. (2021). Organizational change management for sustainability in higher education institutions: A systematic quantitative literature review. *Sustainability*, *13*(13), 7299.

Rietbergen, T., Spoon, D., Brunsveld-Reinders, A. H., Schoones, J. W., Huis, A., Heinen, M., ... & van Bodegom-Vos, L. (2020). Effects of de-implementation strategies aimed at reducing low-value nursing procedures: A systematic review and meta-analysis. *Implementation Science*, *15*, 1–18.

Rodríguez-Saldaña, J. (2004). Challenges and opportunities in border health. *Preventing Chronic Disease*, *2*(1), A03.

Rogers, E. M. (1962/2003). *Diffusion of Innovations* (5th ed.). Free Press.

Rogers, E. M. (2004). A prospective and retrospective look at the diffusion model. *Journal of Health Communication*, *9*(S1), 13–19.

Rogers, E. M., Singhal, A., & Quinlan, M. M. (2014). Diffusion of innovations. In D. W. Stacks, M. B. Salwen, & K. C. Eichhorn (Eds.), *An Integrated Approach to Communication Theory and Research* (pp. 432–448). Routledge.

Ropovik, I., Adamkovic, M., & Greger, D. (2021). Neglect of publication bias compromises meta-analyses of educational research. *PloS One*, *16*(6), e0252415.

Rosen, G. (1983/2016). *The Structure of American Medical Practice, 1875-1941*. University of Pennsylvania Press.

Rosenbusch, N., Brinckmann, J., & Bausch, A. (2011). Is innovation always beneficial? A meta-analysis of the relationship between innovation and performance in SMEs. *Journal of Business Venturing*, *26*(4), 441–457.

Ross, F. (2007). Questioning path dependence theory: The case of the British NHS. *Policy & Politics*, *35*(4), 591–610.

Roth, P. L., Thatcher, J. B., Bobko, P., Matthews, K. D., Ellingson, J. E., & Goldberg, C. B. (2020). Political affiliation and employment screening decisions: The role of similarity and identification processes. *Journal of Applied Psychology*, *105*(5), 472.

Rothstein, H. R., & Hopewell, S. (2009). Grey literature. *The Handbook of Research Synthesis and Meta-Analysis*, *2*, 103–125.

Rubio, D. M., Schoenbaum, E. E., Lee, L. S., Schteingart, D. E., Marantz, P. R., Anderson, K. E., ... & Esposito, K. (2010). Defining translational research: Implications for training. *Academic Medicine*, *85*(3), 470–475.

Ruis, A. R., & Golden, R. N. (2008). The schism between medical and public health education: A historical perspective. *Academic Medicine*, *83*(12), 1153–1157.

Ruiz, J. G., Mintzer, M. J., & Leipzig, R. M. (2006). The impact of e-learning in medical education. *Academic Medicine*, *81*(3), 207–212.

Ruttan, V. W. (1997). Induced innovation, evolutionary theory and path dependence: Sources of technical change. *The Economic Journal*, *107*(444), 1520–1529.

Ruttan, V. W. (2000). *Technology, Growth, and Development: an Induced Innovation Perspective*. Oxford University Press.

Rycroft, R. W., & Kash, D. E. (2002). Path dependence in the innovation of complex technologies. *Technology Analysis & Strategic Management*, *14*(1), 21–35.

Saigh, P. A., & Bremner, J. D. (1999). *The History of Posttraumatic Stress Disorder. Posttraumatic Stress Disorder: A Comprehensive Text*. Allyn & Bacon.

Salerno, M. S., de Vasconcelos Gomes, L. A., Da Silva, D. O., Bagno, R. B., & Freitas, S. L. T. U. (2015). Innovation processes: Which process for which project? *Technovation*, *35*, 59–70.

Salge, T. O. (2012). The temporal trajectories of innovative search: Insights from public hospital services. *Research Policy*, *41*(4), 720–733.

Sanami, M., Flood, T., Hall, R., Kingscott, F., Jayne, D., & Culmer, P. (2017). Translating healthcare innovation from academia to industry. *Advances in Mechanical Engineering*, *9*(3), 1687814017694114.

Saviotti, P. P. (2013). Innovation systems and evolutionary theories. In Edquist, C. (Ed.), *Systems of Innovation* (pp. 180–199). Routledge.

Schiekirka, S., Anders, S., & Raupach, T. (2014). Assessment of two different types of bias affecting the results of outcome-based evaluation in undergraduate medical education. *BMC Medical Education*, *14*, 1–9.

Schoenherr, J. R. (2020). Black boxes of the mind: From psychophysics to explainable artificial intelligence. *Proceedings of Fechner Day*, *2020*, 46–51.

Schoenherr, J. R. (2021). Designing ethical agency for adaptive instructional systems: The FATE of learning and assessment. In *International Conference on Human-Computer Interaction* (pp. 265–283). Springer International Publishing.

Schoenherr, J. R. (2021). Trust and explainability in A/IS-mediated healthcare: Operationalizing the therapeutic alliance in a distributed system. In *2021 IEEE International Symposium on Technology and Society (ISTAS)* (pp. 1–8). IEEE.

Schoenherr, J. R. (2022). Learning engineering is ethical. In J. Goodell (Ed.) *Learning Engineering Toolkit* (pp. 201–228). Routledge.

Schoenherr, J. R. (2022a). Vaccination, values, and health information search behaviour in the new folk medicine. In *2022 IEEE International Symposium on Technology and Society (ISTAS)* (Vol. *1*, pp. 1–10). IEEE.

Schoenherr, J. R. (2022b). Folkmedical technologies and the sociotechnical systems of healthcare. *IEEE Technology and Society Magazine*, *41*(3), 38–49.

Schoenherr, J. R. (2025). The translational research process. In A. E. M. Eltorai, et al. (Eds.), *Translational Neurosurgery*. Elsevier.

Schoenherr, J. R. (2027a). Human-centered artificial intelligence in health professions education and decision-making: A sociotechnical systems perspective. In J. R. Schoenherr (Ed.), *Fundamentals and Frontiers of Medical Education and Decision-Making: Innovation, Implementation, and Translational Research* (pp. 1–76). Routledge.

Schoenherr, J. R. (2027b). The development and dynamics of heterarchical structure in Mayan medical education and healthcare ecosystems. In J. R. Schoenherr (Ed.), *Fundamentals and Frontiers of Medical Education and Decision-Making: Innovation, Implementation, and Translational Research* (pp. 359–411). Routledge.

Schoenherr, J. R. (in preparation a). Cognitive offloading and responsibility in AI-mediated learning: Explainability, metacognition, and automation bias in Higher Education. In *Generative AI in Higher Education: Discourses on Policy, Pedagogy, and Innovation.*

Schoenherr, J. R. (in preparation b). War against systems: Healthcare infrastructure and irregular warfare during the total war in Ukraine. In *Ukraine, Competitive Statecraft, and Irregular Warfare*.

Schoenherr, J. R. & Beaudoin, J. (2027). The evolving landscape of health professions education in East Asia: Heterarchies in East Asian medicine and medical education. In J. R. Schoenherr (Eds.), *Fundamentals and Frontiers of Medical Education and Decision-Making: Innovation, Implementation, and Translational Research* (pp. 462–509). Routledge.

Schoenherr, J. R., & DeFalco, J. (2021). Moral education and A/IS standardization: Responsible and ethical design through education. In *2021 IEEE International Symposium on Technology and Society (ISTAS)* (pp. 1–8). IEEE.

Schoenherr, J. R., & Hamstra, S. J. (2016). Psychometrics and its discontents: An historical perspective on the discourse of the measurement tradition. *Advances in Health Sciences Education*, *21*, 719–729.

Schoenherr, J. R., & Hamstra, S. J. (2017). Beyond fidelity: Deconstructing the seductive simplicity of fidelity in simulator-based education in the health care professions. *Simulation in Healthcare*, *12*(2), 117–123.

Schoenherr, J. R., & Hamstra, S. J. (2024). Validity in health professions education: From assessment instruments to program innovation and evaluation. In *Fundamentals and Frontiers of Medical Education and Decision-Making* (pp. 80–107). Routledge.

Schoenherr, J. R., & Lacroix, G. L. (2020). Performance monitoring during categorization with and without prior knowledge: A comparison of confidence calibration indices with the certainty criterion. *Canadian Journal of Experimental Psychology/Revue canadienne de psychologie expérimentale*, 74(4), 302.

Schoenherr, J. R., & Laschuk, M. (2017). Scientific communication in medical education: Modeling the adoption rate in multiple peer networks. *Proceedings of the International Conference on Social Computing, Behavioral-Cultural Modeling & Prediction and Behaviour Representation in Social Modeling and Simulation.* Washington, USA.

Schoenherr, J. R., & Le-Bouar, C. (2024). Representing and communicating health information: Fundamentals of persuasive health communication. In J. R. Schoenherr & M. M. McConnell (Eds.), *Fundamentals and Frontiers of Medical Education and Decision-Making* (pp. 270–312). Routledge.

Schoenherr, J. R., & McConnell, M. M. (2024a). *Fundamentals and Frontiers of Medical Education and Decision-Making*. Routledge.

Schoenherr, J. R., & McConnell, M. M. (2024b). Human-centered design in health professions education: Informing competency-based education with psychological science. In J. R. Schoenherr & M. M. McConnell (Eds.), *Fundamentals and Frontiers of Medical Education and Decision-Making* (pp. 3–36). Routledge.

Schoenherr, J. R., & Williams-Jones, B. (2016). Early contributions to the evolution of the Canadian Scientific integrity system: Institutional and governmental interaction in the policy diffusion process. *Canadian Journal of Higher Education*, *46*(1), 57–75.

Schoenherr, J. R., Abbas, R., Michael, K., Rivas, P., & Anderson, T. D. (2023). Designing AI using a human-centered approach: Explainability and accuracy toward trustworthiness. *IEEE Transactions on Technology and Society*, *4*(1), 9–23.

Schoenherr, J. R., Chiou, E., & Goldshtein, M. (2024). Building trust with the ethical affordances of education technologies: A sociotechnical systems perspective. In P. Dasgupta, J. Llinas, T. Gillespie, S. Fouse, W. Lawless, R. Mittu, & D. Sofge (Eds.), *Putting AI in the Critical Loop* (pp. 127–165). Academic Press.

Schoenherr, J. R., Waechter, J., & Lee, C. H. (2024). Quantifying expertise in the healthcare professions: Cognitive efficiency and metacognitive calibration. In J. R. Schoenherr & M. M. McConnell (Eds.), *Fundamentals and Frontiers of Medical Education and Decision-Making* (pp. 213–244). Routledge.

Schoenherr, J. R., Waechter, J., & Millington, S. J. (2018). Subjective awareness of ultrasound expertise development: Individual experience as a determinant of overconfidence. *Advances in Health Sciences Education*, *23*(4), 749–765.

Schoonheim-Klein, M., Walmsley, A. D., Habets, L. L. M. H., Van Der Velden, U., & Manogue, M. (2005). An implementation strategy for introducing an OSCE into a dental school. *European Journal of Dental Education*, *9*(4), 143–149.

Schuch, H. S., Haag, D. G., Bastos, J. L., Paradies, Y., & Jamieson, L. M. (2021). Intersectionality, racial discrimination and oral health in Australia. *Community Dentistry and Oral Epidemiology*, *49*(1), 87–94.

Schulman, L. (1987). Knowledge and teaching: Foundations of the new reform. *Harvard Educational Review*, *57*(1), 1–23.

Schully, S. D., Benedicto, C. B., Gillanders, E. M., Wang, S. S., & Khoury, M. J. (2010). Translational research in cancer genetics: The road less traveled. *Public Health Genomics*, *14*(1), 1–8.

Schwartzman, E., Hsu, D. I., Law, A. V., & Chung, E. P. (2011). Assessment of patient communication skills during OSCE: Examining effectiveness of a training program in minimizing inter-grader variability. *Patient Education and Counseling*, *83*(3), 472–477.

Sein-Echaluce, M. L., Fidalgo-Blanco, Á., & Alves, G. (2017). *Technology Behaviors in Education Innovation* (No. ART-2017-98966).

Serdyukov, P. (2017). Innovation in education: What works, what doesn't, and what to do about it? *Journal of Research in Innovative Teaching & Learning*, *10*(1), 4–33.

Seyyed-Kalantari, L., Zhang, H., McDermott, M. B., Chen, I. Y., & Ghassemi, M. (2021). Underdiagnosis bias of artificial intelligence algorithms applied to chest radiographs in under-served patient populations. *Nature Medicine*, *27*(12), 2176–2182.

Shahawy, S., & Diamond, M. B. (2018). Perspectives on induced abortion among Palestinian women: Religion, culture and access in the occupied Palestinian territories. *Culture, Health & Sexuality*, *20*(3), 289–305.

Shankel, S. W., & Mazzaferri, E. L. (1986). Teaching the resident in internal medicine: Present practices and suggestions for the future. *Journal of the American Medical Association*, *256*, 725–729.

Shavers, V. L., Fagan, P., Jones, D., Klein, W. M., Boyington, J., Moten, C., & Rorie, E. (2012). The state of research on racial/ethnic discrimination in the receipt of health care. *American Journal of Public Health*, *102*(5), 953–966.

Shea, C. M., Jacobs, S. R., Esserman, D. A., Bruce, K., & Weiner, B. J. (2014). Organizational readiness for implementing change: A psychometric assessment of a new measure. *Implementation Science*, *9*, 1–15.

Shellah, D. (2022, May 15). Medical education in Palestine: Studying under occupation. in-Training. https://in-training.org/medical-education-in-palestine-studying-under-occupation-23892

Shellah, D., Alkhaldi, M., Najjar, S., & AbuQamar, M. (2025). The imperative of a ceasefire for the recovery of public health education in Gaza. *Eastern Mediterranean Health Journal*, *31*(4), 298–299.

Shulman, L. (1987). Knowledge and teaching: Foundations of the new reform. *Harvard Educational Review*, *57*(1), 1–23.

Simionato de Assis, I., Arcoverde, M. A. M., Ramos, A. C. V., Alves, L. S., Berra, T. Z., Arroyo, L. H., ... & Arcêncio, R. A. (2018). Social determinants, their relationship with leprosy risk and temporal trends in a tri-border region in Latin America. *PLoS Neglected Tropical Diseases*, *12*(4), e0006407.

Simons, D. J., & Chabris, C. F. (1999). Gorillas in our midst: Sustained inattentional blindness for dynamic events. *Perception*, *28*(9), 1059–1074.

Simons, R. C., & Hughes, C. C. (Eds.). (2012). *The Culture-Bound Syndromes: Folk Illnesses of Psychiatric and Anthropological Interest* (Vol. 7). Springer Science & Business Media.

Simpson, P. M., Siguaw, J. A., & Enz, C. A. (2006). Innovation orientation outcomes: The good and the bad. *Journal of Business Research*, *59*(10-11), 1133–1141.

Sinclair, S. (1997). *Making Doctors: An Institutional Apprenticeship*. Routledge.

Slappendel, C. (1996). Perspectives on innovation in organizations. *Organization Studies*, *17*(1), 107–129.

Smith, J. L. (2004). Understanding the process of stereotype threat: A review of mediational variables and new performance goal directions. *Educational Psychology Review*, *16*, 177–206.

Smith, R. (2005). Medical journals are an extension of the marketing arm of pharmaceutical companies. *PLoS Medicine*, *2*, e138

Spears, R., & Otten, S. (2012). Revisiting Tajfel's minimal group studies. In R. Smith & S. A. Haslam (Eds.), *Social Psychology: Revisiting the Classic Studies* (pp. 160–177). Sage.

Spencer, S. J., Steele, C. M., & Quinn, D. M. (1999). Stereotype threat and women's math performance. *Journal of Experimental Social Psychology*, *35*(1), 4–28.

Spielman, A. I., & Sunavala-Dossabhoy, G. (2021). Pandemics and education: A historical review. *Journal of Dental Education*, *85*(6), 741–746.

Spielmans, G. I., & Parry, P. I. (2010). From evidence-based medicine to marketing-based medicine: Evidence from internal industry documents. *Bioethical Inquiry*, *7*, 13–29.

Ssengooba, F., Tuhebwe, D., Ssendagire, S., Babirye, S., Akulume, M., Ssennyonjo, A., ... & Nangami, M. (2021). Experiences of seeking healthcare across the border: lessons to inform upstream policies and system developments on cross-border health in East Africa. *BMJ Open*, *11*(12), e045575.

Starr, P. (1982). *The Social Transformation of American Medicine: The Rise of a Sovereign Profession and the Making of a Vast Industry*. Basic Books.

Steele, C. M., & Aronson, J. (1995). Stereotype threat and the intellectual test performance of African Americans. *Journal of Personality and Social Psychology*, *69*(5), 797.

Steinke, A., & Hövelmann, S. (2020). Whose health matters: trust and mistrust in humanitarian crisis and global health interventions. In R. Haring, I. Kickbusch, D. Ganten, & M. Moeti (Eds.), *Handbook of Global Health* (pp. 1–31). Springer International Publishing.

Strauss, A., Schatzman, L., Ehrlich, D., Bucher, R., & Sabshin, M. (1963). The hospital and its negotiated order. In E. Freidson, E. (Ed.), *The Hospital in Modern Society* (pp. 147–169). Free Press.

Sultan, F., Farley, J. U., & Lehmann, D. R. (1990). A meta-analysis of diffusion models. *Journal of Marketing Research, 27*(1), 70–77.

Supe, A. (2016). Evolution of medical education in India: The impact of colonialism. *Journal of Postgraduate Medicine, 62*(4), 255–259.

Swanson, E. B. (1994). Information systems innovation among organizations. *Management Science, 40*(9), 1069–1092.

Swanwick, T., Forrest, K., & O'Brien, B. C. (2018). *Understanding Medical Education: Evidence, Theory, and Practice* (3rd ed.). Wiley-Blackwell.

Syed, I. B. (2002). Islamic Medicine: 1000 years ahead of its times. *JISHIM, 2*, 2–9.

ten Cate, O. (2017). Competency-based medical education and its competency frameworks. In *Competence-based Vocational and Professional Education: Bridging the Worlds of Work and Education* (pp. 903–929).

Thai, K. P., Craig, S. D., Goodell, J., Lis, J., Schoenherr, J. R., & Kolodner, J. (2022). Learning engineering is human-centered. In *Learning Engineering Toolkit* (pp. 83–123). Routledge.

Thomas, A., & Ellaway, R. H. (2021). Rethinking implementation science for health professions education: A manifesto for change. *Perspectives on Medical Education, 10*(6), 362–368.

Thomson, R., & Schoenherr, J. R. (2020). *Knowledge-to-Information Translation Trainer (KITT): An Adaptive Approach to Explainable Artificial Intelligence*. HCII 2020. Copenhagen, Denmark.

Thrane, S., Blaabjerg, S., & Møller, R. H. (2010). Innovative path dependence: Making sense of product and service innovation in path dependent innovation processes. *Research Policy, 39*(7), 932–944.

Titler, M. G. (2008). The evidence for evidence-based practice implementation. In R. G. Hughes (Ed.), *Patient Safety and Quality: An Evidence-Based Handbook for Nurses*. Agency for Healthcare Research and Quality (US).

Tremonti, L. P., Biddle, W. B. (1982). Teaching behaviors of residents and faculty members. *Journal of Medical Education, 57*, 894–899.

Troncon, L. E. D. A. (2004). Clinical skills assessment: limitations to the introduction of an" OSCE"(Objective Structured Clinical Examination) in a traditional Brazilian medical school. *Sao Paulo Medical Journal, 122*, 12–17.

Turner, B. S. (1987/1995). *Medical Power and Social Knowledge* (2nd ed.). Sage.

Turner, J. L., & Dankoski, M. E. (2008). Objective structured clinical exams: A critical review. *Family Medicine, 40*(8), 574–578.

Valeggia, C. R., & Snodgrass, J. J. (2015). Health of indigenous peoples. *Annual Review of Anthropology, 44*, 117–135.

Valente, T. W. (2010). *Social Networks and Health: Models, Methods, and Applications*. Oxford University Press.

Valente, T. W., & Fosados, R. (2006). Diffusion of innovations and network segmentation: the part played by people in promoting health. *Sexually Transmitted Diseases*, S23–S31.

Valente, T. W., & Pitts, S. R. (2017). An appraisal of social network theory and analysis as applied to public health: Challenges and opportunities. *Annual Review of Public Health, 38*(1), 103–18.

Van Aert, R. C., Wicherts, J. M., & Van Assen, M. A. (2019). Publication bias examined in meta-analyses from psychology and medicine: A meta-meta-analysis. *PloS One, 14*(4), e0215052.

Van den Bulte, C., & Lilien, G. L. (2001). Medical innovation revisited: Social contagion versus marketing effort. *American Journal of Sociology, 106*(5), 1409–1435.

van der Aa, J. E., Aabakke, A. J., Ristorp Andersen, B., Settnes, A., Hornnes, P., Teunissen, P. W., ... & Scheele, F. (2020). From prescription to guidance: A European framework for generic competencies. *Advances in Health Sciences Education, 25*, 173–187.

van Middendorp, J. J., Sanchez, G. M., & Burridge, A. L. (2010). The Edwin Smith papyrus: A clinical reappraisal of the oldest known document on spinal injuries. *European Spine Journal*, *19*, 1815–1823.

Van Rossum, L., Aij, K. H., Simons, F. E., van der Eng, N., & Ten Have, W. D. (2016). Lean healthcare from a change management perspective: The role of leadership and workforce flexibility in an operating theatre. *Journal of Health Organization and Management*, *30*(3), 475–493.

Van Way III, C. (2016). War and Trauma: A History of Military Medicine-Part II. *Missouri Medicine*, *113*(5), 336–340.

Varma, S. (2020). *The Occupied Clinic: Militarism and Care in Kashmir*. Duke University Press.

Venosa, A. R., Baroneza, J. E., & Fernandes, R. A. F. (2027). Medical education in Brazil: A history of an evolving pluralistic healthcare system. In J. R. Schoenherr (Ed.), *Fundamentals and Frontiers of Medical Education and Decision-Making: Innovation, Implementation, and Translational Research* (pp. 310–335). Routledge.

Verghese, A., Charlton, B., Kassirer, J. P., Ramsey, M., & Ioannidis, J. P. A. (2015). Inadequacies of physical examination as a cause of medical errors and adverse events: A collection of vignettes. *American Journal of Medicine*, *128*(12), 1322–1324.e3.

Vogt, L. A., Jordan, C., & Tharp, R. G. (1987). Explaining school failure, producing school success: Two cases. *Anthropology & Education Quarterly*, *18*(4), 276–286.

von Weizsäcker, C. C. (1962/2010). A new technical progress function. *German Economic Review*, *11*(3), 248–265.

Vozenilek, J., Huff, J. S., Reznek, M., & Gordon, J. A. (2004). See one, do one, teach one: advanced technology in medical education. *Academic Emergency Medicine*, *11*(11), 1149–1154.

Wager, E., & Williams, P. (2013). "Hardly worth the effort"? Medical journals' policies and their editors' and publishers' views on trial registration and publication bias: Quantitative and qualitative study. *British Medical Journal*, *347*, 1–9.

Wald, A. (1943). *A Method of Estimating Plane Vulnerability Based on Damage of Survivors*. Statistical Research Group, Columbia University.

Wald, H. S., McFarland, J., & Markovina, I. (2019). Medical humanities in medical education and practice. *Medical Teacher*, *41*(5), 492–496.

Walsh-Bailey, C., Tsai, E., Tabak, R. G., Morshed, A. B., Norton, W. E., McKay, V. R., ... & Gifford, S. (2021). A scoping review of de-implementation frameworks and models. *Implementation Science*, *16*, 1–18.

Walshe, K., & Rundall, T. G. (2001). Evidence-based management: from theory to practice in health care. *The Milbank Quarterly*, *79*(3), 429–457.

Wang, J., Cheng, G. H. L., Chen, T., & Leung, K. (2019). Team creativity/innovation in culturally diverse teams: A meta-analysis. *Journal of Organizational Behavior*, *40*(6), 693–708.

Weinberg, M., Waterman, S., Lucas, C. Á., Falcon, V. C., Morales, P. K., Lopez, L. A., ... & Border Infectious Disease Surveillance Project Working Group. (2003). The US-Mexico border infectious disease surveillance project: Establishing binational border surveillance. *Emerging Infectious Diseases*, *9*(1), 97.

Wells, L., & Gowda, A. (2020). A legacy of mistrust: African Americans and the US healthcare system. *Proceedings of UCLA Health*, *24*, 1–3.

Westfall, J. M., Mold, J., & Fagnan, L. (2007). Practice-based research—"Blue Highways" on the NIH roadmap. *JAMA*, *297*(4), 403–406.

Whitehead, C. R. (2016). On gunboats and grand pianos: medical education exports and the long shadow of colonialism. *Advances in Health Sciences Education, 21*, 1–4.

Wiemers, M., Nadeau, M., Tysinger, J., & Fernandez Falcon, C. (2018). Annual program review process: An enhanced process with outcomes. *Medical Education Online, 23*(1), 1527626.

Wilby, K. J., & Diab, M. (2016). Key challenges for implementing a Canadian-based objective structured clinical examination (OSCE) in a Middle Eastern context. *Canadian Medical Education Journal, 7*(3), e4.

Wilk, P., Maltby, A., & Cooke, M. (2017). Residential schools and the effects on Indigenous health and well-being in Canada—A scoping review. *Public Health Reviews, 38*, 1–23.

Williams, K. N., Ramani, S., Fraser, B., & Orlander, J. D. (2008). Improving bedside teaching: findings from a focus group study of learners. *Academic Medicine, 83*(3), 257–264.

Willis, E, Reynolds, L., & Keleher, H. (2016). *Understanding the Australian Health Care System*. Elsevier Health Sciences.

Wilsford, D. (1994). Path dependency, or why history makes it difficult but not impossible to reform health care systems in a big way. *Journal of Public Policy, 14*(3), 251–283.

Wismar, M., Palm, W., Figueras, J., Ernst, K., & Ginneken, E. V. (2011). *Cross-border Health Care in the European Union: Mapping and Analysing Practices and Policies*. World Health Organization.

Woodman, R. W., & Wayne, S. J. (1985). An investigation of positive-findings bias in evaluation of organization development interventions. *Academy of Management Journal, 28*(4), 889–913.

Woolford, A. (2015). *This Benevolent Experiment: Indigenous Boarding Schools, Genocide, and Redress in Canada and the United States*. University of Nebraska Press.

World Federal for Medical Education (WFME) (2020). *WFME Global Standards for Quality Improvement: Basic Medical Education*. WFME.

World Health Organization (WHO) (2002). *WHO Traditional Medicine Strategy 2002-2005*. World Health Organization.

World Health Organization (WHO) (2013). *WHO Traditional Medicine Strategy 2014-2023*. World Health Organization.

World Health Organization (WHO). (2019). *WHO Global Report on Traditional and Complementary Medicine 2019*. World Health Organization.

World Health Organization (WHO) (2022). *Global Competency and Outcomes Framework for Universal Health Coverage*. WHO.

World Health Organization (WHO). (2023). *Global Competency Framework for Regulators of Medicines*. World Health Organization.

Wu, A., Choi, E., Diderich, M., Shamim, A., Rahhal, Z., Mitchell, M., ... & DeWit, H. (2022). Internationalization of medical education—motivations and formats of current practices. *Medical Science Educator, 32*(3), 733–745.

Zartman, I. W. (Ed.). (2010). *Understanding Life in the Borderlands: Boundaries in Depth and in Motion*. University of Georgia Press.

Zheng, K., Padman, R., Krackhardt, D., Johnson, M. P., & Diamond, H. S. (2010). Social networks and physician adoption of electronic health records: Insights from an empirical study. *Journal of the American Medical Informatics Association, 17*(3), 328–336.

Ziltener, P., & Künzler, D. (2013). Impacts of colonialism–A research survey. *Journal of World-Systems Research, 19*(2), 290–311.

2

COLLECTIVE COMPETENCE IN THE HEALTH PROFESSIONS

Learning, Thinking, and Deciding in Groups

Jordan Richard Schoenherr, Yumi Mahias-Ito, and Xin Yi Li

Healthcare is a collective responsibility. Whether we consider informal social networks of peers within communities or the formal networks of healthcare delivery systems, people must share knowledge, coordinate diverse skill sets, and (share) relevant health experience (Bae et al., 2015; Griffith et al., 2012; Smith & Christakis, 2008; Tasselli, 2014). Patients, family, community members, and healers can only understand a subset of the relevant information necessary for effective healthcare delivery. The dynamic nature of healthcare teams adds an additional layer of complexity in the delivery of care, that can produce both positive and negative outcomes. For instance, members of a healthcare team can bring new perspectives, insight, knowledge, and skills (i.e., *functional diversity*) but the likelihood of miscommunications can arise during knowledge translation and clinical handover, roles might be ambiguous, and an absence of trust can affect patient safety (Dinh et al., 2020; Dreachslin et al., 2000; Johnson et al., 2018; Tang et al., 2013).

Effective and efficient healthcare delivery requires integrating the knowledge, skills, resources, and methods of a diverse group of family members, community members, and healthcare practitioners that can be widely geographically distributed. Rather than focusing exclusively on healthcare professionals (HCPs), we must consider the shared responsibility for healthcare decision-making. Shared decision-making (SDM) requires understanding patient preferences, fostering awareness of choice and treatment alternatives, and facilitating response selection (Elwyn et al., 2017; Kunneman et al., 2109; Makoul & Clayman, 2006; Stiggelbout et al., 2015). Recognizing that this approach to decision-making occurs in a network, we must assess the collective competence of the therapeutic network.

By shifting our focus from individual competency to the capabilities and capacities of networks of practitioners and patients, we introduce new pathways

DOI: 10.4324/9781003498155-2

to delivering care (Rosen et al., 2018). Despite interest in further integration of nonhuman agents such as artificial intelligence (AI) into healthcare settings (Schoenherr, 2027), strengthening human teams with human-centered design approaches will remain a priority for the foreseeable future (Schoenherr & McConnell, 2024). Learning to effectively collaborate and coordinate with other HCPs and patients reflects a distinctive competence addressing factors that affect human performance (e.g., stress, emotions, fatigue, impression formation), health literacy and health beliefs (e.g., disease models), and how – and to whom – that information is communicated (Schoenherr & Le-Bouar, 2024). Healthcare and health professions education must develop assessment methods that account for the fundamental structures and dynamics of groups, providing greater specificity to roles of 'collaborator', 'communicator', etc.

As a step toward a firmer theoretical foundation, this chapter provides a social cognitive framework of collective competence in healthcare delivery and health professions education. Drawing on research in psychological science, the chapter identifies basic principles and processes that are associated with the development of collective competence and distributed situational awareness within teams. Following a review of the concept of collective competence, models of social processes and social learning are reviewed. They highlight the need to understand SDM as a network, requiring the adoption of different assessment and evaluation options. The chapter then reviews evidence in health professions education that demonstrate the properties of interprofessional education (IPE) programs.

2.1 Collective Competence

When a healthcare team is viewed as a *unit*, we can assess its collective competence. *Collective competence* represents the extent to which a group of individuals can effectively and efficiently identify, structure, coordinate, and solve problems (Boreham, 2004, 2011). The sum of the individual competencies does not necessarily equate to collective competence.

Individually, each member of a healthcare team might be capable of performing their duties effectively and have a certain level of situational awareness. Collectively, a group might outperform – or underperform – its individual members. Members of healthcare teams might have unique insight into specific aspects of a clinical case, they might compensate for lapses in attention or knowledge or consider alternative diagnoses and treatment that stem from their own experiences in healthcare delivery. However, a healthcare team might underperform due to communication failures at critical decision points, disagreements and interpersonal discord, or engaging in self-censorship (Bosk, 2003). For instance, information might not be explicitly provided during clinical handover due to assumptions that another clinician is aware of the patient's history, role ambiguity, fatigue impacting the recollection of the need to relate certain information, or the division of attention at an inopportune time, leading to critical oversights. Like individual expertise, collective efficacy is context-dependent: if members of a healthcare team are familiar with the specific kinds of cases and their diagnostic features, available material resources of the delivery setting, and the competencies of members of the healthcare team, collective efficacy will likely be observed.

2.1.1 Collectivism as a Paradigm for Competency

When it was originally formulated, collective competence drew on a cross-cultural comparison based on collectivism–individualism (Hofstede, 1980). Whereas individualistic societies focus on autonomy and individuation of persons within a group, collectivistic societies focus on interdependency, clearly defined roles and responsibilities, and collective action (Brewer & Chen, 2007; Hofstede, 2011; Hui, 1988; Triandis, 2001). Similarly, while self-directed goals and initiatives are encouraged in individualistic societies, group harmony, deference to authority, and cooperation are prioritized in collectivistic societies (Boreham, 2004).[1] Subsequent research has demonstrated the multidimensional nature of collectivism–individualism. For instance, groups can be described in terms of horizontal (equality) and vertical (hierarchical) relationships (Singelis et al., 1995; Sivadas, 2008), which are associated with the exchange norms that guide the roles, responsibilities, and allocation of resources within a group.

The extent to which individual autonomy and collaboration influence performance can be directly applied in the healthcare professions. Supporting the relevance of a collective social paradigm to healthcare delivery, studies have suggested that patterns of healthcare communication and decision-making differ between individualistic and collectivistic societies (Alden et al., 2018; Pun et al., 2018). Responsibility and accountability are also perceived in these terms, with outcomes attributable to the competencies of an individual or a team, respectively (Choi et al., 1999; Mezulis et al., 2004; Yan & Gaier, 1994). These divergent perspectives will necessarily affect the focus of, and receptivity to, members of the healthcare team.

In parallel with research on collectivism, cognitive science has emphasized the importance of *distributed cognition* (Hollan et al., 2000; Hutchins, 1991; Perry, 2003).[2] Rather than the individual being the locus of learning, reasoning, and decision-making, they are situated in a larger, collaborative network that encodes, processes, stores, retrieves, and uses information. When each of these functions is divided and effectively organized across multiple individuals, complicated tasks can be completed faster and more accurately than if they were completed by a single individual. Recognizing the utility of this framework, HCPs have suggested that it can be used to inform clinical decision-making (Boyle et al., 2023a; Wilson et al., 2023) and health professions education (Boyle et al., 2023b; Pimmer et al., 2013). By examining performance at the level of a healthcare team and situating this in the context of the resources, values, conventions, and attitudes of health seekers and society, health professions education can create more effective models of training and decision-making.

The concept of collective competence has important implications for learning outcomes that inform health professions education and the delivery of care. For Boreham (2004), members of a team engage in a process of *sensemaking*. To comprehend a situation, they must construct and share a collective knowledge base through dynamic interactions and develop a sense of interdependency and a shared mental model of the health seeker and environment (Blatt et al., 2006; Hultin & Mahring, 2017; Jordan et al., 2009). By developing a common mental model or causal narrative, the extent to which a collective representation is complete, accurate, and overlaps will ensure that a task is completed in a cohesive manner, i.e., distributed situational awareness. However, this also requires knowledge of perspective-taking, cultural competence, communication skills, and conflict resolution. Prior to reviewing the specific processes which can support collective competence, we consider the use of collective competence in health professions.

2.1.2 Collective Competence in the Healthcare Professions

Health professions education has largely embraced the notion of collective-, team-, and systems-based accounts of competency, while the construct itself is only loosely defined and rarely operationalized (Boyle et al., 2023a, 2023b; Leggat, 2007; Lingard, 2012; Pimmer et al., 2013; Wilson et al., 2023). Nevertheless, the importance assigned to social learning (e.g., see one, do one, teach one), the impact of the social environment, and collaborative care demonstrate a long-term interest in collective competence in the health professions. For instance, Young (1983) notes that

> a practitioner's knowledge ... is determined by (a) whether [they] get to examine and treat a relatively large number of patients who fall into a single diagnostic domain (e.g. common infectious diseases), (b) [their] ability to learn the outcomes of the cases [they] treat, (c) [their] technical means for recording and *communicating [their] clinical findings* and (d) *[their] opportunities for pooling and comparing [their] findings with those of other practitioners.*
>
> *(p. 1206; italics added)*

Absent from this description are the many requisite skills required to communicate and the diversity of healthcare teams. It also fails to include the health seekers' knowledge, beliefs, and communication abilities. Regardless of these limitations, Young clearly emphasizes the distributed nature of clinical reasoning in terms of inter- and intraprofessional communication and collaboration. Defined as 'an active relationship between two or more health or social care professionals who work together to solve problems or provide services' (Zwarenstein & Reeves, 2006; p. 48), interprofessional collaboration is a critical skill. Interprofessional

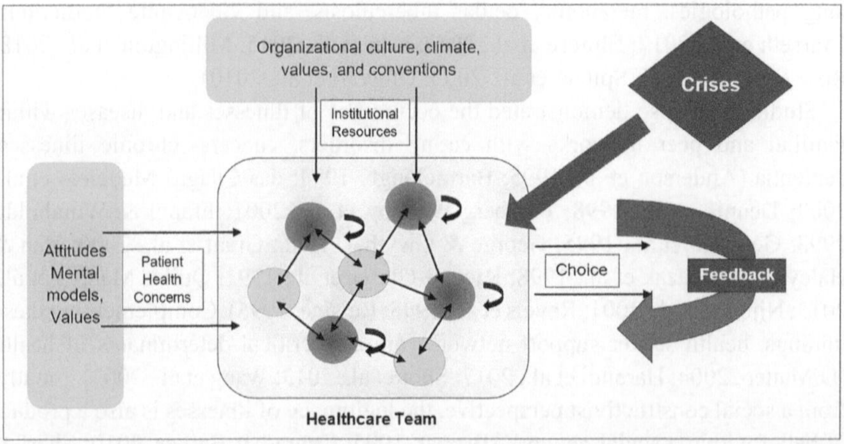

FIGURE 2.1 Collective competence in the distributed network of healthcare teams. Rather than HCPs (dark gray), the unit of analysis is the healthcare team and its ability to interact, utilize feedback, technology (gray circles), and institutional resources to address patients' health concerns. Externalities affect these processes.

interactions are affected by multiple factors including role ambiguity, professional socialization, the amount of time allocated to team building, and differences in leadership and management (Baxter & Brumfitt, 2008; Engestrom et al., 1999; Reeves & Lewin, 2004). Representing collective competence also requires that we move beyond the healthcare team and consider the environments of education and practice and lived experiences of patients and professionals (Figure 2.1).

2.1.3 Illness as a Property of Social Networks

Beyond recognizing that individuals are part of a healthcare team, the need for collective competence stems from how illnesses are presented within a social network. As epidemiological studies reinforce, individual health is embedded within a social environment. Differences in *diagnostic* traditions and training can affect what diseases are detected. Many studies have examined how illness becomes *medicalized* in communities of practice (Schoenherr, 2022a) and differs across cultures (Lupton, 2012). For instance, Fink-Anthe (1992) found international differences in the daily consumption of prescriptions for the UK and Germany, with German health seekers consuming more cardiovascular medication daily compared to UK health seekers. Visser et al. (2014) demonstrated regional differences with the diagnosis of – and medication prescription for – ADHD within the US. This can partially be attributed to differences in diagnosis, with the 'subtypes' of ADHD remaining a matter of some debate (e.g., Geurts et al., 2005; Milich et al., 2001; Milich et al., 2002). Similar results have been observed in diagnoses of concussions, lung pathologies, melanoma, ocular tuberculosis, and videogame 'addictions' (Aarseth et al., 2017; Elmore et al., 2017; Lou et al., 2015; Millington et al., 2018; Rose et al., 2015; cf. Spitzer et al., 2005; Ungvari et al., 2010).

Studies have also demonstrated the occurrence of illnesses and diseases within familial and peer networks with eating disorders, cancers, chronic illnesses, dementia (Anderson et al., 1995; Barraclough, 1994; das Chagas Medeiros et al., 2000; Dennis et al., 1998; Forsberg-Warleby et al., 2001; Franel & Wmaboldt, 1998; Germino et al., 1995; George & Gwyther, 1986; Grant et al., 2000; Han & Haley, 1999; Kazak et al., 1998; Kiecolt-Glaser et al., 1991; Quiles Marcos et al., 2013; Nijboer et al., 2001; Raveis et al., 1998; Reisine, 1995). Complementing these findings, health seeker support networks are also critical determinants of health (DiMatteo, 2004; Harandi et al., 2017; Shor et al., 2013; Wang et al., 2003). Finally, from a social constructivist perspective, the legitimacy of illnesses is also a product of belief within a social network (Brown, 1995; Conrad & Barker, 2010; Sharf & vanderfor, 2003; Ware, 1992).This is evident, in that the western biomedicine has historically ignored psychological and social determinants of health.

Members of a support network provide a variety of resources including information, motivation, emotional support, and financial resources. For instance, studies of first responders and healthcare workers have demonstrated that their receipt of social support is a critical determinant of their resiliency in dealing with the stress and trauma associated with their job (Barth, 2010; Prati & Pietrantoni, 2010; Donnelly et al., 2016; Alnazly, 2021; Labrague, 2021). The effects of support are not uniformly beneficial. Research has also revealed that family members and caregivers of patients with chronic health issues (e.g., autoimmune disease, asthma, cancer, dementia, diabetes, stroke) also experience anxiety, depression, and emotional distress (e.g., Gonzalez-Salvador et al., 1999; Holmes & Deb, 2003; Livingston et al., 2014; Loh et al., 2017; Lowery et al., 2000; Sallim et al., 2015). The distress can exceed that of the patient (Barraclough, 1994; Germino et al., 1995).

Indirect experiences will also impact our health (Hopwood & Schutte, 2017; Houston et al., 2018). Healthcare workers can experience secondary traumatic stress or vicarious stress/trauma when they are indirectly exposed to trauma (Cieslak et al., 2014; Cohen & Collens, 2013). People can also experience collective and generational trauma within a community when members of their group in the present or past were exposed to traumatic events (Cerdeña et al., 2021; Sangalang & Vang, 2017). Even if individuals are not members of a group, knowledge of events can lead to anxiety, stress, and depression due to empathy. For instance, in a meta-analysis of exposure to large-scale violence and disasters, Hopwood and Schutte (2017) found a variety of negative psychological outcomes were associated with people's awareness of these events. Such results can be transparently understood in terms of general empathy, identification with features of the victims, or recognition of the shared humanity of victims. Negative health outcomes in social networks are not restricted to violence or disease. Other systems-based factors include policy structures, health equity, and social influences such as racism and stigma (Lucyk & McLaren, 2017; Mangold et al., 2019).

Differences in diagnostic traditions, prevalence of illnesses within social networks, and how health (issues) can impact a therapeutic network underscore the need for a firm foundation for the study, assessment, and training of collective competence. While the unit of analysis will undoubtedly differ based on available resources and learning objectives, the assessment of collective competence requires understanding the structure and function of teams.

2.2 Social Cognitive Process in Collective Competence

Claiming that competence is a collective property of a social network requires clearly defining what kinds of operations determine collective efficacy of a community, team, or organization. Competency-based education has typically focused on roles such as 'communicator' or 'collaborator'. Although these are necessary features of collective competence, they are not sufficient. Here, we develop a social cognitive framework of collective competence that assumes the knowledge and skills required to complete a task are distributed among the members of a healthcare team or extended network of professionals and community members. Regardless of whether members of a team might share all, some, or none of the same knowledge and skills, they must engage in a process of sensemaking to address the needs of health seekers.

2.2.1 The Foundation of Collective Competence: Sociocultural Approaches to Learning

The sociocultural approach to learning has greatly impacted science (Vygotsky, 1962, 1978; for reviews, see Polly et al., 2017). Rather than focusing on individual cognitive development in relative isolation (Piaget, 1929, 1954; Leach & Scott, 2003), the sociocultural approach focuses on social interactions between learners and educators. Beyond the importance of the availability and use of tools (especially language), Vygotsky's approach emphasized two complementary concepts: social scaffolding and the zone of proximal development (ZPD). Using the analogy of a scaffolding that facilitates the construction of a building, Vygotsky assumed that an educator provides a *social scaffolding* that allows the learner to organize knowledge. Concurrently, educators must also be cognizant that the learner's domain-specific knowledge is limited and must provide them with relevant *novel* information such as facts, relational knowledge, and procedures that can be associated with their current level of competence. This information represents the *ZPD*. Thus, education requires *understanding* the learner's current knowledge and providing them with appropriate cues to enable them to exceed their individual performance. Subsequently, educators must remove these supportive means to allow the learner to perform the task on their own. For instance, educators could provide students with a visual demonstration of how to use a laparoscopic trainer, then shift toward simply providing feedback, and finally leave the learner to practice on their own.

The sociocultural model of learning is apparent even in early educational models in the health professions. Bedside teaching can be understood in terms of social scaffolding, with the learner observing the educators as they perform their rounds. Similarly, the 'see one-do one-teach one' technique attributed to Halstead is consistent with this approach: observing the technique primes the learner, reducing their learning curve if they mentally simulate the behavior of the educators. Teaching the technique to another requires that an instructor take the perspective of the learner. In turn, the learner should take the perspective of the instructor. Social scaffolding can also be observed formally in the concept of entrustable professional activities (EPAs; ten Cate, 2005, 2013): learners are judged relative to the level of supervision required (Ma, 2024; Shorey et al., 2019).

Despite their influence as part of a novel theory of learning, Vygotsky's concepts and proposals were quite general. Subsequent theoretical work has attempted to define the ZPD in terms of accessible knowledge or the kind and number of cues required to learn. However, these models do not specifically address the process of social scaffolding from a social cognitive perspective. For instance, Halstead's approach to education does not suggest *how* learners and educators must perceive, perform, and instruct others.

SDM provides a useful paradigm for understanding how healers and health seekers interact. While there is recognition that the level of patient autonomy differs across healthcare delivery contexts (Kon, 2010; Whitney et al., 2008), SDM is generally defined by an emphasis on empowering patients to collaborate in decision-making, weighting their preferences, and helping them select from among the treatment alternatives (Elwyn et al., 2017; Kunneman et al., 2019; Stiggelbout et al., 2015). Other definitions place additional emphasis on risk assessment, patient education, exchange of information, mutual agreement, and clear definition of roles (for a review, see Makoul & Clayman, 2006). Nevertheless, the processes that define these outcomes are not clearly defined.

In what follows, we identify four basic social cognitive processes associated with collective competence: (a) joint attention processes, (b) transactive memory systems (TMSs) and interactional schemata, (c) empathy and perspective-taking, and (d) conformity biases and groupthink.

2.2.2 Social Learning and Joint Attention Processes

Learning develops expertise by narrowing the focus of attention to a subset of information that is diagnostically relevant (Ericsson, 2007; Norman et al., 2018; for a general demonstration, see Blair et al., 2009). For instance, oncology studies have demonstrated that medical students take longer and look at more features within a display than experienced clinicians (Krupinski, 2010). Social learning facilitates this process. By drawing a learner's attention to diagnostic features of a disease and providing them with feedback, the learner should require markedly fewer events to identify patterns and responses, leading to fewer errors and reducing the time required to acquire knowledge or skill to perform a particular task.

Social scaffolding can be interpreted as the set of verbal and nonverbal cues, learning activities (e.g., task decomposition and reorganization), educational resources (e.g., articles, textbooks), and feedback that facilitate the learner's attention to the subset of affordances in a situation which are known to be relevant to a task. The process of social scaffolding can be operationalized using the concept of a *joint attention process*. A joint attention process occurs when an educator directs the learner's attention to novel features of the environment or more complex (functional) *affordances*. Features represent elements (e.g., colors and shapes), whereas affordances represent ways in which learners can *interact* with objects (e.g., diagnostic features of a pathology, multiple uses for a single instrument, vulnerabilities in interprofessional communication). For the neurological basis of joint attention, see Box 2.1.

BOX 2.1 NEUROSCIENCE OF JOINT ATTENTION

Neuroscientific evidence supports the existence of a distinct set of processes associated with joint attention (e.g., Redcay et al., 2012). For instance, multiple studies have demonstrated the association of joint attention behaviors with the medial prefrontal cortex (mPFC; e.g., Bristow et al., 2007; Williams et al., 2005) a region associated with social cognition more generally (e.g., Krueger et al., 2009; Bzdok et al., 2013). Supporting this, studies of parent–child dyads have found positive associations between the amount of joint attentional behaviors and the vocabulary development of children (e.g., Tomasello & Farrar, 1986; Smith et al., 1988; Carpenter et al., 1998; Markus et al., 2000; Morales et al., 2000). More recently, investigations with adults suggest that activation in areas associated with social cognition (e.g., mPFC) is observed in both the initiator (e.g., teacher) and monitor (e.g., learner) in joint attention episodes.

In a typical joint attention task (Figure 2.2), a learner (Person A) initially (t_1) maintains their own mental model of the problem space [1], distributing their attention across all features of the environment (affordances) because they do not know what is relevant to an expert (Person B). If Person A and Person B want to share the same mental model [2], they must coordinate their attention using a joint attentional process (*a*; e.g., Williams et al., 2005). Using cues and terms that are mutually interpretable and informative (Sperber & Wilson, 1986), the teacher directs the learner's attention to new affordance (t_2). Supporting this, the correspondence between listener's and speaker's eye movement is positively associated with comprehension (Richardson & Dale, 2005; Richardson et al., 2007). Eventually (t_3),

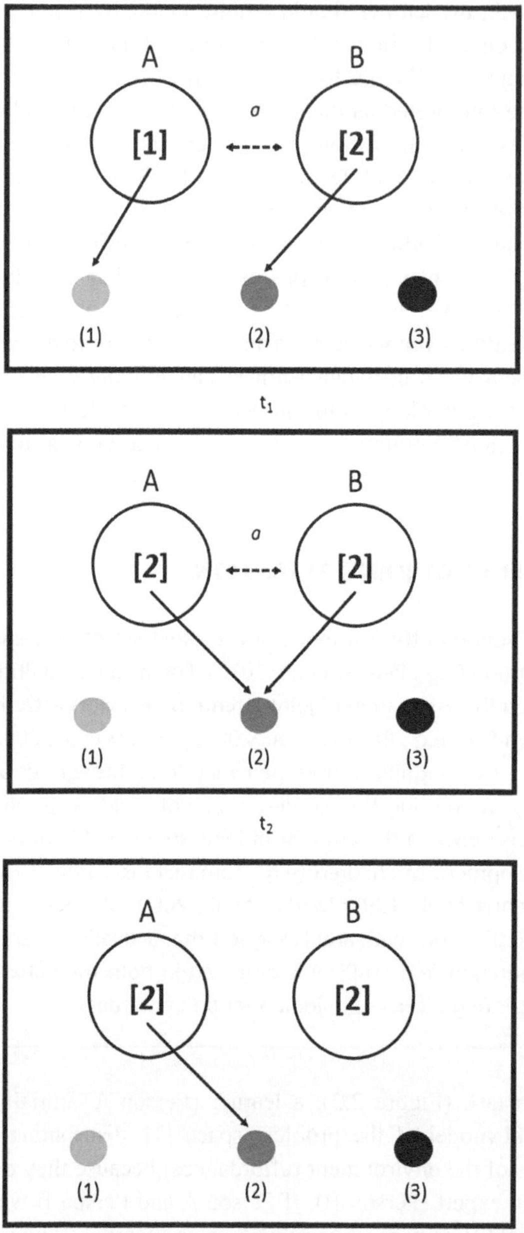

FIGURE 2.2 Simplified joint attentional learning process. Where Person A has a mental representation of the problem space that indicates (1) is a relevant feature of the environment and Person B has a mental representation that indicates (2) is a relevant feature of the environment. Joint attentional processes (a) aid in shifting the learner's focus of attention and mental models by using cues (e.g., gaze, gesticulation).

the learner has internalized the mental model of the teacher [2], no longer requiring a joint attention process to achieve the same level of performance. Such processes are also undoubtedly influenced by affective responses and stressors that define education and practice in the health professions (e.g., McConnell, 2024).

Joint attention allows for information exchange and facilitates cooperation, by promoting the coordination of thoughts and behaviors (Bullowa, 1979; Tomasello, 2009). Thus, joint attention is an important cognitive process in supporting social learning (Mundy, 2003). Within the context of social learning, the notion of shared attention offers a framework in which knowledge can be exchanged. In this attentional level, individuals both follow and intentionally direct others' attention, with the objective to engage in a mutually shared focus of attention (Gilbert, 2007). This shared attention can be used in conjunction with the use of verbal or nonverbal behaviors to communicate that each individual is attending to the same object or modality (Siposova & Carpenter, 2019). For example, a doctor can direct a medical student's attention to a cue both can focus on, by verbally informing the student or by a nonverbal gesture such as pointing and gesturing. Moreover, the learner need not be a passive participant in the learning environment. By sharing their beliefs with a teacher, a learner can facilitate the exchange.

2.2.3 Transactive Memory Systems, Scripts, and Relational Models

The development of collective competence cannot occur in a single episode of interprofessional training or interaction. Learners and educators develop their medical knowledge, understanding of roles and responsibilities, affective and cognitive perspective-taking, and skills over many episodes. In this case, each member of a healthcare team will have to encode, retain, and recall the competencies of other HCPs. Collectively, a team or an organization can be defined as a memory system, with their ability to maintain knowledge of others' competencies referred to as *transactive memory* (Wegner, 1987; for reviews, see Hollingshead, 1998; Moreland & Agote, 2014; Nevo & wand, 2005; Peltokorpi, 2008). Next, we consider properties of TMSs (Figure 2.3).

2.2.3.1 Medical Teams as Transactive Memory Systems

An effective TMS encompasses three aspects: (a) s*pecialization*, which involves understanding each members' specific expertise, (b) *credibility* or trust in the reliability of others' team member's knowledge, and (c) *coordination* defined as the efficient management and sharing of information among team members (Moreland et al., 1996; Moreland, 1999; Nevo & Wand, 2005; Lewis, 2003). Relying on others for specific task-related knowledge allows each team member to focus on their specific expertise rather than allocate time to learning information already known by others. This approach provides the whole team with extensive access to a broad base of relevant knowledge, which can then be applied to interrelated tasks

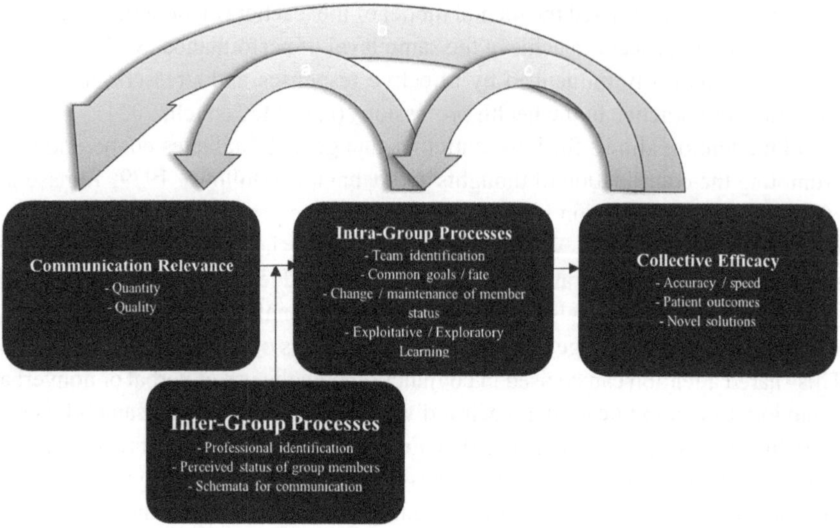

FIGURE 2.3 Dynamic transactive system of collective competence. Communication competencies are used to monitor and regulate intragroup processes that can be affected by differences stemming from inter-group factors. Conjointly, these processes determine collective efficacy. Outcomes of interactions determine collective efficacy. In groups presented tasks over multiple iterations, this creates feedback cycles entailing (a) direct adjustments to communication style within the group prior to task completion (e.g., subtasks or informal interactions), (b) due to global performance on the task or (c) adjustments to intragroup processes, including the change of group member status, learning strategies.

Source: Adapted from Liao et al. (2012) and Li and Huang (2013).

(Moreland, 1999). Studies of TMS have demonstrated that greater efficacy of these processes is related to beneficial outcomes (Moreland & Myakovsky, 2000; Lewis et al., 2005; Michinov & Michinov, 2009).

In healthcare delivery, transactive memory is particularly evident during clinical handovers, which require transferring professional responsibility for a patient from one individual or group to another (Jorm et al., 2009; Jeffcott et al., 2009; Eggins & Slade, 2015). Given that healthcare teams often consist of members from various disciplines (e.g., anesthetists, general practitioners, pharmacists, social workers, and surgeons) and often experience high staff turnover rates, it is unlikely that all team members will know each other personally. Without direct knowledge of each member, HCPs must rely on roles within the TMS to effectively coordinate care (Patel & Arocha, 2001). As TMSs are developed over time through repeated interactions with others, effective communication becomes a critical variable in building successful TMS within a team (Peltokorpi & Hood, 2018).

Rather than formal procedures and protocols, research on medical teams has suggested that performance frequently depends on 'informal coordination processes' and 'side conversations' to gather crucial insights into a patient's condition and treatment plans (Soltani et al., 2019). These verbal exchanges often occur during end-of-shift handovers and can lead to a risk of misunderstandings or omission of crucial details, jeopardizing the patient's health and safety. For instance, a survey conducted in a US hospital including 161 internal medicine and general surgery trainees found that 59% of respondents indicated that inadequate handovers resulted in harm to one or more patients (Kitch et al., 2008). Thus, while transactive memory is a defining feature of healthcare settings, certain factors such as ineffective communication can impede its development and functioning.

2.2.3.2 *Social Scripts and Relational Models in Healthcare*

Rather than perceiving every situation as novel, social interactions tend to be defined by a small set of norms and conventions (Burke & Young, 2011; Reno et al., 1993; Hawkins, 2019). People often refer to *social scripts*, or linear exchange schema for specific kinds of individuals. For instance, when entering a waiting area in a clinic, patients approach the counter, register, wait, are shown to an examination room, wait, and have their exam, followed by an exit. Despite minor variations, this situation is likely familiar to most patients. Adhering to the script ensures efficient communication. However, failing to maintain such a script or violations of the script can cause confusion, frustration, and a failure to provide crucial information (Schoenherr & Le-Bouar, 2024). Box 2.2 provides a classic demonstration.

BOX 2.2 THE DOCTOR–NURSE GAME REVISITED

In the health professions, the 'doctor-nurse game' traditionally defined communication expectations between senior clinicians and subordinates, such that nurses must provide doctors with relevant information, without overtly challenging a clinician's competence as a healthcare professional or creating interpersonal conflict (Stein, 1967). Of course, such asymmetries can stifle opportunities for meaningful dialogue, collaboration, and the exchange of ideas, as subordinates may feel hesitant to voice concerns or offer alternative perspectives (Henriksen & Dayton, 2006). Similarly, the 'sick-role' model describes the position of an ill person relative to a clinician (Parsons, 1951). According to Parsons, when individuals become sick, they temporarily occupy a distinct social role characterized by specific rights and obligations. This includes exemption from normal social roles and responsibilities, granting individuals the right to deviate from typical behavior without full accountability. However, those in the sick role are also expected to actively seek medical help, adhere to treatment regimens, and cooperate with healthcare professionals to regain their health and return to their usual roles and responsibilities as soon as possible (Levine & Kozloff, 1978). If clinicians can understand these expectations, they can adopt strategies to ensure that they address any potential vulnerabilities in the communication and decision process (e.g., Ferretti et al., 2023).

In parallel with specific health-related roles, general relational models (RM) are also evidenced across cultures. Together with collectivism and individualism, horizontal and vertical dimensions define four RM that appear to shape how people remember events and how they interact with others (Fiske, 1991, 1995). For instance, members of a healthcare team might all be perceived as equivalent and interchangeable (i.e., communal sharing of identity and resources) or they might instead be perceived as uniquely qualified to perform a role and have status within an organization based on merit (i.e., proportionality by performance criteria). A failure to conform to these RM could lead to perceptions of incivility or overt disrespect, reducing interpersonal cohesion and creating communication traps wherein relevant information is withheld (Ferretti et al., 2023), necessitating apologies or other forms of contrition. Sharing knowledge of the social scripts and RM that define professional practice is essential for collective competence.

2.2.3.3 Interpersonal Discord and Workplace Incivility

Workplace incivility encompasses minor breaches of group norms, distinguishing it from overtly disrespectful behaviors such as bullying or aggression (Andersson & Pearson, 1999; Pearson et al., 2000). Incivility arises from an appraisal process wherein individuals interpret cues to make social judgments about the intentions behind the instigator's actions (Marchiondo et al., 2018). Uncivil acts are defined as low-intensity deviant behaviors that contravene workplace norms, manifesting in both verbal and nonverbal conduct directed at other group members, often with a goal of status maintenance.

A pernicious feature of incivility is that these behaviors clearly fall short of respectful norms, while not reaching a threshold of disrespect, leading to perceived ambiguity in the intentions of the actor. For instance, if a clinician fails to learn or address their co-workers by name, make eye contact, or return greetings, their co-workers might discount these social cues in the moment. This ambiguity complicates addressing any potential issues, contributing to its cumulative impact on organizational dynamics: colleagues might not want to appear 'sensitive', refraining from discussing the matter directly. In that incivility often perpetuates through direct and indirect reciprocity, it can create a 'spiral of incivility' where minor transgressions escalate into hostile behavior over time (Samosh, 2019).

Workplace incivility is widespread in healthcare settings. Smith et al. (2010) found that 90.4% of novice nurses had experienced some form of incivility during their careers. This behavior frequently evidenced as 'lateral violence', where aggressive actions such as undermining, withholding information, sabotage, infighting, scapegoating, and backstabbing are directed at colleagues within the same group, with nursing being the primary occupation at risk (Duffy, 1995; Farrell, 1997; Carter, 1999; Stanley et al., 2007). Hostile behaviors among co-workers not only inflict emotional distress but also jeopardize the quality of care provided. Laschinger (2014) identified a significant correlation between workplace incivility and nursing quality of care, noting an elevated risk of patient-related errors. Furthermore, Sahay et al. (2015) underscore the association between unsupportive work relationships and unsafe medication administration practices among new graduate nurses, highlighting the imperative of comprehending social scripts and their impact on shaping the workplace environment.

2.2.4 Apology and Conflict Resolution

Individuals are typically inclined to preserve interpersonal relationships, or maintain the status quo (Proudfoot & Kay, 2014; Rego et al., 2018).[3] When friction occurs between individuals, restitution of the relationship often involves the act of making an apology. An apology represents a formal speech act (oral or in writing) that (a) acknowledges the mutual recognition of a violation of a social norm, (b) includes an explicit acknowledgment of wrongdoing, typically in the form of a statement of apology, and (c) elicits a response from the injured party (Tavuchis, 1991). Consequently, intentionality is key in the success of an apology. An apology is more likely to be accepted when there is situational ambiguity surrounding the norm violation or when the transgressor expresses a clear lack of intention to cause harm (Van Dijke & De Cremer, 2011). However, the effectiveness of an apology is undermined if the recipient perceives the transgressor's actions as deliberate or intentional, or the act of apologizing as disingenuous (Struthers et al., 2008; Leunissen et al., 2013; for a comprehensive review, see Fehr et al., 2010).

Studies also suggest that certain demographic factors, such as gender and social status, can influence the likelihood of offering an apology. For instance, males and individuals of higher social status are less inclined to apologize (Walfisch et al., 2013). This observation is particularly pertinent in the medical setting, where hierarchical structures often prevail (Essex et al., 2023). In such contexts, doctors traditionally occupy positions of higher social rank (Elsous et al., 2017). The reluctance to apologize among such individuals can have adverse consequences for professional relationships and the therapeutic alliance, impeding conflict resolution and fostering hostile communication that reduces the collective competence of healthcare teams.

2.2.5 Perspective-Taking and Empathy

Navigating social environments defined by competing RM and individual experiences requires taking the perspective of those within a social network, often referred to as a theory of mind (ToM; Astington & Jenkins, 1995; Frith & Frith, 2005; Gopnik & Wellman, 1992). ToM has been studied extensively in the developmental literature, consisting of the ability to maintain the perspectives including false beliefs, i.e., that someone believes something erroneously. Studies have revealed that ToM development is affected by how many others are in our environment and cultures that prioritize interdependence and can also decrease in adults (Henry et al., 2013).

Perspective-taking is often framed in terms of empathy. Empathy can be defined as two broad sets of processes: affective and cognitive empathy (Baron-Cohen & Wheelwright, 2004; Dvash & Shamay-Tsoory, 2014). *Affective (or emotional) empathy* concerns our ability to experience the affective or emotional states of others. For instance, a clinician's ability to empathize is a critical capability whether interacting with a parent whose infant is critically ill, a young adult experiencing depression and anxiety, or a senior whose partner is receiving end-of-life care.

Cognitive empathy concerns our ability to understand the perceptions, attitudes, beliefs, and values of another. This has often been examined in terms of visual perspective-taking (Piaget & Inhelder, 1967), with some studies suggesting that it is affected by the perceived empowerment of individuals (Galinsky et al., 2006). Research demonstrated that trait-level empathy is associated with improved performance in adults on perspective-taking tasks (Mattan et al., 2016). Crucially, such research has also demonstrated that perspective-taking by people in leadership positions can substantially improve decision-making (Galinsky et al., 2014).

Affective and cognitive aspects of empathy represent distinct abilities (e.g., Cox et al., 2012; Gilin et al., 2013). For instance, in a meta-analysis of workplace studies examining empathic concern (affective empathy) and perspective-taking (cognitive empathy), Longmire and Harrison (2018) found that empathic concern was a stronger predictor of being supportive of co-workers. Studies of negotiation have similarly demonstrated that perspective-taking improves performance, whereas empathic concern reduces performance (Galinsky et al., 2008). Consequently, collective competence not only requires the ability of perspective-taking but also requires an understanding of its limits when people feel disempowered.

2.2.6 Conformity and Groupthink

Despite the benefits of interprofessional collaboration such as enhancing information exchange, knowledge transfer, and decision-making (Morley & Cashell, 2017), collaboration can result in a failure to consider alternative proposals outside one's group or lead to adverse health outcomes if the assumption of a healthcare team goes unchallenged. HCPs must navigate the delicate trade-off presented by conformity within a group, referred to as groupthink.

2.2.6.1 Conformity Bias

Conformity biases are present across all cultures. Studies demonstrate that people will change their responses to what they think others believe (Asch, 1951; Boyd & Richardson, 1985; Zerbe & Paulhus, 1987). This is also present at a societal level in terms of cultural tightness, the extent to which cultural values conform to a set of norms and conventions ('tight') or variability ('loose'; Triandis, 2000; Kondo, 2010; Gelfand et al., 2017). These norms lead to trade-offs in performance. For instance, in healthcare, protocols should be followed for the delivery of care, to ensure the (highest) patient outcomes. However, if there are failures to adequately gather information (e.g., patient history, bloodwork) or assess therapeutic alternatives, and respectfully challenge the assumptions of other members of a healthcare team, this can lead to faulty diagnoses and a failure to consider the consequences of recommending specific treatment options.

2.2.6.2 Organizational Silence

Conformity in healthcare can often lead to a phenomenon known as *organizational silence*, characterized by a collective tendency to say or do very little in response to problems observed within an organization (Henriksen & Dayton, 2006). Rather than being passive, silence is a deliberate and conscious behavior wherein individuals withhold information about critical issues, often due to fear of repercussions or a desire to avoid interpersonal conflict (Morrison & Milliken, 2000; Van Dyne et al., 2003; Alparslan & Kayalar, 2012). When HCPs refrain from voicing their concerns or reporting errors, it prevents the identification and resolution of critical problems that could otherwise compromise patient safety and care. As a result, crucial information about potential hazards or systemic inefficiencies remains unaddressed, which can lead to a decline in the quality of patient care, preventable mistakes, and a loss of public trust in the healthcare system (Altinöz et al., 2011; Yalçin & Baykal, 2012).

Organizational silence can have detrimental effects on employee morale and engagement. When feedback is suppressed, it not only diminishes job satisfaction but can also contribute to higher turnover rates, stifle innovation, and increase workplace incivility (see Section 2.2.3; Aktaş & Şimşek, 2014). The fear of negative consequences, such as punishment, ostracism, or damage to professional relationships, often drives this silence (Premeaux & Bedeian, 2003; Yalçın et al., 2021), with some studies indicating that fewer than 10% of medical staff address clinical practices that are perceived as poor or harmful (Maxfield et al., 2005). Another study indicated that 65.7% of nurses do not talk about issues that concern them, remaining silent due to mistrust in the administration, a perceived lack of experience, and a fear of being ostracized (Erigüç et al., 2014). Consequently, these dynamics perpetuate a cycle of silence that can impede organizational learning and improvement and thereby affect the development of collective competence within a team. Like workplace incivility, this can create maladaptive organizational cultures that are detrimental to the effective delivery of care.

2.2.6.3 Groupthink

Groupthink defines a broad set of problems associated with poor decision-making including self-censorship (silence), conformity, and failures to assess diagnosis alternatives and verify the validity of courses of treatment. One of the primary causes of groupthink is the desire for concordance within a highly cohesive group at the expense of critical thinking or the exploration of alternatives (Janis, 1982).

In addition to self-censorship, members of a group can concurrently attempt to regulate perceived deviation within a group, directing negative feedback to 'deviant' group members. The presence of other distinct antecedents can contribute to the likelihood of the group exhibiting symptoms of groupthink (Janis, 1983; see Table 2.1). Those symptoms in turn influence the group's decision-making processes and lead to suboptimal decisions (Moorhead & Montanari, 1986; Neck & Manz, 1994). In healthcare, groupthink represents a major impediment to the delivery of care, creating significant threats to patient safety (Mannion & Thompson, 2014; Beran et al., 2014).

Groupthink can also be observed at different levels of healthcare organizations ranging from clinical teams delivering care to senior managers and board members

TABLE 2.1 Framework of Groupthink

Features of Groups (Antecedent Conditions)	*Motivation*	*Symptoms of Groupthink*	*Defective Decision-Making and Reduced Performance*
• High group cohesiveness • Insulation of the group • Absence of procedure for judgment and decision-making • Directive leadership • High stress • Few perceived alternatives	• Consensus seeking • Maintenance of status/ group membership	• Perceived invulnerability • Perceived unanimity • Collective rationalization • Perceived morality of group • Stereotypes of outgroup members • Directed pressure on dissenters • Self-censorship	• Incomplete survey of alternatives and outcomes • Poor information search • Failure to consider risk of outcomes • Bias toward available information • Failure to reassess alternatives • Failure to develop contingency plans

Note: Groupthink occurs when situational factors promote concurrence seeking to maintain interpersonal accord within a group. When directive leadership is used, group members might not question the reliability of the process and engage in self-censorship, resulting in faculty decision-making.

overseeing the administration of the organization (Mannion & Thompson, 2014). For instance, a member of a medical team might notice that a patient's symptoms are not consistent with the working diagnosis adopted by others but fail to express their concerns because they assume that other members' judgment must be correct. More generally, the possibility that disagreement might impair a working relationship and the desire to preserve collaborative harmony results in a perceived pressure to conform and might give rise to failures to establish professional exchanges (Srivastava, 2013; Beran et al., 2014).

Despite the lack of formal studies, HCPs have identified many features of groupthink at the level of healthcare teams and organizations (for a recent review, see DiPierro et al., 2022). First, whether at the team- or organizational-level, *group cohesiveness* and *homogeneity* are likely key determinants of groupthink. Cohesion can operate on many levels including members of the team (horizontal cohesion), immediate supervisors or organizational leadership (vertical cohesion), or the organization or profession as a whole (organizational cohesion; Siebold & Kelly, 1988). For instance, studies have found that medical educators are reluctant to fail *their* students, referred to as 'a failure to fail' (Danyluk et al., 2015; Siebert et al., 2006), with other studies observing failures to report lapses in medical students' professionalism (Ziring et al., 2018). Moreover, multiple barriers have also been found for the reporting of critical incidents in hospitals (Bayazidi et al., 2012; Hartnell et al., 2012; Lawton & Parker, 2002; Vrbnjak et al., 2016).

Second, structural features including *leadership* and *hierarchical structure* of healthcare also create barriers (e.g., the doctor–nurse game; Box 2.2) that assumes that nurses must follow a social script that presents information missed by a clinician in a manner that does not violate their status as a leader. More generally, HCPs who have a lower status within an organization (e.g., comparatively junior) might also feel the need to conform to the clinical decisions of higher status clinicians, and to perceive fewer opportunities to engage in group decision-making processes (Beran et al., 2014; Choi et al., 2024; Kaba & Beran, 2016). As we noted above, understanding the RM that are adopted by members of a healthcare team can ensure that social norms are respected, and that relevant information is provided in a timely manner. Depending on the institution or society HCPs are trained in, there might be substantial differences in the perceived role and characteristic of leaders.

Third, a major final impediment concerns *task demands*. Working within emergency or critical care settings necessarily means making decisions quickly to stabilize a patient. In such situations, members of a healthcare team are more likely to rely on heuristics in terms of the available diagnoses and treatment options, often leading to overconfidence (Schoenherr et al., 2024). They will also likely rely on scripts and stereotypes associated with the healthcare team. Acknowledging the potential vulnerabilities associated with teamwork is essential to ensuring collective competency.

2.3 Models of Collaborative Learning and Shared Decision-Making

If teams can be viewed as distributed cognitive systems, then members of a healthcare team must be trained as a unit (Baruah & Paulus, 2008; Singer et al., 2015; Weaver et al., 2014). If training is exclusively focused on developing the competencies of an individual, then HCPs are less likely to be aware of the situational cues that might indicate the need to share information or delegate diagnosis or treatment to another person.

Viewing a healthcare team as a unit is merely the first step. The basic social cognitive processes that facilitate and challenge collective competence must be specified further by identifying key processes and representations that facilitate shared mental models of illness and treatment context between practitioners and patients.

Models of learning define learners' expectations about who, how, and what they should learn. Expectations are in turn derived from an amalgam of cognitive processes associated with past experiences, cultural norms, and social conditioning (Katona, 1946; Markus & Kitayama, 2003; Escandell-Vidal, 2016). In healthcare, these expectations can take the form of the apprenticeship model wherein an individual (apprentice) learns from experienced practitioners through observation, mentorship, and active practice, allowing them to gain clinical skills and knowledge through participation in real-life clinical settings under close supervision (Dennen & Burner, 2008; Mauldin, 2011; Poortman et al., 2011; Schoenherr & McConnell, 2024). Although the apprenticeship model has traditionally been the focus of medical education in western medicine, it is evidenced cross-culturally (Schoenherr, 2021; Schoenherr & McConnell, 2024; Schoenherr & Beaudoin, 2027). For instance, in East Asia, Hsu (1999) differentiates a 'personal mode' of learning defined by a trust-based interpersonal relationship from a 'standardized mode' based on professionalization and standardized exams (Feng, 1994; Gan, 2008).

In this section, we review paradigms for collaborative learning (CL) and decision-making in the healthcare, including simulation-based training, IPE, and collaborative decision-making frameworks. These paradigms highlight the importance of structured debriefing sessions, reflective practice, and real-time feedback in promoting the continuous development of collective competence in healthcare teams.

2.3.1 Collaborative Learning

The traditional apprenticeship model implies an idiosyncratic form of social learning. For instance, in their study of traditional medical practitioners, Adekannbi et al. (2014) found that the reported years of experience of the teacher determined the amount of information shared with apprentices, whereas apprentice learning was positively associated with their marital status and the expected (and actual) length of the apprenticeship. In contrast to an apprenticeship model, CL represents a distributed approach to learning wherein two or more people engage in a learning activity together (Pluta et al., 2013). Given the presence of another learner, this paradigm enables observational learning: both learners can observe the successes and failures of another, with cognitive empathy allowing them to adjust their behavior according to the outcomes and feedback provided to other learners.

Certain kinds of learning tasks might recommend the use of CL, such as problem-based learning (PBL) and team-based learning (TBL). PBL represents a student-centered approach to learning that provides students with specified problems. Problems are provided in small group sessions. Students are randomly assigned to these groups, with an educator acting as a facilitator. During an initial discussion, students must identify issues associated with the problem and engage in self-study to identify solutions. This is followed by a synthesis phase wherein group members combine their work and then explain what they have learned, including any issues they encountered (Barrows & Tamblyn, 1980; Barrows, 1996; Hmelo-Silver, 2004). Similarly, TBL is defined by three phases. First, learners engage in self-directed learning outside the classroom. Second, learners complete an assessment that measures their own knowledge within a domain. Third, once students are deemed to be sufficiently competent, they are then presented with a collaborative problem-solving exercise, the solutions of which are available to other teams within the class. These phases are repeated based on performance and the needs of the program (Thompson et al., 2007).

Hybrid approaches such as case-based collaborative learning (CBCL) combine features of PBL and TBL. Developed largely as a synthesis between PBL, TBL, and case-based learning, CBCL assesses learners' comprehension of material prior to entering the classroom. Students are presented with a new case in class and generate their hypotheses and solutions individually. Unlike PBL, there is a greater focus on problem solving rather than problem finding. Whereas PBL encourages learners to identify issues they believe are most relevant, the cases and questions in CBCL are developed by the instructors in advance. In a direct comparison of PBL and CBCL, Krupat et al. (2016) found that students whose median performance was below their peers in other classes performed better using CBCL compared to PBL. However, these effects were not observed equally across all learners. For instance, the differential impact of instruction method was not observed for learners who performed above the median, possibly suggesting a ceiling effect (Millington et al., 2018).

2.3.1.1 *Benefits of Collaborative Learning*

CL would seem to be consistent with the need to work effectively as members of a healthcare team. Moreover, limited resources (e.g., expensive simulations, limited number of educators, protected time) might make CL a preferable option, as learners can share these resources and obtain feedback. However, CL also presents unique challenges to implementation. The need to coordinate, train, and remove clinicians from service creates unique challenges for implementation including human resources (Schoenherr & Hamstra, 2024). For instance, TBL activities can be discontinued due to the departure of educators who are trained to use these methods (Thompson et al., 2007). Moreover, the validity of these methods will be dependent on learners' and instructors' competence and comfort, and the dynamics that emerge throughout implementation. For instance, early studies investigating surgical knot tying and urinary catheterization found that computer-assisted learning was more effective than peer learning (Rogers et al., 2000; Walsh et al., 2011). Studies of tutors and medical students have also found that feedback (constructive and reflective), respectfulness, active engagements, preparedness, sharing information, and responsibility for outcomes were believed to facilitate CL (Iqbal et al., 2016).

2.3.1.2 Interprofessional Education (IPE)

Healthcare teams are not homogenous groups. Healthcare students are often restricted to the specific curriculum of their respective discipline and might encounter diverse challenges when working with other HCPs, including poor interprofessional communication, ineffective decision-making, stereotyping, and misunderstanding other professionals' competencies (Stadick, 2020; Ateah et al., 2011; Veerapen & Purkis, 2014). With only limited exposure to other healthcare disciplines, traditional hierarchies, stereotypes, and dissatisfaction within working teams can persist (Price et al., 2014; Stadick, 2020).

IPE activities aim to develop interprofessional competencies among students in a wide range of healthcare programs and prepare future health practitioners for learning the intricacy of interprofessional teamwork (Kemp & Brewer, 2023; Stadick, 2020). Five taxonomies of IPE learning strategies include problem-based, exchange-based, simulation-based, observation-based, and practice-based (Freeth et al., 2005). This teaching pedagogy can be supported by the interprofessional classification model, which incorporates six dimensions classifying interprofessional teamwork activities: shared commitment, shared identity, clear team goals, clear roles and responsibilities, interdependence between team members, and integration between work practices (Xyrichis et al., 2018) (Table 2.2).

In line with research on transactive memory, HCPs can collaborate to utilize the collective breadth and depth of their experiences, thereby increasing the likelihood of identifying a correct diagnosis, recognizing vulnerabilities in the decision-making process, improving outcome measures, and providing effective follow-up care. As the foundation of interprofessional collaborative practice, IPE provides the opportunity for two or more HCPs to learn about and from each other to enhance collaboration and quality of care (Green & Johnson, 2015; Stadick, 2020; Reeve et al., 2010).

There is a growing body of evidence that IPE can improve the development of interprofessional knowledge and skills, and attitudes toward collaborative

TABLE 2.2 Summary of Xyrichis et al.'s (2018) Interprofessional Classification Model

Dimension of Interprofessional Activity	*Definition*
Shared commitment	HCPs' perceived attachment toward their team
Shared identity	HCPs' attributed meanings related to their interprofessional team
Clear team goals	Explicit formulation of the goals of the interprofessional team
Clear roles and responsibilities	Distinction of professional roles of members within the interprofessional team
Interdependence between team members	Degree to which the decision-making processes of all team members affect the outcome of interprofessional interactions
Integration between work practices	Contributions of HCPs toward the alignment of professional practice toward the improvement of safety, quality, planning, and efficiency of healthcare

teamwork (Guraya & Barr, 2018; Saragih et al., 2024; Wang et al., 2019). Moreover, such programs can be instrumental in addressing stereotypes within the healthcare system by providing members of the healthcare team with direct experience (Ateah et al., 2011; Oandasan & Reeves, 2005). Health students can retain biased conceptions or understandings of other professions, which can remain as profession-specific ideas if left unchallenged (Turner, 1999). The interdisciplinary nature of IPE promotes CL and allows students to build effective working relationships within the healthcare profession (Barr et al., 2005; Guraya & Barr, 2018).

IPE has also been found to enhance job satisfaction among physicians and nurses working in emergency departments and facilitate complex issue resolution between primary HCPs and their patients (Larivaara & Taanila, 2004; Searle, 2008).

2.3.1.3 IPE Curriculum Development and Implementation

The preceding review underscores the importance of developing IPE programs that align with specific implementation context. Four dimensions of curriculum development framework capture the essential features of IPE programs (e.g., Lee et al., 2013). First, future healthcare practice needs must be identified. IPE development requires the recognition and promotion of necessary educational changes that promote interprofessional collaboration that are aligned with clinical and nonclinical competencies for the effective delivery of care (Meleis, 2016; Thistlethwaite, 2015). Second, curricula must also clearly define competencies that can be operationalized in educational interventions to assess learner outcomes (Thistlethwaite et al., 2014; World Health Organization (WHO), 2010). These can include competencies including interprofessional conflict resolution and communication, team functioning, role clarification, collaborative leadership, ethical practice, and community-centered care (Hepp et al., 2015; Olson et al., 2019; Thistlethwaite & Moran, 2010; van Diggele et al., 2020). Third, practical issues related to teaching, learning, and assessment must also be considered. Simulation activities, healthcare team challenges, and student-led clinics present activities that can be integrated into the curriculum (Anderson & Lennox, 2009; Evans et al., 2020; Moran et al., 2011; Sick et al., 2014; Thistlethwaite, 2015). However, the need to coordinate activities across multiple organizational units, obtaining clinical placements, differences in organizational culture and climate, and coordination with local and national health services all present unique challenges (Anderson et al., 2009; Dunworth, 2007; Rees & Johnson, 2007; Thistlethwaite & Nisbet, 2011). Finally, institutions must ensure that adequate support is provided to deliver programs effectively. Interprofessional faculty discussions are required to initiate and define CL outcomes and establish interprofessional activities to equip students with essential collective competencies, in addition to individual competencies (Orsino & Ng, 2019; Thistlethwaite, 2015). IPE programs can be implemented in a variety of ways, including differences in program delivery planning processes, assessment methods (e.g., attitudes, student and educator competence), diversity of leadership and learners, and learning outcomes (e.g., nontechnical, technical; Aston et al., 2012; Sunguya et al., 2014). All of these facets of program delivery must be acknowledged and addressed.

2.3.2 Collaborative Care

The final facet of collective competence requires an acknowledgment in the shift of the role of HCPs. Rather than placing HCPs in a dominant position in the healthcare setting, there is a growing realization that patient-centered approaches are required for the effective delivery of care. Beyond recognizing healthcare delivery as an exercise in persuasive communication (Schoenherr & Le-Bouar, 2024), collective competence requires that the patient is included as a partner in medical decision-making. Their health literacy, beliefs about illness, roles, and responsibilities are major determinants of whether information is gathered in a timely and complete manner, the flow of interpersonal exchanges, and whether treatment recommendations are adopted. Consequently, medical systems must be viewed as social systems.

2.3.2.1 Models of Doctor–Patient Relationships

The doctor–patient relationship has evolved over time, reflecting a shift from the traditional paternalistic approach to a more patient-centered model that values the patient's autonomy and agency in decision-making (Siegler, 1985). Multiple frameworks have attempted to define the RM (Emanuel & Emanuel, 1992; Szasz & Hollender, 1956). For instance, Szasz and Hollender (1956) delineated three basic models of the doctor–patient relationship that capture these changes. The *Activity–Passivity* model defines a relationship where practitioners wield complete authority and control, with patients playing a passive role as mere recipients of treatment, unable to contribute to decision-making processes. The *Guidance-Cooperation* model acknowledges patient agency to some extent, albeit still within a paternalistic framework. The HCP remains dominant, provides guidance, and assumes that the patient will comply with treatment recommendations. Finally, the *Mutual-Participation* model emphasizes the patient's autonomy in making medical decisions. Here, healthcare providers contribute expertise, while patients actively engage as equal partners in decision-making. This partnership fosters a more personalized relationship, facilitating the development of a therapeutic alliance rooted in mutual trust, respect, and communication (Kaba & Sooriakumaran, 2007; Chipidza et al., 2015).

Care is also situated within the family (Franck & O'Brien, 2019; Hanson et al., 1995; Johnson, 2000; Park et al., 2018; Zhang, 2018). Regardless of the important role of HCPs, family caregivers provide increasingly complicated and sustained support for those experiencing illness. One such approach, *Family-centered model (FCM)*, provides a broad framework that perceives the family as the primary support network for patients. The model was originally focused on infants and youth but has since been extended to other family members, e.g., spouses and children acting as caregivers for parents. Formalizing the FCM approach, Shelton et al. (1987) identify eight core features:

1. While services and HCPs change over time, the family environment remains comparatively constant,
2. Parents and professionals must collaborate at all levels of healthcare,
3. Parents should be provided with complete and unbiased information concerning the health of their child,
4. Emotional and financial support should be at the center of policies and programs,
5. Different methods of coping are valid within the family and within an individual,
6. Developmental needs of the infant, child, adolescent, and their family must be accommodated within the healthcare system,
7. Parent-to-parent (peer) support should be encouraged and facilitated, and
8. Healthcare systems should be designed to be flexible to accommodate the needs of the family during the delivery of care.

Research also supports the importance of family involvement in the delivery of care. For instance, Hanson et al. (1995) demonstrated that low levels of family conflict and high levels of cohesion are positively related to patient outcomes with family stress levels negatively related to patient outcomes. More generally, evidence suggests that how family members perceive the care context, how responsibility is allocated among family members, the extent to which an illness is stigmatized within a family, how family members of those with an illness are stigmatized, and how causal narratives are framed impact health outcomes (Aldersey et al., 2015; Corrigan et al., 2006; Lawton et al., 2007; Lobchuk et al., 2008: Scollan-Koliopoulos et al., 2007; Sunday et al., 2001; Yin et al., 2020).

Contemporary FCM models maintain these same features, identifying four common features in the literature: (a) *consideration of family context* whether immediate or extended, including caregivers and non-caregivers including the cultural norms and conventions and strengths (e.g., coping strategies, competencies, motivation, and resilience), (b) *dedicated policies and procedures* that acknowledge the impact of, and provided by, social organizations and institutions (e.g., national and local, governmental and nongovernmental) to legitimatize family contributions to care, (c) *illness-specific education for family members* including information about the illness, the care provision, and family support needs, and (d) *collaboration between patient, family, and care provider across the time-course of an illness* ensuring that control is maintained by the patient and their family (Kokorelias et al., 2019). Here, communication is seen as central to facilitate each of these elements.

2.3.2.2 Attribution in Healthcare Settings

Attribution is a fundamental psychological process that concerns how an individual perceives a situation or event and attributes causes to outcomes through the basis of their own beliefs and values (Kelley, 1973; Kelley & Michela, 1980; Weiner, 1986; Pollard-Gott, 1993). In the medical context, attributional models provide 'insight into the mechanisms through which health behavior decisions are formed as a function of the sociocultural beliefs, values, and morals' (Lieber et al., 2006, p. 464). Understanding patients' attribution models can inform how health providers approach collaborative care, tailoring interventions and communication strategies to address patients' beliefs and preferences effectively. Multiple models are available for care, most of which are closely associated with the notion of stigma wherein there is a belief that illness can be controlled by a health seeker.

Brickman et al. (1982) proposed four RM of helping and coping based on the attributional beliefs about *who* is responsible for an illness and who is responsible for a solution (Table 2.3). The *Moral Model* assumes an internal attribution where an individual is responsible for the problem and the solution, with internal motivation cited as the key determinant of health promotion and treatment. The *Compensatory*

TABLE 2.3 Attributional Model of Illness Responsibility

		Patient Responsibility for Solution	
		High	*Low*
Patient Responsibility for Problem	High	Moral Model	Enlightenment Model
	Low	Compensatory Model	Medical Model

Source: Adapted from Brickman et al. (1982).

Model assumes an external attribution for problems and an internal attribution for their solutions. An individual experiences illness due to failures of the social environment to provide them with adequate (health) resources. Health seekers must use their agency to (achieve) a solution. The *Enlightenment Model* assumes an internal attribution for health problems and an external attribution for solutions. By providing comparatively ignorant[4] health seekers who are either unwilling or unable to enact a solution with knowledge and insight (enlightenment), healers can heal them. Finally, the *Medical Model* assumes external attribution for both the responsibility of health problems as well as their solutions.

Brickman's attributional models have received some empirical support (Kloss & Lisman, 2003; Karasaki et al., 2013; Palm, 2004; Ronzani et al., 2009). For instance, Ronzani et al. (2009) conducted a study of primary care HCPs in Brazil. When considering substance use (i.e., tobacco, marijuana, and alcohol), clinicians typically held a negative view and maintained that patients were primarily accountable for their own problems and solutions (Moral Model). The adoption of such moral models helps explain why diseases can become stigmatized and why victims are blamed (Martin, 2001; Mantler et al., 2003). Much like RM, different clinicians can maintain different beliefs to the extent to which patients are to blame for their conditions. Kloss and Lisman's study (2003) found that mental health clinicians attributed more blame to the mentally ill, chemically addicted (MICA) patients than addiction clinicians did, suggesting that attributional models shape the way the patients are treated, with differing attributional models leading to potential challenges in compliance.

Despite providing a useful framework, Brickman's attributional models assume that either the patient or the clinicians is responsible for the outcomes of a situation. The model does not consider environmental or contextual factors of systems-level phenomena. For instance, a patient might have developed a disease due to the environment that they inhabit and a limited socioeconomic status that does not afford them the opportunity to live elsewhere (Figure 2.4).

2.3.2.3 Patient-Centered Care: Patient as Priority

Relational Models Theory provide a useful starting point for understanding diverse interpersonal processes within a group. To be effective, collective competence requires that HCPs can take the perspective of patients and family members, understand their values and expectations, provide relevant information, and involve them in the decision-making process (Lipkin, 1984; Grol et al., 1990; Winefield et al., 1996; Epstein et al., 2005; Stacey et al., 2008). For instance, a patient-centered approach requires exploring the patients' experience of the illness and disease, perceiving the patient-as-person (e.g., biography, identity, motivations, values), identifying common ground for disease management, incorporating health promotion and illness prevention activities, building the doctor–patient relationship, and acknowledging the limited resources (e.g., time, treatment options) that are

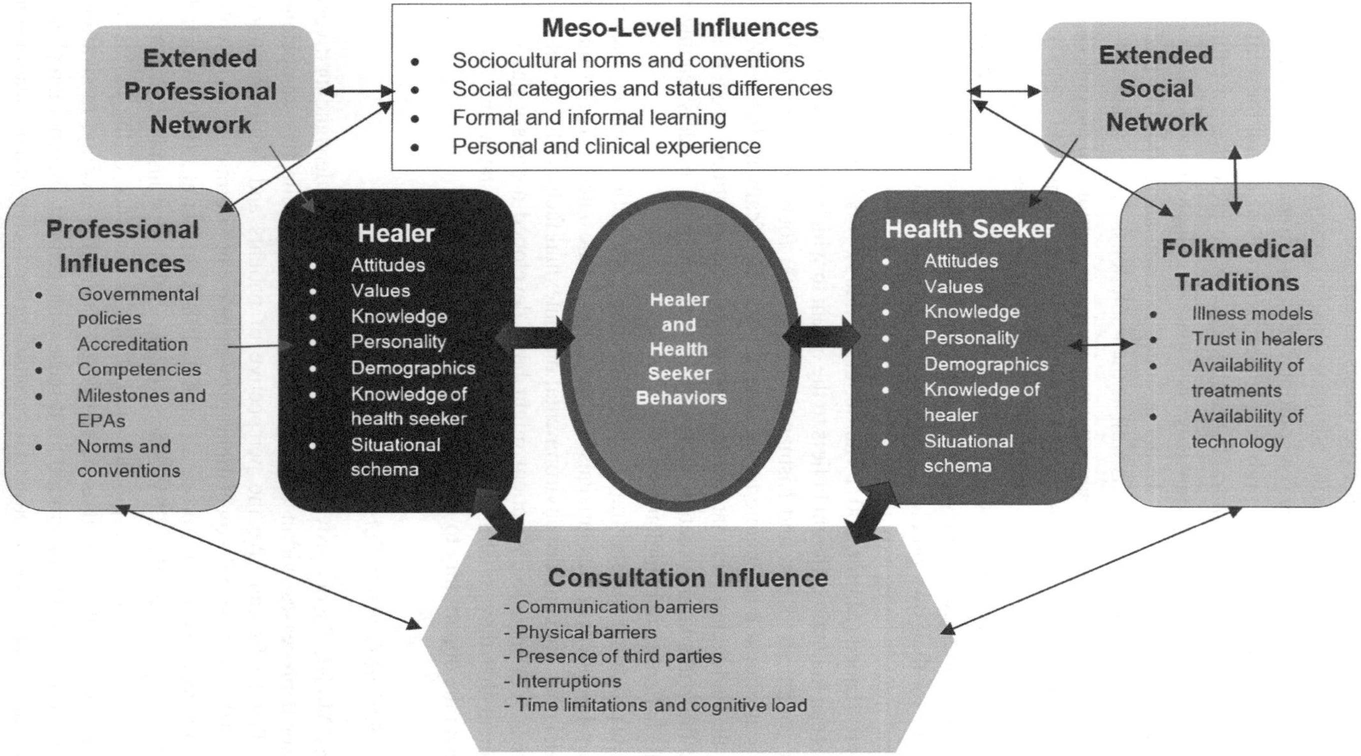

FIGURE 2.4 Model of patient-centered healthcare delivery.

Source: Adapted from Mead and Bower's (2000).

available (Stewart et al., 1995). Such an approach emphasizes the importance of the therapeutic alliance and understanding the mental models of illness maintained by the patients (Schoenherr & Le-Bouar, 2024).

Rather than assuming that clinical decision-making is restricted to HCPs (e.g., McConnell, 2024; Monteiro et al., 2024), the diagnosis and treatment of illness is best formatted as a process of SDM (cf. for discussion of definitional issues, see Charles et al., 1997; Makoul & Clayman, 2006; Moumjid et al., 2007). Depending on the characteristics of the situation (e.g., availability of multiple treatment alternatives), healthcare delivery can be viewed along a continuum: varying patient- or agent-driven healthcare delivery occurs when patients have maximum autonomy and clinicians can provide them with multiple therapeutic alternatives to physician-driven healthcare delivery, which occurs when clinicians must make the decisions (e.g., adjustment to surgical procedures when patient is sedated; Kon, 2010; Whitney et al., 2008).

The adoption of a situation-focused approach provides an effective means to understand how decision-making can be shared between healers and health seekers. For instance, Mead and Bower (2000) discuss five factors that impact patient-centered healthcare delivery. *Shapers* reflect broad influences, such as cultural norms and expectations that can influence individual differences of both the doctor and patient. For instance, gender norms perceiving women as more caring and friendly have encouraged greater patient-centeredness in female physicians (Bertakis & Azaris, 2012). The *professional context* comprises policies, organizational structures, performance incentives and can either support or impede the adoption of patient-centered practices. Finally, *consultation-level influences* can include language barriers or time constraints and can hinder patient-centeredness by limiting effective communication and SDM.

Here, we additionally suggest that SDM is also impacted by specific social networks for HCPs (*professional networks*) and health seekers (*social networks*), with health seekers additionally having access to alternative healthcare traditions such as folkmedical traditions (e.g., Schoenherr, 2021; Schoenherr & Beaudoin, 2027) and technologies (Schoenherr, 2022b, 2022c, 2027b). The inclusion of these components is critical in that HCPs might adopt practices based on their prevalence in *their* professional network, rather than on the basis of evidence. Similarly, health seekers might have multiple therapeutic alternatives that are more comprehensible, familiar, and accessible to them, leading to an increased trust and preference for these options over 'compliance' with the HCP recommendations. These observations also reinforce the need to view diagnostic and treatment recommendations as an instance of persuasive communication.

2.3.2.4 Community-Centered Care: Therapy Management Groups

Discourses concerning the evolution of the 'doctor-patient' relationships ignore alternative models present in other societies. Research in medical anthropology and ethnography have demonstrated that rather than placing a healer or health seeker at the center of an encounter, sets of individuals can define a therapeutic unit. Therapy management groups represent a social network that are directly or indirectly involved in the diagnosis, selection, and evaluation of treatment efficacy or the advocacy between those persons who are ill and the HCPs (Clark, 1993; Genest, 1985; Janzen, 1987, 1987; Nichter, 2003). Critically, the role of members of the therapy network goes beyond simple social support in that they are active participants in the process. In his original summary of health-seeking behavior in Zaire, Janzen (1978) describes it as (a situation):

> whenever an individual or set of individuals becomes ill or is confronted with overwhelming problems. Various maternal and paternal kinsmen, and occasionally their friends and associates, rally for the purpose of sifting information, lending moral support, making decisions, and arranging details of therapeutic consultation. The therapy managing group thus exercises a brokerage function between the sufferer and the specialist.
>
> *(p. 68)*

In Guatemala, Harvey (2011) characterizes healthcare as 'multivocal', with peers and members of the community each contributing their perspective on the illness experience of any given patient. A key component of this approach is the agency of the members of the therapy management group. Rather than being subordinate to HCPs, they were equal actors in the adoption of therapeutic practices. In therapy management groups, illness and disease are seen as a collective experience and responsibility. The impact and consequences of the illness affect the ill person as much as they affect the people surrounding them. For instance, when a person undergoes a cancer treatment or has a limb amputated, this can change the patient's social role, altering the dynamics within a group: friends, family, and community might alter their behavior to compensate and accommodate the patient. Rather than being altruistic, therapy management considers how resources should be distributed to address the illness based on the status of the ill person.

In these settings, medical decision-making occurs collectively, making consensus a vital part of a therapy management group. While in some societies full consensus must be reached for medical teams to act, in others (e.g., Kongo) partial consensus is sufficient to enact a treatment plan. However, in those cases, an individual's status and authority within the group often influences the strength of their opinion, potentially shifting the direction of the discussion, and subsequently treatment plans, away from its original course (see Section 2.3.2) (Janzen, 1987). As therapy management groups encompass both cognitive and social elements, understanding both the sickness and healing experience involves being aware of how social interactions influence and shape knowledge.

2.4 Recommendations for Education and Practice

This chapter has focused on developing a general social cognitive framework for the development of health professions education practices that can be used to train and assess collective competence. Our review demonstrates that the creation of educational activities and assessment instruments to address these demands is daunting. The social networks, interaction dynamics, relational models, and emergent group-level effects are substantial, and any competency-based program will be challenged to assess and address all of these features. In this final section, we review basic recommendations for education and practice in the health professions that can facilitate the development of collective competence.

2.4.1 The Need of Interprofessional Education

Healthcare is often managed by experts providing services across various specialities, and patients seldom receive comprehensive health services from an individual health practitioner, leading to a need to focus on *collective competence* (Lingard et al., 2012). Collaborative success is contingent on both the aggregated competence of individual members, and the cooperative processes within the team (Wagner et al., 2020).

IPE remains a central element in many health professional curricula, in which members from diverse vocations learn about, with, and from each other (Centre for the Advancement of Interprofessional Education, 2016). Research has emphasized that IPE initiatives should be implemented using practice-based learning opportunities such as during clinical placements or incorporated in workplace-based teaching and pedagogies (Guraya, 2015; Lapkin et al., 2013). Although IPE has the potential to enhance students' attitudes and insight toward interprofessional cooperation and clinical decision-making, further investigations are needed to examine the effectiveness of this program in advancing learning outcomes (Lapkin et al., 2013; Reeves et al., 2010).

Overall, the success and benefits of IPE programs have been reported in the literature (Buckley et al., 2014; Frakes et al., 2014; Kickett et al., 2014; Valachovic, 2019). However, IPE has not been emphasized in health curricula and professional settings (Awan et al., 2018; Green & Johnson, 2015). The administration of IPE approaches might be challenging for institutions without concurrent programs such as medicine, nursing, and pharmacy (Lapkin et al., 2013). Other logistical barriers to the implementation of IPE include course design, scheduling restrictions and coordination among different programs, large student capacity, and resource implications (Breitbach et al., 2013; Hammick et al., 2007; Sheldon et al., 2012). An approach to overcome certain challenges consists of e-learning IPE modules, which seem to offer a cost-effective alternative compared to in-person systems (Lapkin et al., 2013). Other technological means can further support IPE, encompassing telecommunications (e.g., interactive videoconferencing, conference calls) and educational technologies that allow learners to overcome barriers imposed by time and location (Curran et al., 2015; Ward et al., 2018).

Our review of the social cognitive literature on transactive memory also suggests several avenues for curriculum and pedagogical development. When viewed as a TMS, health networks can be assessed on the success of encoding, storage, retrieval, and use of information. As we have noted, the extent to which healers and health seekers share mental models of illness, social scripts and RM, motivation, and emotional cues and establish a therapeutic alliance will determine the collective competence of a therapeutic network. Given the varied assessment methodologies developed in psychological science, operationalizing and assessing these competencies is *relatively* straightforward. By assessing the kind of information that is transmitted, how healers and health seekers perceive the 'gist' of the message, the interpretations and inferences they draw, and how and who they relate information to will provide a principled basis for assessment. These measures can be integrated into existing educational intervention so as not to overburden learners and educators with additional assessment. For instance, simulation studies could assess the accuracy of information (e.g., content, diagnostic information, emotional cues) provided by specific actors in a simulation (e.g., standardized patient, nurses, etc.) to determine whether the learners' attention was focused.

2.4.2 Psychological Safety as a Prerequisite of Collective Competence

High-level recommendations for improvements to IPE must necessarily be supplemented with specific recommendations for the delivery of programs and educational activities that consider the demand of professional practice. As other chapters in this volume have noted (Schoenherr, 2027c; Schoenherr & Beaudoin, 2027), the healthcare professions can be defined as a *heterarchical* structure, wherein each specialist performs a defined role. This requires granting equal weight to information provided by everyone in a therapeutic network. For instance, in addition to the development of a therapeutic alliance with patients, HCPs must also promote *psychological safety* within healthcare teams (Schoenherr & Le-Bouar, 2024).

Psychological safety allows team members to feel comfortable questioning others, giving and receiving feedback, and speaking up about errors (Edmonson, 1999). Roles (e.g., doctor, nurse) should not affect how knowledge is shared. Supporting this, studies of psychological safety have demonstrated that safe environments are associated with more effective information sharing and transactive memory (Kessel et al., 2012; Bergmann & Schaeppi, 2016).

One means to promote psychological safety is by using standardized communication tools, like SBAR, that consider factors related to the Situation, Background, Assessment, and Recommendations. SBAR can promote a shared mental model for knowledge transmission by creating a structured method for conveying information (Foronda et al., 2016; Narayan, 2013). It reduces hierarchies by providing a common communication structure for all team members (De Meester et al., 2013; Donahue et al., 2011; Haig et al., 2006). This approach reduces the risk of overlooking relevant information, enhancing patient safety and continuity of care, especially during handovers.

HCPs must also consider how best to integrate technology into their practice to support collective competence (Schoenherr & Michael, 2026). For instance, integrating clinical decision support systems (CDSS) can enhance medical decision-making. CDSS are computerized programs that assist by matching clinical knowledge to patient characteristics (Shortliffe, 1987; Wyatt & Spiegelhalter, 1991; Sim et al., 2001). Like human agents, these systems perform a variety of functions such as alerting, reminding, critiquing, interpreting, predicting, diagnosing, assisting, and suggesting (Beeler et al., 2014). Research has shown that CDSS use reduces medication errors (Jia et al., 2016; Kaushal et al., 2003; Bates & Gawande, 2003), and a systematic review demonstrated that CDSS significantly improved clinical practice in 68% of trials (Alther & Reddy, 2015). However, more research is needed to understand CDSS's impact on patient outcomes and promote its widespread use. Indeed, concerns have been raised with the use of AI in practice, focusing on issues such as how these systems are trained, validated, and used (Schoenherr, 2027b; Schoenherr, 2022a).

Collective competence is not restricted to HCPs. As HCPs' goal is to *assist* patients, they must put health seekers at the center of their practice. Rather than considering HCPs that are faced with a problem of patient 'compliance', we must view HCP–patient interaction as a process of SDM. Promoting patient-centered communication strengthens the therapeutic relationship and encourages greater patient collaboration (Kleinman et al., 2006; Schoenherr & Le-Bouar, 2024).

SDM optimizes patient-centered care through three steps: choice talk, option talk, and decision talk, allowing patients and providers to make informed decisions together (Elwyn et al., 2013). SDM has been shown to improve patient satisfaction, quality of life, and clinical outcomes (Légaré & Thompson-Leduc, 2014). However, communication can be impeded by differing attributional models for illnesses, shaped by cultural backgrounds and experiences (Kleinman et al., 2006). Healthcare providers must take time and direct more effort to understanding patients' perspectives and tailor messages and treatment plans accordingly. When explanatory models differ, negotiation and respectful accommodation are essential. Aligning treatment recommendations with the patient's perspective can enhance adoption of HCP's recommendations (e.g., Pierre-Victor et al., 2017). Involving the patient's therapy management group, including psychologists and social workers, can further support effective communication and treatment.

2.5 Conclusions

Ensuring collective competence is necessary for optimal patient outcomes. There is no single path to achieving collective competence. Maintaining flexibility in health professions curricula and definitions of competence continues to have merit. However, we must ensure that educational activities and assessment instruments are developed in a systematic manner to provide concrete evidence of collective competence, rather than relying on holistic impressions of the efficacy of a therapeutic network. Restricting our considerations to general competencies of 'communication' and 'collaboration' fails to consider the specific demands of the sociocultural context of practitioners and patients. Similarly, specific bonds such as the therapeutic alliance do not consider the larger sociocultural environment of healthcare delivery. Shifting our focus to therapeutic *networks* as the unit of analysis and examining how information is created, retained, shared, and used allows us to establish specific milestones and further specify EPAs. The social cognitive framework provided here should enable program evaluators, educators, and practitioners to operationalize specific knowledge and skills required of their programs and practice.

Notes

1 Here, groups are considered in terms of specific relationships, often kin-based.
2 Humans are no longer the only members of a healthcare team. Whether viewed as tools that are controlled by humans, or whether they are granted some level of autonomy, technology can be used to supplement the capabilities or capacities, i.e., extended cognition (Clark, 2008; Hazlehurst et al., 2008). The extent to which human or artificial agents can work together to diagnose, treat, monitor, and communicate with health seekers is a product of their collective competence.
3 In extreme negative cases, this represents a sunk cost.
4 This term is meant to represent the beliefs and lay theories of the practitioners within the model.

References

Aarseth, E., Bean, A. M., Boonen, H., Colder Carras, M., Coulson, M., Das, D., ... & Van Rooij, A. J. (2017). Scholars' open debate paper on the World Health Organization ICD-11 Gaming Disorder proposal. *Journal of Behavioral Addictions*, *6*(3), 267–270.

Adekannbi, J., Olatokun, W. M., & Ajiferuke, I. (2014). Predictors of traditional medical knowledge transmission and acquisition in Southwest Nigeria. *Information Development*, *32*(3), 566–578.

Aktaş, H., & Şimşek, E. (2014). Organizational silence and its interaction with the perceived performance, organizational culture and demographic variables. *Akdeniz University Faculty of Economics and Administrative Sciences Journal*, *14*(28), 24–52. (Original work published in Turkish).

Alden, D. L., Friend, J., Lee, P. Y., Lee, Y. K., Trevena, L., Ng, C. J., Kiatpongsan, S., Lim Abdullah, K., Tanaka, M., & Limpongsanurak, S. (2018). Who decides: Me or we? Family involvement in medical decision making in Eastern and Western countries. *Medical Decision Making: An International Journal of the Society for Medical Decision Making*, *38*(1), 14–25.

Aldersey, H. M., & Whitley, R. (2015). Family influence in recovery from severe mental illness. *Community Mental Health Journal*, *51*, 467–476.

Alnazly, E., Khraisat, O. M., Al-Bashaireh, A. M., & Bryant, C. L. (2021). Anxiety, depression, stress, fear and social support during COVID-19 pandemic among Jordanian healthcare workers. *Plos one, 16*(3), e0247679.

Alparslan, A. M., & Kayalar, M. (2012). Organizational silence: Behaviors of silence and their organizational and individual effects. *Mehmet Akif Ersoy University Journal of Social Sciences Institute*, *4*(6), 136–147. (Original work published in Turkish)

Altinöz, M., Çöp, S., & Siğindi, T. (2011). The relationship between perceived organizational commitment and organizational cynicism: A research on four- and five-star residential managements in Ankara. *Journal of Social and Economic*, *21*, 285–315. (Original work published in Turkish)

Alther, M., & Reddy, C. K. (2015). Clinical decision support systems. In C. K. Reddy & C. C. Aggarwal (Eds.), *Healthcare Data Analytics* (1st ed., pp. 626–653). Chapman and Hall.

Anderson, C. S., Linto, J., & Stewart-Wynne, E. G. (1995). A population-based assessment of the impact and burden of caregiving for long-term stroke survivors. *Stroke*, *26*(5), 843–849.

Anderson, E. S., & Lennox, A. (2009). The Leicester model of interprofessional education: Developing, delivering and learning from student voices for 10 years. *Journal of Interprofessional Care*, *23*(6), 557–573.

Anderson, E. S., Cox, D., & Thorpe, L. N. (2009). Preparation of educators involved in interprofessional education. *Journal of Interprofessional Care, 23*(1), 81–94.

Andersson, L. M., & Pearson, C. M. (1999). Tit for tat? The spiraling effect of incivility in the workplace. *Academy of Management Review, 24*(3), 452–471. https://doi.org/10.5465/AMR.1999.2202131

Asch, S. E. (1951). Effects of group pressure upon the modification and distortion of judgments. In H. Guetzkow (Ed.), *Groups, Leadership and Men; Research in Human Relations* (pp. 177–190). Carnegie Press.

Astington, J. W., & Jenkins, J. M. (1995). Theory of mind development and social understanding. *Cognition & Emotion, 9*(2-3), 151–165.

Aston, S. J., Rheault, W., Arenson, C., Tappert, S. K., Stoecker, J., Orzoff, J., Galitski, H., & Mackintosh, S. (2012). Interprofessional education: A review and analysis of programs from three academic health centers. *Academic Medicine*, *87*(7), 949–955.

Ateah, C. A., Snow, W., Wener, P., MacDonald, L., Metge, C., Davis, P., Fricke, M., Ludwig, S., & Anderson, J. (2011). Stereotyping as a barrier to collaboration: Does interprofessional education make a difference? *Nurse Education Today, 31*(2), 208–213.

Awan, A. A., Awan, Z. A., Alshawwa, L., Tekian, A., Park, Y. S., & Altyar, A. (2018). Integrating an interprofessional education initiative: Evidence from King Abdulaziz University. *Medical Teacher*, *40*(sup1), S15–S21.

Bae, S. H., Nikolaev, A., Seo, J. Y., & Castner, J. (2015). Health care provider social network analysis: A systematic review. *Nursing Outlook*, *63*(5), 566–584.

Baron-Cohen, S., & Wheelwright, S. (2004). The empathy quotient: An investigation of adults with Asperger syndrome or high functioning autism, and normal sex differences. *Journal of Autism and Developmental Disorders*, *34*(2), 163–175.

Barr, H., Koppel, I., Reeves, S., Hammick, M., & Freeth, D. (2005). *Effective Interprofessional Education: Argument, Assumption And Evidence*. Blackwell Publishing.

Barraclough, J. (1994). *Cancer and Emotion Chichester.* Wiley.

Barrows, H. S. (1996). Problem-based learning in medicine and beyond: A brief overview. *New Directions for Teaching and Learning*, *1996*(68), 3–12.

Barrows, H. S., & Tamblyn, R. M. (1980). *Problem-Based Learning: An Approach to Medical Education*. Springer Publishing Company.

Barth, J., Schneider, S., & Von Känel, R. (2010). Lack of social support in the etiology and the prognosis of coronary heart disease: A systematic review and meta-analysis. *Psychosomatic Medicine, 72*(3), 229–238.

Baruah, J., & Paulus, P. B. (2008). Effects of training on idea generation in groups. *Small Group Research, 39*(5), 523–541.

Bates, D. W., & Gawande, A. A. (2003). Improving safety with information technology. *New England Journal of Medicine, 348*(25), 2526–2534.

Baxter, S. K., & Brumfitt, S. M. (2008). Professional differences in interprofessional working. *Journal of Interprofessional Care, 22*(3), 239–251.

Bayazidi, S., Zarezadeh, Y., Zamanzadeh, V., & Parvan, K. (2012). Medication error reporting rate and its barriers and facilitators among nurses. *Journal of Caring Sciences, 1*(4), 231.

Beeler, P., Bates, D., & Hug, B. (2014). Clinical decision support systems. *Swiss Medical Weekly, 144*(5152), 14073

Beran, T. N., Kaba, A., Caird, J., & McLaughlin, K. (2014). The good and bad of group conformity: A call for a new programme of research in medical education. *Medical Education, 48*(9), 851–859.

Bergmann, B., & Schaeppi, J. (2016) A data-driven approach to group creativity. *Harvard Business Review, 12*, 43–62.

Bertakis, K. D., & Azari, R. (2012). Patient-centered care: The influence of patient and resident physician gender and gender concordance in primary care. *Journal of Women's Health, 21*(3), 326–333.

Blair, M. R., Watson, M. R., & Meier, K. M. (2009). Errors, efficiency, and the interplay between attention and category learning. *Cognition, 112*(2), 330–336.

Blatt, R., Christianson, M. K., Sutcliffe, K. M., & Rosenthal, M. M. (2006). A sensemaking lens on reliability. *Journal of Organizational Behavior, 27*(7), 897–917.

Boreham, N. (2004). A theory of collective competence: Challenging the neo-liberal individualization of performance at work. *British Journal of Educational Studies, 52*(1), 5–17.

Boreham, N. (2011). Competence as collective process. In R. Catts, I. Falk, & R. Wallace (Eds.), *Vocational Learning. Technical and Vocational Education and Training: Issues, Concerns and Prospects* (pp. 77–91). Springer.

Bosk, C. L. (2003). *Forgive and Remember: Managing Medical Failure*. University of Chicago Press.

Boyd, R., & Richerson, P. J. (1985). *Culture and the Evolutionary Process*. University of Chicago Press.

Boyle, J. G., Walters, M. R., Jamieson, S., & Durning, S. J. (2023a). Reframing context specificity in team diagnosis using the theory of distributed cognition. *Diagnosis, 10*(3), 235–241.

Boyle, J. G., Walters, M. R., Jamieson, S., & Durning, S. J. (2023b). Distributed cognition: Theoretical insights and practical applications to health professions education: AMEE Guide No. 159. *Medical Teacher, 45*(12), 1323–1333.

Breitbach, A. P., Sargeant, D. M., Gettemeier, P. R., Ruebling, I., Carlson, J., Eliot, K., Kienstra, K., & Gockel-Blessing, E. A. (2013). From buy-in to integration: Melding an interprofessional initiative into academic programs in the health professions. *Journal of Allied Health, 42*(3), e67–73.

Brewer, M. B., & Chen, Y.-R. (2007). Where (who) are collectives in collectivism? Toward conceptual clarification of individualism and collectivism. *Psychological Review, 114*(1), 133–151.

Brickman, P., Rabinowitz, V. C., Karuza, J. J., Coates, D., Cohn, E., & Kidder, L. (1982). Models of helping and coping. *American Psychologist, 37*(4), 368–384.

Bristow, D., Rees, G., & Frith, C. D. (2007). Social interaction modifies neural response to gaze shifts. *Social Cognitive and Affective Neuroscience, 2*(1), 52–61.

Brown, P. (1995). Naming and framing: The social construction of diagnosis and illness. *Journal of Health and Social Behavior*, 34–52.

Buckley, E., Vu, T., & Remedios, L. (2014). The REACH project: Implementing interprofessional practice at Australia's first student-led clinic. *Education for Health (Abingdon, England), 27*(1), 93–98.

Bullowa, M. (1979). *Before Speech: The Beginning of Interpersonal Communication.* CUP Archive.

Burke, M. A., & Young, H. P. (2011). Social norms. In *Handbook of Social Economics* (Vol. 1, pp. 311–338). North-Holland.

Bzdok, D., Langner, R., Schilbach, L., Engemann, D. A., Laird, A. R., Fox, P. T., & Eickhoff, S. B. (2013). Segregation of the human medial prefrontal cortex in social cognition. *Frontiers in Human Neuroscience, 7*(232), 1–17.

Carpenter, M., Nagell, K., Tomasello, M., Butterworth, G., & Moore, C. (1998). Social Cognition, joint attention, and communicative competence from 9 to 15 months of age. *Monographs of the Society for Research in Child Development, 63*(4), 1–143.

Carter, R. (1999). High risk of violence against nurses. *Nursing Management UK, 6*(8), 5.

Centre for the Advancement of Interprofessional Education. (2016). *Interprofessional education guidelines 2016*. CAIPE. *Interprofessional education guidelines 2016*. CAIPE. Retrieved December, 2025 from: www.caipe.org/resources/publications/caipe-publications/barr-h-gray-r-helme-m-low-h-reeves-s-2016-interprofessional-education-guidelines

Cerdeña, J. P., Rivera, L. M., & Spak, J. M. (2021). Intergenerational trauma in Latinxs: A scoping review. *Social Science & Medicine, 270*, 113662.

Charles, C., Gafni, A., & Whelan, T. (1997). Shared decision-making in the medical encounter: What does it mean? (or it takes at least two to tango). *Social Science & Medicine, 44*(5), 681–692.

Chipidza, F. E., Wallwork, R. S., & Stern, T. A. (2015). Impact of the doctor-patient relationship. *The Primary Care Companion for CNS Disorders*.

Choi, I., Nisbett, R. E., & Norenzayan, A. (1999). Causal attribution across cultures: Variation and universality. *Psychological Bulletin, 125*(1), 47–63.

Choi, J. J., Mhaimeed, N., Al-Mohanadi, D., & Mahmoud, M. A. (2024). Medical residents' perceptions of group biases in medical decision making: A qualitative study. *BMC Medical Education, 24*(1), 661.

Cieslak, R., Shoji, K., Douglas, A., Melville, E., Luszczynska, A., & Benight, C. C. (2014). A meta-analysis of the relationship between job burnout and secondary traumatic stress among workers with indirect exposure to trauma. *Psychological Services, 11*(1), 75–86.

Clark, A. (2008). *Supersizing the Mind: Embodiment, Action, and Cognitive Extension.* Oxford University Press.

Clark, L. (1993). Gender and generation in poor women's household health production experiences. *Medical Anthropology Quarterly, 7*(4), 386–402.

Cohen, K., & Collens, P. (2013). The impact of trauma work on trauma workers: A metasynthesis on vicarious trauma and vicarious posttraumatic growth. *Psychological Trauma: Theory, Research, Practice, and Policy, 5*(6), 570.

Conrad, P., & Barker, K. K. (2010). The social construction of illness: Key insights and policy implications. *Journal of Health and Social Behavior, 51*(1_suppl), S67–S79.

Corrigan, P. W., Watson, A. C., & Miller, F. E. (2006). Blame, shame, and contamination: The impact of mental illness and drug dependence stigma on family members. *Journal of Family Psychology, 20*(2), 239.

Cox, C. L., Uddin, L. Q., Di Martino, A., Castellanos, F. X., Milham, M. P., & Kelly, C. (2012). The balance between feeling and knowing: Affective and cognitive empathy are reflected in the brain's intrinsic functional dynamics. *Social Cognitive and Affective Neuroscience, 7*(6), 727–737.

Curran, V., Reid, A., Reis, P., Doucet, S., Price, S., Alcock, L., & Fitzgerald, S. (2015). The use of information and communications technologies in the delivery of interprofessional education: A review of evaluation outcome levels. *Journal of Interprofessional Care, 29*(6), 541–550.

Danyluk, P. J., Luhanga, F., Gwekwerere, Y. N., MacEwan, L., & Larocque, S. (2015). Failure to fail in a final pre-service teaching practicum. *Canadian Journal for the Scholarship of Teaching and Learning, 6*(3), 5.

das Chagas Medeiros, M. M., Ferraz, M. B., & Quaresma, M. R. (2000). The effect of rheumatoid arthritis on the quality of life of primary caregivers. *The Journal of Rheumatology, 27*(1), 76–83.

De Meester, K., Verspuy, M., Monsieurs, K. G., & Van Bogaert, P. (2013). SBAR improves nurse-physician communication and reduces unexpected death: A pre and post intervention study. *Resuscitation, 84*(9), 1192–1196.

Dennen, V., & Burner, K. (2008). Cognitive apprenticeship model in educational practice. In M. Spector, M. Driscoll, D. Merrill, & J. Merrienboer (Eds.), *Handbook of Research on Educational Communications and Technology* (pp. 425–439). Routledge.

Dennis, M., O'Rourke, S., Lewis, S., Sharpe, M., & Warlow, C. (1998). A quantitative study of the emotional outcome of people caring for stroke survivors. *Stroke, 29*(9), 1867–1872.

DiMatteo, M. R. (2004). Social support and patient adherence to medical treatment: A meta-analysis. *Health Psychology, 23*(2), 207.

Dinh, J. V., Traylor, A. M., Kilcullen, M. P., Perez, J. A., Schweissing, E. J., Venkatesh, A., & Salas, E. (2020). Cross-disciplinary care: A systematic review on teamwork processes in health care. *Small Group Research, 51*(1), 125–166.

DiPierro, K., Lee, H., Pain, K. J., Durning, S. J., & Choi, J. J. (2022). Groupthink among health professional teams in patient care: A scoping review. *Medical Teacher, 44*(3), 309–318.

Donahue, M., Miller, M., Smith, L., Dykes, P., & Fitzpatrick, J. (2011). A leadership initiative to improve communication and enhance safety. *American Journal of Medical Quality, 26*(3), 206–211. https://doi.org/10.1177/1062860610387410

Donnelly, E. A., Bradford, P., Davis, M., Hedges, C., & Klingel, M. (2016). Predictors of posttraumatic stress and preferred sources of social support among Canadian paramedics. *Canadian Journal of Emergency Medicine, 18*(3), 205–212.

Dreachslin, J. L., Hunt, P. L., & Sprainer, E. (2000). Workforce diversity: Implications for the effectiveness of health care delivery teams. *Social Science & Medicine, 50*(10), 1403–1414.

Duffy, E. (1995). Horizontal violence: A conundrum for nursing. *Collegian, 2*(2), 5–17.

Dunworth, M. (2007). Joint assessment in inter-professional education: A consideration of some of the difficulties. *Social Work Education, 26*(4), 414–422.

Dvash, J., & Shamay-Tsoory, S. G. (2014). Theory of mind and empathy as multidimensional constructs. *Topics in Language Disorders, 34*(4), 282–295.

Edmondson, A. (1999). Psychological safety and learning behavior in work teams. *Administrative Science Quarterly, 44*(2), 350–383. https://doi.org/10.2307/2666999

Eggins, S., & Slade, D. (2015). Communication in clinical handover: Improving the safety and quality of the patient experience. *Journal of Public Health Research, 4*(3), 197–199.

Elmore, J. G., Barnhill, R. L., Elder, D. E., Longton, G. M., Pepe, M. S., Reisch, L. M., ... & Piepkorn, M. W. (2017). Pathologists' diagnosis of invasive melanoma and melanocytic proliferations: Observer accuracy and reproducibility study. *BMJ, 357*, j2813.

Elsous, A., Radwan, M., & Mohsen, S. (2017). Nurses and physicians attitudes toward nurse-physician collaboration: A survey from Gaza Strip, Palestine. *Nursing Research and Practice, 2017*, 1–7.

Elwyn, G., Durand, M. A., Song, J., Aarts, J., Barr, P. J., Berger, Z., ... & Van der Weijden, T. (2017). A three-talk model for shared decision making: Multistage consultation process. *BMJ, 359*, j4891.

Elwyn, G., Tsulukidze, M., Edwards, A., Légaré, F., & Newcombe, R. (2013). Using a 'talk' model of shared decision making to propose an observation-based measure: Observer option5 item. *Patient Education and Counseling, 93*(2), 265–271.

Emanuel, E. J., & Emanuel, L. L. (1992). Four models of the physician-patient relationship. *Jama, 267*(16), 2221–2226.

Engestrom, Y., Engestrom, R., & Vahaaho, T. (1999). When the center does not hold: The importance of knotworking. In S. Chaklin, M. Hedegaard, & U. Jensen (Eds.), *Activity Theory and Social Practice* (pp. 326–374). Aarhus University Press.

Epstein, R. M., Franks, P., Fiscella, K., Shields, C. G., Meldrum, S. C., Kravitz, R. L., & Duberstein, P. R. (2005). Measuring patient-centered communication in patient–physician consultations: Theoretical and practical issues. *Social Science & Medicine, 61*(7), 1516–1528.

Ericsson, K. A. (2007). An expert-performance perspective of research on medical expertise: The study of clinical performance. *Medical Education, 41*(12), 1124–1130.

Erigüç, G., Özer, Ö., Turaç, İ. S., & Songur, C. (2014). The causes and effects of the organizational silence: On which issues the nurses remain silent? *International Journal of Management Economics and Business, 10*(22), 131–153.

Escandell-Vidal, V. (2016). Expectations in interaction. *Perspectives in Pragmatics, Philosophy & Psychology, 9*, 493–503.

Essex, R., Kennedy, J., Miller, D., & Jameson, J. (2023). A scoping review exploring the impact and negotiation of hierarchy in healthcare organisations. *Nursing Inquiry, 30*(4), e12571.

Evans, S., Sonderlund, A., & Tooley, G. (2020). Effectiveness of online interprofessional education in improving students' attitudes and knowledge associated with interprofessional practice. *Focus on Health Professional Education: A Multi-Professional Journal, 14*(2), 12–20.

Farrell, G. A. (1997). Aggression in clinical settings: Nurses' views. *Journal of Advanced Nursing, 25*, 501–508.

Fehr, R., Gelfand, M. J., & Nag, M. (2010). The road to forgiveness: A meta-analytic synthesis of its situational and dispositional correlates. *Psychological Bulletin, 136*(5), 894–914.

Feng, Y. (1994). From the imperial examination to the national college entrance examination: The dynamics of political centralism in China's educational enterprise. *Journal of Contemporary China, 4*(8), 28–56.

Ferretti, E., Schoenherr, J. R., Mattiola, A., & Daboval, T. (2023). Vulnerabilities in clinician–parent exchanges and the cascade of communication traps: A review. *Archives of Disease in Childhood, 108*(2), 86–90.

Fink-Anthe, C. (1992). Kulturell beeinflusste therapie gewohnheiten: Bedeutung für den europäischen markt. *Deutsche Apotheker Zeitung 29*, 1534–1539.

Fiske, A. P. (1991). *Structures of Social Life: The Four Elementary Forms of Human Relations*. Free Press.

Fiske, A. P. (1995). Social schemata for remembering people: Relationships and person attributes in free recall of acquaintances. *Journal of Quantitative Anthropology, 5*, 305–324.

Foronda, C., MacWilliams, B., & McArthur, E. (2016). Interprofessional communication in healthcare: An integrative review. *Nurse Education in Practice, 19*, 36–40.

Forsberg-Wärleby, G., Möller, A., & Blomstrand, C. (2001). Spouses of first-ever stroke patients: Psychological well-being in the first phase after stroke. *Stroke, 32*(7), 1646–1651.

Frakes, K. A., Brownie, S., Davies, L., Thomas, J. B., Miller, M. E., & Tyack, Z. (2014). Capricornia Allied Health Partnership (CAHP): A case study of an innovative model of care addressing chronic disease through a regional student-assisted clinic. *Australian Health Review: A Publication of the Australian Hospital Association, 38*(5), 483–486.

Franck, L. S., & O'Brien, K. (2019). The evolution of family-centered care: From supporting parent-delivered interventions to a model of family integrated care. *Birth Defects Research, 111*(15), 1044–1059.

Frankel, K., & Wamboldt, M. Z. (1998). Chronic childhood illness and maternal mental health--Why should we care?. *The Journal of Asthma: Official Journal of the Association for the Care of Asthma, 35*(8), 621–630.

Freeth, D., Reeves, S., Koppel, I., Hammick, M., & Barr, H. (2005). *Evaluating Interprofessional Education: A Self-Help Guide*. Higher Education Academy Learning and Teaching Support Network for Health Sciences and Practice.

Frith, C., & Frith, U. (2005). Theory of mind. *Current Biology, 15*(17), R644–R645.

Galinsky, A. D., Magee, J. C., Inesi, M. E., & Gruenfeld, D. H. (2006). Power and perspectives not taken. *Psychological Science, 17*(12), 1068–1074.

Galinsky, A. D., Magee, J. C., Rus, D., Rothman, N. B., & Todd, A. R. (2014). Acceleration with steering: The synergistic benefits of combining power and perspective-taking. *Social Psychological and Personality Science, 5*(6), 627–635.

Gan, H. (2008). Chinese education tradition – The imperial examination system in feudal China. *Journal of Management and Social Sciences, 4*(2), 115–133.

Gelfand, M. J., Harrington, J., & Fernandez, J. (2017). Cultural tightness-looseness: Ecological affordances and implications for personality. In A. T. Church (Ed.), *The Praeger Handbook of Personality Across Cultures* (pp. 206–236). Praeger.

Genest, S. (1985). Review of The Quest for Therapy in Lower Zaire by J. M. Janzen. *Canadian Review of Sociology and Anthropology, 21*(3), 348–351.

George, L. K., & Gwyther, L. P. (1986). Caregiver well-being: A multidimensional examination of family caregivers of demented adults. *The Gerontologist, 26*(3), 253–259.

Germino, B. B., Fife, B. L., & Funk, S. G. (1995). Cancer and the partner relationship: What is its meaning? *Seminars in Oncology Nursing, 11*(1), 43–50.

Geurts, H. M., Verté, S., Oosterlaan, J., Roeyers, H., & Sergeant, J. A. (2005). ADHD subtypes: Do they differ in their executive functioning profile? *Archives of Clinical Neuropsychology, 20*(4), 457–477.

Gilbert, M. (2007). *Mutual Recognition, Common Knowledge, and Joint Attention. SSRN*, 1–21.

Gilin, D., Maddux, W. W., Carpenter, J., & Galinsky, A. D. (2013). When to use your head and when to use your heart: The differential value of perspective-taking versus empathy in competitive interactions. *Personality and Social Psychology Bulletin, 39*(1), 3–16.

González-Salvador, M. T., Arango, C., Lyketsos, C. G., & Barba, A. C. (1999). The stress and psychological morbidity of the Alzheimer patient caregiver. *International Journal of Geriatric Psychiatry, 14*(9), 701–710.

Gopnik, A., & Wellman, H. M. (1992). Why the child's theory of mind really is a theory. *Mind & Language, 7*, 145–171.

Grant, J. S., Bartolucci, A. A., Elliot, T. R., & Giger, J. N. (2000). Sociodemographic, physical, and psychosocial characteristics of depressed and non-depressed family caregivers of stroke survivors. *Brain Injury, 14*(12), 1089–1100.

Green, B. N., & Johnson, C. D. (2015). Interprofessional collaboration in research, education, and clinical practice: Working together for a better future. *The Journal of Chiropractic Education, 29*(1), 1–10.

Griffiths, F., Cave, J., Boardman, F., Ren, J., Pawlikowska, T., Ball, R., ... & Cohen, A. (2012). Social networks–the future for health care delivery. *Social Science & Medicine, 75*(12), 2233–2241.

Grol, R., De Maeseneer, J., Whitfield, M., & Mokkink, H. (1990). Disease-centred versus patient-centred attitudes: Comparison of general practitioners in Belgium, Britain and the Netherlands. *Family Practice, 7*(2), 100–103.

Guraya, S. Y. (2015). Workplace-based assessment; applications and educational impact. *The Malaysian Journal of Medical Sciences, 22*(6), 5–10.

Guraya, S. Y., & Barr, H. (2018). The effectiveness of interprofessional education in healthcare: A systematic review and meta-analysis. *The Kaohsiung Journal of Medical Sciences, 34*(3), 160–165.

Haig, K., Sutton, S., & Whittington, J. (2006). SBAR: A shared mental model for improving communication between clinicians. *Joint Commission Journal on Quality & Patient Safety, 32*(3), 167–175.

Hammick, M., Freeth, D., Koppel, I., Reeves, S., & Barr, H. (2007). A best evidence systematic review of interprofessional education: BEME Guide no. 9. *Medical Teacher, 29*(8), 735–751.

Han, B., & Haley, W. E. (1999). Family caregiving for patients with stroke. *Review and analysis. Stroke, 30*(7), 1478–1485.

Hanson, C. L., De Guire, M. J., Schinkel, A. M., & Kolterman, O. G. (1995). Empirical validation for a family-centered model of care. *Diabetes Care, 18*(10), 1347–1356.

Harandi, T. F., Taghinasab, M. M., & Nayeri, T. D. (2017). The correlation of social support with mental health: A meta-analysis. *Electronic Physician, 9*(9), 5212.

Hartnell, N., MacKinnon, N., Sketris, I., & Fleming, M. (2012). Identifying, understanding and overcoming barriers to medication error reporting in hospitals: A focus group study. *BMJ Quality & Safety, 21*(5), 361–368.

Harvey, T. S. (2011). Maya mobile medicine in Guatemala: The "other" public health. *Medical Anthropology Quarterly, 25*(1), 47–69.

Hawkins, R. X. D., Goodman, N. D., & Goldstone, R. L. (2019). The emergence of social norms and conventions. *Trends in Cognitive Sciences, 23*(2), 158–169.

Hazlehurst, B., Gorman, P. N., & McMullen, C. K. (2008). Distributed cognition: An alternative model of cognition for medical informatics. *International Journal of Medical Informatics, 77*(4), 226–234.

Henriksen, K., & Dayton, E. (2006). Organizational silence and hidden threats to patient safety. *Health Services Research, 41*(4p2), 1539–1554.

Henry, J. D., Phillips, L. H., Ruffman, T., & Bailey, P. E. (2013). A meta-analytic review of age differences in theory of mind. *Psychology and Aging, 28*(3), 826.

Hepp, S. L., Suter, E., Jackson, K., Deutschlander, S., Makwarimba, E., Jennings, J., & Birmingham, L. (2015). Using an interprofessional competency framework to examine collaborative practice. *Journal of Interprofessional Care, 29*(2), 131–137.

Hmelo-Silver, C.E. (2004). Problem-based learning: What and how do students learn?. *Educational Psychology Review 16*, 235–266.

Hofstede, G. (1980). *Culture's Consequences: International Differences in Work-Related Values*. Sage.

Hofstede, G. (2011). Dimensionalizing Cultures: The Hofstede model in context. *Online Readings in Psychology and Culture, 2*(1).

Hollan, J., Hutchins, E., & Kirsh, D. (2000). Distributed cognition: Toward a new foundation for human-computer interaction research. *ACM Transactions on Computer-Human Interaction (TOCHI), 7*(2), 174–196.

Hollingshead, A. B. (1998). Retrieval processes in transactive memory systems. *Journal of Personality and Social Psychology, 74*(3), 659.

Holmes, A. M., & Deb, P. (2003). The effect of chronic illness on the psychological health of family members. *Journal of Mental Health Policy and Economics, 6*(1), 13–22.

Hopwood, T. L., & Schutte, N. S. (2017). Psychological outcomes in reaction to media exposure to disasters and large-scale violence: A meta-analysis. *Psychology of Violence, 7*(2), 316.

Houston, J. B., Spialek, M. L., & First, J. (2018). Disaster media effects: A systematic review and synthesis based on the differential susceptibility to media effects model. *Journal of Communication, 68*(4), 734–757.

Hsu, E. (1999). *The Transmission of Chinese Medicine*. Cambridge University Press.

Hui, C. H. (1988). Measurement of individualism-collectivism. *Journal of Research in Personality, 22*(1), 17–36.

Hultin, L., & Mähring, M. (2017). How practice makes sense in healthcare operations: Studying sensemaking as performative, material-discursive practice. *Human Relations, 70*(5), 566–593.

Hutchins, E. (1991). The social organization of distributed cognition. In L. B. Resnick, J. M. Levine, & S. D. Teasley (Eds.), *Perspectives on Socially Shared Cognition* (pp. 283–307). American Psychological Association.

Iqbal, M., Velan, G. M., O'Sullivan, A. J., & Balasooriya, C. (2016). Differential impact of student behaviours on group interaction and collaborative learning: Medical students' and tutors' perspectives. *BMC Medical Education, 16*, 1–11.

Janis, I. L. (1982). *Groupthink: Psychological Studies of Policy Decisions and Fiascoes*. Houghton Mifflin.

Janis, I. L. (1983) *Groupthink*. Houghton Mifflin.

Janzen, J. M. (1987). Therapy management: Concept, reality, process. *Medical Anthropology Quarterly, 1*(1), 68–84.

Jeffcott, S. A., Evans, S. M., Cameron, P. A., Chin, G. S., & Ibrahim, J. E. (2009). Improving measurement in clinical handover. *Quality and Safety in Health Care*, *18*(4), 272–276.

Jia, P., Zhang, L., Chen, J., Zhao, P., & Zhang, M. (2016). The effects of clinical decision support systems on medication safety: An overview. *PloS one*, *11*(12), e0167683.

Johnson, A., Nguyen, H., Groth, M., & White, L. (2018). Reaping the rewards of functional diversity in healthcare teams: Why team processes improve performance. *Group & Organization Management*, *43*(3), 440–474.

Johnson, B. H. (2000). Family-centered care: Four decades of progress. *Families, Systems, & Health*, *18*(2), 137.

Jordan, M. E., Lanham, H. J., Crabtree, B. F., Nutting, P. A., Miller, W. L., Stange, K. C., & McDaniel, R. R. (2009). The role of conversation in health care interventions: Enabling sensemaking and learning. *Implementation Science*, *4*(1), 1–13.

Jorm, C. M., White, S., & Kaneen, T. (2009). Clinical handover: Critical communications. *Medical Journal of Australia*, *190*(S11).

Kaba, A., & Beran, T. N. (2016). Impact of peer pressure on accuracy of reporting vital signs: An interprofessional comparison between nursing and medical students. *Journal of Interprofessional Care*, *30*(1), 116–122.

Kaba, R., & Sooriakumaran, P. (2007). The evolution of the doctor-patient relationship. *International Journal of Surgery*, *5*(1), 57–65.

Karasaki, M., Fraser, S., Moore, D., & Dietze, P. (2013). The place of volition in addiction: Differing approaches and their implications for policy and service provision. *Drug and Alcohol Review*, *32*(2), 195–204.

Katona, G. (1946). Psychological analysis of business decisions and expectations. *The American Economic Review*, *36*(1), 44–62.

Kaushal, R., Shojania, K. G., & Bates, D. W. (2003). Effects of computerized physician order entry and clinical decision support systems on medication safety. *Archives of Internal Medicine*, *163*(12), 1409.

Kazak, A. E., Stuber, M. L., Barakat, L. P., Meeske, K., Guthrie, D., & Meadows, A. T. (1998). Predicting posttraumatic stress symptoms in mothers and fathers of survivors of childhood cancers. *Journal of the American Academy of Child and Adolescent Psychiatry*, *37*(8), 823–831.

Kelley, H. H. (1973). The processes of causal attribution. *American Psychologist*, *28*(2), 107–128.

Kelley, H. H., & Michela, J. L. (1980). Attribution theory and research. *Annual Review of Psychology*, *31*(1), 457–501.

Kemp, S., & Brewer, M. (2023). Early stages of learning in interprofessional education: Stepping towards collective competence for healthcare teams. *BMC Medical Education*, *23*(1), 694.

Kessel, M., J. Kratzer, & C. Schultz. (2012). Psychological safety, knowledge sharing, and creative performance in healthcare teams. *Creativity and Innovation Management 21*(2), 147–157.

Kickett, M., Hoffman, J., & Flavell, H. (2014). A model for large-scale, interprofessional, compulsory cross-cultural education with an indigenous focus. *Journal of Allied Health*, *43*(1), 38–44.

Kiecolt-Glaser, J. K., Dura, J. R., Speicher, C. E., Trask, O. J., & Glaser, R. (1991). Spousal caregivers of dementia victims: Longitudinal changes in immunity and health. *Psychosomatic Medicine*, *53*(4), 345–362.

Kitch, B. T., Cooper, J. B., Zapol, W. M., Hutter, M. M., Marder, J., Karson, A., & Campbell, E. G. (2008). Handoffs causing patient harm: A survey of medical and surgical house staff. *The Joint Commission Journal on Quality and Patient Safety*, *34*(10), 563–570d.

Kleinman, A., Eisenberg, L., & Good, B. (2006). Culture, illness, and care: Clinical lessons from anthropologic and cross-cultural research. *FOCUS*, *4*(1), 140–149.

Kloss, J. D., & Lisman, S. A. (2003). Clinician attributions and disease model perspectives of mentally ill, chemically addicted patients: A preliminary investigation. *Substance Use & Misuse*, *38*(14), 2097–2107.

Kokorelias, K. M., Gignac, M. A., Naglie, G., & Cameron, J. I. (2019). Towards a universal model of family centered care: A scoping review. *BMC Health Services Research*, *19*, 1–11.

Kon, A. A. (2010). The shared decision-making continuum. *JAMA*, *304*(8), 903–904.

Kondo, C., Saito, C., Deguchi, A., Hirayama, M., & Acar, A. (2010). Social conformity and response bias revisited: The influence of "others" on Japanese respondents. *Human Affairs*, *20*(4), 356–363.

Krueger, F., Barbey, A. K., & Grafman, J. (2009). The medial prefrontal cortex mediates social event knowledge. *Trends in Cognitive Sciences*, *13*(3), 103–109.

Krupat, E., Richards, J. B., Sullivan, A. M., Fleenor, T. J., & Schwartzstein, R. M. (2016). Assessing the effectiveness of case-based collaborative learning via randomized controlled trial. *Academic Medicine*, *91*(5), 723–729.

Krupinski, E. A. (2010). Current perspectives in medical image perception. *Attention, Perception, & Psychophysics*, *72*(5), 1205–1217.

Kunneman, M., Henselmans, I., Gärtner, F. R., Bomhof-Roordink, H., & Pieterse, A. H. (2019). Do shared decision-making measures reflect key elements of shared decision making? A content review of coding schemes. *Medical Decision Making*, *39*(7), 886–893.

Labrague, L. J. (2021). Psychological resilience, coping behaviours and social support among health care workers during the COVID-19 pandemic: A systematic review of quantitative studies. *Journal of Nursing Management*, *29*(7), 1893–1905.

Lapkin, S., Levett-Jones, T., & Gilligan, C. (2013). A systematic review of the effectiveness of interprofessional education in health professional programs. *Nurse Education Today*, *33*(2), 90–102.

Larivaara, P., & Taanila, A. (2004). Towards interprofessional family-oriented teamwork in primary services: The evaluation of an education programme. *Journal of Interprofessional Care*, *18*(2), 153–163.

Laschinger, H. K. S. (2014). Impact of workplace mistreatment on patient safety risk and nurse-assessed patient outcomes. *Journal of Nursing Administration*, *44*, 284–290.

Lawton, J., Ahmad, N., Peel, E., & Hallowell, N. (2007). Contextualising accounts of illness: notions of responsibility and blame in white and South Asian respondents' accounts of diabetes causation. *Sociology of Health & Illness*, *29*(6), 891–906.

Lawton, R., & Parker, D. (2002). Barriers to incident reporting in a healthcare system. *BMJ Quality & Safety*, *11*(1), 15–18.

Leach, J., & Scott, P. (2003). Individual and sociocultural views of learning in science education. *Science & Education*, *12*, 91–113.

Lee, A., Steketee, C., Rogers, G., & Moran, M. (2013). Towards a theoretical framework for curriculum development in health professional education. *Focus on Health Professional Education: A Multi-Professional Journal*, *14*(3), 70–83.

Légaré, F., & Thompson-Leduc, P. (2014). Twelve myths about shared decision making. *Patient Education and Counseling*, *96*(3), 281–286.

Leggat, S. G. (2007). Effective healthcare teams require effective team members: Defining teamwork competencies. *BMC Health Services Research, 7*(1).

Leunissen, J. M., De Cremer, D., Reinders Folmer, C. P., & van Dijke, M. (2013). The apology mismatch: Asymmetries between victim's need for apologies and perpetrator's willingness to apologize. *Journal of Experimental Social Psychology, 49*(3), 315–324.

Levine, S., & Kozloff, M. A. (1978). The sick role: Assessment and overview. *Annual Review of Sociology, 4*(1), 317–343.

Lewis, K. (2003). Measuring transactive memory systems in the field: Scale development and validation. *Journal of Applied Psychology, 88*(4), 587e604.

Lewis, K., Lange, D., & Gillis, L. (2005). Transactive memory systems, learning, and learning transfer. *Organization Science, 16*(6), 581–598. https://doi.org/10.1287/orsc.1050.0143

Li, Y. H., & Huang, J. W. (2013). Exploitative and exploratory learning in transactive memory systems and project performance. *Information & Management, 50*(6), 304–313.

Liao, J., Jimmieson, N. L., O'Brien, A. T., & Restubog, S. L. (2012). Developing transactive memory systems: Theoretical contributions from a social identity perspective. *Group & Organization Management, 37*(2), 204–240.

Lieber, E., Li, L., Wu, Z., Rotheram-Borus, M. J., & Guan, J. (2006). HIV/STD stigmatization fears as health-seeking barriers in China. *AIDS and Behavior, 10*(5), 463–471.

Lingard, L. (2012). Rethinking competence in the context of teamwork. In *2. Rethinking Competence in The Context of Teamwork* (pp. 42–69). Cornell University Press.

Lingard, L., McDougall, A., Levstik, M., Chandok, N., Spafford, M. M., & Schryer, C. (2012). Representing complexity well: A story about teamwork, with implications for how we teach collaboration. *Medical Education, 46*(9), 869–877.

Lipkin, M. (1984). The medical interview: A core curriculum for residencies in Internal Medicine. *Annals of Internal Medicine, 100*(2), 277.

Livingston, G., Barber, J., Rapaport, P., Knapp, M., Griffin, M., King, D., Romeo, R., Livingston, D., Mummery, C., Walker, Z., Hoe, J., & Cooper, C. (2014). Long-term clinical and cost-effectiveness of psychological intervention for family carers of people with dementia: A single-blind, randomised, controlled trial. *The lancet. Psychiatry, 1*(7), 539–548.

Lobchuk, M. M., Murdoch, T., McClement, S. E., & McPherson, C. (2008). A dyadic affair: Who is to blame for causing and controlling the patient's lung cancer? *Cancer Nursing, 31*(6), 435–443.

Loh, A. Z., Tan, J. S., Zhang, M. W., & Ho, R. C. (2017). The global prevalence of anxiety and depressive symptoms among caregivers of stroke survivors. *Journal of the American Medical Directors Association, 18*(2), 111–116.

Longmire, N. H., & Harrison, D. A. (2018). Seeing their side versus feeling their pain: Differential consequences of perspective-taking and empathy at work. *Journal of Applied Psychology, 103*(8), 894–915.

Lou, S. M., Larkin, K. L., Winthrop, K., Rosenbaum, J. T., & members of Uveitis Specialists Study Group. (2015). Lack of consensus in the diagnosis and treatment for ocular tuberculosis among uveitis specialists. *Ocular Immunology and Inflammation, 23*(1), 25–31.

Lowery, K., Mynt, P., Aisbett, J., Dixon, T., O'Brien, J., & Ballard, C. (2000). Depression in the carers of dementia sufferers: A comparison of the carers of patients suffering from dementia with Lewy bodies and the carers of patients with Alzheimer's disease. *Journal of Affective Disorders, 59*(1), 61–65.

Lucyk, K., & McLaren, L. (2017). Taking stock of the social determinants of health: A scoping review. *PLOS ONE, 12*(5), e0177306.

Lupton, D. (2012). *Medicine as Culture: Illness, Disease and the Body*. Sage.

Ma, T. (2024). Considerations for implementation of a competency-based education program for preclerkship courses. In J. R. Schoenherr & M. M. McConnell (Eds.), *Fundamentals and Frontiers in Health Professions Education and Decision Making: Educational Theory and Psychological Practice*. Routledge.

Makoul, G., & Clayman, M. L. (2006). An integrative model of shared decision making in medical encounters. *Patient Education and Counseling, 60*(3), 301–312.

Mangold, K. A., Bartell, T. R., Doobay-Persaud, A. A., Adler, M. D., & Sheehan, K. M. (2019). Expert consensus on inclusion of the social determinants of health in undergraduate medical education curricula. *Academic Medicine, 94*(9), 1355.

Mannion, R., & Thompson, C. (2014). Systematic biases in group decision-making: Implications for patient safety. *International Journal for Quality in Health Care, 26*(6), 606–612.

Mantler, J., Schellenberg, E. G., & Page, J. S. (2003). Attributions for serious illness: Are controllability, responsibility and blame different constructs? *Canadian Journal of Behavioural Science / Revue Canadienne Des Sciences Du Comportement, 35*(2), 142–152.

Marchiondo, L. A., Cortina, L. M., & Kabat-Farr, D. (2018). Attributions and appraisals of workplace incivility: Finding light on the dark side? *Applied Psychology: An International Review, 67*(3), 369–400.

Markus, H. R., & Kitayama, S. (2003). Culture, self, and the reality of the social. *Psychological Inquiry, 14*(3-4), 277–283.

Markus, J., Mundy, P., Morales, M., Delgado, C. E., & Yale, M. (2000). Individual differences in infant skills as predictors of child-caregiver joint attention and language. *Social Development, 9*(3), 302–315.

Martin, M. W. (2001). *Journal of Medical Humanities, 22*(2), 95–114.

Mattan, B. D., Rotshtein, P., & Quinn, K. A. (2016). Empathy and visual perspective-taking performance. *Cognitive Neuroscience, 7*(1-4), 170–181.

Mauldin, B. (2011). *Apprenticeships in the Healthcare Industry. Administration for Children and Families.* U.S. Department of Health & Human Services.

Maxfield, D. J. Grenny, R. McMillan, K. Patterson, & A. Switzler. (2005). *Silence Kills—The Seven Crucial Conversations for Healthcare*. VitalSmarts.

McConnell, M. (2024). Emotion and clinical decision-making. In J. R. Schoenherr & M. M. McConnell (Eds.), *Fundamentals and Frontiers in Medical Education and Decision-Making: Educational Theory and Psychological Practice*. Routledge.

Mead, N., & Bower, P. (2000). Patient-centredness: A conceptual framework and review of the empirical literature. *Social Science & Medicine, 51*(7), 1087–1110.

Meleis, A. I. (2016). Interprofessional education: A summary of reports and barriers to recommendations. *Journal of Nursing Scholarship, 48*(1), 106–112.

Mezulis, A. H., Abramson, L. Y., Hyde, J. S., & Hankin, B. L. (2004). Is there a universal positivity bias in attributions? A meta-analytic review of individual, developmental, and cultural differences in the self-serving attributional bias. *Psychological Bulletin, 130*(5), 711–747.

Michinov, N., & Michinov, E. (2009). Investigating the relationship between transactive memory and performance in collaborative learning. *Learning and Instruction, 19*(1), 43–54.

Milich, R., Balentine, A. C., & Lynam, D. R. (2001). ADHD combined type and ADHD predominantly inattentive type are distinct and unrelated disorders. *Clinical Psychology: Science and Practice*, *8*(4), 463.

Milich, R., Balentine, A. C., & Lynam, D. R. (2002). The predominately inattentive subtype—not a subtype of ADHD. *The ADHD Report*, *10*(1), 1–6.

Millington, S. J., Arntfield, R. T., Guo, R. J., Koenig, S., Kory, P., Noble, V., ... & Schoenherr, J. R. (2018). Expert agreement in the interpretation of lung ultrasound studies performed on mechanically ventilated patients. *Journal of Ultrasound in Medicine*, *37*(11), 2659–2665.

Monteiro, S., Keuhl, A., Lee, M., & Chan, T. M. (2024). Rethinking clinical reasoning: A paradigm shift. *Journal of Evaluation in Clinical Practice*, *30*(5), 766–773.

Moorhead, G., & Montanari, J. R. (1986). An empirical investigation of the groupthink phenomenon. *Human Relations*, *39*(5), 399–410.

Morales, M., Mundy, P., Delgado, C. E. F., Yale, M., Messinger, D., Neal, R., & Schwartz, H. K. (2000). Responding to joint attention across the 6- through 24-month age period and early language acquisition. *Journal of Applied Developmental Psychology*, *21*(3), 283–298.

Moran, M., Boyce, R. A. & Nissen, L. (2011). Competition the new collaboration? Employing inter-team competitiveness to motivate health students to learn together. In S. Kitto, J. Chesters, J. Thistlethwaite, & S. Reeves (Eds.), *Sociology of Interprofessional Health Care Practice: Critical Reflections and Concrete Solutions* (pp. 155–168). Nova Science Publishers.

Moreland, R. L. (1999). Transactive memory: Learning who knows what in work groups and organizations. In L. Thompson, D. Messick, & J. Levine (Eds.), *Shared Cognition in Organizations: The Management of Knowledge* (pp. 3–31). Erlbaum.

Moreland, R. L., & Argote, L. (2014). Transactive memory in dynamic organizations. In R. S. Peterson & E. A. Mannix (Eds.), *Leading and Managing People in the Dynamic Organization* (pp. 135–162). Psychology Press.

Moreland, R. L., & Myaskovsky, L. (2000). Exploring the performance benefits of group training: Transactive memory or improved communication? *Organizational Behavior and Human Decision Processes*, *82*(1), 117–133.

Moreland, R. L., Argote, L., & Krishnan, R. (1996). Socially shared cognition at work: Transactive memory and group performance. In J. L. Nye & A. M. Brower (Eds.), *What's Social About Social Cognition? Research on Socially Shared Cognition in Small Groups* (pp. 57–84). Sage.

Morley, L., & Cashell, A. (2017). Collaboration in health care. *Journal of Medical Imaging and Radiation Sciences*, *48*(2), 207–216.

Morrison, E. W., & Milliken, F. J. (2000). Organizational silence: A barrier to change and development in a pluralistic world. *Academy of Management Review, 25*(4), 706–725.

Moumjid, N., Gafni, A., Bremond, A., & Carrere, M. O. (2007). Shared decision making in the medical encounter: Are we all talking about the same thing? *Medical Decision Making*, *27*(5), 539–546.

Mundy, P. (2003). The neural basis of social impairments in autism: The role of the dorsal medial-frontal cortex and anterior cingulate system. *Journal of Child Psychology and Psychiatry*, *44*(6), 793–809.

Narayan, M. C. (2013). Using SBAR communications in efforts to prevent patient rehospitalizations. *Home Healthcare Nurse*, *31*(9), 504–515.

Neck, C. P., & Manz, C. C. (1994). From groupthink to teamthink: Toward the creation of constructive thought patterns in self-managing work teams. *Human Relations*, *47*(8), 929–952.

Nevo, D., & Wand, Y. (2005). Organizational memory information systems: A transactive memory approach. *Decision Support Systems*, *39*(4), 549–562.

Nichter, M. (2003). The social relations of therapy management. In M. Lock & M. Nichter (Eds.), *New Horizons in Medical Anthropology* (pp. 95–124). Routledge.

Nijboer, C., Tempelaar, R., Triemstra, M., van den Bos, G. A., & Sanderman, R. (2001). The role of social and psychological resources in caregiving of cancer patients. *Cancer*, *91*(5), 1029–1039.

Norman, G. R., Grierson, L. E. M., Sherbino, J., Hamstra, S. J., Schmidt, H. G., & Mamede, S. (2018). Expertise in medicine and surgery. In K. A. Ericsson, R. R. Hoffman, A. Kozbelt, & A. M. Williams (Eds.), *The Cambridge Handbook of Expertise and Expert Performance* (2nd ed., pp. 331–355). Cambridge University Press.

Oandasan, I., & Reeves, S. (2005). Key elements of interprofessional education. Part 2: Factors, processes and outcomes. *Journal of Interprofessional Care*, *19 Suppl 1*, 39–48.

Olson, A., Rencic, J., Cosby, K., Rusz, D., Papa, F., Croskerry, P., Zierler, B., Harkless, G., Giuliano, M. A., Schoenbaum, S., Colford, C., Cahill, M., Gerstner, L., Grice, G. R., & Graber, M. L. (2019). Competencies for improving diagnosis: An interprofessional framework for education and training in health care. *Diagnosis*, *6*(4), 335–341.

Orsino, A., & Ng, S. (2019). Can adaptive expertise, reflective practice, and activity theory help achieve systems-based practice and collective competence? *Canadian Medical Education Journal*, *10*, e55–e60.

Palm, J. (2004). The nature of and responsibility for alcohol and drug problems: Views among treatment staff. *Addiction Research & Theory*, *12*(5), 413–431.

Park, M., Lee, M., Jeong, H., Jeong, M., & Go, Y. (2018). Patient-and family-centered care interventions for improving the quality of health care: A review of systematic reviews. *International Journal of Nursing Studies*, *87*, 69–83.

Parsons, T. (1951). *The Social System*. Free Press.

Patel, V. L., & Arocha, J. F. (2001). The nature of constraints on collaborative decision making in health care settings. In E. Salas & G. Klein (Eds.), *Linking Expertise and Naturalistic Decision Making* (pp. 383–405). Lawrence Erlbaum.

Pearson, C. M., Andersson, L. M., & Porath, C. L. (2000). Assessing and attacking workplace incivility. *Organizational Dynamics*, *29*(2), 123–137. https://doi.org/10.1016/S0090-2616(00)00019-X

Peltokorpi, V. (2008). Transactive memory systems. *Review of General Psychology*, *12*(4), 378–394.

Peltokorpi, V., & Hood, A. C. (2018). Communication in theory and research on transactive memory systems: A literature review. *Topics in Cognitive Science*, *11*(4), 644–667.

Perry, M. (2003). Distributed cognition. In J. M. Carroll (Ed.), *HCI Models, Theories, and Frameworks: Toward a Multidisciplinary Science* (pp. 193–223). Morgan Kaufmann.

Piaget, J. (1929). *The Child's Conception of the World*. Routledge.

Piaget, J. (1954). *The Construction of Reality in the Child.* trans. M. Cook. Basic Books, Inc., Publishers.

Piaget, J. & Inhelder, B. (1967) In *The child's conception of space*. New York: Norton & Co.

Pierre-Victor, D., Stephens, D. P., Clarke, R., Gabbidon, K., & Madhivanan, P. (2017). Role of healthcare providers' recommendation style in HPV vaccine decision-making among Haitian parents and female patients. *Californian Journal of Health Promotion*, *15*(3), 68–80.

Pimmer, C., Pachler, N., & Genewein, U. (2013). Reframing clinical workplace learning using the theory of distributed cognition. *Academic Medicine*, *88*(9), 1239–1245.

Pluta, W. J., Richards, B. F., & Mutnick, A. (2013). PBL and beyond: Trends in collaborative learning. *Teaching and Learning in Medicine, 25*(sup1), S9–S16.

Pollard-Gott, L. (1993). Attribution theory and the novel. *Poetics*, *21*(6), 499–524.

Polly, D., Allman, B., Casto, A., & Norwood, J. (2017). Sociocultural perspectives of learning. In R. E. West (Ed.), *Foundations of Learning and Instructional Design Technology*. Press Books.

Poortman, C. L., Illeris, K., & Nieuwenhuis, L. (2011). Apprenticeship: From learning theory to practice. *Journal of Vocational Education & Training*, *63*(3), 267–287.

Prati, G., & Pietrantoni, L. (2010). The relation of perceived and received social support to mental health among first responders: A meta-analytic review. *Journal of Community Psychology, 38*(3), 403–417.

Premeaux, S. F., & Bedeian, A. G. (2003). Breaking the silence: The moderating effects of self-monitoring in predicting speaking up in the work- place. *Journal of Management Studies*, *40*(6), 1537–1562.

Price, S., Doucet, S., & Hall, L. M. (2014). The historical social positioning of nursing and medicine: Implications for career choice, early socialization and interprofessional collaboration. *Journal of Interprofessional Care, 28*(2), 103–109.

Proudfoot, D., & Kay, A. C. (2014). System justification in organizational contexts: How a motivated preference for the status quo can affect organizational attitudes and behaviors. *Research in Organizational Behavior*, *34*, 173–187.

Pun, J. K. H., Chan, E. A., Wang, S., & Slade, D. (2018). Health professional-patient communication practices in East Asia: An integrative review of an emerging field of research and practice in Hong Kong, South Korea, Japan, Taiwan, and Mainland China. *Patient Education and Counseling, 101*(7), 1193–1206.

Quiles Marcos, Y., Quiles Sebastián, M. J., Pamies Aubalat, L., Botella Ausina, J., & Treasure, J. (2013). Peer and family influence in eating disorders: A meta-analysis. *European Psychiatry: The Journal of the Association of European Psychiatrists*, *28*(4), 199–206.

Raveis, V. H., Karus, D. G., & Siegel, K. (1998). Correlates of depressive symptomatology among adult daughter caregivers of a parent with cancer. *Cancer*, *83*(8), 1652–1663.

Redcay, E., Kleiner, M., & Saxe, R. (2012). Look at this: The neural correlates of initiating and responding to bids for joint attention. *Frontiers in Human Neuroscience*, *6*, 169.

Rees, D., & Johnson, R. (2007). All together now? Staff views and experiences of a pre-qualifying interprofessional curriculum. *Journal of Interprofessional Care, 21*(5), 543–555.

Reeves, S., & Lewin, S. (2004). Hospital based interprofessional collaboration: Strategies and meanings. *Journal of Health Services Research and Policy, 9*, 218–225.

Reeves, S., Zwarenstein, M., Goldman, J., Barr, H., Freeth, D., Koppel, I., & Hammick, M. (2010). The effectiveness of interprofessional education: Key findings from a new systematic review. *Journal of Interprofessional Care, 24*(3), 230–241.

Rego, S., Arantes, J., & Magalhães, P. (2018). Is there a sunk cost effect in committed relationships? *Current Psychology*, *37*, 508–519.

Reisine, S. T. (1995). Arthritis and the family. *Arthritis Care and Research: The Official Journal of the Arthritis Health Professions Association*, *8*(4), 265–271.

Reno, R. R., Cialdini, R. B., & Kallgren, C. A. (1993). The transsituational influence of social norms. *Journal of Personality and Social Psychology*, *64*(1), 104–112.

Richardson, D. C., & Dale, R. (2005). Looking to understand: The coupling between speakers' and listeners' eye movements and its relationship to discourse comprehension. *Cognitive Science*, *29*(6), 1045–1060.

Richardson, M. J., Marsh, K. L., Isenhower, R. W., Goodman, J. R., & Schmidt, R. C. (2007). Rocking together: Dynamics of intentional and unintentional interpersonal coordination. *Human Movement Science, 26*(6), 867–891.

Rogers, D. A., Regehr, G., Gelula, M., Yeh, K. A., Howdieshell, T. R., & Webb, W. (2000). Peer teaching and computer-assisted learning: An effective combination for surgical skill training? *Journal of Surgical Research, 92*(1), 53–55.

Ronzani, T. M., Higgins-Biddle, J., & Furtado, E. F. (2009). Stigmatization of alcohol and other drug users by primary care providers in southeast Brazil. *Social Science & Medicine*, *69*(7), 1080–1084.

Rose, S. C., Fischer, A. N., & Heyer, G. L. (2015). How long is too long? The lack of consensus regarding the post-concussion syndrome diagnosis. *Brain Injury*, *29*(7-8), 798–803.

Rosen, M. A., DiazGranados, D., Dietz, A. S., Benishek, L. E., Thompson, D., Pronovost, P. J., & Weaver, S. J. (2018). Teamwork in healthcare: Key discoveries enabling safer, high-quality care. *The American Psychologist, 73*(4), 433–450.

Sahay, A., Hutchinson, M., & East, L. (2015). Exploring the influence of workplace supports and relationships on safe medication practice: A pilot study of Australian graduate nurses. *Nurse Education Today, 35*(5), e21–e16.

Sallim, A. B., Sayampanathan, A. A., Cuttilan, A., & Ho, R. (2015). Prevalence of mental health disorders among caregivers of patients with Alzheimer Disease. *Journal of the American Medical Directors Association, 16*(12), 1034–1041.

Samosh, J. (2019). What is workplace incivility? An investigation of employee relational schemas. *Organization Management Journal, 16*(2), 81–97.

Sangalang, C. C., & Vang, C. (2017). Intergenerational trauma in refugee families: A systematic review. *Journal of Immigrant and Minority Health, 19*, 745–754.

Saragih, I. D., Hsiao, C.-T., Fann, W.-C., Hsu, C.-M., Saragih, I. S., & Lee, B.-O. (2024). Impacts of interprofessional education on collaborative practice of healthcare professionals: A systematic review and meta-analysis. *Nurse Education Today, 136*, 106136. https://doi.org/10.1016/j.nedt.2024.106136

Schoenherr, J. R. (2021). Trust and explainability in A/IS-mediated healthcare: Operationalizing the therapeutic alliance in a distributed system. In *2021 IEEE International Symposium on Technology and Society (ISTAS)* (pp. 1–8). IEEE.

Schoenherr, J. R. (2022a). The essence of AI: Features and functions of autonomous/intelligent systems. In J. R. Schoenherr(Ed.), *Ethical Artificial Intelligence From Popular to Cognitive Science: Trust in the Age of Entanglement.* Routledge.

Schoenherr, J. R. (2022b). Vaccination, values, and health information search behaviour in the new folk medicine. In *2022 IEEE International Symposium on Technology and Society (ISTAS)* (Vol. *1*, pp. 1–10). IEEE.

Schoenherr, J. R. (2022c). Folkmedical technologies and the sociotechnical systems of healthcare. *IEEE Technology and Society Magazine*, *41*(3), 38–49.

Schoenherr, J. R. (2027a). Innovation and implementation in the health professions: Translating research in education and healthcare delivery. In Schoenherr, J. R. (Ed.), *Fundamentals and Frontiers of Medical Education and Decision-Making: Innovation, Implementation, and Translational Research* (pp. p1–76). Routledge.

Schoenherr, J. R. (2027b). Human-centered artificial intelligence in health professions education and decision-making: AsSociotechnical systems perspective. In Schoenherr,

J. R. (Ed.), *Fundamentals and Frontiers of Medical Education and Decision-Making: Innovation, Implementation, and Translational Research* (pp. 132–190). Routledge.

Schoenherr, J. R. (2027c). The Development and Dynamics of Heterarchical Structure in Mayan Medical Education and Healthcare Ecosystems. In Schoenherr, J. R. (Ed.), *Fundamentals and Frontiers of Medical Education and Decision-Making: Innovation, Implementation, and Translational Research* (pp. 359–411). Routledge.

Schoenherr, J. R., & Beaudoin, J. (2027). The evolving landscape of health professions education in East Asia: Heterarchies in East Asian medicine and medical education. In J. R. Schoenherr (Ed.), *Fundamentals and Frontiers of Medical Education and Decision-Making: Innovation, Implementation, and Translational Research* (pp. 462–509). Routledge.

Schoenherr, J. R., & Hamstra, S. J. (2024). Validity in health professions education: From assessment instruments to program innovation and evaluation. In J. R. Schoenherr & M. M. McConnell (Eds.), Fundamentals and Frontiers in Medical Education: Educational Theory and Psychological Practice. Routledge.

Schoenherr, J. R., & Le-Bouar, C. (2024). Representing and communicating health information: Fundamentals of persuasive health communication. In J. R. Schoenherr & M. M. McConnell (Eds.), *Fundamentals and Frontiers of Medical Education and Decision-Making* (pp. 270–312). Routledge.

Schoenherr, J. R., & McConnell, M. M. (2024). Human-centered design in health professions education: Informing competency-based education with psychological science. In *Fundamentals and Frontiers of Medical Education and Decision-Making* (pp. 3–36). Routledge.

Schoenherr, J. R., Waechter, J., Lee, C. H. (2024). Quantifying expertise in the healthcare professions: cognitive efficiency and metacognitive calibration. In J. R. Schoenherr & M. M. McConnell (Eds.), *Fundamentals and Frontiers in Medical Education: Educational Theory and Psychological Practice.* Routledge.

Scollan-Koliopoulos, M., O'Connell, K. A., & Walker, E. A. (2007). Legacy of diabetes and self-care behavior. *Research in Nursing & Health*, *30*(5), 508–517.

Searle, J. (2008). Nurse practitioner candidates: Shifting professional boundaries. *Australasian Emergency Nursing Journal*, *11*(1), 20–27.

Sharf, B. F., & Vanderford, M. L. (2003). Illness narratives and the social construction of health. In T. L. Thompson, A. M. Dorsey, K. Miller, & R. Parrott (Eds.), *The Routledge Handbook of Health Communication* (pp. 23–48). Routledge.

Sheldon, M., Cavanaugh, J. T., Croninger, W., Osgood, W., Robnett, R., Seigle, J., & Simonsen, L. (2012). Preparing rehabilitation healthcare providers in the 21st century: Implementation of interprofessional education through an academic-clinical site partnership. *Work (Reading, Mass.)*, *41*(3), 269–275.

Shelton, T. L., Jeppson, E. S., & Johnson, B. H. (1987). *Family-Centered Care for Children with Special Health Care Needs*. Association for the Care of Children's Health.

Shor, E., Roelfs, D. J., & Yogev, T. (2013). The strength of family ties: A meta-analysis and meta-regression of self-reported social support and mortality. *Social Networks, 35*(4), 626–638.

Shorey, S., Lau, T. C., Lau, S. T., & Ang, E. (2019). Entrustable professional activities in health care education: A scoping review. *Medical Education*, *53*(8), 766–777.

Shortliffe, E. H. (1987). Computer programs to support clinical decision-making reply. *JAMA: The Journal of the American Medical Association*, *258*(17), 2375.

Sick, B., Sheldon, L., Ajer, K., Wang, Q., & Zhang, L. (2014). The student-run free clinic: An ideal site to teach interprofessional education? *Journal of Interprofessional Care*, *28*(5), 413–418.

Siebert, C. J., Clark, A., Kilbridge, A., & Peterson, H., 2006. When preservice teachers struggle or fail: Mentor teachers' perspectives. *Chula Vista, 123*(3), 409–423.

Siebold, G. L., & Kelly, D. R. (1988). *Development of the Combat Platoon Cohesion Questionaire* (Vol. 817). US Army Research Institute for the Behavioral and Social Sciences.

Siegler, M. (1985). The progression of medicine: From physician paternalism to patient autonomy to bureaucratic parsimony. *Archives of Internal Medicine, 145*(4), 713–715.

Sim, I., Gorman, P., Greenes, R. A., Haynes, R. B., Kaplan, B., Lehmann, H., & Tang, P. C. (2001). Clinical decision support systems for the practice of evidence-based medicine. *Journal of the American Medical Informatics Association, 8*(6), 527–34.

Singelis, T. M., Triandis, H. C., Bhawuk, D. P. S., & Gelfand, M. J. (1995). Horizontal and vertical dimensions of individualism and collectivism: A theoretical and measurement refinement. *Cross-Cultural Research, 29*(3), 240–275.

Singer, S. J., Benzer, J. K., & Hamdan, S. U. (2015). Improving health care quality and safety: The role of collective learning. *Journal of Healthcare Leadership, 7*, 91–107.

Siposova, B., & Carpenter, M. (2019). A new look at joint attention and common knowledge. *Cognition, 189*, 260–274.

Sivadas, E., Bruvold, N. T., & Nelson, M. R. (2008). A reduced version of the horizontal and vertical individualism and collectivism scale: A four-country assessment. *Journal of Business Research, 61*(3), 201–210.

Smith, C. B., Adamson, L. B., & Bakeman, R. (1988). Interactional predictors of early language. *First Language, 8*, 143–156.

Smith, K. P., & Christakis, N. A. (2008). Social networks and health. *Annual Review of Sociology, 34*(1), 405–429.

Smith, L., Andrusyszyn, M., & Laschinger, H. (2010). Effects of workplace incivility and empowerment on newly graduated nurses' organizational commitment. *Journal of Nursing Management, 18*, 1004–1015.

Soltani, F., Raeisi, A., & Rarani, M. (2019). Challenges of patient handover process in healthcare services: A systematic review. *Journal of Education and Health Promotion, 8*(1), 173.

Sperber, D., & Wilson, D. (1986). *Relevance: Communication and Cognition*. Blackwell.

Spitzer, R. L., Lilienfeld, S. O., & Miller, M. B. (2005). Rosenhan revisited: The scientific credibility of Lauren Slater's Pseudopatient diagnosis study: 1. *The Journal of Nervous and Mental Disease, 193*(11), 734–739.

Srivastava, R. (2013). Speaking up—When doctors navigate medical hierarchy. *The New England Journal of Medicine, 368*(4), 302–305.

Stacey, D., Samant, R., & Bennett, C. (2008). Decision making in oncology: A review of patient decision aids to support patient participation. *CA: A Cancer Journal for Clinicians, 58*(5), 293–304.

Stadick, J. L. (2020). The relationship between interprofessional education and health care professional's attitudes towards teamwork and interprofessional collaborative competencies. *Journal of Interprofessional Education & Practice, 19*, 100320.

Stanley, K. M., Martin, M. M., Michel, Y., Welton, J. M., & Nemeth, L. S. (2007). Examining lateral violence in the nursing workforce. *Issues in Mental Health Nursing, 28*(11), 1247–1265.

Stein, L. I. (1967). The doctor-nurse game. *Archives of General Psychiatry, 16*(6), 699.

Stewart, M., Brown, J. B., Weston, W. W., McWhinney, I. R., McWilliam, C. L., & Freeman, T. R. (1995). *Patient-Centered Medicine: Transforming the Clinical Method.* Sage.

Stiggelbout, A. M., Pieterse, A. H., & De Haes, J. C. (2015). Shared decision making: Concepts, evidence, and practice. *Patient Education and Counseling*, *98*(10), 1172–1179.

Struthers, C. W., Eaton, J., Santelli, A. G., Uchiyama, M., & Shirvani, N. (2008). The effects of attributions of intent and apology on forgiveness: When saying sorry may not help the story. *Journal of Experimental Social Psychology*, *44*(4), 983–992.

Sunday, J., Eyles, J., & Upshur, R. (2001). Applying Aristotle's doctrine of causation to Aboriginal and biomedical understandings of diabetes. *Culture, Medicine and Psychiatry*, *25*, 63–85.

Sunguya, B. F., Hinthong, W., Jimba, M., & Yasuoka, J. (2014). Interprofessional education for whom? —Challenges and lessons learned from its implementation in developed countries and their application to developing countries: A systematic review. *PloS one*, *9*(5), e96724.

Szasz, T. S., & Hollender, M. H. (1956). A contribution to the philosophy of medicine: The basic models of the doctor-patient relationship. *A.M.A. Archives of Internal Medicine*, *97*(5), 585–592.

Tang, C. J., Chan, S. W., Zhou, W. T., & Liaw, S. Y. (2013). Collaboration between hospital physicians and nurses: An integrated literature review. *International Nursing Review*, *60*(3), 291–302.

Tasselli, S. (2014). Social networks of professionals in health care organizations: A review. *Medical Care Research and Review*, *71*(6), 619–660.

Tavuchis, N. (1991). *Mea Culpa: A Sociology of Apology and Reconciliation*. Stanford University Press.

Ten Cate, O. (2005). Entrustability of professional activities and competency-based training. *Medical Education*, *39*(12), 1176–1177.

Ten Cate, O. (2013). Nuts and bolts of entrustable professional activities. *Journal of Graduate Medical Education*, *5*(1), 157–158.

Ten Cate, O., Balmer, D. F., Caretta-Weyer, H., Hatala, R., Hennus, M. P., & West, D. C. (2021). Entrustable professional activities and entrustment decision making: a development and research agenda for the next decade. *Academic Medicine*, *96*(Supplement_1), S96–S104.

Thistlethwaite, J., & Moran, M. (2010). Learning outcomes for interprofessional education (IPE): Literature review and synthesis. *Journal of Interprofessional Care*, *24*(5), 503–513.

Thistlethwaite, J., & Nisbet, G. (2011). Preparing educators for interprofessional learning: Rationale, educational theory and delivery. In *Sociology of Interprofessional Health Care Practice: Critical Reflections and Concrete Solutions* (pp. 169–184).

Thistlethwaite, J. E. (2015). Interprofessional education: Implications and development for medical education. *Educación Médica*, *16*(1), 68–73.

Thistlethwaite, J. E., Forman, D., Rogers, G., Steketee, C., & Yassine, T. (2014). Interprofessional education competencies and frameworks in health: A comparative analysis. *Acad Med*, *89*(6), 869–874.

Thompson, B. M., Schneider, V. F., Haidet, P., Levine, R. E., McMahon, K. K., Perkowski, L. C., & Richards, B. F. (2007). Team-based learning at ten medical schools: Two years later. *Medical Education*, *41*(3), 250–257.

Tomasello, M. (2009). *The Cultural Origins of Human Cognition*. Harvard University Press.

Tomasello, M., & Farrar, M. J. (1986). Joint attention and early language. *Child Development*, *57*, 1454–1463.

Triandis, H. C. (2000). Culture and conflict. *International Journal of Psychology*, *35*(2), 145–152.

Triandis, H. C. (2001). Individualism-collectivism and personality. *Journal of Personality*, *69*(6), 907–924.

Turner, J. C. (1999). Some current issues in research on social identity and self-categorization theories. *Social Identity: Context, Commitment, Content*, *3*(1), 6–34.

Ungvari, G. S., Xiang, Y. T., Hong, Y., Leung, H. C., & Chiu, H. F. (2010). Diagnosis of schizophrenia: Reliability of an operationalized approach to 'praecox-feeling'. *Psychopathology*, *43*(5), 292–299.

Valachovic, R. W. (2019). Integrating oral and overall health care: Building a foundation for interprofessional education and collaborative practice. *Journal of Dental Education, 83*(2 Suppl), S19–S22.

van Diggele, C., Roberts, C., Burgess, A., & Mellis, C. (2020). Interprofessional education: Tips for design and implementation. *BMC Medical Education, 20* (Suppl 2), 455.

van Dijke, M., & Cremer, D. D. (2011). When social accounts promote acceptance of unfair ultimatum offers: The role of the victim's stress responses to uncertainty and power position. *Journal of Economic Psychology*, *32*(3), 468–479.

Van Dyne, L., Ang, S., & Botero, I. C. (2003). Conceptualizing employee silence and voice as multidimensional constructs. *Journal of Management Studies, 40*(6), 1359–1392.

Veerapen, K., & Purkis, M. E. (2014). Implications of early workplace experiences on continuing interprofessional education for physicians and nurses. *Journal of Interprofessional Care, 28*(3), 218–225.

Visser, S. N., Danielson, M. L., Bitsko, R. H., Holbrook, J. R., Kogan, M. D., Ghandour, R. M., Perou, R., & Blumberg, S. J. (2014). Trends in the parent-report of health care provider-diagnosed and medicated attention-deficit/hyperactivity disorder: United States, 2003–2011. *Journal of the American Academy of Child & Adolescent Psychiatry, 53*(1), 34–46.

Vrbnjak, D., Denieffe, S., O'Gorman, C., & Pajnkihar, M. (2016). Barriers to reporting medication errors and near misses among nurses: A systematic review. *International Journal of Nursing Studies, 63*, 162–178.

Vygotsky, L. S. (1962). *Thought and Language*. MIT Press.

Vygotsky, L. S. (1978). *Mind in Society: The Development of Higher Psychological Processes*. Harvard University Press.

Wagner, M., Dubé, T., & Gomez-Garibello, C. (2020). It takes a team: Generating evidence to define and foster collective competence in health professions education. *Canadian Medical Education Journal*, *11*(5), e109–e111.

Walfisch, T., Van Dijk, D., & Kark, R. (2013). Do you really expect me to apologize? The impact of status and gender on the effectiveness of an apology in the workplace. *Journal of Applied Social Psychology*, *43*(7), 1446–1458.

Walsh, C. M., Rose, D. N., Dubrowski, A., Ling, S. C., Grierson, L. E., Backstein, D., & Carnahan, H. (2011). Learning in the simulated setting: A comparison of expert-, peer-, and computer-assisted learning. *Academic Medicine*, *86*(10), S12–S16.

Wang, H. H., Wu, S. Z., & Liu, Y. Y. (2003). Association between social support and health outcomes: A meta-analysis. *The Kaohsiung Journal of Medical Sciences, 19*(7), 345–350.

Wang, Z., Feng, F., Gao, S., & Yang, J. (2019). A systematic meta-analysis of the effect of interprofessional education on health professions students' attitudes. *Journal of Dental Education, 83*(12), 1361–1369.

Ward, W., Zagoloff, A., Rieck, C., & Robiner, W. (2018). Interprofessional education: Opportunities and challenges for psychology. *Journal of Clinical Psychology in Medical Settings, 25*(3), 250–266.

Ware, N. C. (1992). Suffering and the social construction of illness: The delegitimation of illness experience in chronic fatigue syndrome. *Medical Anthropology Quarterly*, *6*(4), 347–361.

Weaver, S. J., Dy, S. M., & Rosen, M. A. (2014). Team-training in healthcare: A narrative synthesis of the literature. *BMJ Quality & Safety, 23*(5), 359–372.

Wegner, D. M. (1987). Transactive memory: A contemporary analysis of the group mind. In *Theories of Group Behavior* (pp. 185–208).

Weiner, B. (1986). *An Attributional Theory of Motivation and Emotion.* Springer New York.

Whitney, S. N., Holmes-Rovner, M., Brody, H., Schneider, C., McCullough, L. B., Volk, R. J., & McGuire, A. L. (2008). Beyond shared decision making: An expanded typology of medical decisions. *Medical Decision Making, 28*(5), 699–705.

Williams, J. H., Waiter, G.D., Perra, O., Perrett, D.I., & Whiten, A. (2005). An fMRI study of joint attention experience. *Neuroimage, 25*(1), 133–140.

Wilson, E., Daniel, M., Rao, A., Torre, D., Durning, S., Anderson, C., ... & Seifert, C. M. (2023). A scoping review of distributed cognition in acute care clinical decision-making. *Diagnosis, 10*(2), 68–88.

Winefield, H., Murrell, T., Clifford, J., & Farmer, E. (1996). The search for reliable and valid measures of patient-centredness. *Psychology & Health, 11*(6), 811–824.

World Health Organization (WHO) (2010). *Framework for Action on Interprofessional Education & Collaborative Practice.* www.who.int/publications/i/item/framework-for-action-on-interprofessional-education-collaborative-practice

Wyatt, J., & Spiegelhalter, D. (1991) Field trials of medical decision-aids: Potential problems and solutions. *Proceedings of the Annual Symposium on Computer Application in Medical Care*, 3–7.

Xyrichis, A., Reeves, S., & Zwarenstein, M. (2018). Examining the nature of interprofessional practice: An initial framework validation and creation of the InterProfessional Activity Classification Tool (InterPACT). *Journal of Interprofessional Care, 32*(4), 416–425.

Yalçın, B., & Baykal, Ü. (2012). The subjects of and reasons for nurses' remaining silent in private hospitals and relative factors. *Journal of Education and Research in Nursing, 9*(2), 42–50. (Original work published in Turkish)

Yalçın, B., Baykal, Ü., & Türkmen, E. (2021). Why do nurses choose to stay silent? A qualitative study. *International Journal of Nursing Practice, 28*(1), e13010.

Yan, W., & Gaier, E. L. (1994). Causal attributions for college success and failure: An Asian-American comparison. *Journal of Cross-Cultural Psychology, 25*(1), 146–158.

Yin, M., Li, Z., & Zhou, C. (2020). Experience of stigma among family members of people with severe mental illness: A qualitative systematic review. *International Journal of Mental Health Nursing, 29*(2), 141–160.

Young, A. (1983). The relevance of traditional medical cultures to modern primary health care. *Social Science & Medicine, 17*(16), 1205–1211.

Zerbe, W. J., & Paulhus, D. L. (1987). Socially desirable responding in organizational behavior: A preconception. *Academy of Management Review, 12*(2), 250–264.

Zhang, Y. (2018). Family functioning in the context of an adult family member with illness: A concept analysis. *Journal of Clinical Nursing, 27*(15-16), 3205–3224.

Ziring, D., Frankel, R. M., Danoff, D., Isaacson, J. H., & Lochnan, H. (2018). Silent witnesses: Faculty reluctance to report medical students' professionalism lapses. *Academic Medicine, 93*(11), 1700–1706.

Zwarenstein, M., & Reeves, S. (2006). Knowledge translation and interprofessional collaboration: Where the rubber of evidence-based care hits the road of teamwork. *Journal of Continuing Education in the Health Professions, 26*(1), 46–54.

3

HUMAN-CENTERED ARTIFICIAL INTELLIGENCE IN HEALTH PROFESSIONS EDUCATION AND DECISION-MAKING

A Sociotechnical Systems Perspective[1]

Jordan Richard Schoenherr

3.1 Introduction to Human-Centered Artificial Intelligence

Healthcare depends on collaboration. No single individual can acquire the skills, competencies, and experience needed to manage the complexity of modern care (Berman et al., 2023; Lingard, 2012; Manser, 2009; Schoenherr et al., 2026). Expertise and situational awareness are distributed across teams, healthcare professions (HCPs), and technologies. Artificial intelligence (AI)[2] has been rapidly adopted in health professions education, clinical practice, and public healthcare delivery. From adaptive learning systems that personalize feedback to diagnostic tools that synthesize complex datasets to public health surveillance platforms that monitor, predict, and coordinate responses to outbreaks, AI technologies are now influencing HCPs' education, clinical decision-making, and public health systems worldwide (Greenhalgh et al., 2017; Kelly et al., 2019; Obermeyer & Emanuel, 2016; Rajkomar et al., 2019; Topol, 2019a; Wartman & Combs, 2018; World Health Organization (WHO), 2021, 2025).

AI status in healthcare has become increasingly ambiguous in recent years (Mittelstadt, 2019; Ghassemi et al., 2021; Morley & Floridi, 2024). While these technologies were introduced as isolated, elementary tools for decision support, they have emerged as agents of care (Coeckelbergh, 2020; Fjeld et al., 2020; Michael et al., 2024; Mittelstadt, 2019; Schoenherr, 2022). This has provoked intense ethical debate, professional resistance, and institutional caution (Char et al., 2018; Michael et al., 2025). Yet AI's value depends on how effectively they are implemented in the classroom, clinical workflows, and healthcare delivery. HCPs, educators, and administrators must understand the validity of algorithms used in learning and care and ensure their application follows ethical and professional

DOI: 10.4324/9781003498155-3

standards (Amann et al., 2020a; Schoenherr & Michael, 2026; Schoenherr, 2022; Schoenherr & Hamstra, 2024; Shortliffe & Sepúlveda, 2018).

AI can structure deliberate practice and individualized assessment, though its capacity to promote specific facets of reflection remains underexamined (Chen et al., 2023; Chan & Zary, 2019; Daniel et al., 2021; Masters, 2019; Wartman & Combs, 2018). AI can also improve early detection and consistency in specific diagnostic tasks. However, whether these systems can support clinician reasoning in conditions of uncertainty is less well-established (Jiang et al., 2017; Liu et al., 2019; Obermeyer & Emanuel, 2016; Rajkomar et al., 2019; Topol, 2019a; Shortliffe & Sepúlveda, 2018). When implemented in both educational and clinical contexts, systems must remain transparent, interpretable, and accountable (Bernstam et al., 2022; Mittelstadt, 2019; Morley & Floridi, 2024; World Health Organization (WHO), 2024a; UNESCO, 2025a).

Technology in healthcare and education should strengthen healthcare delivery and educational practice rather than create obstacles (Amann et al., 2020; Norman & Stappers, 2015; Shneiderman, 2020a, 2020b). However, the introduction of technology often involves trade-offs. Organizations must reskill educators and HCPs, reallocate resources to acquire, maintain, and retire supporting systems (e.g., learning management systems (LMS), electronic health records (EHR), and simulation platforms), and adapt the structure of teams to new workflows. The friction and failures found in technology adoption often stem from limited understanding of how individuals and teams respond to change (Argyris & Schön, 1978; Fullan, 2001; Lewin, 1947). These frameworks were later operationalized to explain why digital tools frequently fail to achieve intended organizational changes without cultural alignment, reflective practice, and participatory design (Kotter, 1996; Mumford, 2006; Schein, 1985). If systems are not designed and implemented with their human users in mind, competence, communication, and trust decline, reducing the quality of learning and care.

3.1.1 A Human-Centered Approach to AI and Sociotechnical Systems

Healthcare must place patients, students, HCPs, and the public at its center, with learning and clinical technologies enhancing the connections between these stakeholders. If their requirements are not addressed, assessments will be invalid, programs fail, and resources are wasted. More troubling, patient outcomes might decline. Inasmuch as credibility can be gained by adopting validated technologies (Schoenherr, 2016), it can also be lost if those technologies are unsupported or poorly aligned with human needs. The authority of the professions depends on aligning technological and institutional change with the values, roles, and competences of practitioners and the healthcare and innovation ecosystem (Leydesdorff & Etzkowitz, 1998; Starr, 1982; Freidson, 2001; Hughes, 1958). If innovations in education or care establish systems without reinforcing human relationships, professional identity, and the social structures that enable trust, the social dimensions of healthcare will erode (Bowker & Star, 1999; Mumford, 1983; Cherns, 1976; Orlikowski, 1992).

A human-centered approach to AI design and implementation must ensure that AI supports patient and learner needs and enhances HCPs' capabilities rather than replacing or subordinating them to systems (Michael et al., 2024; Schoenherr & Michael, 2026; Xu & Gao, 2025). In healthcare delivery and health professions education, technologies must respect health seeker's[3] autonomy, clinical judgment and identity, and institutional responsibility. This approach defines AI as an instrument for improving learning, reasoning, and care, rather than a substitute for human expertise (Ericsson, 2007; Norman & Stappers, 2015; Shneiderman, 2020a, 2020b). Human-centered approaches emphasize understanding the cognitive processes and biases of users, the development and breakdown of collective competence and interpersonal dynamics over time, and how these processes scale from local teams to institutions and health systems (see Table 3.1; Croskerry, 2003; Greenhalgh et al., 2004; Hutchins, 1995; Lingard, 2012; Norman, 1983; Schoenherr et al., 2023; Schoenherr & McConnell, 2024). General approaches such as human-centered design (HCD) and specific formulations such as human-centered AI (HCAI) require focusing on transparency, usability, and accountability throughout development and implementation (see Table 3.1; International Organization for Standardization, 2019; Shneiderman, 2020a, 2020b; Xu & Gao, 2025).

Sociotechnical systems (STSs) theory provides a complementary foundation for HCAI in healthcare delivery and education by adopting a systems-level approach. It recognizes the interdependence between people, organizations, and technologies within complex environments (Baxter & Sommerville, 2011; Bowker & Star, 1999; Cherns, 1976; Emery & Trist, 1960; Mumford, 1983; Orlikowski, 1992; Star & Ruhleder, 1996; Trist & Bamforth, 1951; Shortliffe & Sepúlveda, 2018). AI-based technologies are one subsystem that is interdependent with human agents at multiple levels. This chapter reviews the micro-level interactions between users and systems, the meso-level organizational structures that affect implementation, and the macro-level regulatory and cultural contexts that influence how AI is developed, adopted, and sustained (Carayon et al., 2006; Greenhalgh et al., 2017; Hollnagel, 2017; Sittig & Singh, 2010; Timmermans & Berg, 2003).

In these systems, learners, educators, HCPs, patients, institutions, professional organizations, and regulators all interact. From an STS perspective, the performance of AI depends on how it mediates communication, promotes trust in the healthcare professions and communities which they serve, associated with entrustable professional activities, and the culture of learning within human social networks (Greenhalgh et al., 2017; Hollnagel, 2017).

Improvements in individual components do not guarantee better system performance. The STS approach recognizes that trade-offs emerge as people and institutions adopt, adapt, reject, and de-implement technologies. Changes in

TABLE 3.1 Human-Centered Design Dimensions for AI Systems in the Health Professions

Dimension	*Definition and Focus*	*Primary Responsibility*
Technical/model validity	Accuracy, sensitivity, and specificity of algorithmic outputs; correspondence between model predictions and ground-truth data.	Developers/data scientists
Reliability and robustness	System stability with variable data and operating conditions; accommodates data drift, adversarial inputs, and over-trust.	IT/data science
Security and privacy	Data integrity, confidentiality, access control, and regulatory compliance (e.g., HIPAA/GDPR).	Security/compliance team
Construct/clinical validity	Relevance of algorithmic outputs to intended learners, patients, or public; alignment with domains and constructs.	Health professionals/ educators/institutions/ administrators
Usability and cognitive fit	Interface congruent with user workflow, cognitive load, and situational awareness; visualization and interaction.	Human-factors teams
Interpretability, explainability, and contestability	Interpretable, transparent, and explainable; meaningful human control to contest or override output.	Clinical leads/IT governance
Relationship development and maintenance	Facilitates communication, coordination, trust, and development/ maintenance of professional identity among HCPs, learners, and health seekers.	Administrators/educators
Institutional	Effective and efficient distribution of resources, healthcare delivery, and minimizing medical errors.	Administrators/ institution
Sustainability and lifecycle management	Long-term maintenance, retraining/ reskilling, avoidance of never-skilling, de-implementation, and vendor accountability.	Administrators/vendor/ institution
Ethical and equity review	Fairness across sub-groups, mitigation of bias and harm, ethical oversight and equity monitoring.	Administrators/ethics committee

workload, skill distribution, coordination with AI, and professional autonomy can strengthen or weaken overall performance (Carayon et al., 2011; Kremer et al., 2022). Designing and evaluating AI with human-centered principles can help ensure that innovations support collaboration, sustain therapeutic relationships, improve patient outcomes, and reinforce the institutional structures essential to effective healthcare delivery and education.

In parallel, we must also recognize that there are multiple translational pathways for an innovation to be adopted and adapted from science to clinical practice, from clinical practice to institutional or societal levels, or from societal levels to inform theory and research directions (Schoenherr, 2027b). AI systems that are developed at one level might not scale in an obvious manner, as the field of social forces[4] that define each level can be fundamentally altered depending on the use case and social network properties, e.g., organizational culture, professional values.

3.1.2 AI Use Cases in the Health Professions

Evaluating AI in medicine requires criteria beyond accuracy. AI tools must demonstrate implementation validity: they must perform reliably within the educational or clinical contexts for which they are intended (Cresswell & Sheikh, 2013; Gama et al., 2022; Schoenherr & Hamstra, 2024). A system that functions well in one setting can fail in another when workflow, data quality, infrastructure, expertise, institutional support, or user acceptance differ (Cresswell & Sheikh, 2013; Greenhalgh et al., 2017; Rahimi et al., 2024; Wong et al., 2021). Assessing AI therefore involves determining not only whether it works but whether it works appropriately for specific learners, HCPs, and social and physical environments (Cresswell & Sheikh, 2013; Greenhalgh et al., 2017; Rahimi et al., 2024; World Health Organization (WHO), 2024).

AI applications in healthcare can be grouped by use case, functional properties, and the required level of human oversight within educational, clinical, or public health workflows (Shneiderman, 2020a, 2020b; Topol, 2019a). For instance, educational systems provide structured feedback, deliberate practice, and assessment. Clinical decision-support systems (CDSS) process data to support reasoning, diagnosis, and treatment planning. Administrative and analytic tools manage documentation, scheduling, and quality assurance, indirectly influencing how HCPs and students learn and make decisions. Each AI use case is associated with distinct advantages and challenges (Luxton, 2016; Paranjape et al., 2019; Schwalbe & Wahl, 2020; Topol, 2019a). However, if the challenges are not addressed, they introduce unnecessary risks for their users and data subjects (learners).

When adopting AI-based technologies, stakeholders must weigh system accuracy, efficiency, scalability, and reliability against potential bias, over-reliance and over-trust along with reductions in transparency and explainability (Amann et al., 2020; Matheny et al., 2025; Michael et al., 2024; Schoenherr et al., 2023; Sendak et al., 2020). Systematic evaluation across these criteria is essential. For practitioners and educators, this means examining potential trade-offs at each stage of implementation within a workflow between accuracy and explainability, efficiency and oversight, and automation and awareness (Han et al., 2024; Shortliffe & Sepúlveda, 2018; Tikhomirov et al., 2024). Ideally, this requires the engagement of many stakeholders to understand how they perceive the capabilities and capacities of AI. This chapter focuses on the affordances of AI in healthcare and highlights general implementation considerations.

3.1.3 *Overview*

By adopting a sociotechnical perspective, this chapter examines how AI's affordances impact how HCPs and educators learn, decide, and collaborate within educational institutions and healthcare systems. It provides a concise review and guidance for designing and implementing AI-based systems that enhance competency, safety, and trust in health professions education and clinical decision-making. Section 3.2 outlines the informational, inferential, relational, and organizational affordances of AI and their implications for implementation validity. These basic features define AI's utility in the healthcare professions. Section 3.3 considers these affordances in health professions education in the development of clinical competencies. Section 3.4 examines AI in medical decision-making, including diagnostic reasoning, risk prediction, and collaborative support systems that support clinical judgment and healthcare delivery. Section 3.5 describes the integrative framework by considering how AI has been implemented at scale, examining design and implementation frameworks as well as cybersecurity. The chapter concludes by identifying how HCD and STS principles can be used to ensure that AI adoption remains human-centered.

3.2 Affordances of Artificial Intelligence

When new technologies are introduced into healthcare or education, their value depends on the capabilities they provide and the constraints they impose on the educators and HCPs who use them. Ideally, technologies are adopted because of the utility of their functional affordances relative to human needs (Schoenherr, 2022) and capabilities rather than the prestige (Schoenherr, 2016).

Affordances describe the actions that a technology enables, restricts, or requires (Gibson, 1979; Leonardi, 2011; Norman, 1988; Majchrzak & Markus, 2013). They are not fixed properties of a technology but are the result of interaction between tools, their user, and the environmental. For medical educators and HCPs, recognizing an AI system's affordances is essential for understanding where and when it can support judgment, streamline workflow, or improve feedback, and what systems, processes, or individuals might be affected by organizational change (Cabitza et al., 2017; Ghassemi et al., 2021).

Like all technologies, AI were developed with specific goals in mind. The first generation of artificial neural networks (NN) were developed to process information (McCulloch & Pitts, 1943; Rosenblatt, 1958). In contrast, contemporary AI prioritizes prediction, connection, and adaptation to other systems (Jordan & Mitchell, 2015; LeCun et al., 2015). Despite the many possible functions of AI, they provide social cognitive affordances[5] that are relevant to the health professions (see also Schoenherr

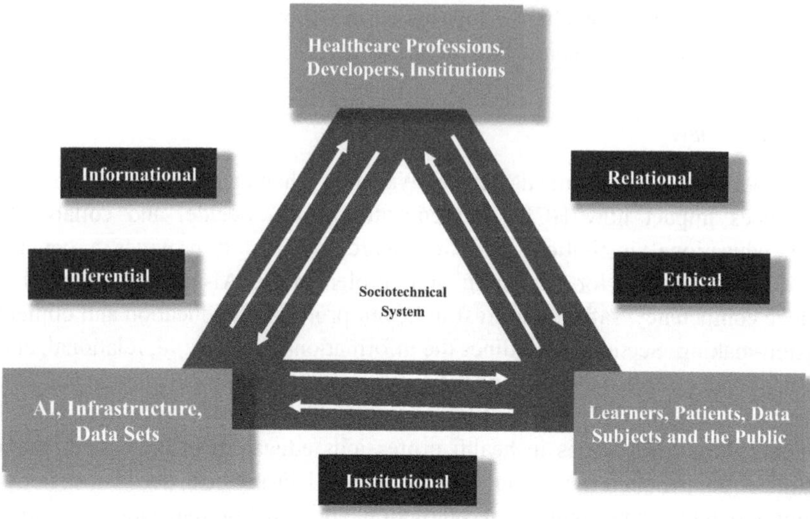

FIGURE 3.1 Affordances with the sociotechnical systems of healthcare. Each human or technological system is associated with its own level of intelligence (I) and granted a level of autonomy (A) by the interactional context. Agents have varying levels of connectivity (C) to each other. Each connection can be unidirectional (independent) or bidirectional (interdependent). Connections define an affordance (informational, inferential, relational, organizational, or ethical) to the agents.

& Michael, 2026; Schoenherr, 2026; Schoenherr, 2027a; Schoenherr, 2027b). These affordances address functional aspects of the STS approach by considering how interaction occurs across different levels (i.e., micro-, macro-, and meso-levels; Baxter & Sommerville, 2011; Carayon et al., 2006). At a general level, four primary affordances can be defined (For their relationship, see Figure 3.1).[6]

Informational Affordances. Informational affordances define how AI systems collect, organize, and present data. In education, adaptive learning platforms can identify performance trends and support students toward targeted practice. In clinical care, AI systems integrate laboratory, imaging, and historical data to create patient records and profiles. These affordances can reduce information overload but are dependent on data quality, timeliness, and model validity (Cabitza et al., 2017; Ghassemi et al., 2021; Judd & Kennedy, 2011; Rajkomar et al., 2019; Sendak et al., 2020).

Inferential Affordances. Inferential affordances define a system's capacity to detect patterns and generate predictions (Caruana et al., 2015; Ribeiro et al., 2016; Amann et al., 2020). In education, AIs can identify learning needs and provide simulation feedback. In clinical decision support, such systems can assist in differential diagnosis, triage, or risk assessment. However, inference without transparency and explainable they can obscure uncertainty and inferential processes and limit user understanding (Caruana et al., 2015; Ghassemi et al., 2021; Ribeiro et al., 2016; Thomson & Schoenherr, 2020).

Relational Affordances. Relational affordances define how AI technologies affect collaboration, authority, and responsibility. In education, AI tutors or dashboards can mediate instructor–student interactions, redistributing the source of feedback, experience, and expertise. In clinical care, AI recommendations can determine how team members discuss diagnoses, assign responsibility, or develop professional relationships and therapeutic alliances. Recognizing these relational effects can promote and maintain human relationships, prevent over-reliance on systems, preserve professional accountability, and reduce the risk of misconduct, including inappropriate reuse or misattribution of AI-generated content (Alam et al., 2023; Benda et al., 2023; Morley & Floridi, 2024; Morris et al., 2018; Nouis et al., 2025; Okamoto et al., 2025; UNESCO, 2025).

Organizational Affordances. Organizational affordances define how AI systems affect workflow, institutional processes, and professional and patient autonomy. Automated documentation, scheduling, and performance-monitoring tools can be used to reduce administrative burden and improve operational consistency (Meskó & Göröget, 2020; Rajkomar et al., 2019). Yet automation can also influence how labor is distributed, how expertise is recognized, and how work is evaluated (Cresswell & Sheikh, 2013; Greenhalgh et al., 2017; Kremer et al., 2022). Integrating predictive analytics or digital documentation can increase cognitive and administrative load if these systems are incongruent with local routines or infrastructure (Cabitza et al., 2017; Rahimi et al., 2024). Effective implementation requires governance and feedback systems that link AI deployment to institutional priorities, workforce well-being, and regulatory frameworks (Matheny et al., 2025; Michael et al., 2024; Sendak et al., 2020). From a sociotechnical perspective, organizational affordances can strengthen individual and collective autonomy, fairness and equity, and sustainability in healthcare and education (Taddeo et al., 2023). For instance, if we recognize that cognitive, social, and technical affordances can lead to institutional discrimination (Schoenherr, 2027a), social or algorithmic processes can be used to mitigated these negative outcomes.

Within AI use cases in health professions education and healthcare delivery, the task for educators, HCPs, and public health professionals is to identify which affordances support or conflict with professional norms, patient safety, institutional efficiency, and learning objectives. HCD principles can support this process by testing systems in relevant contexts, incorporating stakeholder feedback, and refining design through iterative evaluation (Schoenherr &

McConnell, 2024b). To provide evidence for implementation validity, the affordances of AI must be understood within complex, interdependent systems of learning and care (Greenhalgh et al., 2017; Michael et al., 2025; Schoenherr & Hamstra, 2024; Schoenherr & Michael, 2026). In the next section, current and future use cases are identified based on current requirements of competency-based medical education (CBME) and medical decision-making.

3.3 Artificial Intelligence in Health Professions Education

AI-based technologies have been used in healthcare education to support learning, assessment, and curriculum design across disciplines and levels of training (Berman et al., 2023; Feigerlova et al., 2025; Lewis & Sedgwick, 2015; Masters, 2019; Mahmood, 2023; Navarro-Bringas et al., 2020; Özkan & Göl, 2024; Sadiq et al., 2025; Steel et al., 2025; Strielkowski, 2025) (Figure 3.2; see Table 3.2 for an overview). When implemented using HCD principles, these systems can increase educators' and learners' capacity to observe, analyze, practice, and reflect through adaptive feedback and simulation tools (Cant & Cooper, 2021; Cook et al., 2010; Dawson et al., 2022; Zary et al., 2019). The redistribution of information processing tasks between educators and learners can improve feedback and efficiency but can also create reasoning biases if users misunderstand how people think and learn individually or in groups (Croskerry, 2013; Norman et al., 2017; Schoenherr, in preparation a). AI in education must therefore be assessed for both technical accuracy along with its capacity to support human judgment, reflection, and collective decision-making (Frank et al., 2010; Holmboe et al., 2010; van der Vleuten et al., 2012).

3.3.1 *Supporting Learning and Feedback*

AI is used in health professions education to improve learning, assessment, and program evaluation (Guze, 2015; Han et al., 2022; Moran et al., 2018; Ruiz et al., 2006; Vozenilek et al., 2004). Simulation and clinical rehearsal remain the most established applications (Cant & Cooper, 2021; Cook et al., 2010; Dawson et al., 2022; Zary et al., 2019). Intelligent simulation systems and virtual patients allow learners to rehearse complex cases under educator supervision in safe, controlled settings. Algorithms adjust difficulty, vary presentations, and deliver individualized feedback through adaptive modeling and automated assessment (García-Torres et al., 2024; Khakpaki et al., 2025).

Within CBME, these simulations can map observed actions to performance milestones and competencies, supporting entrustment decisions and personalized learning trajectories (Frank et al., 2010; Holmboe et al., 2010; ten Cate & Taylor, 2020).

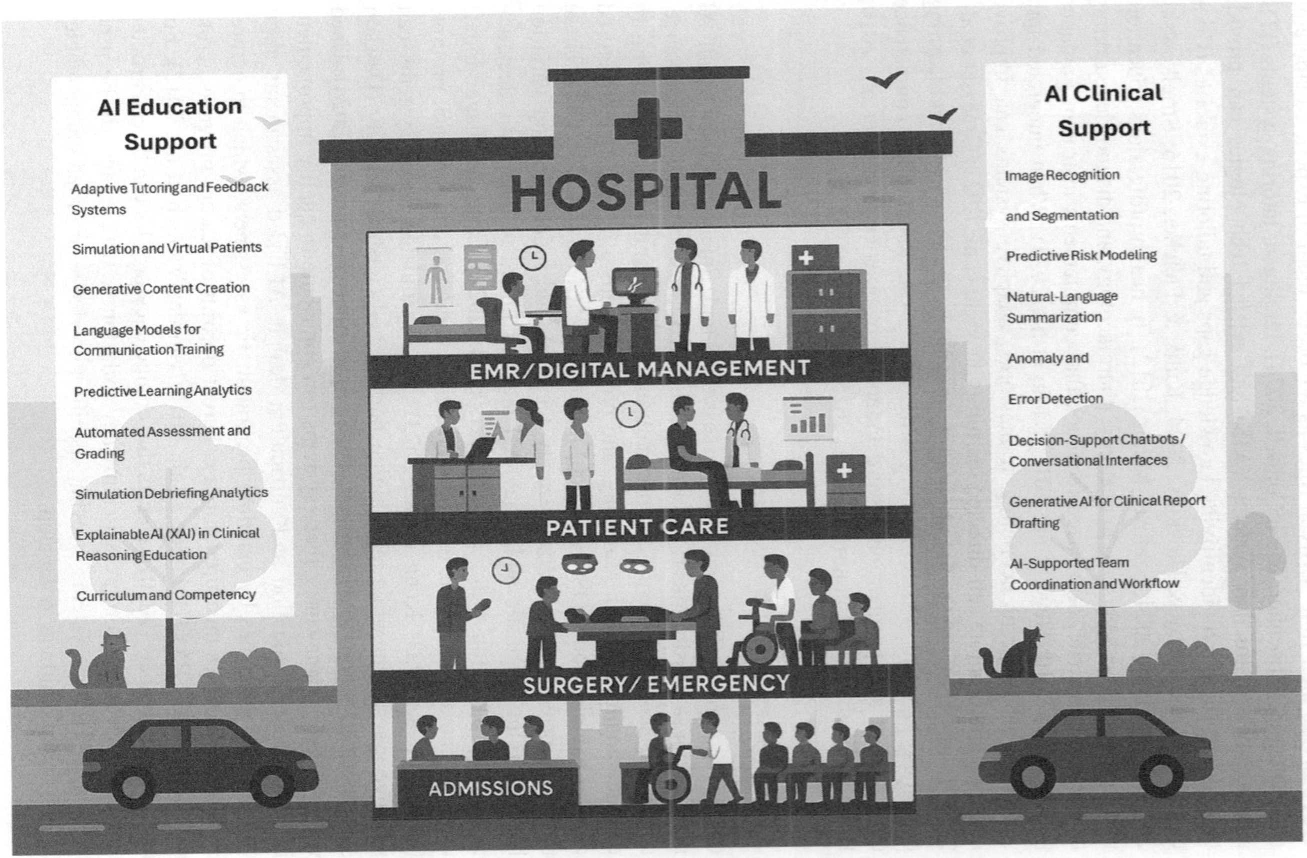

FIGURE 3.2 AI support functions have affected healthcare professionals' education and delivery.

3.3.1.1 Simulation and Adaptive Learning

HCPs divide their time between roles as advocate, medical expert, collaborator, and educator (Schoenherr & McConnell. 2024). Intelligent tutoring systems (ITS) and adaptive instruction systems (AIS) and related technologies can provide targeted instruction by identifying knowledge gaps and tailoring exercises (Cook et al., 2013; du Plooy & Hawkins, 2024; Kulik & Fletcher, 2016; Strielkowski, 2025; Schoenherr, 2024; Szafir & Mutlu, 2012). In health professions education, these systems have been used in anatomy, pharmacology, and diagnostic reasoning to deliver immediate, data-based feedback that complements instructor guidance (Cook et al., 2010; Hege et al., 2011; Sadiq et al., 2025). When integrated into structured feedback or debriefing frameworks, adaptive systems can improve retention and promote self-directed learning (de Melo et al., 2021; Graesser et al., 2018; Lomis et al., 2023). By aligning automated feedback to EPAs and learning outcomes, ITS and AIS reinforce CBME's focus on longitudinal competence development and progression toward independent practice (Frank et al., 2010; Holmboe et al., 2010; Létourneau et al., 2025; Schoenherr, 2024).

3.3.1.2 Assessment and Feedback

CBME requires valid, continuous assessment and timely feedback, with AI providing new possibilities (Feigerlova et al., 2025; Masters, 2019). For instance, automated scoring systems can use natural language and image processing to evaluate communication, reasoning, and professionalism in objective structured clinical examinations (OSCEs; Luordo et al., 2025; Misra et al., 2024). These tools can provide standardized, timely feedback and reduce grading variation by identifying linguistic and behavioral markers linked to diagnostic accuracy and empathy (Cotton et al., 2023; Masters et al., 2024). Large language models used to generate and refine examination items, vignettes, and feedback prompts (Gilson et al., 2023; Kung et al., 2023). When validated, these systems can improve assessment while maintaining fairness and construct validity (Dawson & Sutherland-Smith, 2023; Sallam, 2023; Schoenherr & Hamstra, 2024). Used within CBME frameworks, these systems can contribute to quality improvement in both learner evaluation and curriculum design. AI-based assessments align with CBME principles by enabling programmatic assessment, which integrates multiple low-stakes measures into a coherent portrait of learner progress across milestones and EPAs (Holmboe et al., 2010; van der Vleuten et al., 2012). For instance, Schoenherr (2020) suggests that competency profiles can be constructed to assess a learner's progress toward key milestones, which can also be used to inform ITS/AIS systems on what specific knowledge or broad competencies learners must continue to develop.

TABLE 3.2 Health Professions Education AI Use Cases

Function	*Educational Use Cases*	*Primary Affordance*	*HCD Considerations*
Adaptive tutoring and feedback systems	Intelligent tutoring in anatomy, pharmacology, or procedural skills	Personalized pacing, targeted feedback, and improved retention	Maintain educator oversight; ensure feedback accuracy and fairness
Simulation and virtual patients	Case-based reasoning, diagnostic scenarios, and ethics simulations	Safe, repeatable clinical practice with real-time feedback	Balance fidelity with accessibility; debrief to reinforce reflection
Generative content creation	Automated question/ item generation, case vignettes, and test banks	Expands learning materials efficiently	Require expert review; validate content alignment with objectives
Language models for communication training	Patient interviewing, counseling, and interprofessional dialogue	Realistic conversational practice and feedback	Include empathy cues and cultural sensitivity; clarify model role
Predictive learning analytics	Monitoring learner progress and predicting performance gaps	Early identification of at-risk learners and tailored remediation	Use anonymized data; avoid stigmatization and opaque scoring
Automated assessment and grading	MCQ, OSCE documentation, reflective writing	Consistent, scalable feedback	Maintain transparency; allow instructor override
Simulation debriefing analytics	NLP and video analysis of simulation sessions	Enhances reflection and instructor feedback quality	Prioritize psychological safety; retain human facilitator control
Explainable AI (XAI) in clinical reasoning education	Decision-support teaching tools in diagnostic reasoning courses	Promotes metacognition and understanding of reasoning steps	Present interpretable rationales; encourage learners to challenge outputs
Curriculum and competency mapping tools	Analyzing course objectives, assessment coverage, and alignment	Informs curriculum design and accreditation readiness	Ensure data accuracy; allow manual adjustments by faculty
Generative AI for educational resource design	Synthesizing reading lists, summaries, or visual explanations	Supports educator productivity and access to knowledge	Require source transparency; attribute original materials

3.3.1.3 *Learning Analytics and Curriculum Evaluation*

AI-based learning analytics can support curriculum design and evaluation (Chen et al., 2023; Ifenthaler & Yau, 2020). Aggregated learning data identify competencies requiring reinforcement and inform curricular revisions. Predictive analytics detect learners needing academic or clinical support early in training (Gázquez-García et al., 2025; Khalil & Ebner, 2016; Nguyen et al., 2024). Transparent validation, educator co-design, and fairness auditing are essential to preserve validity, accountability, and learner trust (Abbas et al., 2021a, 2021b; Cross et al., 2024; Ifenthaler & Schumacher, 2016; Michael et al., 2024; Saqr et al., 2023; Schoenherr et al., 2023). Within CBME, learning analytics operationalize evidence-based progress monitoring, linking performance data to defined milestones and entrustment decisions while supporting early remediation and individualized learning plans.

3.3.1.4 *Faculty Development and Digital Professionalism*

The use of AI for instruction and assessment requires explicit inclusion in faculty development and professional competency frameworks (Berman et al., 2023; Coiera, 2019; Ma, 2024; Masters et al., 2024). Educators and learners must interpret AI outputs, identify bias, and understand algorithmic design principles (Long et al., 2020; Ng et al., 2024). These skills reinforce lifelong learning and adaptive expertise within professional development frameworks (Mehta et al., 2025; Shimizu et al., 2023), supporting UNESCO (2025) and World Health Organization (WHO) (2024) calls for AI literacy and ethical integration in health professions education. CBME emphasizes faculty competencies in assessment, feedback, and supervision. AI literacy can support these capabilities by enabling educators to align algorithmic feedback with milestone judgments, reflective practice, and empathic teaching (Chan et al., 2024; Sallam, 2023).

3.3.2 *Cognitive Development and Diagnostic Reasoning*

Traditionally, healthcare competencies are based on the need to develop diagnostic expertise, communication and interpersonal skills, and collaborative care. This requires understanding how HCPs learn the patterns associated with illness, reason about diagnoses and treatment alternatives, identify critical decision points, and can stop to deliberate (Croskerry, 2009; Klein, 1993; Norman & Brooks, 1997; Schmidt & Rikers, 2007).

3.3.2.1 *Pattern Recognition and Diagnostic Expertise*

Pattern recognition is a central feature of medical expertise. It allows clinicians to connect perceptual cues with underlying causal mechanisms and retrieve relevant illness scripts efficiently (Norman et al., 2007; Schmidt & Rikers, 2007). AI can enhance this learning by exposing students to varied, cases in imaging, pathology, and dermatology (Brinker et al., 2022; Cant & Cooper, 2021; Cook et al., 2010; Khosravi et al., 2024; Winkler-Schwartz et al., 2019). Moreover, attentional methods have been proposed to display which image regions influence predictions, though their reliability as explanations of model reasoning remains contested (Rudin, 2019; Ghassemi et al., 2021).

AI-supported modules can combine annotated image libraries with automated feedback on diagnostic accuracy. Moreover, while longitudinal tracking of interpretation development over training is untested (Park et al., 2022; Tun et al., 2025). Repeated exposure assist learners in distinguishing normal from abnormal and recognize atypical findings earlier. Within CBME, these structured experiences provide evidence for diagnostic reasoning milestones. Analytics representing accuracy, biases, response time, and case diversity contribute to programmatic assessment, extending diagnostic training beyond case scarcity while maintaining educator oversight and accountability (Bilgic et al., 2024; Frank et al., 2010; van der Vleuten et al., 2012).

3.3.2.2 Clinical Reasoning and Metacognitive Development

Clinical expertise defines the core of professional competence and identity (Norman, 2005, ten Cate et al., 2016). HCD principles ensure that cognitive capabilities and limitations inform design about how humans and systems interact (Berman et al., 2023; Carayon et al., 2006). Expertise develops through repeated exposure to clinical cases that vary in presentation and context (Grierson, 2014). Such variability allows learners to build a robust understanding of the diagnostic features, situational factors, and constraints that shape the challenges faced by HCPs in practice (Schmidt & Rikers, 2007). AI can enhance decision-making and diagnostic reasoning by providing structured exposure to cases, feedback, and reflection (Rajkomar et al., 2019). Integrated into CBME, these systems can scaffold learners' progression from novice to proficient levels of entrustment by explicitly mapping diagnostic reasoning to defined EPAs and cognitive milestones.

3.3.2.3 AI-Supported Diagnostic and Group Learning

Case-based environments that embed AI tools can train learners to test hypotheses, compare reasoning with algorithmic outputs, and analyze discrepancies, fostering metacognitive awareness (Norman et al., 2017; Sujan et al., 2023). In small-group and problem-based learning (PBL) curricula, AI-generated patient summaries and diagnostic suggestions can promote collaborative reflection (Hege et al., 2011; Kononowicz et al., 2019). These applications advance CBME goals by supporting observable behaviors across teamwork, communication, and clinical reasoning competencies, enabling educators to make structured entrustment decisions grounded in authentic practice.

3.4 Artificial Intelligence in Medical Decision-Making

AI is also embedded within workflows directly and indirectly across healthcare systems, from private practices to hospitals and public health settings (Jiang et al., 2017; Topol, 2019a, 2019b). Its capacity to collect, integrate, and analyze data enables personalized care, risk prediction, and outcome monitoring (Kelly et al., 2019; Rajkomar et al., 2019). Effective implementation requires that professional competencies are strengthened, ethical standards are upheld, and AI systems support the therapeutic relationship between HCPs and patients (Amann et al., 2020; Beil et al., 2019; Coiera, 2021; Morley et al., 2020). As in education, AI should not replace human reasoning, moral judgment, or communication. In settings where resources are constrained or access to care is limited, AI can improve precision, efficiency, and continuity of care within and beyond the clinical environment if created and implemented with HCD principles (Cascella et al., 2023; Jha et al., 2008). Table 3.3 summarizes current applications of AI in medical decision-making.

3.4.1 AI for Individual Clinical Reasoning and Decision Support

HCD requires that we consider what individual patients, practitioners, and technological artifacts independently contribute to performance, to identify how their interaction can be organized to improve clinical outcomes and avoid cognitive overload. Effective integration requires understanding the cognitive limitations and decision points that define clinical procedures and recognizing when information supports decision-making while avoiding the introduction of extraneous cognitive overload (Schoenherr et al., 2024; see Schoenherr, 2027b).

3.4.1.1 Early Detection and Screening

Retrospective evaluations report AI matching or exceeding expert accuracy in diabetic retinopathy, breast cancer, and tuberculosis screening (Khosravi et al., 2024; McKinney et al., 2020). However, such results have limited reproducibility (Haibe-Kains et al., 2020), and prospective multi-system evaluations show more variable performance. They can act as triage aids that prioritize high-risk cases and reduce clinician workload (Rodriguez-Ruiz et al., 2019; Ting et al., 2017). Performance varies across populations and data sources, requiring independent validation and recalibration (Adamson & Smith, 2018; Ghassemi et al., 2021; Kelly et al., 2019; Lekadir et al., 2025; Rajkomar et al., 2019; World Health Organization (WHO), 2024).

Early detection tools must be designed around HCPs' diagnostic workflow, patients' values, and the organizational context in which they are used. Following HCD principles (Carayon et al., 2006; Shneiderman, 2020a, 2020b; Sittig & Singh,

2010), developers should co-design interfaces with radiologists and technologists to fit routine reading sequences, minimize cognitive load, and make model confidence and rationale explicit, i.e. chain-of-thought. System outputs should demonstrate why a case was flagged and how confidence is affected by properties of images or sound, to promote explainability and contestability. Implementation requires iterative usability testing, feedback loops for model accuracy and confidence calibration, and post-deployment monitoring to ensure performance remains safe, transparent, and equitable (World Health Organization (WHO), 2024).

3.4.1.2 Development of Models for Scaffolding in Tissue Engineering

In addition to processing information, AI can be used to design, optimize, and fabricate three-dimensional scaffolds that replicate anatomical architecture. Recent reviews have examined how AI supports scaffold design, bioprinting processes, materials selection, and performance prediction for multiple tissues (Gharibshahian et al., 2024; Jeznach et al., 2024; Kolomenskaya et al., 2023; Wu et al., 2024). AI-based design can generate patient-specific structures based on clinicians' goals, reducing trial-and-error and improving model fidelity (Liu et al., 2023). While promising, these approaches require high-quality multimodal datasets (e.g., imaging, materials testing, and bioprinting telemetry) and rigorous experimental and clinical validation before routine use (Jammalamadaka & Tappa, 2018; Kolomenskaya et al., 2023) (Box 3.1).

BOX 3.1 AFFORDANCES OF HUMAN–DIGITAL TWINS

A human–digital twin is a dynamic computational model of an individual that integrates genomic, physiological, behavioral, and environmental data to simulate and forecast health trajectories (Bruynseels et al., 2018; Björnsson et al., 2020; Schoenherr, in press). These models enable continuous risk estimation and virtual testing of therapeutic strategies, allowing clinicians to anticipate treatment response, reduce adverse events, and support precision dosing (Corral-Acero et al., 2020; Ammar et al., 2023). On a larger scale, population-level twins are used in critical and chronic care to predict sepsis or heart failure by comparing real-time data with simulated trajectories from similar cases (Viceconti et al., 2021).

HDTs illustrate key affordances of AI in medicine. Their *informational affordances* integrate multimodal data into a coherent representation of patient state. Their *inferential affordances* support real-time prediction and simulation. Their *relational affordances* connect clinicians, patients, and models in continuous dialogue. Finally, their *institutional affordances* affect how public health surveillance collects and uses data and how this data informs policy, affects governance structures, and integrates with the wider healthcare system.

HCD principles require that we consider how HDTs are used by HCPs and health seekers (Bruynseels et al., 2018; Viceconti et al., 2021). Based on their affordances, four broad sets of concerns are apparent. Excessive or poorly structured data can overload working memory, making it harder to identify clinically relevant patterns. Opaque reasoning processes limit users' ability to evaluate and calibrate judgments, reducing trust in model outputs. The outputs of HDT must be explainable to the individuals assessing the data and to those who are the targets of HDTs. As agents with limited attentional and working memory capacities, constant alerts and interactive interfaces can divide attention, adversely affecting situational awareness and impairing sustained clinical reasoning if not well designed. Health seekers might also choose to rely on HDTs when HCPs are available due to comparative convenience. Unclear governance and accountability can lead to diffusion of responsibility, weakening reflective practice and learning from biases and errors (Amann et al., 2020; Morley & Floridi, 2024; for psychological processes, see Schoenherr & Thomson, 2024).

Regenerative medicine exemplifies HCD by integrating the expertise of software and materials engineers, HCPs, and patients throughout the innovation process. Material properties such as mechanical strength and implantability must be design for specific patient needs, including health beliefs, compliance, pain tolerance, and immune responsiveness. These factors influence both procedural outcomes and long-term compatibility. Effective implementation depends on the collective competence of multidisciplinary surgical teams, who translate computational models and bioprinted constructs into safe, reproducible clinical interventions (Carayon et al., 2006; Kolomenskaya et al., 2023).

3.4.1.3 Diagnostic Reasoning and Decision Support

Studies have frequently demonstrated that algorithmic decision-making can be equivalent to or exceed unaided clinical judgment, with an average ~10% accuracy advantage in meta-analysis (Ægisdóttir et al., 2006; Goldberg, 1970; Grove et al., 2000; Meehl, 1954), supporting the use of AI in diagnostic reasoning. CDSS are among the earliest algorithmic tools used in medicine, designed to help HCPs synthesize data and generate diagnostic hypotheses (Berner & La Lande, 2007; Gorry & Barnett, 1968; Gorry, 1973; Sutton et al., 2020). These systems integrate structured and unstructured information such as laboratory results, imaging data, and clinical notes to improve clinicians' diagnostic accuracy and treatment planning (Ouanes et al., 2024; Rajkomar et al., 2019). In time sensitive practices such as emergency medicine, CDSS can rapidly analyze patient data to identify conditions that might otherwise be overlooked, such as sepsis or myocardial infarction (Henry

TABLE 3.3 Healthcare Delivery AI Use Cases

Function	*Clinical/Public Health Use Case*	*Primary Benefit*	*HCD Considerations*
Image recognition and segmentation	Radiology, dermatology, pathology	Early anomaly detection, faster screening	Display uncertainty; allow annotation and override
Predictive risk modeling	ICU triage, sepsis alerts, readmission prediction	Early warning and prioritization	Provide reasoning trace; avoid alarm fatigue
Natural-language summarization	Electronic health records, discharge summaries	Reduce documentation time	Support clinician review and correction
Anomaly and error detection	EHR data integrity, drug interactions	Identifies incomplete or contradictory entries	Display flagged data with context, not hard stops
Decision-support chatbots/ conversational interfaces	Primary care triage, telemedicine	Accessible symptom assessment and guidance	Provide clear disclaimers, escalation pathways
Generative AI for clinical report drafting	Radiology, pathology	Increased reporting speed, standardization	Retain human sign-off; flag uncertain findings
AI-supported team coordination and workflow optimization	Predictive scheduling, patient-flow management, and interdisciplinary handover support	Improves collective competence, reduces delays, and enhances communication across care teams	Co-design dashboards with frontline staff; ensure transparency of resource-allocation logic; preserve accountability and shared situational awareness
Mobile and decentralized health platforms	Community screening, rural telemedicine, mHealth for maternal and chronic-disease care	Extends reach of care to low-resource and remote settings; supports continuity and equity of access	Design for offline use and low bandwidth; co-design with community health workers; ensure data privacy and ethical governance
Multimodal data fusion	Imaging, labs, and EHR	Comprehensive view of patient state	Clarify data provenance and update logic
Explainable AI (XAI) interfaces	All diagnostic contexts	Transparency and trust calibration	Tailor explanations to mental models

et al., 2015; Nemati et al., 2018). In internal medicine, CDSS can assist with differential diagnoses, by suggesting next diagnostic steps, and recommending evidence-based interventions (Cabitza et al., 2017; Shortliffe & Sepúlveda, 2018).

The value and risks of AI in healthcare were recognized early in the development of decision-support systems, representing one of the first discussions of what is now termed explainable AI (Gorry & Barnett, 1968; Gorry, 1973; Schoenherr, 2024). Explainable AI techniques can make model reasoning apparent through reasoning traces ('chain-of-thought'), saliency mapping, confidence scores, or ranked evidence lists that parallel clinical reasoning steps (Hoffman et al., 2018; Mohseni et al., 2023; Schoenherr, 2021). When integrated into EHRs, these systems can provide context-specific prompts and alerts that reinforce adherence to evidence-based guidelines (Benda et al., 2023; Sendak et al., 2020). However, caution is required, as explanations can create unwarranted confidence when they are incomplete or misleading (Gilpin et al., 2018; Rudin, 2019; Sun et al., 2025; Thomson & Schoenherr, 2020). Generative AI models are particularly prone to 'hallucinations', producing plausible but inaccurate explanations that can distort clinical judgment (Ji et al., 2023; Schoenherr, 2026c).

Effective CDSS must integrate seamlessly into individual cognitive and organizational workflows. Human attentional and working memory limitations necessitate interfaces that are simple, use adjustable alert thresholds, and provide results and recommendations in a manner consistent with clinical competencies. The automaticity that defines expertise (Schoenherr et al., 2024) also requires that we identify which decision points in a procedure information can be provided during that will not interfere with reasoning. Outside of this critical period, shifts in attention caused by alerts, information, or recommendations might be disregarded or discounted or distract a clinician during a critical event (Schoenherr, 2027b). Usability testing with diverse clinician groups should be used to identify gaps between real and perceived accuracy and reduce over-reliance by aligning AI support with the needs of HCPs (Shneiderman, 2020a, 2020b; Sittig & Singh, 2010).

3.4.1.4 Prognosis and Risk Prediction

Predictive analytics are a critical tool of AI in medical decision-making. Machine learning models can estimate outcomes such as mortality, readmission, or disease progression using longitudinal data from health records, imaging, and wearable biosensors (Kelly et al., 2019; Rajkomar et al., 2019). In intensive-care settings, AI-based early warning systems can continuously monitor vital signs and detect clinical deterioration hours before conventional scoring systems (Henry et al., 2015; Singh et al., 2024). In chronic-disease management, risk-prediction algorithms can identify patients who might benefit from early intervention or follow-up (Bertsimas et al., 2018; Nakayama et al., 2023; Rahimi et al., 2024) (Box 3.2).

BOX 3.2 BEYOND FOLKMEDICAL TECHNOLOGIES DECENTRALIZED AUTONOMOUS HEALTHCARE PROVISIONS

Mobile phone applications, digital platforms, and AI-based systems represent a largely unregulated form of 'new folk medicine' (Schoenherr, 2021a, 2022c). When properly regulated and integrated within public health frameworks, decentralized autonomous healthcare systems can provide an accessible means of extending essential services to underserved populations or residents of remote regions. Rather than depending exclusively on centralized infrastructure, this approach combines mobile devices, AI-enabled decision support, and community-based providers to form local health nodes that operate semi-autonomously yet remain connected through federated learning, data exchange protocols, and collaborative oversight. While not yet implemented on a large integrated scale, such systems could address care delivery gaps in resource-scarce contexts, including low- and middle-income countries and conflict-affected regions (Schoenherr & Ginsburg, submitted).

Applications of Mobile and AI-Enabled Health Tools

In sub-Saharan Africa, AI-enhanced mobile diagnostic tools have demonstrated feasibility for decentralized screening. For instance, a multi country initiative used federated learning on chest-radiography datasets to improve tuberculosis detection while maintaining patient privacy in limited bandwidth conditions (Fabila et al., 2025). Similarly, AI-assisted smartphone ophthalmoscopy in Kenya and Ghana increased diabetic-retinopathy screening coverage and referral accuracy compared with conventional community screening (Daniel et al., 2021). In India, rural telemedicine networks employ AI algorithms for ECG and ultrasound interpretation to assist non-specialist providers. Mobile maternal health platforms such as *Swasthya Slate* and *Sakhi* have improved early detection of pregnancy complications and reduced unnecessary referrals (Nagraj et al, 2023; Pérez et al., 2025). In the Pacific Islands, hybrid offline and online mHealth systems that integrate satellite links and AI-assisted diagnostics, such as the *CommCare Pacific* pilot, have maintained continuity of care for dispersed populations with intermittent connectivity (Were, 2022; World Health Organization (WHO), 2023).

Implementation and Policy Implications

Examined across these initiatives, three priorities are apparent. First, edge usability and inclusivity ensure that mobile and AI tools can be used effectively by community health workers with varying levels of digital literacy. Second, contextual adaptation and governance must embed co-design, feedback loops, and ethical data sharing agreements to preserve local autonomy. Third, sustainability and oversight link algorithmic transparency with model retraining and integration into national health-information systems where feasible. For medical educators and practitioners, these decentralized architectures exemplify a human-centered approach to AI: technologies that enhance decision-making, sustain continuity of care, and promote equitable access while preserving professional accountability.

However, the practical value of prediction depends on the congruence of training data and the target population, how these tools are integrated into workflow, and communication protocols. Alerts must reach individuals and teams that can act in a timely manner, be configured to limit false positives, and avoid alarm fatigue that can promote complacency (Benda et al., 2023; Ratwani et al., 2018; Sendak et al., 2020). Predictive systems should also present an explanation that reduces uncertainty, mitigates overconfidence bias, and eliminates misinterpretation (Leslie et al., 2021; World Health Organization (WHO), 2024). Training and simulation exercises can assess cognitive load and trust calibration, ensuring that predictions support individual and team situational awareness and coordination (Carayon et al., 2006; Schoenherr, in preparation b; Sittig & Singh, 2010).

3.4.1.5 Surgical Preparation and Planning

In surgical preparation and planning, AI systems can generate patient-specific 3D reconstructions, perform automated segmentation, and predict perioperative risk (Bagaria & Chaudary, 2017; Chen et al., 2025; Fadero et al., 2014; van Leeuwen et al., 2022). Systematic reviews demonstrate that AI-driven planning tools can improve anatomical visualization, shorten planning time, and enhance implant or prosthetic alignment over specialties including orthopedics, spine surgery, and cranio-maxillofacial reconstruction (Johnson et al., 2022; Geda et al., 2024; Varghese et al., 2024). Machine learning models can process preoperative imaging, evaluate anatomical complexity, and suggest optimal surgical approaches or instrument configurations, allowing surgeons to focus on judgment, practice, and execution. Effective use requires transparent reliability metrics, interpretability, and integration with existing imaging and navigation workflows to maintain clinical safety and professional accountability (Lin & Kuo, 2023; Nguyen et al., 2024).

Previous studies have demonstrated that surgical ability is associated with visuospatial and mental rotation ability, which in turn are linked to short-term and working memory capacity (Hegarty & Sims, 1994; Keehner et al., 2004; Wanzel et al., 2002; cf. Millington et al., 2017; Schoenherr et al., 2018). To be effective tools for preparation and planning, we must consider how the process of mental model construction, bias, and change is affected by feedback and reflection during task performance (Gentner & Stevens, 1983; Norman, 1983). Interfaces should present confidence intervals, allow user adjustments and overrides, and capture feedback on prediction accuracy to support metacognitive calibration (Koriat, 2012; Schoenherr et al., 2018; Schoenherr et al., 2024). Physical ergonomics and time pressure must be considered alongside algorithmic reliability (Carayon et al., 2006; Carayon et al., 2021; Holden et al., 2013; Kaplan et al., 2023).

3.4.2 AI for Team-Based, Organizational, and Population-Level Systems

An AI-STS approach in healthcare requires that we look beyond individual patients, practitioners, and technological artifacts to consider the social subsystems within general practices, hospitals, and public health settings. These subsystems function at the meso- (e.g., groups, teams, and organizational units) and macro-level (e.g., institutional, regulatory, and societal domains). Each level has its own conventional goals (e.g., interpersonal accord, organizational efficiency), constraints (e.g., time pressure, workflows), and feedback mechanisms (e.g., quick and *ad hoc*, systematic and cyclical). Importantly, the ways in which competencies are defined, trained, and measured can differ across institutional and cultural contexts, influencing how AI is designed, implemented, evaluated, and de-implemented (Carayon et al., 2006; Schoenherr & Michael, 2026).

3.4.2.1 Collaborative Systems Supporting Collective Competence

Healthcare delivery depends on teamwork rather than individual expertise. Most clinical care is provided by interdisciplinary teams whose coordination relies on effective information management, overlapping mental models and situational awareness, and collective decision-making (Lingard, 2012; Manser, 2009). AI systems can facilitate collaboration by improving data sharing, communication, and workflow coordination (Carayon et al., 2014; Lee et al., 2025; Sittig & Singh, 2010; Tun et al., 2025). Shared dashboards can integrate data from radiology, laboratory, pharmacy, and nursing documentation into unified, updated patient profiles (Khosravi et al., 2024; Rahimi et al., 2024). Predictive analytics can identify patients who require multidisciplinary review or early intervention (Lee et al., 2025; Sendak et al., 2020). In oncology, integrated AI systems have enhanced tumor-board preparation and treatment planning by combining imaging, genomic, and clinical data (Khosravi et al., 2024).

AI systems can also be used during clinical handover, a persistent source of communication failures and medical errors (Abraham et al., 2022; Starmer et al., 2014). Summarization tools can create structured handover reports highlighting key changes in condition, treatment, and follow-up needs prospectively improving the completeness, clarity, and efficiency in AI-mediated reports (Jin et al., 2023;

Wang & Zhang, 2024). Moreover, at the organizational level, predictive scheduling systems optimize resource allocation and team composition (Birkhoff et al., 2023; Gupta et al., 2025).

HCD can facilitate collaboration as a sociotechnical process that integrates human communication, information systems, and organizational structure. Co-design with frontline HCPs ensures that dashboards and handover tools can facilitate typical conversational practices and respect professional roles (Abbas et al., 2021a, 2021b). This requires understanding the social scripts and formal procedures used to communicate (Schoenherr & LeBouar, 2025). Evaluation should examine shared mental models, workload, and the distribution of situational awareness among team members (for broader discussions, see Schoenherr, under review; Schoenherr & Michael, 2026). Professional societies and regulatory bodies must ensure that verification procedures clearly define how responsibility is allocated between practitioners, administrators, and AI systems (Carayon et al., 2006; Morley et al., 2020; Sittig & Singh, 2010).

3.4.2.2 Organizational Efficiency and Change Management

In addition to cognitive efficiency of individual HCPs, HCPs must also ensure the efficient use of organizational resources (Schoenherr et al., 2024). Institutional process such as workforce optimization, patient-flow management, and administrative decision support have also been a recent focus of systems development (Rajkomar et al., 2019; Meskó et al., 2023). Predictive scheduling and logistics models can forecast patient admissions, optimize staff assignments, and bed allocation, contributing to measurable efficiency gains and reduced waiting times (Birkhoff et al., 2023; Gupta et al., 2025). In parallel, intelligent documentation and triage systems have been used to automate repetitive administrative tasks, freeing HCPs for delivering care (Kelly et al., 2019; Topol, 2019b).

Such affordances suggest that AI-driven operational management systems can improve workflow coordination, shorten turnaround times, and influence efficiency and care quality. For instance, a recent hospital-wide implementation in Saudi Arabia demonstrated that AI-supported operations management improved process visibility, interdepartmental communication, and patient care coordination, particularly when paired with staff training and leadership engagement (Abbasi et al., 2024).

Integration of AI at an institutional level requires mapping existing workflows and identifying points of friction that automation can likely improve (Carayon et al., 2006; Sittig & Singh, 2010). Co-design with managers, HCPs, and administrative personnel is critical to align algorithmic recommendations with organizational culture and accountability structures (Abbas et al., 2025; Shneiderman, 2022; World Health Organization (WHO), 2024). Change-management research shows that leadership involvement, stakeholder engagement, and feedback loops determine whether AI systems are adopted or abandoned (Fullan, 2001; Kotter, 1996; Schein, 1985; Yildiz et al., 2025). When used appropriately, AI can become an instrument for organizational learning, enabling systematic monitoring, feedback, and adaptation within complex healthcare systems (Carayon et al., 2006; Sittig & Singh, 2010).

3.4.2.3 Public Healthcare

Public health appears to be the best possible use case for AI, with large, diverse populations and datasets, limited resources, and a critical need to promote equitable, timely interventions and preventative care. When implemented with transparent governance and human oversight, AI can strengthen surveillance, triage, and resource allocation improving population-level outcomes (da Silva Jr et al., 2024; Miller, 2024; Panteli, 2025; World Health Organization (WHO), 2024). AI supports epidemiologic surveillance and chronic-disease monitoring by integrating imaging, laboratory, environmental, and behavioral data streams (Esteva et al., 2017; Lowe et al., 2023; Madhi et al., 2024; Rajkomar et al., 2019). Population-level modelling can lead to earlier outbreak detection and resource prioritization (Nguyen et al., 2024; Wong et al., 2025). Predictive analytics can be used to forecast hospital demand, optimize staffing, and anticipate medication shortages (Meskó et al., 2023; Rahimi et al., 2024).

Public health has the greatest need for co-design processes within HCD, bringing together local health workers, end users, health agencies, non-governmental organizations (NGOs), and developers to ensure accessibility, language appropriateness, and contextual fit (Schoenherr & Grubesic, in preparation). Transparency, data-literacy support, and participatory governance reinforce legitimacy and trust. Implementation frameworks such as NASSS (Greenhalgh et al., 2017) and World Health Organization (WHO) (2024) guidance emphasize adaptability, sustainability, and equitable impact across demographic and infrastructural contexts.

3.5 Implementation Considerations

The preceding sections demonstrate that AI is, or can be, embedded in many areas of healthcare. Understanding AI's informational, inferential, relational, and organizational affordances reveals both its potential benefits and risks. However, these affordances emerge only through human–AI interaction. Improvements in diagnosis, coordination, and access to care require evaluation of each system's implementation validity within its intended context. Beyond model validity or the construct validity of assessment and pedagogical practices, implementation validity requires explicit assessment of how well a technology fits the people, workflows, and institutions that rely on it (Messick, 1989; Schoenherr & Hamstra, 2024). This final section considers case studies and validation frameworks.

3.5.1 Lessons from Early Implementations

Technologies are adopted based on their affordances. The history of AI adoption can also be understood in these terms, with affordances defining the primary unit of selection (Schoenherr, 2027a). Healthcare was among the first processional to adopt AI into its workflows. Whether in clinical decision-making (Gorry & Barnett, 1968) or mental health (ELIZA; Weizenbaum, 1966), early systems demonstrated both promise and limitations. However, recent case studies in epidemiology and decision support in hospitals identify factors for the success and failure of these systems.

3.5.1.1 Google Flu Trends: Usability without Data Integrity

Google Flu Trends (GFT) was developed to rapidly estimate influenza activity by analyzing aggregated search queries related to flu symptoms and treatments. Early evaluations suggested that GFT could detect increases in influenza-like illness before traditional surveillance systems, highlighting the promise of search-based epidemiological monitoring (Ginsberg et al., 2009). However, subsequent analyses revealed substantial overestimations of flu prevalence, attributed to shifts in search behavior, media influence, and the absence of model recalibration (Lazer et al., 2014; Olson et al., 2013).

Subsequent evaluations of GFT revealed a gradual drift toward overestimation of flu prevalence. During the 2012–2013 influenza season, GFT's estimates were roughly double Centers for Disease Control and Prevention (CDC) reports at their peak (Lazer et al., 2014; Olson et al., 2013; Santillana et al., 2014). The discrepancy was attributed to several design and implementation issues. First, GFT relied on correlations between search frequency and disease incidence without incorporating epidemiological context or causal modeling. Second, the model was trained on data from a narrow time window and failed to adapt to changes in search behavior and media coverage, resulting in data drift. Finally, the use of proprietary algorithms limited external validation and prevented timely recalibration (Boyd & Crawford, 2012; Ginsberg et al., 2009; Kandula & Shaman, 2019).

Although GFT was presented as a contribution to population-level surveillance, it was not designed for use by HCPs or epidemiologists. The system functioned primarily as a demonstration of large-scale, data-driven forecasting rather than a decision-support tool integrated within public health infrastructure. A focus on HCD might have improved interpretability and usability, but without a valid and adaptive underlying model, such improvements could not ensure practical or epidemiological value.

3.5.1.2 IBM Watson for Oncology: The Limits of Transferability

IBM Watson for Oncology demonstrates how early optimism in AI implementation can outpace practical reality. The system was designed to generate evidence-based treatment recommendations by analyzing patient data in combination with findings from the medical literature. The training corpus was drawn primarily from Memorial Sloan Kettering and included synthetic patient cases generated by a small group of MSKCC oncologists, limiting generalizability to other institutional contexts and patient populations (Ross & Swetlitz, 2018). Despite extensive collaborations with major health institutions, evaluations revealed inconsistent performance, mismatched recommendations, and limited clinician confidence (Keikes et al., 2018; Strickland, 2019).

The failure of IBM Watson for Oncology has been attributed to several interrelated factors. The training dataset used to develop the system was drawn primarily from a single academic institution, limiting generalizability to other clinical environments and patient populations (Ross & Swetlitz, 2018; Zou & Schiebinger, 2018). The system's reasoning process lacked transparency and explainability, making it difficult for HCPs to assess whether recommendations were valid (Amann et al., 2020). Implementation teams underestimated the variability in local guidelines, treatment availability, terminology, and record structures. When Watson Oncology was implemented within geographically and institutionally diverse settings, substantial localization challenges were reported (Ross & Swetlitz, 2018; Zou et al., 2020).

One reason for these implementation issues undoubtedly stems from the fact that HCPs were not fully engaged in the design or workflow adaptation processes, resulting in a decision-support tool that was misaligned with oncologists' reasoning patterns, institutional decision-making norms, and the interaction practices of tumor boards (Höfflinger & Amann, 2020). Because Watson's model of decision-making was incongruent with clinicians' cognitive and communicative practices, adoption remained limited due to representational translation issues (Schoenherr & Michael, 2026). The system's eventual disuse underscores a broader lesson: neglecting the sociotechnical context of AI and its integration within human, organizational, and institutional systems can undermine even technically advanced innovations (Höfflinger & Amann, 2020).

3.5.1.3 COVID-19 Prediction Models: Overfitting and Validation Gaps

During the COVID-19 pandemic, hundreds of AI models were developed to predict infection, disease severity, and patient outcomes. The period represented the most stringent test of AI's capabilities in healthcare due to the need for rapid, large-scale deployment in an ongoing public health emergency. Many models were created from small or non-representative datasets, were insufficiently tested, and failed when applied to new populations. Systematic reviews found that nearly all models were biased, poorly validated, or unsuitable for clinical use (Robertshaw et al., 2023; Wynants et al., 2020). The rush to implement tools without adequate governance frameworks was largely defined by wasted effort, confusion, and false hope. However, this pattern has the appearance of evolutionary processes suggesting that it should not have been entirely unexpected (Schoenherr, 2027a).

Nevertheless, without structured validation processes that account for population diversity and institutional context, AI systems cannot be assumed to generalize or prove useful in crisis conditions.

3.5.1.4 AI-Enabled Radiology and Pathology: Gradual Success

In contrast to the foregoing examples, the gradual integration of AI into radiology and pathology has produced more sustainable benefits. Tools for triaging chest X-rays, identifying lung nodules, and detecting diabetic retinopathy have improved efficiency and diagnostic accuracy when deployed under careful human supervision (Kelly et al., 2019; Khosravi et al., 2024). The success of these systems can largely be attributed to incremental implementation, with repeated testing and validation against well-defined oversight procedures in a localized setting, and clear role boundaries.

3.5.2 Cybersecurity: A Sociotechnical Affordance (A Special Case)

The distribution of healthcare digital infrastructure across hospitals, organizations, and connected medical devices creates persistent cybersecurity vulnerabilities (Dameff et al., 2023; Kruse et al., 2017; Williams & Woodward, 2015). System connectivity enables data integration and coordination but also creates affordances that can be exploited by cybercriminals and state actors (Cybersecurity and Infrastructure Security Agency (CISA), 2024; European Union Agency for Cybersecurity (ENISA), 2023; Schoenherr, 2027b). Between 2014 and 2022, the U.S. Department of Health and Human Services recorded 1,138 data breaches involving protected health information that collectively exposed the records of more than 164 million patients, with the largest breach involving 3.3 million patient records (HHS, 2023). In several instances, the scale of these breaches prompted national concern. In 2015, Anthem Inc. reported a data breach compromising the data of 78.8 million individuals, including names, birth dates, home addresses, Social Security numbers, employment information, and medical IDs (HHS, 2016; Office of Personnel Management, 2016). In 2023, the FBI's Internet Crime Complaint Center (IC3) received 249 cybercrime complaints from healthcare and public health organizations—the highest number across all U.S. critical-infrastructure sectors (FBI IC3, 2024). These incidents underscore that cybersecurity in healthcare is a sociotechnical affordance, requiring coordination between technical systems, professional practices, and institutional governance structures (Dameff et al., 2023; Kruse et al., 2017; Ronquillo et al., 2018; Stanberry, 1997a, 1997b; Williams & Woodward, 2015). In some case, cyberattacks against healthcare infrastructure are tactics used in warfare (e.g., Ukraine; see Schoenherr, 2027c).

While compartmentalization can contain intrusions, such fragmented security architectures leave institutions unevenly protected, especially in mixed public–private systems (Blanke & McGrady, 2016; Kruse et al., 2017; Li et al., 2016; Mansfield-Devine, 2017; Smith, 2019). To that end, if healthcare is understood as an STS vulnerable to cyberattacks, we must identify and address the interdependent vulnerabilities that define these systems.

Recent ransomware and supply-chain attacks demonstrate how cybersecurity failures can disrupt both clinical care and education. In 2023, the MOVEit and SolarWinds breaches exposed vulnerabilities in widely used vendor software, allowing attackers to infiltrate multiple hospitals, universities, and government agencies through trusted third-party channels (Cybersecurity and Infrastructure Security Agency (CISA), 2024; European Union Agency for Cybersecurity (ENISA), 2023). In the MOVEit incident, attackers exploited a zero-day vulnerability[7] in a file-transfer program to exfiltrate large volumes of data undetected. In the SolarWinds breach, hackers inserted malicious code into a routine software update that subsequently spread to thousands of hospitals, universities, and government systems. Once inside, attackers used tactics such as credential theft, social engineering, and lateral movement to gain access to sensitive patient and institutional information (Cybersecurity and Infrastructure Security Agency (CISA), 2024; European Union Agency for Cybersecurity (ENISA), 2023).

These incidents compromised protected health information and research data, forcing temporary shutdowns of electronic health record systems and delaying patient services. Similarly, large-scale ransomware attacks on hospitals in the United States and United Kingdom paralyzed imaging and laboratory networks, diverted emergency cases, and cost institutions millions in recovery and legal penalties (HHS, 2024; NHS, 2023).

3.5.2.1 *Common Attack Vectors: From Technical to Social*

Healthcare systems face diverse cyber threats that exploit both technical vulnerabilities and human error (European Union Agency for Cybersecurity (ENISA), 2023). *Data breaches* remain the most frequent, exposing protected health information, learner records, and institutional data, often resulting in regulatory penalties and reputational damage (IBM Security & Ponemon Institute, 2024; HHS, 2023). Increasingly, *ransomware attacks* are used to encrypt critical systems such as EHRs, imaging platforms, or connected devices, halting operations and threatening data release (Check Point Software Technologies, 2024; Mansfield-Devine, 2017). Medical equipment can also be attacked individually, or collectively in *medical device and Internet-of-Medical-Things (IoMT) intrusions* exploit weak authentication or outdated software in networked pumps, monitors, and wearables, potentially disrupting therapy or data integrity (FDA, 2024; Kumar et al., 2025). ON an equally broad scale, *supply-chain compromises* gain access to third-party vendor systems to infiltrate institutional networks (European Union Agency for Cybersecurity (ENISA), 2023; Cybersecurity and Infrastructure Security Agency (CISA), 2024).

Traditionally, cybersecurity has focused on the hardware and software that defines systems, with human factors remaining a secondary set of concerns. However, specific cyberattacks are focused on human biases to trust, share, and help others. As an STS, HCPs must be aware that the workarounds that are used to bypass security controls (e.g., selecting a weak password, sharing passwords, failure to log out) can place learner and patient records and colleagues at risk. Human-targeted threats such as *phishing and social engineering* account for most healthcare cyber incidents by manipulating trust to harvest credentials or deliver malware (Proofpoint & Ponemon Institute, 2024). Finally, *insider threats* bypass perimeter defenses and require behavioral monitoring, continuous training, strong access control, and conversational and behavioral monitoring to detect and differentiate unintentional security policy violations and intentional ones (Schoenherr, 2027d; Schoenherr et al., 2022).

3.5.3 Validation and Evaluation

As the failures and successes of AI described in the preceding sections demonstrate, validation and evaluation are essential to ensure both model validity and implementation validity. These processes must be guided by human-centered co-design that includes all relevant stakeholders (Abbas et al., 2021a, 2021b; Michael et al., 2024; Schoenherr et al., 2023). HCPs should be involved early in development to ensure that systems reflect critical decision points, collaborative workflows, documentation practices, and decision priorities. Models must be validated on representative datasets before deployment and continued monitoring in real-world settings. Evaluation should follow emerging standards such as the FDA's *Good Machine Learning Practice* (2025), the *NICE Evidence Standards Framework* (2022), and the British Standard *BS 30440: Validation Framework for the Use of AI in Healthcare*. To ensure valid implementation, evaluation frameworks must apply rigorous evidentiary standards that assess not only technical performance but also usability, integ

3.5.3.1 Learning Health System (LHS) and Learning Education System (LES) Models

The Learning Health System (LHS) model developed for continuous quality improvement in clinical care has been extended to AI-supported healthcare. LHS frameworks conceive of clinical environments as adaptive systems that continuously learn from practice, data, and feedback (Friedman et al., 2017; World Health Organization (WHO), 2024). In AI implementation, each deployment is accompanied by structured monitoring of outcomes, bias, and user experience, with data from routine use informing retraining and recalibration. A similar approach is evident in the Learning Education System (LES) model within health professions education, which uses data from simulations, assessments, and feedback analytics to update instructional strategies (Ellaway et al., 2014; Feigerlova et al., 2025). Both models emphasize cyclical learning involving measurement, adaptation, (re)evaluation, and redesign. When applied together, they can promote alignment between clinical performance and educational design, ensuring that insights from care directly inform training.

3.5.3.2 Human-Centered Sociotechnical Systems (HCAI/iSTS) Models

Human-centered sociotechnical models have been adapted for healthcare delivery and health professions education to manage the complexity of human–AI interaction. Xu and Gao (2025) introduced the *Intelligent Sociotechnical Systems (iSTS)* framework, which defines four interdependent levels of assessment: individual, team, organization, and ecosystem. This structure reflects both clinical practice and professional education, where outcomes depend on coordination among people, processes, and technologies. When applied to education, the framework ensures that learners, faculty, and system designers collaborate in co-design and that human oversight is maintained throughout AI integration. In clinical care, it can support transparent workflows, explicit sign-off procedures, and alignment between technical systems and institutional policy.

3.5.3.4 Co-Design and Participatory Implementation in Health Professions Education

In health professions education, implementation should adopt participatory co-design principles (Abbas et al., 2021a, 2021b). Programs in the United Kingdom, Canada, and Europe have employed iterative design cycles to integrate AI tools into simulation, assessment, and feedback. Co-design brings together educators, learners, HCPs, and data scientists to define learning objectives, evaluate usability, and adapt algorithms to maintain validity and educational relevance (Tolsgaard et al., 2021; Sujan et al., 2023). This approach assumes that acceptance and sustained use are based on principled trust and perceived educational value, rather than technical accuracy alone. Early evaluations indicate that participatory models improve uptake, ensure contextual alignment, and reduce misuse by embedding reflective practice and feedback throughout implementation (Dantas et al., 2026).

3.5.3.5 Implementation Validity Framework

Developed for assessment and evaluation instruments regardless of their modality, the Implementation Validity Framework adopts an explicit empirical approach that identifies six sources of evidence to determine whether an innovation is well adapted to its implementation context. These include financial support, program support, material resources, task dependencies, relationships to other educational or clinical innovations, and program integration (Schoenherr & Hamstra, 2024). For instance, hospitals and learning institutions must ensure that they have sustainable funding and personnel to monitor and regulate AI-based technologies, understand how their use affects learners' and educators' relationships, and whether these technologies provide unique value to the institutions that adopt them over and above traditional pedagogical and non-AI-based technologies (e.g., LMSs, paper-based testing). The adoption of 'workarounds' by student learners and prospective never-skilling present real concerns (Ke et al., 2026; Schoenherr, in preparation). When combined with model validity, high levels of implementation validity indicate an ecologically optimized system. Continuous monitoring of resource use, system performance, and user engagement provides feedback for incremental adjustments or de-implementation when necessary. This approach is consistent with the principles of LHS and LES, embedding evaluation and adaptation into routine operations. By basing implementation in empirical evidence and institutional context, organizations can integrate AI tools in a valid and efficient manner that allows meaningful comparison with other systems.

3.6 Conclusions

AI-based technologies are not a solution that can be evaluated in isolation. They are components of evolving human-centered systems that mediate learning, diagnostic and clinical decision-making, and delivery of care. From this perspective, design, validation, and regulation determine whether AI strengthens or challenges the relationships that define professional practice in the HCPs. AI design and implementation must remain accountable to human values, institutional norms, and professional oversight, ensuring that systems support and enhance human expertise and collaboration. HCD also requires that we understand differences in implementation context, cultural biases, and the representativeness of data sets used to train models.

3.6.1 Perceiving AI's Affordances

The value of AI in health professions education and healthcare delivery depends on understanding its affordances: what it allows, constrains, and requires of learners, educators, HCPs, and institutions. This chapter has identified four affordances in healthcare derived from the social cognitive functions that support, supplement, or supplant: informational, inferential, relational, and organizational. These affordances determine how AI systems influence detection, reasoning, collaboration, and institutional performance. In each case, a system should be adopted or rejected on the basis of whether and how they achieve these ends.

These affordances align with the HCD approach to AI, with the ability to perceive them a critical feature of situational awareness (Schoenherr & Michael, 2026). At a low level of situational awareness, individuals might only recognize AI's basic functions: processing data (informational) and making basic predictions (inferential). However, when evaluation is limited to these functions alone,

AI becomes denatured and decoupled from the HCP, designers and developers, communities, and institutional systems that sustain it, and the students, data subjects, and health seekers that populate its data sets and use it. Understanding cognitive offloading, never-skilling, and deskilling remains important (Schoenherr, in preparation a), but an exclusive focus on these phenomena neglects the broader social and physical ecology that these systems are embedded within.

At a higher level of situational awareness, we must perceive the immediate and meso-level relational and institutional affordances that define AI. By adopting a learning management system to mediate assessment or adaptive/intelligent instruction systems to teaching and provide feedback, we can fundamentally alter downstream affordances such as the information that is exchanged and inferences that are made between human agents now shift toward AI. As interdependence increases between educators, learners, HCPs, and patients, the institutions that control and monitor AI take on increasing importance and power. Educators and HCPs must recognize the inherently relational nature of AI to identify tools that improve learning, safety, and judgment while avoiding those that create unnecessary dependence or risk to learners and patients.

Affordances are not fixed properties of a technology. HCPs, learners, and health seekers must actively perceive them. They are the result of interaction between people, systems, and environments (Schoenherr & Hamstra, 2024). This conforms to the main assumptions of implementation validity: the evidence that supports the use of a technology or an instructional practice must be continuously renewed. Social and technical systems are constantly evolving. HCPs adapt to new standards, while the learners who become clinicians and public healthcare workers bring their own values, priorities, and histories. We cannot take it for granted that developers, distributors, or users of AI have actively reflected on how AI use impacts the current educational or clinical environments. They will most likely trust that someone has assessed the safety, validated, and reliability of technologies used to provide instruction and care. Without an awareness of the affordances, we run the risk of systems exerting an unwelcome influence on us and are adopted without considering the individual and social consequences of their use.

3.6.1.1 Relational and Organizational Affordances in the STS of Healthcare

A sociotechnical perspective situates AI within the interaction of people, organizations, and infrastructures. At the micro-level, it examines how learners and practitioners use AI tools in their daily work. At the meso-level, it considers interpersonal dynamics, human-systems integration, and workflow management. At the macro-level, it addresses broader regulatory, cultural, and ethical contexts (Schoenherr & Michael, 2026). Attention to these levels, their respective affordances, and the associated design and ethical issues ensure that the evaluation of AI systems considers the trust, adaptability, and sustainability associated with these systems within healthcare and educational environments.

Relational and organizational affordances are comparatively neglected. From the perspective of HCD, understanding how therapeutic alliances are created, maintained, improved, and damaged when AI is used as a mediator between HCPs and patients is critical. Similarly, organizational affordance engender trust, while trust as a cognitive (rational) and affective (intuitive) influence can have significant ramification in terms of whether health seekers come to rely on the HCPs, i.e., complimentary care, or folk medical technologies (Schoenherr, 2022b; Schoenherr, 2026d; Schoenherr & Beaudoin, 2027).

To address these needs, HCD in healthcare AI adoption must adopt explainability as a minimal standard. First, this approach continues the long tradition of professional values to understand how systems work (Gorry, 1973). As a profession, healthcare is only granted a special status in society because of the integrity of its services. Were this integrity to be undermined by opaque algorithms or were systems' reasoning not transparent and contextualized, it would adversely impact public trust and threaten the legitimacy of professional judgment. HCPs must also acknowledge that their status will change with the introduction of AI. The healthcare professions have been continuously redefined, increasing the scope of the expected competencies of practitioners. It is unrealistic to expect one HCP to be competent in all domains. The need for AI literacy challenges traditional health professions education in terms of pedagogical and assessment practices, academic integrity, and the validation of AI-assisted learning, as well as what kinds of competency profiles are required for responsible use, oversight, and interpretation of AI systems. The constant evolution of these technologies demands its own dedicated professionals with specific competencies to interpret, explain, challenge, and present the products of these systems.

Second, if health seekers understand these systems and how they are integrated, trust can be built on a foundation of reliability and accuracy. Doing so strengthens the therapeutic alliance that is essential for adherence and engagement. Patients must also be capable of accessing, contesting, and requesting principled corrections to their health data. If the opacity of AI systems or the STS in which they are embedded is too great, HCPs and health seekers cannot be said to possess the autonomy that is ethically guaranteed them. This also means that HCPs must be prepared to engage in knowledge translation. Without the requisite competencies to explain what data are used to train a model, which elements of a health record are linked to diagnostic or treatment recommendations, and how that information is protected or shared within and beyond healthcare institutions, patients will be unlikely to develop or sustain trust in the HCPs. If the health professions are placed on a par with folk medical technologies, social proof might dominate science.

3.6.1.2 The Missing Half of Clinical AI Evaluation

Most evaluations of AI systems in healthcare delivery and the health professions focus exclusively on data quality, model validity and accuracy, or predictive validity (Kelly et al., 2019; Rajkomar et al., 2019; Topol, 2019a). These metrics measure technical performance but do not address how AI adoption changes the social and institutional infrastructure of care. In his work on construct validity, Messick (1989) highlighted the need to accumulate multiple sources of evidence to make a validity argument. In addition to considering how learning and assessment sampled a domain and used comparable response processes, he also emphasized the need to understand the social consequences of testing: how the act of test-taking influenced the learner and the validity of the test itself. This same concern must be extended to AI implementation in healthcare, where the use of systems alters communication, trust, accountability, and decision authority across professionals and institutions.

An HCD perspective requires that we understand the relational and organizational affordances that determine whether systems build or undermine trust, support or interfere with communication, and how they redistribute responsibility among HCPs, educators, patients, and AI systems. By altering the flow of information, AI affects social interaction at both small and large scales. On a small scale, learners and HCPs might drift away from consulting with peers and preceptors, choosing instead to rely on AI for the immediacy of its responses. Patients might follow a similar pattern, preferring an AI chatbot that will not judge their health choices or disclose embarrassing information. Designers, developers, and administrators of AI in educational, clinical, and public health contexts must ensure that they understand how responsibility is distributed and who is accountable for the recommendations and actions of such systems.

Organizational affordances matter as much as relational ones. AI systems can redistribute workload, reconfigure decision hierarchies, or amplify inequities in who bears cognitive or ethical responsibility (Michael et al., 2024; Schoenherr et al., 2023). If competency-based milestones and entrustable professional activities are delegated to AI, the health professions must clearly define where and when humans must remain in the loop. Defining the necessary intelligence, autonomy, and connectivity of AI systems in healthcare requires careful assessment of workflows, the social-cognitive limitations of individuals and teams, and criteria for evaluating how medical errors made by AI can be compared to those of human practitioners. While current evidence suggests that humans and AI work best in combination (Sendak et al., 2020), it is foreseeable that in some circumstances AI might perform better autonomously, such as in allocating finite resources during multiattribute decision-making or managing clinical handovers after extended shifts. Regardless of when, where, or how this occurs, it remains clear that both relational and institutional affordances must be evaluated to ensure safety, accountability, and equity.

Notes

1 This chapter was an experiment (Section 3.3–3.4). In the spirit of the subject, I *attempted* to use an LLM to edit, create, and conduct research. I knew from countless student papers that LLMs (at present) have substantial vulnerabilities. My hope was that modest

use (typo checking, citation insertion, reference suggestions, and constructing a figure) would prove easy. They did not. I was impressed that I could see different structures of my paper simulated almost instantly, that I could obtain summaries quickly, and that logical gaps could even be seen by the system, but there was a trade-off. After prompting the system to 'correct typos and identify grammatical errors', I found swathes of text transformed into heterogeneous slop (I almost gave up the em-dash!). Nearly half of the suggested references were made up—a few of my own—although, it pointed me in novel directions, many of which were blind alleys. Citations were equally bad, creating new references on the fly, changing dates, and misplacing citations. Other than causing an existential crisis (is my writing that bad?), it demonstrated how prompts and context rot are ubiquitous within the generation of models which I used. This chapter almost didn't appear in this volume. Later, when I came back to it, I disentangled these errors after almost two months of—'undo' wasn't available and I clearly did not save my document enough. I was able to revise the chapter. Apparently, identifying my own 'slop' from 'AI slop' is harder than I suspected. At the very least, I was able to research, analyze, and document these issues into something more constructive (Schoenherr, 2027c). I hope by the time you read this, these systems will be much improved. I leave this for the historical record so that other generation can understand what we sacrificed for their sociotechnical system. If it doesn't work out: sorry.

2 Here, I use AI as a general term rather than machine learning (ML), neural networks (NN), or autonomous intelligent systems (AIS). However, specific terms are used when references use cases and evidence provided in the literature.

3 Here, I use the term health seeker to identify individuals who are motivated to preserve health while not necessarily using the formal social networks of healthcare institutions. Patient is any individual who is directly engaged with the health professions community to receive diagnoses, recommendations, or care. Data subject is used to refer to individuals whose attributes in whole or part have been converted into records available to AI with or without their knowledge.

4 Lewin (1947) draws an analogy with physics, noting that we live in a field of (social) forces that bias human behavior.

5 According to Schoenherr (2022), the primary affordances are intelligence, autonomy, and connectivity. For instance, informational affordance would concern how intelligent a system is in terms of performing its task, how much human intervention is required, and the extent to which a system is integrated with others during the performance of its task. Similarly, relational affordance would concern the ability to understand human relational models, whether a system requires coupling with other agents, and the social network the system is embedded within.

6 Ethical affordances have been included in the table but are discussed elsewhere at length (Schoenherr, 2022).

7 Zero-day vulnerabilities are software flaws that are unknown to the vendor or user that can be exploited by attackers before fixes (patches) are available. The name suggests that developers have 'zero days' to fix the issue.

Bibliography

Abbas, R., Hamdoun, S., Abu-Ghazaleh, J., Chhetri, N., Chhetri, N., & Michael, K. (2021a). Co-designing the future with public interest technology. *IEEE Technology and Society Magazine*, *40*(3), 10–15.

Abbas, Q., Jeong, W., & Lee, S. W. (2025). Explainable AI in clinical decision support systems: A meta-analysis of methods, applications, and usability challenges. *Healthcare, 13*(17), 2154.

Abbas, R., Pitt, J., & Michael, K. (2021b). Socio-technical design for public interest technology. *IEEE Transactions on Technology and Society, 2*(2), 55–61.

Abbasgholizadeh Rahimi, S., Légaré, F., Sharma, G., Archambault, P., Zomahoun, H. T. V., Chandavong, S., ... & Légaré, J. (2021). Application of artificial intelligence in community-based primary health care: Systematic scoping review and critical appraisal. *Journal of Medical Internet Research, 23*(9), e29839.

Abbasi, M., Rahman, M., & Zainal, A. (2024). Artificial intelligence in hospital resource management: Evidence from a multicenter efficiency study. *Health Care Management Science, 27*(1), 55–69.

Abraham, J., Kannampallil, T., & Patel, V. L. (2022). Addressing handoff communication failures with AI-based summarization tools: Early evaluation and design recommendations. *JAMA Network Open, 5*(11), e2240792.

Ackoff, R. L., & Warfield, J. N. (1977). Redesigning the future: A systems approach to societal problems. *IEEE Transactions on Systems, Man, and Cybernetics, 7*(10), 759–759.

Adamson, A. S., & Smith, A. (2018). Machine learning and health care disparities in dermatology. *JAMA Dermatology, 154*(11), 1247–1248.

Adlung, L., Cohen, Y., Mor, U., & Elinav, E. (2021). Machine learning in clinical decision making. *Med, 2*(6), 642–665.

Ægisdóttir, S., White, M. J., Spengler, P. M., Maugherman, A. S., Anderson, L. A., Cook, R. S., ... & Rush, J. D. (2006). The meta-analysis of clinical judgment project: Fifty-six years of accumulated research on clinical versus statistical prediction. *The Counseling Psychologist*, 34(3), 341–382.

Ahmed, K., Khan, R., Patel, V., Nagpal, K., Priest, O., Ashrafian, H., Athanasiou, T., & Darzi, A. (2015). Training and safety in robotic surgery: A review of adverse events. *Annals of Surgery, 261*(5), 830–839.

Ahsan, Z. (2025). Integrating artificial intelligence into medical education: A narrative systematic review of current applications, challenges, and future directions. *BMC Medical Education, 25*(1), 1187.

Alam, A., Anderson, T., & Tay, Y. H. (2023). Generative AI in higher education: Risks of academic misconduct and approaches for prevention. *Computers & Education, 194*, 104692.

Ali, M. S., Ahsan, M. M., Tasnim, L., Afrin, S., Biswas, K., Hossain, M. M., ... & Raman, S. (2024). Federated learning in healthcare: Model misconducts, security, challenges, applications, and future research directions—A systematic review. *arXiv Preprint*, arXiv:2405.13832. https://arxiv.org/abs/2405.13832

Alves, M., et al. (2024). Use of artificial intelligence tools in supporting decision-making in hospital management. *BMC Health Services Research, 24*, Article 1282.

Amann, J., Blasimme, A., Vayena, E., Freitag, M., & Kieslich, K. (2020a). Responsible AI in healthcare: Translating principles into practice. *Journal of Medical Internet Research, 22*(7), e16214.

Amann, J., Blasimme, A., Vayena, E., Frey, D., & Madai, V. I. (2020b). Explainability for artificial intelligence in healthcare: A multidisciplinary perspective. *BMC Medical Informatics and Decision Making, 20*(1), 310.

Ammar, A., Khachfe, H. H., & Khachfe, H. A. (2023). Digital twin applications in healthcare: A scoping review. *Journal of Medical Systems, 47*(1), 67.

Argyris, C., & Schön, D. A. (1978). *Organizational learning: A theory of action perspective.* Addison-Wesley.

Bagaria, V., & Chaudhary, K. (2017). A paradigm shift in surgical planning and simulation using 3Dgraphy: experience of first 50 surgeries done using 3D-printed biomodels. *Injury*, *48*(11), 2501–2508.

Batra, U., Nathany, S., Nath, S. K., Jose, J. T., Sharma, T., Pasricha, S., ... & Rawal, K. (2024). AI-based pipeline for early screening of lung cancer: Integrating radiology, clinical, and genomics data. *The Lancet Regional Health – Southeast Asia*, *24*, 100352.

Baxter, G., & Sommerville, I. (2011). Socio-technical systems: From design methods to systems engineering. *Interacting with Computers*, *23*(1), 4–17.

Beil, M., Proft, I., van Heerden, D., Sviri, S., & van Heerden, P. V. (2019). Ethical considerations about artificial intelligence for prognostication in intensive care. *Intensive Care Medicine Experimental*, *7*(1), 70.

Bellemo, V., Lim, Z. W., Lim, G., Nguyen, Q. D., Xie, Y., Yip, M. Y., ... & Ting, D. S. (2019). Artificial intelligence using deep learning to screen for referable and vision-threatening diabetic retinopathy in Africa: A clinical validation study. *The Lancet Digital Health*, *1*(1), e35–e44.

Benda, N. C., Das, L. T., & Ratwani, R. M. (2023). Designing trustworthy clinical decision support systems: Human factors and explainability considerations. *Journal of the American Medical Informatics Association*, *30*(3), 516–525.

Benke, K., & Benke, G. (2018). Artificial intelligence and big data in public health. *International Journal of Environmental Research and Public Health*, *15*(12), 2796.

Berman, S., Khosravi, P., & Daniel, M. (2023). Artificial intelligence in competency-based medical education: Applications and implications. *Medical Teacher*, *45*(8), 765–772.

Berman, S., Schoenherr, J. R., & Hamstra, S. J. (2023). Cognitive foundations of adaptive expertise in health professions education. *Advances in Health Sciences Education*, *28*(3), 421–440.

Berner, E. S., & La Lande, T. J. (2007). Overview of clinical decision support systems. In E. S. Berner (Ed.), *Clinical decision support systems: Theory and practice* (2nd ed., pp. 1–22). Springer.

Bernstam, E. V., Shireman, P. K., Meric-Bernstam, F., Zozus, M. N., Jiang, X., Brimhall, B. B., ... & Becich, M. J. (2022). Artificial intelligence in clinical and translational science: Successes, challenges, and opportunities. *Clinical and Translational Science*, *15*(2), 309–321.

Bertsimas, D., Dunn, J., Pawlowski, C., Zhuo, Y. D., Silberholz, J., & Weinstein, A. M. (2018). Applied informatics using machine learning to predict outcomes in heart failure. *JACC: Heart Failure*, *6*(2), 155–164.

Bertsimas, D., Orfanoudaki, A., & Weiner, R. B. (2020). Personalized treatment for coronary artery disease patients: A machine learning approach. *Health Care Management Science*, *23*(4), 482–506.

Bilgic, E., Chen, D. M., & Chan, T. (2024). Implementation of learning analytics in medical education: Practical considerations. In *Fundamentals and frontiers of medical education and decision-making* (pp. 108–136). Routledge.

Birkhoff, S. D., Green, M. J., & Patel, S. R. (2023). Machine-learning approaches to workforce optimization and predictive scheduling in hospital operations. *Health Systems*, *12*(2), 147–162.

Bittle, K., & El-Gayar, O. (2025). Generative AI and academic integrity in higher education: A systematic review and research agenda. *Information*, *16*(4), 296.

Björnsson, B., Borrebaeck, C., Elander, N., Gasslander, T., Gawel, D. R., Gustafsson, M., ... & Stenfelt, S. (2020). Digital twins to personalize medicine. *Genome Medicine*, *12*(1), 4.

Blanke, S. J., & McGrady, E. (2016). When it comes to securing patient health information from breaches, your best medicine is a dose of prevention: A cybersecurity risk assessment checklist. *Journal of Healthcare Risk Management*, *36*(1), 14–24.

Bowker, G. C., & Star, S. L. (1999). *Sorting things out: Classification and its consequences*. MIT Press.

Boyd, D., & Crawford, K. (2012). Critical questions for big data: Provocations for a cultural, technological, and scholarly phenomenon. *Information, Communication & Society*, *15*(5), 662–679.

Brinker, T. J., Hekler, A., Enk, A. H., Klode, J., Hauschild, A., Berking, C., Schilling, B., Haferkamp, S., Schadendorf, D., Holland-Letz, T., Utikal, J. S., & von Kalle, C. (2022). Deep learning outperformed 136 of 157 dermatologists in a head-to-head dermoscopic melanoma image classification task. *European Journal of Cancer*, *113*, 47–54.

Bruynseels, K., Santoni de Sio, F., & van den Hoven, J. (2018). Digital twins in health care: Ethical implications of an emerging engineering paradigm. *Frontiers in Genetics*, *9*, 31.

Cabitza, F., Rasoini, R., & Gensini, G. F. (2017). Unintended consequences of machine learning in medicine. *JAMA*, *318*(6), 517–518.

Cant, R., & Cooper, S. (2021). Simulation-based learning in nurse education: Systematic review. *Nurse Education Today*, *104*, 104985.

Carayon, P., Hancock, P. A., Leveson, N., Noy, I., Sznelwar, L., & van Hootegem, G. (2021). Advancing a sociotechnical systems approach to workplace safety: Integrating human factors and organizational design. *Applied Ergonomics*, *95*, 103453.

Carayon, P., Schoofs Hundt, A., Karsh, B.-T., Gurses, A. P., Alvarado, C. J., Smith, M., & Flatley Brennan, P. (2006). Work system design for patient safety: The SEIPS model. *Quality & Safety in Health Care*, *15*(Suppl 1), i50–i58.

Carayon, P., Wetterneck, T. B., Rivera-Rodriguez, A. J., Hundt, A. S., Hoonakker, P., Holden, R., & Gurses, A. P. (2014). Human factors systems approach to healthcare quality and patient safety. *Applied Ergonomics*, *45*(1), 14–25.

Caruana, R., Lou, Y., Gehrke, J., Koch, P., Sturm, M., & Elhadad, N. (2015). Intelligible models for healthcare: Predicting pneumonia risk and hospital 30-day readmission. In *Proceedings of the 21st ACM SIGKDD international conference on knowledge discovery and data mining* (pp. 1721–1730). ACM.

Cascella, M., Montomoli, J., Bellini, V., & Bignami, E. (2023). Evaluating the feasibility of ChatGPT in healthcare: An analysis of multiple clinical and research scenarios. *Journal of Medical Systems*, *47*(1), 33.

Chan, T., Sebok-Syer, S., & Sherbino, J. (2024). Teaching with AI: Developing assessment literacy and feedback practices in CBME. *Medical Education*, *58*(4), 392–400.

Chan, K. S., & Zary, N. (2019). Applications and challenges of implementing artificial intelligence in medical education: Integrative review. *JMIR Medical Education*, *5*(1), e13930.

Char, D. S., Shah, N. H., & Magnus, D. (2018). Implementing machine learning in health care—Addressing ethical challenges. *New England Journal of Medicine*, *378*(11), 981–983.

Check Point Software Technologies. (2024). *Cyber security report 2024*. www.checkpoint.com

Chen, X., Dai, C., Peng, M., Wang, D., Sui, X., Duan, L., ... & Yang, F. (2025). Artificial intelligence driven 3D reconstruction for enhanced lung surgery planning. *Nature Communications*, *16*(1), 4086.

Chen, P.-H., Lundberg, S. M., & Lee, S.-I. (2023). Explainable AI for healthcare educators: Applications and implications. *Academic Medicine*, *98*(9), 1123–1130.

Cheng, A., Calhoun, A., & Reedy, G. (2025). Artificial intelligence-assisted academic writing: Recommendations for ethical use. *Advances in Simulation*, *10*(1), 22.

Cherns, A. (1976). The principles of sociotechnical design. *Human Relations*, *29*(8), 783–792.

Ciecierski-Holmes, T., Singh, R., Axt, M., Brenner, S., & Barteit, S. (2022). Artificial intelligence for strengthening healthcare systems in low- and middle-income countries: A systematic scoping review. *NPJ Digital Medicine*, *5*(1), 162.

Coeckelbergh, M. (2020). *AI Ethics*. MIT Press.

Coiera, E. (2019). The last mile: Where artificial intelligence meets reality. *Journal of Medical Internet Research*, *21*(11), e16323.

Coiera, E. (2021). The science of implementation: Designing AI for real-world healthcare. *BMJ*, *372*, n312.

Cook, D. A., Brydges, R., Hamstra, S. J., Zendejas, B., Szostek, J. H., Wang, A. T., Erwin, P. J., & Hatala, R. (2013). Comparative effectiveness of technology-enhanced simulation versus other instructional methods: A systematic review and meta-analysis. *Simulation in Healthcare*, *7*(5), 308–320.

Cook, D. A., Hatala, R., Brydges, R., Zendejas, B., Szostek, J. H., Wang, A. T., ... & Hamstra, S. J. (2010). Technology-enhanced simulation for health professions education: A systematic review and meta-analysis. *JAMA*, *306*(9), 978–988.

Corral-Acero, J., Margara, F., Marciniak, M., Rodero, C., Loncaric, F., Feng, Y., ... & Lamata, P. (2020). The 'Digital Twin' to enable the vision of precision cardiology. *European Heart Journal*, *41*(48), 4556–4564.

Cotton, D. R. E., Cotton, P. A., & Shipway, J. R. (2023). Chatting and cheating: Ensuring academic integrity in the era of ChatGPT. *Innovations in Education and Teaching International*, *61*(2), 228–239.

Cresswell, K. M., & Sheikh, A. (2013). Organizational issues in the implementation and adoption of health information technology innovations: An interpretative review. *International Journal of Medical Informatics*, *82*(5), e73–e86.

Croskerry, P. (2003). The importance of cognitive errors in diagnosis and strategies to minimize them. *Academic Emergency Medicine*, *10*(11), 1130–1132.

Croskerry, P. (2009). A universal model of diagnostic reasoning. *Academic Medicine*, *84*(8), 1022–1028.

Croskerry, P. (2013). From mindless to mindful practice—Cognitive bias and clinical decision making. *New England Journal of Medicine*, *368*(26), 2445–2448.

Cross, J. L., Jamison, T. J., & Patel, S. M. (2024). Bias in medical artificial intelligence: Implications for clinical decision-making. *Frontiers in Artificial Intelligence*, *7*, 11542778.

Cybersecurity and Infrastructure Security Agency (CISA). (2024). *Stop ransomware guide*. U.S. Department of Homeland Security. www.cisa.gov/stopransomware

da Silva Jr, C. A., Rodrigues, F. R., & Santos, L. M. (2024). Artificial intelligence in public health: Opportunities, challenges, and regulatory implications. *Frontiers in Public Health*, *12*, 1376029.

Dameff, C., Tully, J., Chan, T. C., Castillo, E. M., Savage, S., Maysent, P., ... & Longhurst, C. A. (2023). Ransomware attack associated with disruptions at adjacent emergency departments in the U.S. *JAMA Network Open*, *6*(5), e2312270.

Daniel, M., Gordon, M., Patricio, M., Hider, A., Pawlik, C., Bhatt, N., ... & Brydges, R. (2021). An evidence synthesis of competency-based time-variable undergraduate medical education. *Medical Teacher*, *43*(S2), S8–S80.

Dantas, C., Reigada, C., Cabrita, M., Mitsis, A., Ghiţă, C., Geanta, M., ... & Costa, E. (2026). Co-research in the development of AI and digital health tools for cancer management and care: a systematic review. *BMC Health Services Research, 26*, 844.

Dawson, P., & Sutherland-Smith, W. (2023). Generative AI and assessment integrity in medical education. *Medical Teacher, 45*(3), 312–320.

Dawson, S., Poquet, O., Colvin, C., Rogers, T., Pardo, A., & Gašević, D. (2022). The role of artificial intelligence in education: Promises and implications for teaching and learning. *Computers and Education: Artificial Intelligence, 3*, 100068.

Deng, R., Jiang, M., Yu, X., Lu, Y., & Liu, S. (2024). Does ChatGPT enhance student learning? A systematic review and meta-analysis of experimental studies. *Computers & Education, 227*, 105224.

Di Martino, F., & Delmastro, F. (2023). Explainable AI for clinical and remote health applications: A survey on tabular and time-series data. *Artificial Intelligence Review, 56*(6), 5261–5315.

du Plooy, E., & Hawkins, M. (2024). Personalized adaptive learning in higher education: A systematic review. *Higher Education Research & Development*. Advance online publication.

Drakoulas, G., Stavroulakis, T., Michalopoulos, G., Vavourakis, V., & Drikakis, D. (2024). ExplainNet: Towards explainable AI for scaffold design in tissue engineering. *Biofabrication, 16*(2), 025034.

El Arab, R. A., Abu-Mahfouz, M. S., Abuadas, F. H., Alzghoul, H., Almari, M., Ghannam, A., & Seweid, M. M. (2025). Bridging the gap: From AI success in clinical trials to real-world healthcare implementation—A narrative review. *Healthcare, 13*(7), 701.

Ellaway, R. H., Pusic, M. V., Galbraith, R. M., & Cameron, T. (2014). Developing the role of big data and analytics in health professional education. *Medical Teacher, 36*(3), 216–222.

Emery, F. E., & Trist, E. L. (1960). Socio-technical systems. In C. W. Churchman & M. Verhulst (Eds.), *Management science, models, and techniques* (Vol. 2, pp. 83–97). Pergamon.

Endsley, M. R. (2012). Situation awareness. In G. Salvendy (Ed.), *Handbook of human factors and ergonomics* (pp. 553–568). Wiley.

Ericsson, K. A. (2007). An expert-performance perspective of research on medical expertise: The study of clinical performance. *Medical Education, 41*(12), 1124–1130.

Esteva, A., Kuprel, B., Novoa, R. A., Ko, J., Swetter, S. M., Blau, H. M., & Thrun, S. (2017). Dermatologist-level classification of skin cancer with deep neural networks. *Nature, 542*(7639), 115–118.

European Union Agency for Cybersecurity (ENISA). (2023). *ENISA Threat Landscape: Health Sector*. ENISA. www.enisa.europa.eu/publications

Fazlollahi, A. M., Bakhaidar, M., Alsayegh, A., Yilmaz, R., Winkler-Schwartz, A., Mirchi, N., ... & Del Maestro, R. F. (2022). Effect of artificial intelligence tutoring vs expert instruction on learning simulated surgical skills among medical students: A randomized clinical trial. *JAMA Network Open, 5*(2), e2149008.

Fabila, J., Garrucho, L., Campello, V. M., Martín-Isla, C., & Lekadir, K. (2025). Federated learning in low-resource settings: A chest imaging study in Africa – Challenges and lessons learned. *arXiv preprint arXiv:2505.14217*.

Federal Bureau of Investigation, Internet Crime Complaint Center (IC3). (2024). *2023 internet crime report*. FBI. www.ic3.gov/Media/PDF/AnnualReport/2023_IC3Report.pdf

Fadero, P. E., & Shah, M. (2014). Three dimensional (3D) modelling and surgical planning in trauma and orthopaedics. *The Surgeon, 12*(6), 328–333.

Feigerlova, E., Perrot, N., & Dahan, M. (2025). Artificial intelligence in medical education: A systematic review. *BMC Medical Education, 25*(1), 141.

Fjeld, J., Achten, N., Hilligoss, H., Nagy, A., & Srikumar, M. (2020). *Principled artificial intelligence: Mapping consensus in ethical and rights-based approaches to principles for AI.* Berkman Klein Center Research Publication, 2020-1.

Flanagin, A., Bibbins-Domingo, K., Berkwits, M., & Christiansen, S. L. (2023). Nonhuman "authors" and implications for the integrity of scientific publication and medical knowledge. *JAMA, 329*(8), 637–639.

Frank, J. R., Snell, L., & Ten Cate, O. (2010). Competency-based medical education: Theory to practice. *Medical Teacher, 32*(8), 638–645.

Friedman, C. P., Allee, N. J., Delaney, B. C., Flynn, A. J., Silverstein, J. C., Sullivan, K. J., & Tcheng, J. E. (2017). The science of learning health systems: Foundations for a new journal. *Learning Health Systems, 1*(1), e10020.

Freidson, E. (2001). *Professionalism: The third logic.* University of Chicago Press.

Fullan, M. (2001). *The new meaning of educational change* (3rd ed.). Teachers College Press.

Gama, F., Tyskbo, D., Nygren, J., Barlow, J., Reed, J., & Svedberg, P. (2022). Implementation frameworks for artificial intelligence translation into health care practice: Scoping review. *Journal of Medical Internet Research, 24*(1), e32215.

García-Torres, D., Vicente Ripoll, M. A., Fernández Peris, C., & Mira Solves, J. J. (2024). Enhancing clinical reasoning with virtual patients: A hybrid systematic review combining human reviewers and ChatGPT. *Healthcare, 12*(22), 2241.

Gazquez-Garcia, J., Sánchez-Bocanegra, C. L., & Sevillano, J. L. (2025). AI in the health sector: Systematic review of key skills for future health professionals. *JMIR medical education, 11*(1), e58161.

Geda, M. W., Tang, Y. M., & Lee, C. K. M. (2024). Applications of artificial intelligence in Orthopaedic surgery: A systematic review and meta-analysis. *Engineering Applications of Artificial Intelligence, 133*, 108326.

Gentner, D., & Stevens, A. L. (Eds.). (1983). *Mental models.* Lawrence Erlbaum Associates.

Gharibshahian, M., Salibian, A. A., Veiga, N., Kantor, N., Menon, N., da Silva, P. R., ... & Evans, G. R. D. (2023). The role of 3D bioprinting in the development of next-generation tissue models. *Frontiers in Bioengineering and Biotechnology, 11*, 1240258.

Ghassemi, M., Oakden-Rayner, L., & Beam, A. L. (2021). The false hope of current approaches to explainable artificial intelligence in health care. *The Lancet Digital Health, 3*(11), e745–e750.

Gibson, J. J. (1979). *The ecological approach to visual perception.* Houghton Mifflin.

Gilpin, L. H., Bau, D., Yuan, B. Z., Bajwa, A., Specter, M., & Kagal, L. (2018). Explaining explanations: An overview of interpretability of machine learning. In *Proceedings of the 5th IEEE international conference on data science and advanced analytics* (pp. 80–89). IEEE.

Gilson, A., Safranek, C. W., Huang, T., Socrates, V., Chi, L., Taylor, R. A., Chartash, D., & Liebovitz, D. M. (2023). How does ChatGPT perform on the United States Medical Licensing Examination? *JMIR Medical Education, 9*, e45312.

Ginsberg, J., Mohebbi, M. H., Patel, R. S., Brammer, L., Smolinski, M. S., & Brilliant, L. (2009). Detecting influenza epidemics using search engine query data. *Nature, 457*(7232), 1012–1014.

Goldberg, L. R. (1970). Man versus model of man: A rationale, plus some evidence, for a method of improving on clinical inferences. *Psychological Bulletin, 73*(6), 422–432.

Gorry, G. A. (1973). Computer-assisted clinical decision making. *Methods of Information in Medicine, 12*(1), 45–51.

Gorry, G. A., & Barnett, G. O. (1968). Experience with a model of sequential diagnosis. *Computers and Biomedical Research, 1*(5), 490–507.

Graesser, A. C., Hu, X., & Sottilare, R. (2018). Intelligent tutoring systems. In F. Fischer, C. E. Hmelo-Silver, S. R. Goldman, & P. Reimann (Eds.), *International handbook of the learning sciences* (pp. 246–255). Routledge.

Greenhalgh, T., Robert, G., Macfarlane, F., Bate, P., & Kyriakidou, O. (2004). Diffusion of innovations in service organizations: Systematic review and recommendations. *Milbank Quarterly, 82*(4), 581–629.

Greenhalgh, T., Wherton, J., Papoutsi, C., Lynch, J., & Hughes, G. (2017). Beyond adoption: A new framework for theorizing and evaluating nonadoption, abandonment, scale-up, spread, and sustainability of health and care technologies (NASSS). *Journal of Medical Internet Research, 19*(11), e367.

Grierson, L. E. (2014). Information processing, specificity of practice, and the transfer of learning: considerations for reconsidering fidelity. *Advances in Health Sciences Education*, 19(2), 281–289.

Grove, W. M., Zald, D. H., Lebow, B. S., Snitz, B. E., & Nelson, C. (2000). Clinical versus mechanical prediction: A meta-analysis. *Psychological Assessment, 12*(1), 19–30.

Gupta, S., Wan, F., Bhatt, D. L., & Carter, R. E. (2025). Artificial intelligence in hospital operations: A systematic review. *NPJ: Digital Medicine, 8*(1), 47.

Guze, P. A. (2015). Using technology to meet the challenges of medical education. *Transactions of the American Clinical and Climatological Association, 126*, 260–270.

Hamilton, A. (2024). Artificial intelligence and healthcare simulation: The shifting landscape of medical education. *Cureus, 16*(5), e59747.

Han, J., Davids, J., Ashrafian, H., Darzi, A., Elson, D. S., & Sodergren, M. (2022). A systematic review of robotic surgery: From supervised paradigms to fully autonomous robotic approaches. *The International Journal of Medical Robotics and Computer Assisted Surgery, 18*(2), e2358.

Han, S., Kim, T., Lee, J., & Park, Y. (2024). Balancing automation and accountability in AI-assisted clinical decision making: A systematic review. *Frontiers in Artificial Intelligence, 7*, 138412.

Hegarty, M., & Sims, V. K. (1994). Individual differences in mental animation during mechanical reasoning. *Memory & Cognition, 22*(4), 411–430.

Hege, I., Owens, T., Bhargava, A., & Schuvighoff, E. (2011). The challenge of creating content for problem-based learning cases: Where should AI fit? In *Proceedings of the 2011 IEEE 11th international conference on advanced learning technologies* (pp. 176–178). IEEE.

Henry, K. E., Hager, D. N., Pronovost, P. J., & Saria, S. (2015). A targeted real-time early warning score (TREWScore) for septic shock. *Science Translational Medicine, 7*(299), 299ra122.

Heller, F. (1997). Sociotechnology and the environment. *Human Relations, 50*(5), 605–624.

Hoff, K. A., & Bashir, M. (2015). Trust in automation: Integrating empirical evidence on factors that influence trust. *Human Factors, 57*(3), 407–434.

Hoffman, R. R., Mueller, S. T., Klein, G., & Litman, J. (2018). Metrics for explainable AI: Challenges and prospects. *AI Magazine, 39*(4), 56–68.

Holden, R. J., Carayon, P., Gurses, A. P., Hoonakker, P., Hundt, A. S., Ozok, A. A., & Rivera-Rodriguez, A. J. (2013). SEIPS 2.0: A human factors framework for studying and improving the work of healthcare professionals and patients. *Ergonomics*, *56*(11), 1669–1686.

Hollnagel, E. (2017). *Safety-II in practice: Developing the resilience potentials.* Routledge.

Holmboe, E. S., Sherbino, J., Long, D. M., Swing, S. R., & Frank, J. R. (2010). The role of assessment in competency-based medical education. *Medical Teacher*, *32*(8), 676–682.

Hughes, E. C. (1958). *Men and their work.* Free Press.

Hutchins, E. (1995). *Cognition in the wild.* MIT Press.

IBM Security & Ponemon Institute. (2024). *Cost of a data breach report 2024.* IBM Corporation. www.ibm.com/reports/data-breach

Ifenthaler, D., & Schumacher, C. (2016). Student perceptions of privacy principles for learning analytics. *Educational Technology Research and Development*, *64*(5), 923–938.

Ifenthaler, D., & Yau, J. Y.-K. (2020). Utilising learning analytics to support study success in higher education: A systematic review. *Educational Technology Research and Development*, *68*(4), 1961–1990.

International Organization for Standardization. (2019). *ISO 9241-210:2019: Ergonomics of human–system interaction—Part 210: Human-centred design for interactive systems.* ISO. www.iso.org/standard/77520.html

Jammalamadaka, U., & Tappa, K. (2018). Recent advances in biomaterials for 3D printing and tissue engineering. *Journal of Functional Biomaterials*, *9*(1), 22.

Jeznach, A., Nakielski, P., & Pierini, F. (2024). Artificial intelligence for designing scaffolds for tissue engineering: Systematic review. *ACS Biomaterials Science & Engineering*, *10*(7), 4345–4365.

Jha, A. K., Doolan, D., Grandt, D., Scott, T., & Bates, D. W. (2008). The use of health information technology in seven nations. *International Journal of Medical Informatics*, *77*(12), 848–854.

Ji, Z., Lee, N., Frieske, R., Yu, T., Su, D., Xu, Y., ... & Fung, P. (2023). Survey of hallucination in natural language generation. *ACM Computing Surveys*, *55*(12), 1–38.

Jiang, F., Jiang, Y., Zhi, H., Dong, Y., Li, H., Ma, S., Wang, Y., Dong, Q., Shen, H., & Wang, Y. (2017). Artificial intelligence in healthcare: Past, present and future. *Stroke and Vascular Neurology*, *2*(4), 230–243.

Jin, Y., Cui, Y., Luo, T., Tang, H., Tang, L., Zhu, L., ... & He, B. (2023). Application of artificial intelligence in clinical medical handover: A systematic review. *Frontiers in Medicine*, *10*, 1202165.

Jordan, M. I., & Mitchell, T. M. (2015). Machine learning: Trends, perspectives, and prospects. *Science*, *349*(6245), 255–260.

Judd, T., & Kennedy, G. (2011). Expediency-based practice? Medical students' reliance on Google and Wikipedia for biomedical inquiries. *British Journal of Educational Technology*, *42*(2), 351–360.

Kamel Rahimi, A., Pienaar, O., Ghadimi, M., Canfell, O. J., Pole, J. D., Shrapnel, S., ... & Sullivan, C. (2024). Implementing AI in hospitals to achieve a learning health system: Systematic review of current enablers and barriers. *Journal of Medical Internet Research*, *26*, e49655.

Kandula, S., & Shaman, J. (2019). Near-term forecasts of influenza-like illness: An evaluation of autoregressive time-series approaches. *Epidemics*, *27*, 41–51.

Kaplan, A. D., Kessler, T. T., Brill, J. C., & Hancock, P. A. (2023). Trust in artificial intelligence: Meta-analytic findings. *Human Factors*, *65*(2), 337–359.

Karwowski, W. (2012). A review of human factors challenges of complex adaptive systems: Discovering and understanding chaos in human performance. *Human Factors*, *54*(6), 983–995.

Ke, Y., Jin, L., Ong, J. C. L., Thirunavukarasu, A. J., Car, J., Cheung, C. Y., ... & Liu, N. (2026). AI-induced never-skilling in medical education. *Nature Medicine*, 1–10.

Keehner, M., Tendick, F., Meng, M. V., Anwar, H. P., Hegarty, M., Stoller, M. L., & Shafer, D. M. (2004). Spatial ability, experience, and skill in laparoscopic surgery. *The American Journal of Surgery*, *188*(1), 71–75.

Keikes, L., Medlock, S., van de Berg, D. J., Zhang, S., Guicherit, O. R., Punt, C. J., & van Oijen, M. G. (2018). The first steps in the evaluation of a "black-box" decision support tool: a protocol and feasibility study for the evaluation of Watson for Oncology. *Journal of Clinical and Translational Research*, *3*(Suppl 3), 411.

Kellman, P. J. (2013). Adaptive and perceptual learning technologies in medical education and training. *Military Medicine*, *178*, 98–106.

Kelly, C. J., Karthikesalingam, A., Suleyman, M., Corrado, G., & King, D. (2019). Key challenges for delivering clinical impact with artificial intelligence. *BMC Medicine*, *17*(1), 195.

Khakpaki, A. (2025). Advancements in artificial intelligence transforming medical education: a comprehensive overview. *Medical Education Online*, *30*(1), 2542807.

Khalil, M., & Ebner, M. (2016). Learning analytics: Principles and constraints. In *Proceedings of the 27th annual conference of the society for information technology and teacher education* (pp. 1178–1185). Association for the Advancement of Computing in Education.

Khosravi, M., Zare, Z., Mojtabaeian, S. M., & Izadi, R. (2024). Artificial intelligence and decision-making in healthcare: A thematic analysis of a systematic review of reviews. *Health Services Research and Managerial Epidemiology*, *11*, 23333928241234863.

King, A. C., Doueiri, Z. N., Kaulberg, A., & Rosas, L. G. (2025). The promise and perils of artificial intelligence in advancing participatory science and health equity in public health. *JMIR Public Health and Surveillance*, *11*(1), e65699.

Klein, G. A. (1993). A recognition-primed decision (RPD) model of rapid decision making. In G. A. Klein, J. Orasanu, R. Calderwood, & C. E. Zsambok (Eds.), *Decision making in action: Models and methods* (pp. 138–147). Ablex.

Kolomenskaya, E., Vulf, M., Amend, K., & Nikonova, A. (2023). The imposition of artificial intelligence at stages of scaffold design for tissue engineering. *Biomedicines*, *11*(8), 2048.

Kononowicz, A. A., Woodham, L. A., Edelbring, S., Stathakarou, N., Davies, D., Saxena, N., ... & Zary, N. (2019). Virtual patient simulations in health professions education: Systematic review and meta-analysis by the Digital Health Education Collaboration. *Journal of Medical Internet Research*, *21*(7), e14676.

Koriat, A. (2012). The self-consistency model of subjective confidence. *Psychological Review*, *119*(1), 80–113.

Kotter, J. P. (1996). *Leading change*. Harvard Business School Press.

Kremer, I., Schultz, T. J., & Cannon, J. (2022). Sociotechnical perspectives on AI adoption in healthcare. *BMJ Health & Care Informatics*, *29*(1), e100519.

Kruse, C. S., Frederick, B., Jacobson, T., & Monticone, D. K. (2017). Cybersecurity in healthcare: A systematic review of modern threats and trends. *Technology and Health Care*, *25*(1), 1–10.

Kulik, J. A., & Fletcher, J. D. (2016). Effectiveness of intelligent tutoring systems: A meta-analytic review. *Review of Educational Research*, *86*(1), 42–78.

Kumar, R., Singh, A., Subahi, A., Humaida, M., Joshi, S., & Sharma, M. (2025). Leveraging artificial intelligence to achieve sustainable public healthcare services in Saudi Arabia: A systematic literature review of critical success factors. *Computer Modeling in Engineering & Sciences*, *142*(2), 1289.

Kung, T. H., Cheatham, M., Medenilla, A., Sillos, C., De Leon, L., Elepaño, C., ... & Tseng, V. (2023). Performance of ChatGPT on USMLE: Potential for AI-assisted medical education using large language models. *PLOS Digital Health*, *2*(2), e0000198.

Land, F., & Hirschheim, R. (1983). Participative systems design: Rationale, tools, and techniques. *Journal of Applied Systems Analysis*, *10*(10), 15–18.

Lazer, D., Kennedy, R., King, G., & Vespignani, A. (2014). The parable of Google Flu: Traps in big data analysis. *Science*, *343*(6176), 1203–1205.

LeCun, Y., Bengio, Y., & Hinton, G. (2015). Deep learning. *Nature*, *521*(7553), 436–444.

Lee, D., & Yoon, S. N. (2021). Application of artificial intelligence-based technologies in the healthcare industry: Opportunities and challenges. *International Journal of Environmental Research and Public Health*, *18*(1), 271.

Lekadir, K., et al. (2025). FUTURE-AI: International consensus guideline for trustworthy AI in healthcare. *Nature Machine Intelligence*, *7*(1), 1–13.

Leonardi, P. M. (2011). When flexible routines meet flexible technologies: Affordance, constraint, and the imbrication of human and material agencies. *MIS Quarterly*, *35*(1), 147–167.

Létourneau, A., Deslandes Martineau, M., Charland, P., Karran, J. A., Boasen, J., & Léger, P. M. (2025). A systematic review of AI-driven intelligent tutoring systems (ITS) in K–12 education. *NPJ Science of Learning*, *10*(1), 29.

Leslie, D., Mazumder, A., Peppin, A., Wolters, M. K., & Hagerty, A. (2021). Does "AI" stand for augmenting inequality in the era of COVID-19 healthcare? *BMJ*, *372*, n304.

Lewin, K. (1947). Frontiers in group dynamics. *Human Relations*, *1*(1), 5–41.

Lewis, J. H., & Sedgwick, M. (2015). Using technology to meet the challenges of medical education. *Transactions of the American Clinical and Climatological Association*, *126*, 260–270.

Li, X., Allmendinger, R., Uyarra, E., & Mercer, J. *Bridging Fragmentation in Cybersecurity Governance: A SocioTechnical Analysis of Expert Consensus on Problems, Solutions, and Adoption Barriers. Solutions, and Adoption Barriers.*

Liu, X., Faes, L., Kale, A. U., Wagner, S. K., Fu, D. J., Bruynseels, A., Mahendiran, T., Moraes, G., Shamdas, M., Kern, C., Ledsam, J. R., Schmid, M. K., Balaskas, K., Topol, E. J., Bachmann, L. M., Keane, P. A., & Denniston, A. K. (2019). A comparison of deep learning performance against health-care professionals in detecting diseases from medical imaging: A systematic review and meta-analysis. *The Lancet Digital Health*, *1*(6), e271–e297.

Lomis, K., Durning, S. J., & Santen, S. A. (2023). Artificial intelligence for health professions educators. *NAM Perspectives*. Advance online publication. https://doi.org/10.31478/202109a

Leydesdorff, L., & Etzkowitz, H. (1998). Triple helix of innovation: Introduction. *Science and Public Policy*, *25*(6), 358–364.

Liawrungrueang, W., Cho, S. T., Sarasombath, P., Kim, I., & Kim, J. H. (2023). Current trends in artificial intelligence-assisted spine surgery: A systematic review. *Asian Spine Journal*, *18*(1), 146.

Lingard, L. (2012). Rethinking competence in the context of teamwork. *Perspectives on Medical Education*, *1*(2), 75–82.

Loftus, T. J., Tighe, P. J., Filiberto, A. C., Efron, P. A., Brakenridge, S. C., Mohr, A. M., ... & Bihorac, A. (2020). Artificial intelligence and surgical decision-making. *JAMA Surgery*, *155*(2), 148–158.

Long, D., & Magerko, B. (2020). What is AI literacy? Competencies and design considerations. In *Proceedings of the 2020 CHI conference on human factors in computing systems* (pp. 1–16).

Luordo, D., Torres Arrese, M., Tristán Calvo, C., Shani Shani, K. D., Rodríguez Cruz, L. M., García Sánchez, F. J., ... & Villena Garrido, M. V. (2025). Application of artificial intelligence as an aid for the correction of the objective structured clinical examination (OSCE). *Applied Sciences, 15*(3), 1153.

Luxton, D. D. (Ed.). (2016). *Artificial intelligence in behavioral and mental health care*. Academic Press.

Ma, Y., Nguyen, A., & Han, J. (2024). Promoting artificial intelligence competencies for medical students: A scoping review on frameworks, programs, and tools. *arXiv preprint arXiv:2407.18939.*

Mahmood, Z. (2023). Looking back on digital medical education over the last 25 years: A narrative review. *Journal of Medical Internet Research, 26*, e60312.

Majchrzak, A., and Markus, M. 2013. "Technology Affordances and Constraints Theory (of MIS)," in Encyclopedia of Management Theory, E. Kessler (ed.), Thousand Oaks, CA: SAGE Publications, pp. 832–836.

Manser, T. (2009). Teamwork and patient safety in dynamic domains of healthcare: A review of the literature. *Acta Anaesthesiologica Scandinavica, 53*(2), 143–151.

Mansfield-Devine, S. (2017). Ransomware: Taking businesses hostage. *Network Security, 2017*(10), 8–17.

Markus, M. L., & Silver, M. S. (2008). A foundation for the study of IT Effects: A new look at DeSanctis and Poole's concepts of structural features and spirit. *Journal of the Association for Information Systems*, 9(10), 609–632.

Masters, K. (2019). Artificial intelligence in medical education. *Medical Teacher*, *41*(9), 976–980.

Masters, K., Benjamin, J., Agrawal, A., MacNeill, H., Pillow, M. T., & Mehta, N. (2024). Twelve tips on creating and using custom GPTs to enhance health professions education. *Medical Teacher*, *46*(6), 752–756.

Matheny, M. E., Goldsack, J. C., Saria, S., Shah, N. H., Gerhart, J., Cohen, I. G., ... & Horvitz, E. (2025). Artificial intelligence in health and health care: Priorities for action. *Health Affairs*, *44*(2), 163–170.

McCulloch, W. S., & Pitts, W. (1943). A logical calculus of the ideas immanent in nervous activity. *Bulletin of Mathematical Biophysics*, *5*(4), 115–133.

McKinney, S. M., Sieniek, M., Godbole, V., Godwin, J., Antropova, N., Ashrafian, H., ... & Shetty, S. (2020). International evaluation of an AI system for breast cancer screening. *Nature*, *577*(7788), 89–94.

Meehl, P. E. (1954). *Clinical versus statistical prediction: A theoretical analysis and a review of the evidence.* University of Minnesota Press.

Mehta, N., Mehta, S., Rubenstein, A., & Wood, S. K. (2025). Not replaced, but reinvented: AI education pathways to prepare future physicians to lead healthcare transformation. *Perspectives on Medical Education*, *14*(1), 849.

Meskó, B., & Görög, M. (2020). A short guide for medical professionals in the era of artificial intelligence. *NPJ Digital Medicine*, *3*(1), 126.

Meskó, B., Hetényi, G., & Győrffy, Z. (2023). Will artificial intelligence solve the human resource crisis in healthcare? *BMJ Health & Care Informatics*, *30*(1), e100692.

Messick, S. (1989). Validity. In R. L. Linn (Ed.), *Educational measurement* (3rd ed., pp. 13–103). American Council on Education/Macmillan.

Michael, K., Schoenherr, J. R., & Vogel, K. M. (2024). Failures in the loop: Human leadership in AI-based decision-making. *IEEE Transactions on Technology and Society*, *5*(1), 2–13.

Michael, K., Vogel, K. M., Pitt, J., & Zafeirakopoulos, M. (2024). Artificial intelligence in cybersecurity: A socio-technical framing. *IEEE Transactions on Technology and Society*, *6*, 15–30.

Millington, S. J., Arntfield, R. T., Guo, R. J., Koenig, S., Kory, P., Noble, V., ... & Schoenherr, J. R. (2017). The Assessment of Competency in Thoracic Sonography (ACTS) scale: validation of a tool for point-of-care ultrasound. *Critical Ultrasound Journal*, *9*(1), 25.

Mirchi, N., Bissonnette, V., Yilmaz, R., Ledwos, N., Winkler-Schwartz, A., & Del Maestro, R. F. (2020). The virtual operative assistant: An explainable artificial intelligence tool for simulation-based training in surgery and medicine. *PLOS ONE*, *15*(2), e0229596.

Mishra, G. V., Luharia, A. A., Naqvi, W., & Sood, A. (2024). Artificial intelligence in OSCE: innovations and implications for medical education assessment–a systematic review. In *2024 2nd DMIHER International Conference on Artificial Intelligence in Healthcare, Education and Industry (IDICAIEI)* (pp. 1–5). IEEE.

Mittelstadt, B. (2019). Principles alone cannot guarantee ethical AI. *Nature Machine Intelligence*, *1*(11), 501–507.

Moglia, A., Georgiou, K., Georgiou, E., Satava, R. M., & Cuschieri, A. (2021). A systematic review on artificial intelligence in robot-assisted surgery. *International Journal of Surgery*, *95*, 106151.

Mohseni, S., Zarei, N., Ragan, E. D., & Fern, A. (2023). A framework for designing and evaluating explainable AI systems. *Journal of Human-Centered AI*, *4*(2), 35–47.

Moran, J., Briscoe, G., & Peglow, S. (2018). Current technology in advancing medical education: perspectives for learning and providing care. *Academic psychiatry*, *42*(6), 796–799.

Morley, J., Cowls, J., Taddeo, M., & Floridi, L. (2020). Ethical guidelines for COVID-19 tracing apps. *Nature*, *582*(7810), 29–31.

Morley, J., & Floridi, L. (2024). *The ethics of AI in health care: An updated mapping review*. SSRN. https://ssrn.com

Morris, R. R., Kouddous, K., Kshirsagar, R., & Schueller, S. M. (2018). Towards an artificially empathic conversational agent for mental health applications: System design and user perceptions. *Journal of Medical Internet Research*, *20*(6), e10148.

Mumford, E. (1983). *Designing human systems for new technology: The ETHICS method.* Manchester Business School.

Mumford, E. (2006). The story of socio-technical design: Reflections on its successes, failures, and potential. *Information Systems Journal*, *16*(4), 317–342.

Nair, M., Svedberg, P., Larsson, I., & Nygren, J. M. (2024). A comprehensive overview of barriers and strategies for AI implementation in healthcare: Mixed-method design. *PLOS ONE*, *19*(8), e0305949.

Nagraj, S., Kennedy, S., Jha, V., Norton, R., Hinton, L., Billot, L., Rajan, E., Mohammed Abdul, A., Phalswal, A., Arora, V., Praveen, D., & Hirst, J. (2023). A mobile clinical decision support system for high-risk pregnant women in rural India (SMARThealth Pregnancy): Pilot cluster randomized controlled trial. *JMIR Formative Research*, *7*, e44362.

Nakayama, L. F., Zago Ribeiro, L., Novaes, F., Miyawaki, I. A., Miyawaki, A. E., de Oliveira, J. A. E., ... & Silva, P. S. (2023). Artificial intelligence for telemedicine diabetic retinopathy screening: A review. *Annals of Medicine*, *55*(2), 2258149.

National Health Service (NHS). (2023). *Cyber security guidance for healthcare professionals procuring and deploying connected medical devices.* NHS England. www.england.nhs.uk

National Institute for Health and Care Excellence (NICE). (2022). *Evidence standards framework for digital health technologies* (updated to include AI). NICE. www.nice.org.uk/about/what-we-do/our-programmes/evidence-standards-framework-for-digital-health-technologies

National Institute of Standards and Technology (NIST). (2023). *AI risk management framework (AI RMF 1.0).* U.S. Department of Commerce. www.nist.gov/itl/ai-risk-management-framework

Navarro-Bringas, E., González-Camarillo, A., & Rodríguez-Méndez, R. (2020). Sociotechnical learning systems in higher education. *Computers & Education*, *149*, 103806.

Nemati, S., Holder, A., Razmi, F., Stanley, M. D., Clifford, G. D., & Buchman, T. G. (2018). An interpretable machine learning model for accurate prediction of sepsis in the ICU. *Critical Care Medicine*, *46*(4), 547–553.

Ng, D. T. K., Wu, W., Leung, J. K. L., Chiu, T. K. F., & Chu, S. K. W. (2024). Design and validation of the AI literacy questionnaire: The affective, behavioural, cognitive and ethical approach. *British Journal of Educational Technology*, *55*(3), 1082–1104.

Nguyen, N. B. C., & Karunaratne, T. (2024). Learning analytics with small datasets—State of the art and beyond. *Education Sciences*, *14*(6), 608.

Norman, D. A. (1983). Some observations on mental models. In D. Gentner & A. L. Stevens (Eds.), *Mental models* (pp. 7–14). Lawrence Erlbaum Associates.

Norman, D. A. (1988). *The psychology of everyday things*. Basic Books.

Norman, D. A. (1999). Affordance, conventions, and design. *Interactions*, *6*(3), 38–43.

Norman, D. A., & Stappers, P. J. (2015). DesignX: Complex sociotechnical systems. *She Ji: The Journal of Design, Economics, and Innovation, 1*(2), 83–106.

Norman, G., Sherbino, J., Dore, K., Wood, T., Young, M., Gaissmaier, W., Kreuels, B., & Monteiro, S. (2017). The etiology of diagnostic errors: A controlled trial of system 1 versus system 2 reasoning. *Academic Medicine*, *89*(2), 277–284.

Norman, G. R. (2005). Research in clinical reasoning: Past history and current trends. *Medical Education*, *39*(4), 418–427.

Norman, G. R., & Brooks, L. R. (1997). The non-analytical basis of clinical reasoning. *Advances in Health Sciences Education*, *2*(2), 173–184.

Norman, G. R., Grierson, L. E. M., Sherbino, J., Hamstra, S. J., Schmidt, H. G., & Mamede, S. (2018). Expertise in medicine and surgery. In K. A. Ericsson, R. R. Hoffman, A. Kozbelt, & A. M. Williams (Eds.), *The Cambridge handbook of expertise and expert performance* (2nd ed., pp. 331–355). Cambridge University Press.

Norman, G. R., Young, M., & Brooks, L. (2007). Non-analytical models of clinical reasoning: The role of experience. *Medical Education*, *41*(12), 1140–1145. https://doi.org/10.1111/j.1365-2923.2007.02914.x

Nouis, S. C., Uren, V., & Jariwala, S. (2025). Evaluating accountability, transparency, and bias in AI-assisted healthcare decision-making: a qualitative study of healthcare professionals' perspectives in the UK. *BMC Medical Ethics*, *26*(1), 89.

Obermeyer, Z., & Emanuel, E. J. (2016). Predicting the future—Big data, machine learning, and clinical medicine. *New England Journal of Medicine*, *375*(13), 1216.

Office of Personnel Management, U.S. (2016). *Cybersecurity resource center*. OPM. www.opm.gov/cybersecurity

Okamoto, K., Miyata, T., Nagayama, T., Sannomiya, Y., Hashimoto, A., Nishiki, H., ... & Takamura, H. (2025). Current status and future applications of robotic surgery in upper gastrointestinal surgery: A narrative review. *Cancers*, *17*(12), 1933.

Olson, D. R., Konty, K. J., Paladini, M., Viboud, C., & Simonsen, L. (2013). Reassessing Google Flu Trends data for detection of seasonal and pandemic influenza: A comparative epidemiological study at three geographic scales. *PLOS Computational Biology*, *9*(10), e1003256.

Orlikowski, W. J. (1992). The duality of technology: Rethinking the concept of technology in organizations. *Organization Science*, *3*(3), 398–427.

Ouanes, S., et al. (2024). AI-assisted clinical decision-making: A systematic review. *The Lancet Digital Health*, *6*(2), e85–e98.

Özkan, O., & Göl, S. (2024). Incorporating technology adoption in medical education: A systematic review. *Medical Education Online*, *29*(1), 2260718.

Panteli, D., Adib, K., Buttigieg, S., Goiana-da-Silva, F., Ladewig, K., Azzopardi-Muscat, N., ... & McKee, M. (2025). Artificial intelligence in public health: Promises, challenges, and an agenda for policymakers and public health institutions. *The Lancet Public Health*, *10*(5), e428–e432.

Paranjape, K., Schinkel, M., Panday, R. N., Car, J., & Nanayakkara, P. (2019). Introducing artificial intelligence training in medical education. *JMIR Medical Education*, *5*(2), e16048.

Park, J. J., Tiefenbach, J., & Demetriades, A. K. (2022). The role of artificial intelligence in surgical simulation. *Frontiers in Medical Technology*, *4*, 1076755.

Park, S. H., & Lee, S. P. (1998). EMG pattern recognition based on artificial intelligence techniques. *IEEE Transactions on Rehabilitation Engineering*, *6*(4), 400–405.

Pérez-Osorio, K. C., Jiménez-Nieto, Y. A., González-Diaz, J. E., Rodríguez-Vásquez, G., Rodríguez-Parada, A., & Juárez-Rivera, O. (2025). Mobile apps to improve diabetes mellitus self-care: A scoping review. *New Challenges in Software Engineering: Volume 1*, 405–431.

Pierce, R. L., Van Biesen, W., Van Cauwenberge, D., Decruyenaere, J., & Sterckx, S. (2022). Explainability in medicine in an era of AI-based clinical decision support systems. *Frontiers in Genetics*, *13*, 903600.

Pore, A., Li, Z., Dall'Alba, D., Hernansanz, A., De Momi, E., Menciassi, A., ... & Vander Poorten, E. (2023). Autonomous navigation for robot-assisted intraluminal and endovascular procedures: A systematic review. *IEEE Transactions on Robotics*, *39*(4), 2529–2548.

Proofpoint & Ponemon Institute. (2024). *Cyber insecurity in healthcare: The cost and impact on patient safety and care*. Proofpoint. www.proofpoint.com

Rahimi, S. A., Légaré, F., Sharma, G., Archambault, P., Zomahoun, H. T. V., Chandavong, S., ... & Légaré, J. (2021). Application of artificial intelligence in community-based primary health care: Systematic scoping review. *Journal of Medical Internet Research*, *23*(9), e29839.

Rahimi, S. A., Vimarlund, V., & Timpka, T. (2024). Contextual determinants of artificial intelligence implementation in healthcare: A scoping review. *Journal of the American Medical Informatics Association*, *31*(2), 257–270.

Rajkomar, A., Dean, J., & Kohane, I. (2019). Machine learning in medicine. *New England Journal of Medicine*, *380*(14), 1347–1358.

Ratwani, R. M., Savage, E., Will, A., Arnold, R., Khairat, S., Miller, K., ... & Guttag, J. (2018). A usability and safety analysis of electronic health records: A multi-center study. *Journal of the American Medical Informatics Association, 25*(9), 1197–1201.

Ratti, E., Morrison, M., & Jakab, I. (2025). Ethical and social considerations of applying artificial intelligence in healthcare: A two-pronged scoping review. *BMC Medical Ethics, 26*(1), 68.

Reddy, S. (2024). Generative AI in healthcare: An implementation-science-informed translational path on application, integration, and governance. *Implementation Science, 19*, 27.

Reeves, S., Xyrichis, A., & Zwarenstein, M. (2018). Teamwork, collaboration, coordination, and networking. *Journal of Interprofessional Care, 32*(1), 1–3.

Ribeiro, M. T., Singh, S., & Guestrin, C. (2016). "Why should I trust you?": Explaining the predictions of any classifier. In *Proceedings of the 22nd ACM SIGKDD international conference on knowledge discovery and data mining* (pp. 1135–1144). ACM.

Robertshaw, H., Karstensen, L., Jackson, B., Sadati, H., Rhode, K., Ourselin, S., ... & Booth, T. C. (2023). Artificial intelligence in the autonomous navigation of endovascular interventions: A systematic review. *Frontiers in Human Neuroscience, 17*, 1239374.

Rodenburg, D., Hungler, P., Etemad, S. A., Howes, D., Szulewski, A., & Mclellan, J. (2018). Dynamically adaptive simulation based on expertise and cognitive load. In *2018 IEEE games, entertainment, media conference (GEM)* (pp. 1–6). IEEE.

Rodriguez-Ruiz, A., Lång, K., Gubern-Merida, A., Broeders, M., Gennaro, G., Clauser, P., ... & Sechopoulos, I. (2019). Stand-alone artificial intelligence for breast cancer detection in mammography. *Annals of Internal Medicine, 170*(11), 794.

Rosenblatt, F. (1958). The perceptron: A probabilistic model for information storage and organization in the brain. *Psychological Review, 65*(6), 386–408.

Ronquillo, J. G., Winterholler, J. E., Cwikla, K., Szymanski, R., & Levy, C. (2018). Health IT, hacking, and cybersecurity: National trends in data breaches of protected health information. *JAMIA Open, 1*(1), 15–19.

Ross, C., & Swetlitz, I. (2018, September 5). IBM pitched its Watson supercomputer as a revolution in cancer care. It's nowhere close. *STAT News*. www.statnews.com/2017/09/05/watson-ibm-cancer/

Rudin, C. (2019). Stop explaining black-box machine learning models for high-stakes decisions and use interpretable models instead. *Nature Machine Intelligence, 1*(5), 206–215.

Ruiz, J. G., Mintzer, M. J., & Leipzig, R. M. (2006). The impact of e-learning in medical education. *Academic Medicine, 81*(3), 207–212.

Sadiq, F., Khan, A., & Ahmed, M. U. (2025). Impact of technology on human behaviours in medical education: Editorial overview. *Frontiers in Medicine, 12*, 1546296.

Saif-Ur-Rahman, K. M., Islam, M. S., Alaboson, J., Ola, O., Hasan, I., Islam, N., ... & Joarder, T. (2023). Artificial intelligence and digital health in improving primary health care service delivery in LMICs: A systematic review. *Journal of Evidence-Based Medicine, 16*(3), 303–320.

Sallam, M. (2023). ChatGPT utility in healthcare education, research, and practice: Systematic review on the promising perspectives and valid concerns. *Healthcare, 11*(6), 887.

Salmon, P. M., & Plant, K. L. (2022). Distributed situation awareness: From awareness in individuals and teams to the awareness of technologies, sociotechnical systems, and societies. *Applied Ergonomics, 98*, 103599.

Santillana, M., Zhang, D. W., Althouse, B. M., & Ayers, J. W. (2014). What can digital disease detection learn from (an external revision to) Google Flu Trends? *American Journal of Preventive Medicine, 47*(3), 341–347.

Saqr, M., López-Pernas, S., Jovanović, J., & Gašević, D. (2023). Intense, turbulent, or wallowing in the middle: A longitudinal study of cross-course online tactics, strategies, and trajectories. *Internet and Higher Education, 57*, 100902.

Schein, E. H. (1985). *Organizational culture and leadership.* Jossey-Bass.

Schmidt, H. G., & Rikers, R. M. J. P. (2007). How expertise develops in medicine: Knowledge encapsulation and illness script formation. *Medical Education, 41*(12), 1133–1139.

Schoenherr, J. R. (2016). Prestige technology in the evolution and social organization of early psychological science. *Theory and Psychology*, 1–28.

Schoenherr, J. R. (2017). Prestige technology in the evolution and social organization of early psychological science. *Theory & Psychology, 27*(1), 6–33.

Schoenherr, J. R. (2020). Adapting the zone of proximal development to the wicked environments of professional practice. *HCII 2020*. Copenhagen, Denmark.

Schoenherr, J. R. (2021). Trust and explainability in A/IS-mediated healthcare: Operationalizing the therapeutic alliance in a distributed system. In *2021 IEEE international symposium on technology and society (ISTAS)* (pp. 1–8). IEEE.

Schoenherr, J. R. (2022). Learning engineering is ethical. In J. Goodall & J. Kolodner (Eds.), *Learning engineering toolkit* (pp. 201–228). Routledge.

Schoenherr, J. R. (2022a). *Ethical artificial intelligence: From popular to cognitive science.* Routledge.

Schoenherr, J. R. (2022b). Folkmedical technologies and the sociotechnical systems of healthcare. *IEEE Technology and Society Magazine, 41*(3), 38–49.

Schoenherr, J. R. (2022c). Vaccination, values, and health information search behaviour in the New Folk Medicine. In *2022 IEEE international symposium on technology and society (ISTAS)* (pp. 1–10). IEEE.

Schoenherr, J. R. (2027b). *Insider threat and organizational decision-making: An interdisciplinary approach.* Cambridge University Press.

Schoenherr, J. R. (2026b). The translational research process. In Eltorai, A. E. M., et al. (Eds.), *Translational neurosurgery* (pp. 3–7). Elsevier.

Schoenherr, J. R. (2026c). From Realism to Relevance: Rethinking Simulator Fidelity in the Era of Generative AI. *IEEE Transactions on Technology and Society*, 7(2), 91–100.

Schoenherr, J. R. (2026d). The development and dynamics of heterarchical structure in Mayan medical education and healthcare ecosystems. In J. R. Schoenherr (Ed.), *Fundamentals and frontiers of medical education and decision-making*. Routledge.

Schoenherr, J. R. (2027a). Evolutionary theory and the affordances of AI sociotechnical systems: Group selection and collective memory systems. Dwivedi, Y. K. & Wade, M. R. (Eds.), *Information systems theory: Digital society in the era of artificial intelligence* Vol. 3. Springer Nature.

Schoenherr, J. R. (2027b). Application in Sociotechnical Systems in AI for Meaningful Human Control: Criteria for MHC of AWS using Cognitive Load Theory. In Dwivedi, Y. K. & Wade, M. R. (Eds.), *Information systems theory: digital society in the era of artificial intelligence* Vol. 3. Springer Nature.

Schoenherr, J. R. (2027c). War against systems: Healthcare infrastructure and irregular warfare during the total war in Ukraine. In *Ukraine, competitive statecraft, and irregular warfare*.

Schoenherr, J. R. (in press). Developing agency in human digital twins: Defining minimal agentic capabilities. *IEEE Transactions on Technology and Society*.

Schoenherr, J. R., Abbas, R., Michael, K., Rivas, P., & Anderson, T. D. (2023). Designing AI using a human-centered approach: Explainability and accuracy toward trustworthiness. *IEEE Transactions on Technology and Society*, *4*, 9–23.

Schoenherr, J. R., & Grubesic, R. (submitted). AI as community technologies: Building autonomous healthcare infrastructures for rural, low-income, and Indigenous contexts. *IEEE Transactions on Technology and Society.*

Schoenherr, J. R., & Hamstra, S. J. (2024). Validity in health professions education: From assessment instruments to program innovation and evaluation. In J. R. Schoenherr & M. M McConnell (Eds.), *Fundamentals and Frontiers of medical education and decision-making* (pp. 80–107). Routledge.

Schoenherr, J. R. & Beadoin, J. (2026). The evolving landscape of health professions education in East Asia: Heterarchies in East Asian medicine and medical education. In J. R. Schoenherr (Ed.), *Fundamentals and Frontiers of medical education and decision-making.* Routledge.

Schoenherr, J. R., & LeBouar, S. (2025). Communication and cognitive coordination in AI-enabled clinical teams. In J. R. Schoenherr (Ed.), *Handbook of human-centered AI* (pp. 531–549). Springer.

Schoenherr, J. R., Månsson, K., & Gioe, D. V. (2022). Multiple approach paths to insider threat (MAP-IT): Intentional, ambivalent, and unintentional pathways to insider threats. *Counter-Insider Threat Research and Practice*, *1*, 1–23.

Schoenherr, J. R., & Michael, K. (2026). Multi-level sociotechnical systems approach to human-centered AI. In W. Xu (Ed.), *Handbook of human-centered artificial intelligence* (pp. 1–74).

Schoenherr, J. R., & McConnell, M. M. (2024a). Human-centered design in health professions education: Informing competency-based education with psychological science. In J. R. Schoenherr & M. McConnell (Eds.), *Fundamentals and Frontiers of medical education and decision-making* (pp. 3–36). Routledge.

Schoenherr, J. R., & McConnell, M. (Eds.). (2024b). *Fundamentals and Frontiers of medical education and decision-making: Educational theory and psychological practice.* Routledge.

Schoenherr, J. R., & Thomson, R. (2024). When AI fails, who do we blame? Attributing responsibility in human–AI interactions. *IEEE Transactions on Technology and Society*, *5*(1), 61–70.

Schoenherr, J. R., Waechter, J., & Lee, C. H. (2024). Quantifying expertise in the healthcare professions: Cognitive efficiency and metacognitive calibration. In J. R. Schoenherr & M. McConnell (Eds.), *Fundamentals and Frontiers of medical education and decision-making* (pp. 213–244). Routledge.

Schoenherr, J. R., Waechter, J., & Millington, S. J. (2018). Subjective awareness of ultrasound expertise development: Individual experience as a determinant of overconfidence. *Advances in Health Sciences Education*, *23*(4), 749–765.

Schwaeke, J., Gerlich, C., Nguyen, H. L., Kanbach, D. K., & Gast, J. (2025). Artificial intelligence (AI) for good? Enabling organizational change towards sustainability. *Review of Managerial Science*, *19*, 3013–3038.

Schwalbe, N., & Wahl, B. (2020). Artificial intelligence and the future of global health. *The Lancet*, *395*(10236), 1579–1586.

Sendak, M. P., Elish, M. C., Gao, M., Futoma, J., Ratliff, W., Nichols, M., & Balu, S. (2020). The human body is a black box: Supporting clinical decision-making with deep learning.

In *Proceedings of the 2020 Conference on Fairness, Accountability, and Transparency* (pp. 99–109).

Shimizu, I., Kasai, H., Shikino, K., Araki, N., Takahashi, Z., Onodera, M., ... & Kawakami, E. (2023). Developing medical education curriculum reform strategies to address the impact of generative AI: qualitative study. *JMIR medical education*, *9*(1), e53466.

Shneiderman, B. (2020a). Human-centered artificial intelligence: Reliable, safe & trustworthy. *International Journal of Human–Computer Interaction*, *36*(6), 495–504.

Shneiderman, B. (2020b). Human-centered artificial intelligence: Three fresh ideas. *AIS Transactions on Human–Computer Interaction*, *12*(3), 109–124.

Shneiderman, B. (2022). *Human-centered AI*. Oxford University Press.

Shortliffe, E. H., & Sepúlveda, M. J. (2018). Clinical decision support in the era of artificial intelligence. *JAMA*, *320*(21), 2199–2200.

Singh, H., Sittig, D. F., & Wilson, L. (2024). Early warning systems in clinical practice: Balancing automation and human oversight. *NPJ Digital Medicine*, *7*(1), 38.

Sittig, D. F., & Singh, H. (2010). A new sociotechnical model for studying health information technology in complex adaptive healthcare systems. *Quality & Safety in Health Care*, *19*(Suppl 3), i68–i74.

Smith, W. (2019). *A comprehensive cybersecurity defense framework for large organizations* (Doctoral dissertation, Nova Southeastern University).

Sparrow, B., Liu, J., & Wegner, D. M. (2011). Google effects on memory: Cognitive consequences of having information at our fingertips. *Science*, *333*(6043), 776–778.

Stanberry, B. (1997a). The legal and ethical aspects of telemedicine: Confidentiality and the patient's rights of access. *Journal of Telemedicine and Telecare*, *3*(4), 179–187.

Stanberry, B. (1997b). The legal and ethical aspects of telemedicine: Data protection, security, and European law. *Journal of Telemedicine and Telecare*, *4*(1), 18–24.

Stanney, K. M., Archer, J., Skinner, A., Horner, C., Hughes, C., Brawand, N. P., ... & Perez, R. S. (2022). Performance gains from adaptive extended reality training fueled by artificial intelligence. *The Journal of Defense Modeling and Simulation*, *19*(2), 195–218.

Stanton, N. A. (2016). Distributed situation awareness. *Theoretical Issues in Ergonomics Science*, *17*(1), 1–7.

Stanton, N. A., Salmon, P. M., Walker, G. H., Salas, E., & Hancock, P. A. (2017). State-of-science: Situation awareness in individuals, teams, and systems. *Ergonomics*, *60*(4), 449–466.

Star, S. L., & Ruhleder, K. (1996). Steps toward an ecology of infrastructure: Design and access for large information spaces. *Information Systems Research*, *7*(1), 111–134.

Starmer, A. J., Spector, N. D., Srivastava, R., Allen, A. D., Landrigan, C. P., & Sectish, T. C. (2014). I-PASS, a mnemonic to standardize verbal handoffs. *Pediatrics*, *129*(2), 201–204.

Starr, P. (1982). *The social transformation of American medicine*. Basic Books.

Steel, P. A. D., Jenkins, R. A., & Lee, S. (2025). Learning health system strategies in the AI era. *NPJ Digital Medicine*, *8*(1), 29.

Strickland, E. (2019, April 2). How IBM Watson overpromised and underdelivered on AI health care. *IEEE spectrum*. https://spectrum.ieee.org/how-ibm-watson-overpromised-and-underdelivered-on-ai-health-care

Strielkowski, W. (2025). AI-driven adaptive learning for sustainable educational development. *Sustainable Development*, *33*(2), 451–463.

Sujan, M., Smith-Frazer, C., Malamateniou, C., Connor, J., Gardner, A., Unsworth, H., & Husain, H. (2023). Validation framework for the use of AI in healthcare: overview of the new British standard BS30440. *BMJ Health & Care Informatics*, *30*(1), e100749.

Sun, Q., Akman, A., & Schuller, B. W. (2025). Explainable artificial intelligence for medical applications: A review. *ACM Transactions on Computing for Healthcare*, *6*(2), 1–31.

Sutton, R. T., Pincock, D., Baumgart, D. C., Sadowski, D. C., Fedorak, R. N., & Kroeker, K. I. (2020). An overview of clinical decision support systems: Benefits, risks, and strategies for success. *NPJ Digital Medicine*, *3*(1), 17.

Susnjak, T., & McIntosh, T. R. (2024). ChatGPT: The end of online exam integrity? *Education Sciences*, *14*(6), 656.

Szafir, D., & Mutlu, B. (2012). Pay attention! Designing adaptive agents that monitor and improve user engagement. In *Proceedings of the SIGCHI conference on human factors in computing systems* (pp. 11–20).

Taddeo, M., Jones, P., Abbas, R., Vogel, K., & Michael, K. (2023). Socio-technical ecosystem considerations: An emergent research agenda for AI in cybersecurity. *IEEE Transactions on Technology and Society*, *4*(2), 112–118.

ten Cate, O., Hart, D., Ankel, F., Busari, J., Englander, R., Glasgow, N., ... & Touchie, C. (2016). Entrustment decision making in clinical training. *Academic Medicine*, *91*(2), 191–198.

Thomson, R., & Schoenherr, J. R. (2020). Knowledge-to-information translation training (KITT): An adaptive approach to explainable artificial intelligence. In *International conference on human–computer interaction* (pp. 187–204). Springer International Publishing.

Tihan, T., Canbulat, N., Aktaş, C., Ölmez, S., Oflaz, F., Abacıoğlu, H., ... & Participants of the First Symposium on Healthcare Academic Professionals Education 2024. (2025). Critical issues and the impact of technology in healthcare professional education in low- and middle-income countries: A call for transformation. *Medical Science Educator*, *35*, 2657–2665.

Tikhomirov, D., Schoenherr, J. R., & Sauer, J. (2024). Automation bias and complacency in AI-assisted clinical decision-making. *Frontiers in Artificial Intelligence*, *7*, 1394826.

Timmermans, S., & Berg, M. (2003). *The gold standard: The challenge of evidence-based medicine and standardization in health care*. Temple University Press.

Ting, D. S. W., Cheung, C. Y.-L., Lim, G., Tan, G. S. W., Quang, N. D., Gan, A., ... & Wong, T. Y. (2017). Development and validation of a deep learning system for diabetic retinopathy and related eye diseases using retinal images from multiethnic populations with diabetes. *JAMA*, *318*(22), 2211–2223.

Tolsgaard, M. G., Boscardin, C. K., Park, Y. S., Cuddy, M. M., & Sebok-Syer, S. S. (2021). The role of data science and machine learning in health professions education: Practical applications, theoretical contributions, and epistemic injustices. *Advances in Health Sciences Education*, *28*(1), 237–258.

Topol, E. J. (2019a). *Deep medicine: How artificial intelligence can make healthcare human again.* Basic Books.

Topol, E. J. (2019b). High-performance medicine: The convergence of human and artificial intelligence. *Nature Medicine*, *25*, 44–56.

Trist, E. L., & Bamforth, K. W. (1951). Some social and psychological consequences of the longwall method of coal-getting. *Human Relations*, *4*(1), 3–38.

Tun, H. M., Naing, L., Malik, O. A., & Rahman, H. A. (2025). Artificial Intelligence (AI)-based tools in the diagnosis and management of prostate cancer: a systematic review and meta-analysis. *Prostate Cancer and Prostatic Diseases*, 1–15.

UNESCO. (2025a). *AI competency and ethics in health education: A global policy framework.* United Nations Educational, Scientific and Cultural Organization.
UNESCO. (2025b). *AI and the future of education: Disruptions, dilemmas and directions.* UNESCO Publishing. https://unesdoc.unesco.org
U.S. Department of Health and Human Services, Office for Civil Rights (HHS). (2023). *Annual report to Congress on breaches of unsecured protected health information for calendar year 2022.* HHS. www.hhs.gov/sites/default/files/breach-report-to-congress-2022.pdf
U.S. Department of Health and Human Services. (2023/2024). *Healthcare sector cybersecurity: Introduction to the HHS strategy.* ASPR. https://aspr.hhs.gov/cyber/Documents/Health-Care-Sector-Cybersecurity-Dec2023-508.pdf
U.S. Department of Health and Human Services. (2024). *Healthcare and public health (HPH) cybersecurity performance goals.* HHS.
U.S. Food and Drug Administration. (2023). *Cybersecurity in medical devices: Quality system considerations and content of premarket submissions.* FDA.
van der Vegt, A. H., Scott, I. A., Dermawan, K., Schnetler, R. J., Kalke, V. R., & Lane, P. J. (2023). Implementation frameworks for end-to-end clinical AI: Derivation of the SALIENT framework. *Journal of the American Medical Informatics Association, 30*(9), 1503–1515.
van der Vleuten, C. P. M., Schuwirth, L. W. T., Driessen, E. W., Dijkstra, J., Tigelaar, D., Baartman, L. K. J., & van Tartwijk, J. (2012). A model for programmatic assessment fit for purpose. *Medical Teacher, 34*(3), 205–214.
van Leeuwen, F. W., & van der Hage, J. A. (2022). Where robotic surgery meets the metaverse. *Cancers, 14*(24), 6161.
Vasey, B., Lippert, K. A., Khan, D. Z., Ibrahim, M., Koh, C. H., Horsfall, H. L., ... & McCulloch, P. (2023). Intraoperative applications of artificial intelligence in robotic surgery: A scoping review of current development stages and levels of autonomy. *Annals of Surgery, 278*(6), 896–903.
Velez, M., & Rister, A. (2025). Beyond academic integrity: Navigating institutional and disciplinary anxieties about AI-assisted authorship in technical and professional communication. *Journal of Business and Technical Communication, 39*(1), 115–132.
Viceconti, M., Hernandez Herrero, D., Rochette, M., & Pappalardo, F. (2021). In silico trials: Verification, validation and uncertainty quantification of predictive models used in the regulatory evaluation of biomedical products. *Methods, 185*, 120–127.
Vincent, C., Moorthy, K., Sarker, S. K., Chang, A., & Darzi, A. W. (2004). Systems approaches to surgical quality and safety: From concept to measurement. *Annals of Surgery, 239*(4), 475–482.
von Borzyskowski, I., Mazumder, A., Mateen, B., & Wooldridge, M. (2021). *Data science and AI: Reflections on the response of the U.K.'s data science and AI community to the COVID-19 pandemic.* Alan Turing Institute.
Vozenilek, J., Huff, J. S., Reznek, M., & Gordon, J. A. (2004). See one, do one, teach one: Advanced technology in medical education. *Academic Emergency Medicine, 11*(11), 1149–1154.
Wang, D., & Zhang, S. (2024). Large language models in medical and healthcare fields: applications, advances, and challenges. *Artificial Intelligence Review, 57*(11), 299.
Wanzel, K. R., Hamstra, S. J., Anastakis, D. J., Matsumoto, E. D., & Cusimano, M. D. (2002). Effect of visual-spatial ability on learning of spatially-complex surgical skills. *The Lancet, 359*(9302), 230–231.

Wartman, S. A., & Combs, C. D. (2018). Medical education must move from the information age to the age of artificial intelligence. *Academic Medicine*, *93*(8), 1107–1109.
Wei Gao, Z. (2025). Human-centered AI frameworks and sociotechnical integration. *IEEE Transactions on Human-Machine Systems*, *55*(3), 1–12.
Were, M. C. (2022). Challenges in digital medicine applications in under-resourced settings. *Nature Communications*, *13*(1), 3020.
Williams, P. A., & Woodward, A. J. (2015). Cybersecurity vulnerabilities in medical devices: A complex environment and multifaceted problem. *Medical Devices: Evidence and Research*, *8*, 305–316.
Winkler-Schwartz, A., Bissonnette, V., Mirchi, N., Ponnudurai, N., Yilmaz, R., Ledwos, N., ... & Del Maestro, R. F. (2019). Artificial intelligence in medical education: Best practices using machine learning to assess surgical expertise in virtual reality simulation. *Journal of Surgical Education*, *76*(6), 1681–1690.
Wong, A., Plasek, J. M., Montecalvo, S. P., & Zhou, L. (2021). Natural language processing and its implications for the future of medication safety: A narrative review of recent advances and challenges. *Pharmacotherapy*, *41*(2), 187.
Wong, Z. S.-Y., Zhou, J., & Zhang, Q. (2019). Artificial intelligence for infectious disease big data analytics. *Infection, Disease & Health*, *24*(1), 44–48.
World Health Organization (WHO). (2021). *Ethics and governance of artificial intelligence for health.* World Health Organization.
World Health Organization. (2023). *Advancing health information and digital transformation in the health sector* [Paper for the Fifteenth Pacific Health Ministers Meeting, 20–22 September 2023, Tonga]. WHO Western Pacific Region. Retrieved Dec 10, 2025 from: https://cdn.who.int/media/docs/default-source/wpro---documents/dps/phmm-phoh-documents/15th-phmm/advancing-health-information-and-digital-transformation-phmm-paper.pdf
World Health Organization (WHO). (2024a). *Global guidance on the ethics and governance of artificial intelligence for health.* World Health Organization.
World Health Organization (WHO). (2024b). *Harnessing artificial intelligence for health: Governance, risk management and ethical considerations.* World Health Organization. www.who.int/publications/i/item/9789240097720
World Health Organization (WHO). (2025). *Global strategy on digital health 2025–2030.* World Health Organization.
Wynants, L., Van Calster, B., Collins, G. S., Riley, R. D., Heinze, G., Schuit, E., ... & van Smeden, M. (2020). Prediction models for diagnosis and prognosis of Covid-19: Systematic review and critical appraisal. *BMJ*, *369*, m1328.
Xu, W., & Gao, W. (2024). Intelligent sociotechnical systems: A hierarchical human-centered AI framework. *arXiv Preprint*, arXiv:2409.13770. https://arxiv.org/abs/2409.13770
Xu, W., & Gao, Z. (2025). An intelligent sociotechnical systems (iSTS) framework: Enabling a hierarchical human-centered AI (hHCAI) approach. *IEEE Transactions on Technology and Society*, *6*(1), 31–46.
Yang, J., Blount, Y., & Amrollahi, A. (2024). Artificial intelligence adoption in a professional service industry: A multiple case study. *Technological Forecasting and Social Change*, 201, 123251.
Yang, S. J., Ogata, H., Matsui, T., & Chen, N. S. (2021). Human-centered artificial intelligence in education: Seeing the invisible through the visible. *Computers and Education: Artificial Intelligence*, *2*, 100008.

Yildiz, E., Çetin Gürkan, G., & Şahin Dağli, F. (2025). AI-supported organizational change management in healthcare institutions. *BMC Health Services Research*, *25*(1), 212.

Young, A. T., Amara, D., Bhattacharya, A., & Wei, M. L. (2021). Patient and general public attitudes towards clinical artificial intelligence: A mixed methods systematic review. *The Lancet Digital Health*, *3*(9), e599–e611.

Yusuf, A., Pervin, N., & Román-González, M. (2024). Generative AI and the future of higher education: A threat to academic integrity or reformation? Evidence from multicultural perspectives. *International Journal of Educational Technology in Higher Education*, *21*(1), 21.

Zary, N., Johnson, G., Boberg, J., & Fors, U. (2019). Development, implementation, and pilot evaluation of a web-based virtual patient case simulation environment—Web-SP. *BMC Medical Education*, *19*, 325.

Zou, J., & Schiebinger, L. (2018). Design AI so that it's fair. *Nature*, *559*(7714), 324–326.

SECTION 2

Implementation Case Studies

Institutional and Nations Perspectives

4

COMMUNICATION IN ETHICALLY SENSITIVE SITUATIONS

Implementing a Training Program in Neonatology

Thierry Daboval, Emanuela Ferretti, and Alexandra Barkova

The high mortality rates, medical complexity, uncertainty in prognosis, rapid advancements in life-sustaining medical technologies to support life, and elevated parental expectations in our modern society make ethically sensitive situations a ubiquitous feature of neonatal and perinatal medicine (NPM). Consequently, NPM training programs must prioritize education in communication skills when situations are ethically ambiguous, wherein multiple values, norms, conventions, and perspectives can complement and conflict in time-constrained decision-making environments where errors are costly. Such complexity also underscores the need for iterative adaptation and contextual alignment during program design. These are key features of implementation validity in educational innovation (Schoenherr & Hamstra, 2024).

Practitioners face many challenges in the delivery of care, including interprofessional coordination, triaging cases based on patient need, managing limited resources, and delivering care in a time-limited environment. Ethical dilemmas are of critical importance to the health-care professions but are not always given explicit consideration. As an interdisciplinary field, ethics presents many challenges, including identifying the objects of analysis (e.g., sanctity of life v. quality of health v. dignity of death), the agency of patients and family members, and the appropriate ethical framework (e.g., consequences, principles, or ethical communication and sensemaking). Unsurprisingly, there are also major disagreements between educators and practitioners regarding what and how ethically ambiguous situations should be taught, the appropriate means to assess outcomes, and the efficacy of assessment tools (de la Garza et al., 2017; Giubilini et al., 2016; Goldie et al., 2002; Hafferty & Franks, 1994; Self et al., 1989; Watts et al., 2017). Many NPM training programs implemented the model of Entrustable Professional Activities (EPAs) to provide educational approaches with feedback,

DOI: 10.4324/9781003498155-4

but specific competencies and milestones are yet to be defined, particularly during ethically challenging clinical scenarios.

Communication of prospective consequential negative outcomes, such as the likelihood of the presence of a disability or the passing of a newborn ("bad news"), and providing compassionate and empathetic support to the infant and families, although included, seem lost in the overwhelming framework of learning ethically oriented objectives (Cummings, 2016)

4.1 Communication in Medical Field: Developing a Therapeutic Alliance

Effective communication is a necessary feature of any clinical encounter (Greenhalgh et al., 2018; Schoenherr & LeBouar, 2024; Vermeir et al., 2015; Wanzer et al., 2004). Many studies have suggested that medical errors are largely attributable to a lack of effective communication among intervention-team members (Alvarez & Coiera, 2006; Greenberg et al., 2007; Schaefer et al., 1994; Sutcliffe et al., 2004; Varpio et al., 2008; cf. McDonald et al., 2000). Complementing these observations, contemporary medicine has also adopted the concept of a therapeutic alliance, requiring that clinicians and patients understand, collaborate in decision-making, and select and monitor the efficacy of therapy (Figure 4.1; i.e., a form of collective competence; see Schoenherr et al., 2026).

NPM is defined by complex interpersonal dynamics, where a binary clinician–patient model of communication does not hold. The patients of NPM are neonates (infants), who cannot advocate for themselves or express preferences, opinions, or make informed choices. As such, an effective communication model must acknowledge the perspective of multiple stakeholders beyond the patient or legal guardians within the window of what is best for the neonates defined by contextually accepted options in such situation. As the number and diversity of stakeholders' preferences increase, the complexity of communication and delivery of care will rapidly increase. Fostering agency and mindfulness in shared patient–clinician decision-making requires identifying effective means to teach and empower these stakeholders in situations where time and information are limited.

4.2 The Family-Centered Communication

Neonatal intensive care units (NICUs) are stressful environments for parents. To address the demands of this situation, a Family-Centered Model (FCM) based on the principle that parental involvement in their child's care can reduce stress and increase satisfaction has been proposed (Franck & O'Brien, 2019; Hanson et al., 1995; Johnson, 2000; Kokorelias et al., 2019). In contrast to Healthcare Provider-centered approaches, FCM represents an extension of models of collective competence, viewing the therapeutic network (family) as the basic unit of analysis

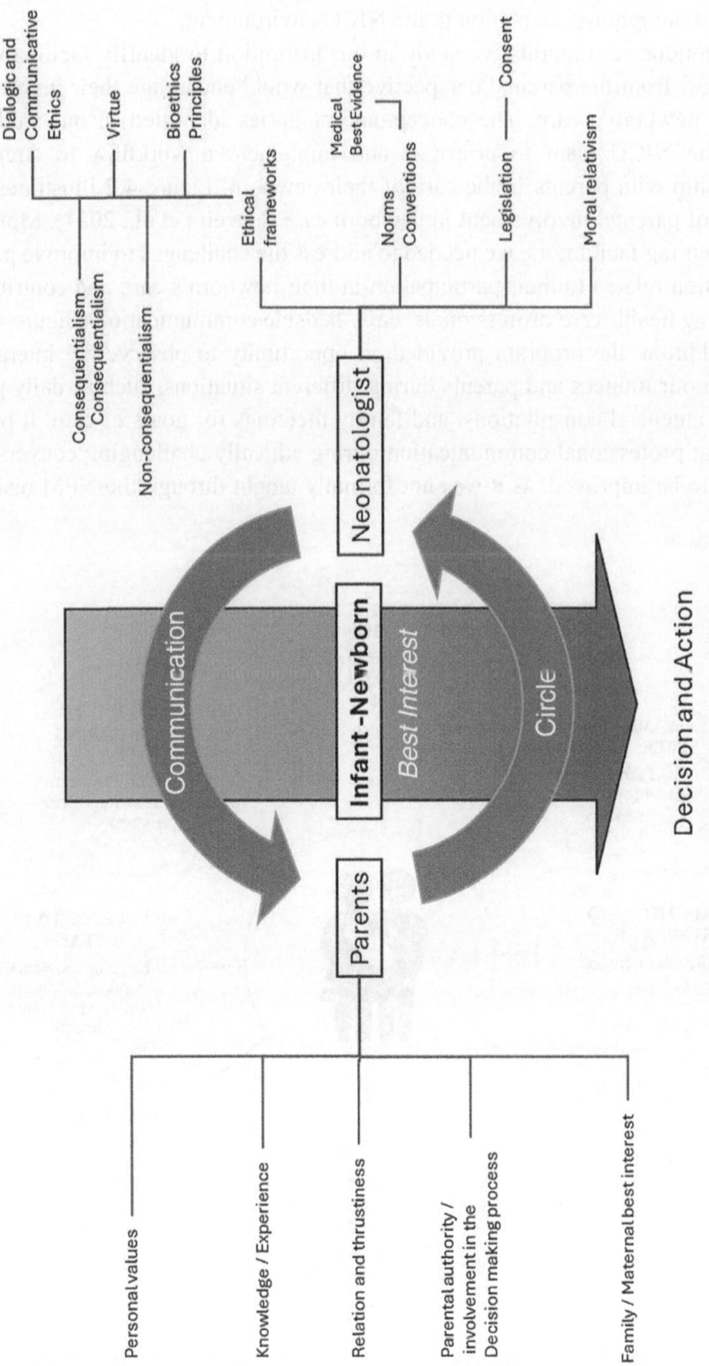

FIGURE 4.1 Communication in a shared decision-making (SDM) process model.

(Schoenherr et al., 2026). Other Parenting Unit models in neonatology have been proposed but require adaptation to the NICU environment.

We conducted a qualitative study in our institution to identify facilitators and challenges from the parents' perspective that would encourage their involvement in their newborn's care. The conceptual categories identified in our study will allow the NICU team to prioritize and implement a workflow to strengthen partnership with parents in the care of their newborn. Figure 4.2 illustrates these themes of parental involvement in newborn care (Ferreira et al., 2021). More than implementing facilitators, we needed to address the challenges to improve parents' satisfaction related to their participation in their newborn's care and contribute to improving health-care professionals' daily bedside communication (Figure 4.2).

In addition, the program provided an opportunity to observe the interactions between our trainees and parents during different situations, such as daily patient rounds, antenatal consultations, and family meetings for goals of care. It became clear that professional communication during ethically challenging conversations needed to be improved, as it was not formally taught through the NPM residency

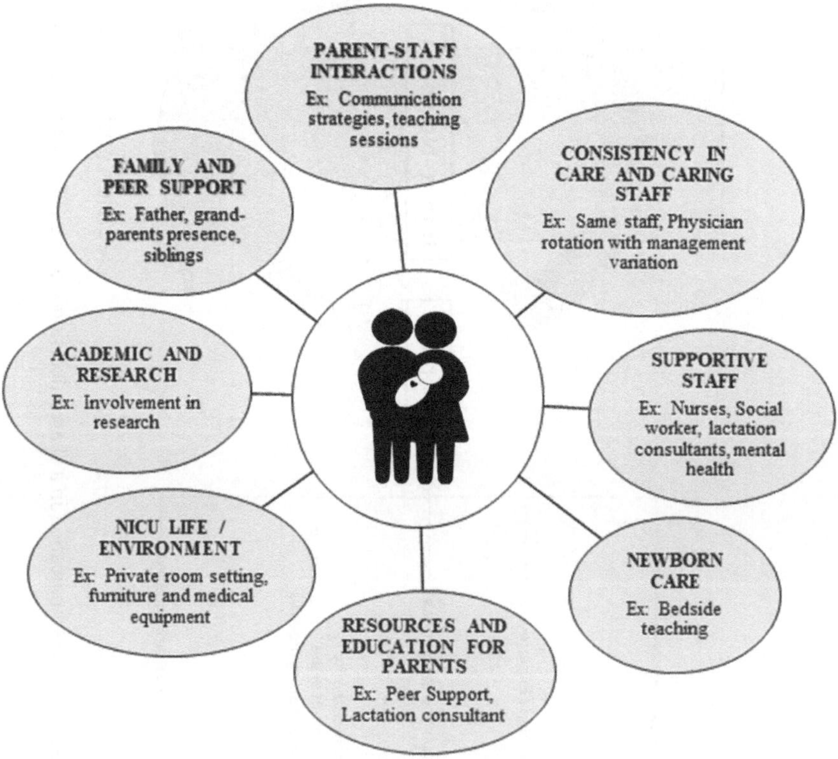

FIGURE 4.2 The dynamic themes of parental involvement in newborn care (Ferreira et al, 2021).

program at the University of Ottawa (located in Ontario, Canada). We adapted our residency training program (Daboval et al., 2013) to align it with the NPM training objectives discussed in the 2007 publication by the Royal College of Physicians and Surgeons of Canada (RCPSC). These objectives, as well as the introduction of competency-based CanMEDS roles, prompted Canadian NPM residency program directors to reassess their approaches to ethics education. With the current lack of literature directly addressing the topic, a nation-wide survey investigated ethics teaching methods, standards, and assessments in other Canadian NPM residency programs (Daboval et al., 2014a, 2014b). Below is a schematic summary of the skills needed to competently navigate challenging conversations (Table 4.2).

4.3 Communication Ethics Education in Medicine: Adult and Pediatrics

Ethical frameworks provide a useful point of reference for the development of ethics training programs. The principles of autonomy, beneficence, non-maleficence, and justice form the foundational pillars of biomedical ethics and remain central to ethics education in medicine (Beauchamp, 2019). However, these principles alone do not encompass the full spectrum of critical thinking and professional interactions required in contemporary health care (Norman et al., 2018; Patel et al., 2005; Schwartz & Griffin, 2012; for a review, see Schoenherr & McConnell, 2024). While essential for teaching ethically grounded approaches, these principles often fall short in addressing how diverse perspectives, rooted in valid ethical concepts, can be harmonized in therapeutic decisions—especially within the framework of shared decision-making (Daboval & Shidler, 2014).

Shared decision-making is intrinsically tied to effective communication (Altin & Stock, 2016; Edwards & Elwyn, 2009; Land et al., 2017; Roodbeen et al., 2020; Schoenherr et al., 2026). Ethical decision-making requires open, honest, and unfettered communication that builds trust and ensures that decisions are ethically justified (Daboval & Shidler, 2014; Kon, 2009). Furthermore, in today's diverse societies that strive for inclusivity, ethics education must integrate empathy and cultural competence to foster meaningful doctor–patient relationships and provide sensitive, patient-centered care (Betancourt, 2006).

Ethics education in medicine should be multifaceted, blending theoretical understanding, case-based application, bedside approach, and self-reflection. Pedagogical approaches must emphasize the dynamic interplay between ethical theory and real-world scenarios (Figure 4.3). These approaches align with principles of adaptive implementation, which are defined as innovations cycles of design, testing, and feedback (Damschroder et al., 2009; Schoenherr & Hamstra, 2024).

To bridge the gap between theory and practice, case-based learning with complex and realistic scenarios is widely recommended in medical education literature. Experiential learning techniques, such as simulations and role-playing, further prepare trainees by building confidence and competence while promoting critical self-reflection before facing real-world challenges (Boyd & Fales, 1983; McLean, 2004). Programs should also encourage open dialogue about personal biases, fostering self-awareness and a commitment to equitable, unbiased patient care. Such an approach is consistent with educational paradigms that promote culturally sensitive and relevant pedagogy (Schoenherr, 2027).

Experienced preceptors and mentors play a pivotal role in shaping trainees' ethical decision-making abilities by guiding them through nuanced real-life situations. Additionally, the integration of technology, including interactive modules, virtual discussions, and global collaboration, has revolutionized ethics education, making it more accessible and engaging for today's learners. Collectively, these approaches nurture critical thinking, effective communication, and collaborative decision-making. Ethics education in medicine frequently emphasizes professionalism and communication in contexts such as delivering bad news, acknowledging mistakes, and understanding research ethics (Oljeski et al., 2004). These aspects are crucial in pediatrics, and even more so in NPM, due to the unique complexities of caring for children and newborns. The physician's primary responsibility to the infant's best interests adds another layer of complexity to the ethical considerations in this field (Table 4.1; Coughlin, 2018; Ross, 1998).

Unlike adult medicine—where the paradigm shift from paternalism to respect for patient autonomy occurred in the 1980s (McCullough & Cross, 1985; Rothman, 2001)—pediatrics presents unique challenges. The balance between respecting parental authority and ensuring the infant's best interests introduces ethical tensions not commonly encountered in adult care. In newborn care, the transition from paternalistic models is particularly nuanced, as physicians must balance dual obligations within a framework of shared decision-making and ethical integrity.

4.4 SOLE Program Development, Implementation, and Evaluation through ACT4ETHICS

The program was developed within the Ottawa Hospital Network (OHN) in coordination with the University of Ottawa's Department of Medicine. The OHN consists of multiple hospitals and health-care facilities, integrating patient care, education, and research for the Ottawa Valley region. As part of the OHN, the Children's Hospital of Eastern Ontario (CHEO) serves as a regional center providing comprehensive medical care to children, youth, and their families—ranging from emergency services to specialized treatments in cardiology, surgery, oncology, neurology, and neonatology.

4.4.1 Phase 1—Developing and Implementing the SOLE Program

The updated pilot teaching program (Table 4.1) was implemented from July 2009 to June 2011. It ran on a bi-monthly schedule for the two-year residency in NPM, totaling 14 hours of formal instruction. This period included 6 hours of workshop

TABLE 4.1 Current Outline of the Neonatal Ethics Teaching Program

Phase	*Educational Activities*	
First year	1. Steps to Obtain Consent: How to Conduct an Ethical Neonatal Consultation 2. Legislative and Normative Frameworks in Neonatology 3. Bioethical Principles 4. Workshop: Ethical Models of the Physician–Patient Relationship 5. Scenario-Oriented Learning in Ethics: Limit of Viability	Portfolio and mentorship meetings
Second year	6. Reflection on Death 7. Workshop: How to Break Bad News 8. Resolving Ethical Conflict Using Communication 9. Scenario-Oriented Learning in Ethics: Unexpected Birth Malformation	

TABLE 4.2 List of the Principal and Key Competencies of the Neonatal Ethics Teaching Program at the University of Ottawa

Principal competency	Work in partnership with parents of a sick newborn to plan the newborn's care. *("Sick newborn" refers to a child with a high risk of mortality and/or morbidity that might impair his/her long-term quality of life.)*
Key competency C1	Effectively facilitate the doctor–patient relationship and the dynamic exchanges with parents that occur before, during, and after the birth of their baby. This must occur in order to plan the care of their newborn while respecting the ethical principles and values of each participant involved in the decision-making process (parents, physician, and other health professionals).
Key competency C2	Appropriately recognize and manage the ethical conflicts of interest that might arise during a consultation for the planning of care of a newborn.
Key competency C3	Generate self-reflection on the interaction with the parents and other professionals in order to improve his/her efficiency in communication and collaboration.

Source: Adapted from Daboval et al. (2013).

simulations using standardized patients (SPs) and 2 hours of mentorship focused on reviewing self-reflection portfolios based on personal experience.

First, we identified the competencies to be acquired by trainees completing the NPM residency. These skills were determined following a review with all practicing neonatologists at the University of Ottawa. The principal competency and associated key competencies outlined in Table 4.2 emphasize the CanMEDS roles—communicator, professional, collaborator, and health advocate. The phased rollout reflects principles of staged implementation, beginning with feasibility testing, stakeholder alignment, and adaptation to local resources before broader dissemination (Damschroder et al., 2009; Schoenherr, 2026).

We analyzed existing seminars from the 1992 ethics teaching program. Several seminars were modified or refined, and new interactive sessions were added, such as *Steps to Obtain Consent: How to Conduct an Ethical Neonatal Consultation*, and workshops on *Ethical Models of the Physician–Patient Relationship* and *How to Break Bad News*.

A major accomplishment in renewing our Neonatal Ethics Teaching Program was the gradual implementation of simulation sessions based on a recognized Problem-Based Learning Exercise teaching model (Martineau & Girard, 2010a, 2010b). Over 13 years, we developed formal teaching and interactive workshops in accordance with our students' needs—validated through a national survey—culminating in an assessment instrument (Daboval et al., 2019). These sessions evolved into small-group teaching designed to facilitate communication during ethically sensitive conversations, called *Scenario-Oriented Learning in Ethics (SOLE)*, where trainees practice communication skills with SPs acting as parents.

The SOLEs became keystones of the updated program (Ferretti et al., 2015), as interactive teaching—role-playing with SPs, focused debriefing, and feedback—proved highly effective for developing communication and professionalism (Johnston et al., 2011; McManus et al., 1993).

4.4.1.1 Scenarios

The SOLEs were implemented to allow trainees to practice communication skills and integrate ethical thinking in a structured setting across five typical challenging clinical scenarios encountered in NPM. These included parents requesting non-standard medical care, expressing overwhelming emotions, or posing difficult questions such as, "*What would you do, doctor, if it were your child?*". The scenarios mirrored the most frequent and complex situations in neonatology: infants at risk of premature birth and limited viability, unexpected congenital anomalies, severe illness in the NICU, and postnatal communication of suspected Trisomy 21. Each provided a safe, controlled learning environment for skill development.

4.4.1.2 Feedback and Debriefing

During SOLEs, two or more trained facilitators—faculty in neonatology, obstetrics, maternal–fetal medicine, genetics, palliative care, or law—observed trainees directly and conducted guided "mini-debriefing" feedback sessions. Although SOLEs share some features with Objective Structured Clinical Examinations (OSCEs), they differ by permitting interruptions for safety or real-time feedback rather than end-of-session comments. Built on real-case situations, SOLE sessions aimed to recognize where and why communication mistakes arise and to transform these into constructive learning opportunities (Figure 4.3).

To accomplish these learning objectives, we developed a concurrent guided debriefing-feedback model in which communication errors in simulation become valuable learning opportunities (Ferretti et al., 2019). *Figure 4.3 illustrates this dynamic interaction scheme used during SOLE workshops.*

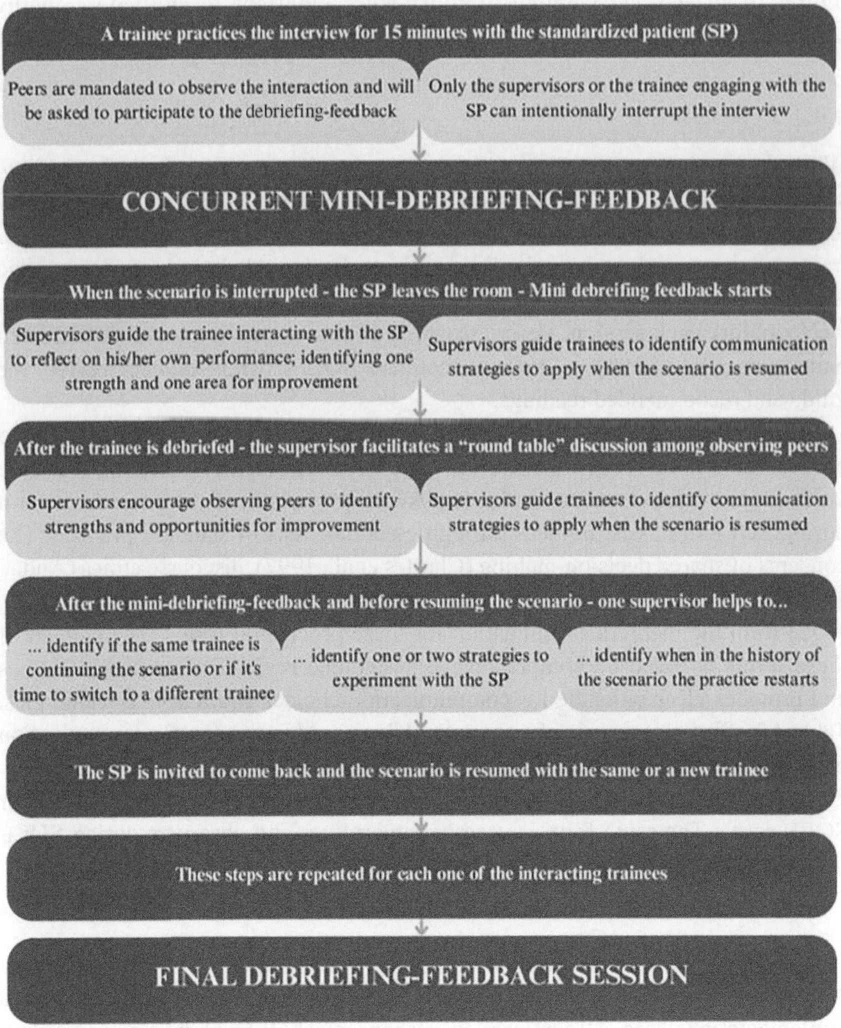

FIGURE 4.3 Dynamic interaction scheme of the mini debriefing-feedback during a SOLE workshop.

Source: Adapted from Ferretti et al. (2019).

Communication is an applied science; in-person learning can be aligned with adult learners' experience, creating more effective communicators. To promote ethical sense-making, open dialogue encourages students to learn from one another when confronting gaps in experience during SOLEs. Facilitators provide targeted resources to help trainees integrate new communication concepts into practice. An important component of self-reflection in trainees across specialties is the use of narrative reflection (Ferretti et al., 2022). Therefore, at the close of each SOLE workshop, standardized patients employ figures of speech and labeling of "unspoken" emotions to cultivate empathy and professionalism.

4.4.1.3 Assessment

While developing the SOLE, we did not find any valid or reliable tools for guiding, supervising, and evaluating performance in simulated scenarios to support ethics learning in NPM. We therefore developed a series of SOLE-specific guides for trainees, supervisors, and standardized patients. Each guide introduces content and logistics for all participants (see Appendix) and is distributed approximately two weeks before each session. Before teaching begins, supervisors and standardized patients receive training on how to facilitate SOLEs, while trainees review the guide and recommended readings.

Within both the trainee and supervisor guides, we created an evidence-based procedural form derived from literature reviews of each scenario, offering cognitive guidance for supervisors and trainees alike. Supervisors use the procedural form during SOLEs to assist trainees through essential steps of standard practice. The concepts of shared decision-making (Charles et al., 1997), discourse ethics (Audet, 1995; Habermas, 2004), and the axioms of communication (Watzlawick et al., 1972) form the theoretical foundation for these procedural forms. The content of these forms is based on comprehensive systematic reviews of empirical studies and provides clear rationale for communication choices and teaching techniques. Table 4.3 offers an example of a procedural form used for postnatal communication of an unexpected diagnosis of Trisomy 21.

The procedural form outlines elements of competency before trainees encounter SOLE cases. The same form is used by supervisors and observers during SOLE training to assess and provide constructive feedback.

4.4.1.4 Trainees' Evaluation of the Program

Analyzing Trainees' Feedback. Learners' feedback was integral to the program's implementation phase. All seminars, workshops, and SOLEs of the new curriculum received highly positive evaluations from trainees using a standardized Likert-scale survey after each session. Overall satisfaction averaged 5.8 out of 7. Based on trainee feedback, certain program elements were modified. For example, the

Ethics Models of the Physician–Patient Relationship module was converted from a seminar to a workshop format, increasing satisfaction from 4.8 to 6.3 out of 7.

Our SOLE model for teaching communication in small groups continues to receive excellent evaluations from participants. During workshop sessions with SPs, trainees are encouraged to test communication theories and observe responses from individuals of diverse cultural backgrounds. In a supportive atmosphere, they share ideas, ask questions, and move beyond their comfort zones—where genuine learning takes place.

Trainee Performance and Self-Reflection. In addition to written and oral feedback during SOLE training, trainees maintain a personal portfolio that promotes self-reflection in their roles as communicators, professionals, and health advocates. Each trainee identifies ethically challenging situations they have encountered, analyzes their strengths and weaknesses, and reviews these analyses biannually during mentorship meetings with an academic neonatologist (Buckley et al., 2009; Tochel et al., 2009). A subsequent survey indicated that combining portfolios with one-on-one mentorship was preferred over either approach alone (Daboval et al., 2019).

Portfolios for trainees across health professions were also expanded as broader tools for assessment and reflection. One-on-one mentorship sessions improved learning outcomes and evaluation consistency. The results of this pilot study were presented at the Pediatric Academic Societies International meeting, where we concluded that integrating portfolios into mentorship sessions helps identify gaps in trainees' competencies during antenatal consultations.

4.4.2 Phase 2—Developing a Comprehensive Communication Assessment Tool for Ethically Sensitive Situations: ACT4Ethics

Defining what constitutes improved communication remains challenging. Many facets appear to be related to such outcomes—demonstration of techniques within a communication framework, greater situational awareness, improved rapport with family members, and increased trainee confidence during clinical encounters. Without a well-designed assessment instrument specifically adapted to ethically sensitive situations, evaluation of communication relies heavily on subjective interpretation (O'Donnell et al., 2011).

In 2019, our research team developed an assessment tool focused on distinguishing among ethical judgment and decision-making, respect and empathy, and both basic and advanced communication competencies during ethically sensitive clinical encounters. Although this instrument was initially developed in the context of NPM, the *Assessment of Communication Tool for Ethics (ACT4Ethics)* can be applied across diverse medical specialties. ACT4Ethics incorporates key elements of the competencies required for medical communication, professionalism, and collaboration (Daboval et al., 2019).

It encompasses competencies in both verbal and nonverbal communication tailored to medical interviews, adaptive communication techniques for delivering bad news, and the ability to recognize the ethical dimensions of a situation, including aspects of virtue ethics, bioethical principles, and communicative ethics. Additionally, it involves assessing ethical judgment and decision-making skills while actively engaging patients and families in the decision-making process.

Communication. The communication subscale assesses both verbal and nonverbal communication skills, as well as complex elements such as conversational pragmatics that arise during clinical interactions (Kurtz et al., 2003; Makoul, 2001). Recognizing the knowledge gap between patients and physicians, this subscale also evaluates the use of techniques such as closing verbal communication "loops," which involve seeking explicit confirmation of mutual understanding during critical points of discussion (Brindley & Reynolds, 2011).

Ethically sensitive conversations often involve affectively charged information that requires an empathetic approach (Baile et al., 2000). This includes addressing the recipients' values and beliefs (Andersson & Pearson, 1999; Cortina et al., 2001) while adapting to the specific clinical setting (Guidroz et al., 2010; Hutton & Gates, 2008; Papastavrou et al., 2012).

Civility and Respect. Not all difficulties encountered by clinicians can be attributed to the clinical or ethical facets of a situation. The civility subscale differentiates incivility from disrespect, focusing on behaviors where intentions are unclear but may lead to long-term adverse consequences (Andersson & Pearson, 1999). Empathy—a core component of civility—is conceptualized along two dimensions, cognitive and affective, with the addition of a third dimension, empathy for diversity:

- *Cognitive empathy:* The ability to understand another's thoughts and beliefs, enabling predictions of their behavior (Eslinger, 1998).
- *Affective empathy:* The capacity to share emotional experiences, encompassing both joy and sorrow (Davis, 1994).
- *Empathy for diversity:* Sensitivity to differing perspectives, recognizing and respecting diversity in cultural, social, and individual contexts.

Research has identified distinct neurological bases for these dimensions. In clinical practice, a perceived lack of respect for patients' emotions, beliefs, or choices can lead to reluctance in disclosing vital information or considering alternative treatments.

Judgment and Decision-Making. Beyond building a therapeutic alliance, the information gathered through verbal and nonverbal communication is essential for

TABLE 4.3 Example of a Procedural Form Guiding the Trainees during Difficult Conversations

Key Components for the Communication of a T21 Diagnosis

**Note: this is a guideline of steps to facilitate communication. They do not necessarily need to be performed in the order provided. Many steps may occur or re-occur throughout the whole encounter.*

Suggested Communication Strategies	*Rationale*
• *Greet the parents and introduce yourself* • *Inquire about father's/partner's presence or absence (if applicable)*	Clarify your role to establish trustful relationship. Work to inform parents together as this promoted a greater satisfaction with the overall process.
• *Choose a setting that is quiet to minimize disruptions (remember to turn your phone and/or pager to vibrate)* • *Encourage unknown or additional people to leave the room (i.e. RN, acquaintances)*	Promotes safe and therapeutic space for what may be a challenging or sensitive conversation. Allows parents to freely express themselves without feeling rushed, interrupted, or judged by others.
• *Be sure that the parent(s) have seen their baby and that s/he is in the room with you* • *Refer to the baby by his/her name and look at him/her as appropriate*	Destigmatize the diagnosis as early as possible to promote attachment. Parents should see you role modelling natural interactions with them as well as with the baby.
• *Sit down so that you are on the same level as the parents throughout the discussion* • *Make eye-contact with the parents and maintain a calm but confident demeanor*	Reinforces that you are equals and minimize feelings of paternalistic communication. Promotes a therapeutic alliance and decreases the anxiety that can be bred by uncertainty.
• *After congratulating parents on the birth of their baby, if you have not already done so, you should deliver a "warning sign"* 1. *"I've been asked to see you because the OB team has some concerns about your baby's [ex. overall lower muscular tone]..."* 2. *"While examining [name of baby/your baby], I noticed some features that make me think of Down syndrome [ex. flat nasal bridge, upslanting eyes]..."* • *Clarify whether parents have noticed anything "unusual" or "unexpected" about their baby and, if so, what they observed*	Recognizing that the delicate nature of this conversation may trigger a variety of emotions, parents should begin by receiving congratulations on the birth of their baby as this prepares them to receive unexpected new in an optimistic manner. Mothers frequently report noticing something "different" about their baby even before the diagnosis of T21 is given. Clarify for identified features whether they are typical to T21 or unrelated.
• *Clarify how parents understand T21 so that you may build off their existing knowledge base (pay attention to their language)* 1. *"What have you heard about Down syndrome?"* 2. *"Have you ever had any personal experience with someone who has Down syndrome?"* • *Pay attention to the language they use so that you may match the complexity of your explanations to their own understanding*	T21 is a relatively common diagnosis so it is important to appreciate parents' baseline knowledge. Studies have shown that only ½ of parents felt information conveyed was easy to understand.

clinical decision-making. The judgment and decision-making subscale evaluates the integration of clinical and ethical considerations. This includes situational awareness—the ability to understand the environment and anticipate future events (Endsley, 1995); evidence gathering and analysis to form unbiased diagnoses (Kahneman, 2011); and decision-making within the constraints of real clinical contexts (Klein, 1999). Effective decision-making requires synthesizing diverse sources of information, including contributions from patients, families, and other health-care professionals. Clinicians must combine respect, empathy, and effective communication to optimize clinical encounters and ensure that ethical and clinical considerations remain harmoniously balanced.

The ACT4Ethics scale is composed of 12 competencies distributed among these three main domains (Figure 4.4). Responses for each competency are organized along a five-point Likert scale. Examples of milestones and stages—aligned with the continuum defined by the "entrustability" stages of competency (Frank et al., 2015)—are provided alongside each domain.

If an assessing clinician identifies concerns sufficient to suggest that the trainee should be limited in their permission to communicate with patients or family members without supervision, this may be indicated under the *red flag* option adjacent to the rating scale.

The second part of the assessment tool captures relevant situational factors that might impact ethical judgment and decision-making. Clear examples are included to guide assessors and account for variability arising from the diverse, unpredictable elements of real-life clinical encounters. These qualifications help contextualize evaluations and allow assessors to note whether a concern arose due to context or competency.

ACT4Ethics concludes with an overall assessment scale, whose score should positively correlate with the mean scores across the three subscales.

Furthermore, this assessment tool evaluates whether the educational program provides adequate preparation and employs appropriate teaching methods to achieve the goal of supporting trainees' learning. It helps ensure that trainees begin independent practice with refined communication skills. This tool enables clinician-teachers to assess and monitor the development of trainees' judgment and communication skills during ethically sensitive conversations, aligning with the Canadian national framework *Competence by Design* (CBD) for competency-based medical education in residency training and specialty practice. Finally, it guides the provision of meaningful feedback to ensure that trainees develop specific communication, empathy, decision-making, and ethical competencies.

4.5 Current Status of the NPM Ethics Program

Since the beginning of our program, participants' evaluations have been overwhelmingly positive, and we continue to integrate feedback from trainees, supervisors, and external reviewers into ongoing improvements.

Our observations indicate that the more frequently trainees make communication or socio-behavioral errors the more intense their desire becomes to interrupt the scenario to allow them to learn by exploring their own feelings and misunderstandings. Essentially, recognizing the "mistake" in a constructive process becomes a positive stepping stone from which to learn and implement change (Ferretti et al., 2019).

Since 2008, the SOLE training has been running two to four times per year within the NPM program of the Department of Pediatrics at the University of Ottawa. It is still directed by its original creators, although new supervisors are undergoing training in educational principles applicable to observing sensitive conversations and reinforcing the program's core values. SOLE has also received strong approval from the most recent Royal College Internal Accreditation Evaluation. Four universities—Limerick University in Ireland, the University of Bologna in Italy, Warsaw University in Poland, and McMaster University in Canada—have incorporated or are working toward incorporating the program into their curricula.

Nevertheless, certain challenges must be recognized. One such issue concerns trainee commitment and participation. We have noted a lack of preparation among trainees before the workshop, which may have several causes, such as fatigue, disengagement due to a "know-it-all" attitude, or simple lack of motivation. Investigating trainees' commitment to the program might be useful; however, in our experience, they still benefit from the sessions, as evidenced by their constructive feedback.

Another challenge concerns the impact that ACT4Ethics feedback might have on trainees. Although it is important to highlight inadequate skills, receiving a "red flag" note may be demoralizing and undermine trainees' desire to learn and improve.

Challenges also arise from the supervisors' perspective, including a lack of protected time and limited encouragement or incentives for teaching. One of Guskey's levels emphasizes the importance of organizational support. Although the University of Ottawa, the Department of Innovation in Medical Education (DIME), and the Royal College have recognized and funded the implementation of the program, larger systemic factors may still be at play. Historically, in Canada, there has been no formal mandate for physicians to teach (Khamisa et al., 2016). Consequently, there is no dedicated or protected time for academic physicians to educate trainees. Physicians must therefore conduct training on their own time and cover their own expenses, which do not favor prioritizing these endeavors. Additional institutional support might allow for better training in professional competencies in medicine such as ethical decision-making and communication.

Another limitation concerns the evaluation metrics of the SOLE program. For the moment, we have used a Likert scale to measure trainees' satisfaction. However, it is important to recognize that such questionnaires may not yield honest answers. Students may fall victim to response bias—either extreme responding (e.g., selecting "satisfied" for all questions to save time) or social-desirability bias (selecting "satisfied" to appear competent; Edwards & Horst, 1953). In addition, student satisfaction does not necessarily imply successful training. For example, a trainee may feel satisfied by an easy lesson because it was simple to perform but fail to realize that they did not learn new material. A long-term assessment of the program's effectiveness is crucial and should include insights from alumni who have already been in the workforce for some time.

The knowledge test was intended to provide such a measurement of the program's effectiveness (Moore et al., 2017). However, it is no longer used, as it proved both time-consuming and logistically demanding. On the other hand, it could be employed to test the validity and reliability of the SOLE tool. Given that only three to five trainees are admitted to the NPM program at the University of Ottawa each year, it would take many cohorts to obtain a sample size large enough to conduct meaningful statistical analysis (Moore et al., 2017). Although experts in the field have been contacted to provide input on the program's validity, a separate peer-reviewed quantitative study incorporating a larger participant sample might prove beneficial. Conducting the knowledge test in combination with the ACT4Ethics evaluation for each cohort therefore presents questionable utility.

The ACT4Ethics tool also poses certain challenges. As the current program is subject to the Canadian Royal College of Physicians, it must abide by their rules and regulations. While the current EPAs for NPM consider communication competencies, there remains a need for a validated scale to assess them. We have conducted a pilot study to assess the reliability and validity of the ACT4Ethics tool (Daboval et al., 2019); however, a complete external validation is still underway and has faced difficulties engaging medical-education experts to complete the process. Once this step is complete, the assessment communication tool will be submitted to the Royal College for approval and may eventually be applied during training and examinations, such as the national OSCE, across multiple medical specialties and subspecialties.

Another limitation of the ACT4Ethics tool lies in its reliance on supervisors. The integration of more than one evaluator to assess trainees' communication skills has been instrumental in exposing trainees to diverse expertise and perspectives. However, by relying on ratings from multiple supervisors, issues of inter-rater reliability must be addressed. In addition, no selection criteria have been established for identifying professionals who provide feedback. For future practice, it may be best to ensure that supervisors themselves recognize their own bias and risk for discrimination. Such adverse cases could, in fact, lead to deterioration in trainees' ethical reasoning and undermine the purpose of the training. It is particularly important to consider stereotypes that persist in medicine—for instance, female patients, especially elderly women—are often perceived by physicians as hypochondriacs, creating an additional communication barrier (Root, 1987). As it is impossible for any individual to fully rid themselves of bias or preconception, the program should be approached from a perspective that values clear communication and open-mindedness regarding all ethical components at stake during decision-making. Training works well only if the feedback is good, therefore, it is essential that future supervisors safeguard the program's central ideology of acceptance, a respectful, inclusive, non-judgmental approach.

The overall political and social environment—both in ethics and in medicine—continues to evolve, requiring us to adapt the teaching program accordingly. Although the program addresses ethically ambiguous situations, it does not aim to teach specific "right or wrong" ideologies but rather focuses on fostering honest, human communication and ethically grounded judgment towards the decision-making process. Over time, developing minimal assessment criteria for evaluators may prove essential.

With changing times, we anticipate that the SOLE scenarios may eventually need to adapt to the cultural, ideological, and socio-demographic changes over time. The emergence of artificial intelligence (AI) will likely revolutionize medical training, as virtual-reality simulations may be conducted with virtual patients instead of actors. More broadly, AI, machine learning, and related technologies will profoundly affect how medical education is delivered (Michael & Schoenherr, 2026). As with any pedagogical or assessment innovation, the adoption of AI and its integration within medical curricula will require a clear understanding of learner competencies, desired professional outcomes, the technology's development and validation process, and how it is used to assess performance (Schoenherr, 2025). The use of such technologies will also introduce new ethical considerations that educators must recognize (Schoenherr, 2021, 2022; Schoenherr & DeFalco, 2021; Schoenherr et al., 2024). For now, our trainees have expressed a strong preference for face-to-face training, as it allows a better understanding of nonverbal cues and full engagement in realistic conversations.

In the meantime, we have encountered unanticipated interest in our SOLE workshops. We now include members of the neonatal transport team, as well as trainees from other disciplines, including pediatric intensive care, obstetrics and gynecology, maternal–fetal medicine, palliative care, and genetics.

4.6 Conclusion

Education in NPM and in the medical fields more generally requires further training on how to handle ethically challenging and ambiguous situations, fully including the interests of the child, the parents, and other stakeholders. Our program aims to give trainees the opportunity to improve their communication skills during sets of safe SOLE practice rounds while simultaneously receiving feedback. The ACT4Ethics evaluation aims to guide trainees toward individualized areas of improvement including genuine communication skills, empathy, and ethically grounded judgment and decision making.

The implementation of the program has been met with multiple challenges, such as a lack of dedicated training, protected time, and incentives for supervisors. This, in turn, has slowed the implementation of the program through deficiencies in knowledge translation—such as raising awareness about the program and conducting validation studies.

The implementation of educational innovations such as SOLE and ACT4Ethics must also consider the contextual and organizational factors that influence their success. As noted in implementation science frameworks, even well-designed programs may face challenges if they are not aligned with available institutional resources, faculty time, and cultural dynamics (Schoenherr & Hamstra, 2024). Sustainable adoption depends on how effectively the innovation is adapted to the local environment, integrated into existing training structures, and supported through leadership engagement and resource allocation (Damschroder et al., 2009; Schoenherr & McConnell, 2024). Ongoing evaluation, stakeholder collaboration, and responsiveness to user feedback will therefore be critical to ensure that the program continues to meet evolving clinical and educational needs.

Overall, the program has been perceived positively by trainees and evaluated favorably by the Royal College of Physicians' Accreditation. Further work will allow the program to become a core tool in any area of medicine for training communication skills during encountered ethically sensitive situations.

All references for SOLE scenarios can be found in Appendix.

Altin, S. V., & Stock, S. (2016). The impact of health literacy, patient-centered communication and shared decision-making on patients' satisfaction with care received in German primary care practices. *BMC Health Services Research*, *16*, 1–10.

Alvarez, G., & Coiera, E. (2006). Interdisciplinary communication: An uncharted source of medical error? *Journal of Critical Care*, *21*(3), 236–242.

Andersson, L., & Pearson, C. (1999). Tit for tat? The spiraling effect of incivility in the workplace. *Academic Management Review*, *24*(3), 452–471.

Audet, M. (1995). Jürgen Habermas: L'éthique de la discussion. In M. H. Parizeau (Ed.), *Hopital & ethique: Roles et defis des comites d'ethiques cliniques* (pp. 167–175). Les presses de l'Université Laval.

Baile, W. F., Buckman, R., Lenzi, R., et al. (2000). SPIKES—A six-step protocol for delivering bad news: Application to the patient with cancer. *Oncologist*, *5*(4), 302–311.

Beauchamp, C. (2019). *Principles of Biomedical Ethics*. 8th ed. Oxford University Press.

Betancourt, J. R. (2006). Cultural competence and medical education: Many names, many perspectives, one goal. *Academic Medicine*, *81*(6), 499–501.

Boyd, E. M., & Fales, A. W. (1983). Reflective learning key to learning from experience. *Journal of Humanistic Psychology*, *23*(2), 99–117.

Brindley, P. G., & Reynolds, S. F. (2011). Improving verbal communication in critical care medicine. *Journal of Critical Care*, *26*(2), 155–159.

Buckley, S., Coleman, J., Davison, I., Khan, K. S., Zamora, J., Malick, S., ... & Sayers, J. (2009). The educational effects of portfolios on undergraduate student learning: A Best Evidence Medical Education (BEME) systematic review. BEME Guide No. 11. *Medical Teacher*, *31*(4), 282–298.

Charles, C., Gafni, A., & Whelan, T. (1997). Shared decision-making in the medical encounter: What does it mean? (or it takes at least two to tango). *Social Science & Medicine*, *44*(5), 681–692.

Cortina, L. M., Magley, V. J., Williams, J. H., & Langhout, R. D. (2001). Incivility in the workplace: Incidence and impact. *Journal of Occupational Health Psychology*, *6*(1), 64–80.

Coughlin, K. W. (2018). Medical decision-making in paediatrics: Infancy to adolescence. *Paediatrics & Child Health*, *23*(2), 138–146.

Cummings, C. L. (2016). Teaching and assessing ethics in the newborn ICU. *Seminars in Perinatology*, *40*(4), 261–269.

Daboval, T., Ferretti, E., & Moore, G. P. (2014a). Innovative holistic teaching in a Canadian neonatal perinatal residency program. *Hastings Center Report*, *44*(6), 21–25.

Daboval, T., Ferretti, E., Moussa, A., van Manen, M., Moore, G., Srinivasan, G., Moldovan, A., Agarwal, A., & Albersheim, S. (2019). Needs assessment of Ethics and Communication Teaching for Perinatal Medicine Programs in Canada. *Paediatrics & Child Health*, *24*(3), e116–e124. https://doi.org/10.1093/pch/pxy108

Daboval, T., Moore, G. P., & Ferretti, E. (2013). How we teach ethics and communication during a Canadian neonatal perinatal medicine residency: An interactive experience. *Medical Teacher*, *35*(3), 194–200.

Daboval, T., Moore, G. P., Rohde, K., Moreau, K., & Ferretti, E. (2014b). Teaching ethics in neonatal and perinatal medicine: What is happening in Canada? *Paediatrics & Child Health*, *19*(1), e6–e10.

Daboval, T., & Shidler, S. (2014). Ethical framework for shared decision makin in the neonatal intensive care unit: Communicative ethics. *Journal of Paediatrics & Child Health*, *19*(6), 302–304.

Daboval, T., Ward, N., Schoenherr, J. R., Moore, G. P., Carew, C., Lambrinakos-Raymond, A., & Ferretti, E. (2019). Testing a communication assessment tool for ethically sensitive scenarios: Protocol of a validation study. *JMIR Research Protocols*, *8*(5), e12039.

Damschroder, L. J., Aron, D. C., Keith, R. E., Kirsh, S. R., Alexander, J. A., & Lowery, J. C. (2009). Fostering implementation of health services research findings into practice: A consolidated framework for advancing implementation science. *Implementation Science*, *4*(1), 50.

Davis, M. (1994). *Empathy: A Social Psychological Approach*. Taylor & Francis.

de la Garza, S., Phuoc, V., Throneberry, S., Blumenthal-Barby, J., McCullough, L., & Coverdale, J. (2017). Teaching medical ethics in graduate and undergraduate medical education: A systematic review of effectiveness. *Academic Psychiatry*, *41*, 520–525.

Edwards, A., & Elwyn, G. (Eds.). (2009). *Shared Decision-Making in Health Care: Achieving Evidence-Based Patient Choice*. Oxford University Press.

Edwards, A. L. (1953). The relationship between the judged desirability of a trait and the probability that the trait will be endorsed. *Journal of Applied Psychology*, *37*(2), 90.

Endsley, M. R. (1995). Toward a theory of situation awareness in dynamic systems. *Human Factors*, *37*(1), 32–64.

Eslinger, P. J. (1998). Neurological and neuropsychological bases of empathy. *European Neurology*, *39*(4), 193–199.

Ferreira, A. C. F. M., Eveloff, R. J., Freire, M., & Santos, M. T. B. R. (2021). The impact of oral-gut inflammation in cerebral palsy. *Frontiers in Immunology*, *12*, 619262.

Ferretti, E., Rohde, K., Moore, G., & Daboval, T. (2015). The birth of scenario-oriented learning in ethics. *Med Educ*, *49*(5), 517–518. https://doi.org/10.1111/medu.12706.

Ferretti, E., Rohde, K., Moore, G. P., & Daboval, T. (2019). Catch the moment: The power of turning mistakes into 'precious' learning opportunities. *Paediatrics & Child Health, 24*(3), 156–159.

Ferretti, E., Schoenherr, J. R., Mattiola, A., & Daboval, T. (2022). Vulnerabilities in clinician–parent exchanges and the cascade of communication traps: A review. *Archives of Disease in Childhood, 108*(2), 86–90.

Franck, L. S., & O'Brien, K. (2019). The evolution of family-centered care: From supporting parent-delivered interventions to a model of family integrated care. *Birth Defects Research, 111*(15), 1044–1059.

Frank, J. R., Snell, L., & Sherbino, J., (Eds.). (2015). CanMEDs 2015 physician competency framework. In *CanMEDS 2015 Physician Competency Framework* (pp. 1–30). Royal College of Physicians and Surgeons of Canada.

Giubilini, A., Milnes, S., & Savulescu, J. (2016). The medical ethics curriculum in medical schools: Present and future. *The Journal of Clinical Ethics, 27*(2), 129–145.

Goldie, J., Schwartz, L., McConnachie, A., & Morrison, J. (2002). The impact of three years' ethics teaching, in an integrated medical curriculum, on students' proposed behaviour on meeting ethical dilemmas. *Medical Education, 36*(5), 489–497.

Greenberg, C. C., Regenbogen, S. E., Studdert, D. M., Lipsitz, S. R., Rogers, S. O., Zinner, M. J., & Gawande, A. A. (2007). Patterns of communication breakdowns resulting in injury to surgical patients. *Journal of the American College of Surgeons, 204*(4), 533–540.

Greenhalgh, J., Gooding, K., Gibbons, E., Dalkin, S., Wright, J., Valderas, J., & Black, N. (2018). How do patient reported outcome measures (PROMs) support clinician-patient communication and patient care? A realist synthesis. *Journal of Patient-Reported Outcomes, 2*, 1–28.

Guidroz, A. M., Burnfield-Geimer, J. L., Clark, O., et al. (2010). The nursing incivility scale: Development and validation of an occupation-specific measure. *Journal of Nursing Measurement, 18*(3), 176–200.

Habermas, J. (2004). Discourse ethics. In H. Gensler, E. Spurgin, & J. Swindal (Eds.), *Ethics: Contemporary Readings* (pp. 146–153). Routledge.

Hafferty, F. W., & Franks, R. (1994). The hidden curriculum, ethics teaching, and the structure of medical education. *Academic Medicine, 69*(11), 861–71.

Hanson, C. L., De Guire, M. J., Schinkel, A. M., & Kolterman, O. G. (1995). Empirical validation for a family-centered model of care. *Diabetes Care, 18*(10), 1347–1356.

Hutton, S., & Gates, D. (2008). Workplace incivility and productivity losses among direct care staff. *AAOHN Journal, 56*(4), 168–175.

Johnson, B. H. (2000). Family-centered care: Four decades of progress. *Families, Systems, & Health, 18*(2), 137.

Kahneman D. (2011). *Thinking, Fast and Slow*. Anchor Canada.

Khamisa, K., Bandeali, S., & Fellus, I. (2016). The development of a novel medical education elective for fourth-year medical students. *International Journal of Medical Education, 7*, 342.

Klein G. (1999). *Sources of Power: How People Make Decisions*. The MIT Press

Kokorelias, K. M., Gignac, M. A., Naglie, G., & Cameron, J. I. (2019). Towards a universal model of family centered care: A scoping review. *BMC Health Services Research, 19*, 1–11.

Kon, A. A. (2009). The "window of opportunity:" Helping parents make the most difficult decision they will ever face using an informed non-dissent model. *American Journal of Bioethics*, *9*(4), 55–56.

Kurtz, S., Silverman, J., Benson, J., & Draper, J. (2003). Marrying content and process in clinical method teaching: Enhancing the Calgary-Cambridge guides. *Academic Medicine*, *78*(8), 802–809.

Land, V., Parry, R., & Seymour, J. (2017). Communication practices that encourage and constrain shared decision making in health-care encounters: Systematic review of conversation analytic research. *Health Expectations*, *20*(6), 1228–1247.

Makoul, G. (2001). Essential elements of communication in medical encounters: The Kalamazoo consensus statement. *Academic Medicine*, *76*(4), 390–393.

Martineau, B., & Girard, G. (2010a). *Cahier du mentor ICP I*. 8th ed. Universite′ de Sherbrooke.

Martineau, B., & Girard, G. (2010b). *Cahier du mentor ICP II*. 8th ed. Universite de Sherbrooke.

McCullough, L. B., & Cross, A. W. (1985). Respect for autonomy and medical paternalism reconsidered. *Theoretical Medicine*, *6*, 295–308.

McDonald, C. J., Weiner, M., & Hui, S. L. (2000). Deaths due to medical errors are exaggerated in Institute of Medicine report. *JAMA*, *284*(1), 93–95.

McLean, M. (2004). Does the curriculum matter in ethics education? *Medical Education*, *38*(8), 916–917.

McManus, I. C., Vincent, C. A., Thom, S., & Kidd, J. (1993). Teaching communication skills to clinical students. *British Medical Journal*, *306*(6888), 1322–1327.

Michael, K., & Schoenherr, J. R. (2026). Multi-level sociotechnical systems approach to human-centered AI. In *Handbook of Human-Centered Artificial Intelligence* (pp. 1–74). Springer Nature Singapore.

Moore, G. P., Ferretti, E., & Daboval, T. (2017). Developing a knowledge test for a neonatal ethics teaching program. *Cureus*, *9*(12), e1971.

Norman, G. R., Grierson, L. E., Sherbino, J., Hamstra, S. J., Schmidt, H. G., & Mamede, S. (2018). Expertise in medicine and surgery. In K. A. Ericsson, R. R. Hoffman, A. Kozbelt & A. M. Williams (Eds.), *The Cambridge Handbook of Expertise and Expert Performance* (2nd ed., pp. 331–355). Cambridge University Press.

O'Donnell, J. A., Oakley, M., Haney, S., O'Neill, P. N., & Taylor, D. (2011). Rubrics 101: A primer for rubric development in dental education. *Journal of Dental Education*, *75*(9), 1163–1175.

Oljeski, S. A., Homer, M. J., & Krackov, W. S. (2004). Incorporating ethics education into the radiology residency curriculum: A model. *American Journal of Roentgenology*, *183*(3), 569–571.

Papastavrou, E., Efstathiou, G., Tsangari, H., et al. (2012). Patients' and nurses' perceptions of respect and human presence through caring behaviours: A comparative study. *Nursing Ethics*, *19*(3), 369–379.

Patel, V. L., Arocha, J. F., & Zhang, J. (2005). Thinking and reasoning in medicine. In K. J. Holyoak & R. G. Morrison (Eds.), *The Cambridge Handbook of Thinking and Reasoning* (Vol. *14*, pp. 727–750). Cambridge University Press.

Roodbeen, R., Vreke, A., Boland, G., Rademakers, J., van den Muijsenbergh, M., Noordman, J., & van Dulmen, S. (2020). Communication and shared decision-making with patients with limited health literacy; helpful strategies, barriers and suggestions for improvement reported by hospital-based palliative care providers. *PLOS ONE*, *15*(6), e0234926.

Root, M. J. (1987). Communication barriers between older women and physicians. *Public Health Reports*, *102*(4 Suppl), 152.

Ross, L. F. (1998). *Children, Families, and Health Care Decision Making.* Oxford University Press.

Rothman, D. J. (2001). The origins and consequences of patient autonomy: A 25-year retrospective. *Health Care Analysis*, *9*(3), 255–264.

Schaefer, H. G., Helmreich, R. L., & Scheidegger, D. (1994). Human factors and safety in emergency medicine. *Resuscitation*, *28*(3), 221–225.

Schoenherr, J. R. (2021). Designing ethical agency for adaptive instructional systems: The FATE of learning and assessment. In *International Conference on Human-Computer Interaction* (pp. 265–283). Springer International Publishing.

Schoenherr, J. R. (2022). Learning engineering is ethical. In J. Goodale & J. Kolodner (Eds.), *Learning Engineering Toolkit* (pp. 201–228). Routledge.

Schoenherr, J. R. (2027). Innovation, implementation, and translational research in health professions education and healthcare delivery. In J. R. Schoenherr (Eds.), *Fundamentals and Frontiers of Medical Education and Decision-Making: Innovation, Implementation, and Translational Research* (pp. 1–76). Routledge.

Schoenherr, J. R., Chiou, E., & Goldshtein, M. (2024). Building trust with the ethical affordances of education technologies: A sociotechnical systems perspective. In P. Dasgupta, J. Llinas, T. Gillespie, S. Fouse, W. Lawless, R. Mittu & D. Sofge (Eds.), *Putting AI in the Critical Loop* (pp. 127–165). Academic Press.

Schoenherr, J. R., & DeFalco, J. (2021, October). Moral education and A/IS standardization: Responsible and ethical design through education. In *2021 IEEE International Symposium on Technology and Society (ISTAS)* (pp. 1–8). IEEE.

Schoenherr, J. R., & Hamstra, S. J. (2024). Validity in health professions education: From assessment instruments to program innovation and evaluation. In J. R. Schoenherr & M. M. McConnell (Eds.), *Fundamentals and Frontiers of Medical Education and Decision-Making* (pp. 80–107). Routledge

Schoenherr, J. R., & Le-Bouar, C. (2024). Representing and communicating health information: Fundamentals of persuasive health communication. In J. R. Schoenherr & M. McConnell (Eds.), *Fundamentals and Frontiers of Medical Education and Decision-Making* (pp. 270–312). Routledge.

Schoenherr, J. R., Mahias-Ito, I., & Li, X. (2026). Collective competence in the health professions: Learning, thinking, and deciding in groups. In J. R. Schoenherr (Eds.), *Fundamentals and Frontiers of Medical Education and Decision-Making: Innovation, Implementation, and Translational Research*, Routledge.

Schoenherr, J. R., & McConnell, M. M. (2024). *Fundamentals and Frontiers of Medical Education and Decision-Making*. Routledge.

Schwartz, S., & Griffin, T. (2012). *Medical Thinking: The Psychology of Medical Judgment and Decision Making*. Springer Science & Business Media.

Self, D. J., Wolinsky, F. D., & Baldwin Jr, D. C. (1989). The effect of teaching medical ethics on medical students' moral reasoning. *Academic Medicine*, *64*(12), 755–9.

Sutcliffe, K. M., Lewton, E., & Rosenthal, M. M. (2004). Communication failures: An insidious contributor to medical mishaps. *Academic Medicine*, *79*(2), 186–194.

Tochel, C., Haig, A., Hesketh, A., Cadzow, A., Beggs, K., Colthart, I., & Peacock, H. (2009). The effectiveness of portfolios for post-graduate assessment and education: BEME Guide No 12. *Medical Teacher*, *31*(4), 299–318.

Varpio, L., Hall, P., Lingard, L., & Schryer, C. F. (2008). Interprofessional communication and medical error: A reframing of research questions and approaches. *Academic Medicine*, *83*(10), S76–S81.

Vermeir, P., Vandijck, D., Degroote, S., Peleman, R., Verhaeghe, R., Mortier, E., ... & Vogelaers, D. (2015). Communication in healthcare: A narrative review of the literature and practical recommendations. *International Journal of Clinical Practice*, *69*(11), 1257–1267.

Wanzer, M. B., Booth-Butterfield, M., & Gruber, K. (2004). Perceptions of health care providers' communication: Relationships between patient-centered communication and satisfaction. *Health Communication*, *16*(3), 363–384.

Watts, L. L., Medeiros, K. E., Mulhearn, T. J., Steele, L. M., Connelly, S., & Mumford, M. D. (2017). Are ethics training programs improving? A meta-analytic review of past and present ethics instruction in the sciences. *Ethics & Behavior*, *27*(5), 351–384.

Watzlawick, P., Beavin, J. H., Jackson, D. D., & Morche, J. (1972). *Une logique de la communication*. Edition Points.

Whitehead, C. R., Austin, Z., & Hodges, B. D. (2011). Flower power: The armoured expert in the CanMEDS competency framework? *Advances in Health Sciences Education, 16*, 681–694.

Appendix

Example of SOLE

The following contains an example of one of the guides used in SOLE. Guides are freely available and can be found at: https://www.mededportal.org/doi/10.15766/mep_2374-8265.10044

References

Boggs S, Daboval T, Ben Fadel N, Moore G, Ferretti E. Neonatal Ethics Teaching Program – Scenario Oriented Learning in Ethics: Announcing the Diagnosis of Trisomy 21. *Edition Might 2018. University of Ottawa. Jia, F., & Krettenauer, T.* (2017). *Recognizing moral identity as a cultural construct. Frontiers in psychology, 8, 412.Facilitator Guide, Standardized Patient Guide, Trainee Guide. Ed. Might 2018. University of Ottawa.* URL: http://hdl.handle.net/10393/37944

Daboval T, Ferretti E, Rohde K, Muirhead P, Moore G. Neonatal Ethics Teaching Program – Scenario Oriented Learning in Ethics: Antenatal Consultation at the Limit of Viability. *Ed. January* 2015. *University of Ottawa.*

Daboval T, Ferretti E, Moore G. Neonatal Ethics Teaching Program. Problem Based Learning in Ethics (PBLE): Antenatal Consultation at the Limit of Viability. *Edition Might* 2013. *University of Ottawa.*

Ferretti, E., Daboval, T., & Moore G (2012). Neonatal Ethics Teaching Program. Problem Based Learning in Ethics (PBLE): Unexpected Malformation at Birth. *Edition October 2012.* University of Ottawa.

Ferretti, E., Moore, G., Rohde, K., Muirhead, P., & Daboval, T. (2015). Neonatal Ethics Teaching Program – Scenario Oriented Learning in Ethics: Unexpected Birth Malformation. *Edition January 2015. University of Ottawa. Facilitator Guide, Standardized Patient Guide, Trainee Guide. Ed. Jan 2015.* University of Ottawa.

Moore G, Ferretti E, Daboval T. Neonatal Ethics Teaching Program. Problem Based Learning in Ethics (PBLE): Critically Ill Newborn in the NICU. Ed. Jan 2015. *University of Ottawa.*

Moore G, Ferretti E, Rohde K, Muirhead P, Daboval T. Neonatal Ethics Teaching Program – Scenario Oriented Learning in Ethics: Critically Ill Newborn in the NICU. *Edition January* 2015. *University of Ottawa.* URL: http://hdl.handle.net/10393/32442

Participants	Define the roles of all participants of the encounter (e.g.: caregiver, mother, father, family, friend, trainees and level of training, experienced or novice allied health professionals, subspecialist physician, translator, other...)

Domain	Did the learner ...	1	2	3	4	5	Red flag	Stage	Examples of Behaviours to Support Assessment and Corresponding Stages
Communication	... demonstrate verbal communication skills	☐	☐	☐	☐	☐	☐	Red flag	***Interrupts, uses a forceful voice or dominates conversation, causing patient/caregiver(s) distress***
								1-2	Uses convention: introduces self and explains role with medical team, uses layman's terminology
								3-4	Aligns goals and maintains focus of the meeting with patient/caregiver(s) wishes
								4-5	Builds and maintains rapport with patient/caregiver(s) with constant flow in interactions and exchanges
	... demonstrate non-verbal communication skills	☐	☐	☐	☐	☐	☐	Red flag	***Inappropriately uses nonverbal cues such as closed or aggressive posture, abrupt exit/entrance, restlessness, or inappropriately frowns/smiles***
								1-2	Makes appropriate amount of eye contact, standing vs sitting, leaning toward patient/caregiver(s)
								2-3	Uses adjusted voice intonation, active listening, shows attentiveness
								3-4-5	Responds to nonverbal cues from patient/caregiver(s), uses own nonverbal communication appropriately
	... demonstrate adaptability during the encounter	☐	☐	☐	☐	☐	☐	Red flag	***Strictly adheres to checklist without flexibility***
								1-2-3	Integrates patient/caregiver(s) expectations into agenda of the encounter
								4-5	Adopts dynamic and flexible flow of conversation, following verbal cues from patient/caregiver(s), allows for moments of silence
	... close loops during and at the end of the encounter	☐	☐	☐	☐	☐	☐	Red flag	***Does not answer patient's/caregiver(s)' questions, does not formulate a plan for next steps***
								1-2	Leaves an opening for future discussion
								3-4	Directly/clearly addresses patient's/caregiver(s)' questions
								3-4-5	Periodically summarizes and uses transitions to facilitate patient's/caregiver(s)' understanding
								4-5	Closes encounter leaving patient/caregiver(s) with realistic hope and expectations, but recognizing uncertainty
Civility and Respect	... demonstrate perspective-taking, cognitive empathy	☐	☐	☐	☐	☐	☐	Red flag	***Ignores or misses patient's/caregiver(s)' concerns, queries, disregards differences in values***
								1-2/2-3	Identifies (1 – 2), articulates (2 – 3) patient's/caregiver(s)' concerns
								2-3-4	Solicits and explores patient's/caregiver(s)' values, beliefs, perspectives and preferences
								4-5	Addresses and validates patient's/caregiver(s)' concerns, emotional features, values and norms
	... demonstrate compassion, affective empathy	☐	☐	☐	☐	☐	☐	Red flag	***Ignores patient's/caregiver(s)' emotional reactions, or becomes inappropriately overcome with positive/negative emotion***
								1-2/3-4	Listens (1 – 2), displays genuine emotional responses (3 – 4)
								4-5	Validates and supports patient's/caregiver(s)' feelings and maintains emotional composure
	... demonstrate sensitivity to perspective difference, empathy diversity	☐	☐	☐	☐	☐	☐	Red flag	***Stereotypes patient/caregiver(s) based on culture, religion, gender or sexual identity***
								1-2/3-4	Identifies (1–2), addresses (3–4) differences in perspectives in between physician and other participants
								4-5	In the context of patient's/caregiver(s)' culture, religion, gender or sexual identity; interprets emotions, gestures and facial expressions appropriately
Clinical and Ethical Judgment and Decision-Making	... incorporate standards of practice	☐	☐	☐	☐	☐	☐	Red flag	***Acts in conflict with professional ethics***
								1-2	Identifies the standards of practice
								3-4-5	Acknowledges and appreciates the standards of practice in the context of the encounter
	... appreciate the complexity of the decision	☐	☐	☐	☐	☐	☐	Red flag	***Fails to incorporate patient's/caregiver(s)' needs and perspectives***
								1-2-3	Demonstrates an understanding of the complexity, uncertainty, and ambiguity of the situation
								2-3-4	Acknowledges that patient's/caregiver(s)' choices might not follow guidelines and evidence-based medicine
								4-5	Weighs the evidence and conventions in clinical care with patient's/caregiver(s)' needs
	... engage patient/caregiver(s) in the decision	☐	☐	☐	☐	☐	☐	Red flag	***Deliberately influences patient/caregiver(s) toward a decision without justification***
								1-2	Provides medical information that facilitates patient's/caregiver(s)' participation
								3-4-5	Balances information provided on the specific needs and preferences of the patient/caregiver(s)
								3-4	Incorporates patient's/caregiver(s)' perspectives, values and religious beliefs into the decision-making process
								4-5	Engages and invites silent participants to verbalize their perceptions when appropriate
	... manage disagreements/ethical conflicts	☐	☐	☐	☐	☐	☐	Red flag	***Ignores or fails to address disagreements between participants (e.g. healthcare providers, patient, caregiver(s))***
								1-2/3-4	Recognizes ethical conflicts (1 – 2) and articulates the basis of the conflict (3 – 4)
								5	While facilitating ethical resolution toward an agreement, incorporates the situation's specific characteristics and the patient's/caregiver(s)' best interest, wishes and autonomy; stay open to the involvement of an interdisciplinary team
	... take steps toward an agreement	☐	☐	☐	☐	☐	☐	Red flag	***Fails to obtain agreement on next steps that will lead to a final decision***
								1-2/3-4	Summarizes the critical features of the encounter (1 -2) and obtains agreement on the next steps (3 -4)
								4-5	Leaves encounter with mutual understanding and by identifying common ground

Please refer to the instructions provided in next page to complete the scale

FIGURE 4.4a

Relevant situational factors that interfered with an ethically justified decision-making process	Not a concern	Moderate concern	Major concern
The physical environment of the encounter was not appropriately set-up prior to the meeting	☐	☐	☐
Uncontrollable environment factors (e.g., noise, interruption, lighting, temperature)	☐	☐	☐
Time limitations that were attributable to the clinical context	☐	☐	☐
Physician's physical or mental/cognitive fatigue (e.g.: post call, etc.)	☐	☐	☐
Other: (e.g., patient's/caregiver(s)' emotions, reactions) ________	☐	☐	☐
Concerns and constructive comments for the trainee:			
Comments on positive examples during the encounter:			

OVERALL ASSESSMENT	Stage 1	Stage 2	Stage 3	Stage 4	Stage 5
At what stage of competency did the trainee perform?	☐	☐	☐	☐	☐

	No	Somewhat	Yes
Did the trainee perform at their current stage of training?	☐	☐	☐
Did the trainee perform in a manner that exceeded their expected stage of training?	☐	☐	☐

¶ Entrustability Scale - Definition of stages of competency			
Stage 1	*Entry to residency*	*Requires full supervision* ***(I had to do)***	*Functions at the level of a* ***pre-graduate trainee.***
Stage 2	*Transition to discipline*	*Requires constant direction* ***(I had to talk them through)***	*This stage emphasizes the orientation and assessment of new trainees arriving from different medical schools and programs including outside of Canada. This stage corresponds to the* ***junior resident status in their first 2-3 months*** *of residency.*
Stage 3	*Foundation of discipline*	*Some independence but requires intermittent direction* ***(I had to prompt them from time to time)***	*This stage covers broad-based competencies that every trainee must acquire before moving on to more advanced, discipline-specific competencies. This stage continues to correspond with* ***junior resident status.***
Stage 4	*Core of discipline*	*Independence but still requires supervision just in case* ***(I needed to be in the room just in case)***	*This stage covers the core competencies that make up the majority of a discipline. This stage corresponds to the early stage of* ***senior resident status.***
Stage 5	*Transition to independent practice*	*Complete independence* ***(I did not need to be there)***	*At this stage the trainee should demonstrate readiness to make the transition to autonomous practice. This stage of residency continues to correspond with the later stage of* ***senior resident or junior attending*** *role.*

Instructions to complete the scale provided in previous page

- **Bolded items** flag professional concerns that could be independent of the stage of competency scored: check this box when important concerns arose during the encounter that jeopardized the relationship between the patient/caregiver(s) and the medical team.
- ¶ **Stages of competency evaluated on a scale 1 to 5** where Stage "1" corresponds to entry to residency, Stage 2 to transition to discipline, Stage 3 to foundation of discipline, Stage 4 to core of discipline, and Stage "5" correspond to transition to independent practice (see Table for more details).
- ¶¶ **In parenthesis**, a range of competency developmental stage a rater should observe is provided. The stage at which the behavior should be observed is **bolded**.

FIGURE 4.4b

5

DEVELOPING AND IMPLEMENTING A MEDICAL HUMANITIES CURRICULUM IN THE UNDERGRADUATE MEDICAL CURRICULUM IN NEPAL

Rajesh Nath Gongal and Madhusudan Subedi

5.1 Introduction

As students enter a medical school to start their journey toward becoming a competent clinician, they are asked to dissect a cadaver to identify muscles, organs, nerves, and vessels and to memorize the details of each of these parts. The physiological functions of each of the organ systems are discussed extensively. Who this person was, where he/she might have lived, and how his/her family might feel about the dissection of a loved one are given little consideration (cf. Dixson, 1999; Hallam, 2017; Robbins et al., 2009; Schoenherr, 2022).

Medical students are also bombarded with a vast quantity of patterns: microorganisms, chemical compounds, pathophysiologies, and diagnostic tests. Thereafter, the only explicit goal of healthcare professions is to recognize these diseases (e.g., Montiero et al., 2024) and provide treatment with psychomotor skills (Abdo et al., 2024). Undoubtedly, the core competencies of healthcare professionals concern medical expertise; however, the larger context of healthcare delivery, socio-cultural milieu, and history are left unaddressed.

Even if we are to focus on the cognitive processes of learning, the exclusive focus on diagnosis and treatment fails to consider the emotions (McConnell, 2024), and the therapeutic alliances that develops between practitioners and patients (Elvins & Green, 2008; Kim et al., 2008; Martin et al., 2000; Taccolini et al., 2018; Vasquez, 2007). These failures can also impact practices, creating vulnerabilities in the communication between healthcare professionals and their patients (Ferretti et al., 2023). As a result of the neglect of these professional competencies, it should be unsurprising then that a clinician might have difficulty comforting a mother of a child dying of septicemia, or a young girl with metastatic cancer, or that students

DOI: 10.4324/9781003498155-5

have difficulty discussing the ethicality and morality of foregoing cardiopulmonary resuscitation (CPR).

Medical education institutions must address these deficits, by moving beyond the biomedical model of care toward one that integrates traditional forms of healthcare delivery and acknowledges the attitudes and beliefs of patients, their communities, and the healthcare system itself (e.g., Gago et al., 2024; Schoenherr, 2027; Schoenherr & Beaudoin, 2027). This growing realization has led to increased interest in the medical humanities (MH) (Bleakey, 2015; Brody, 2011; Fitzgerald & Callard, 2016; Ousager & Johannssen, 2010; Shapiro et al., 2009) and developing means to assess learner competencies in these areas (Cerceo & Vasan, 2023; Gago et al., 2024; Lee et al., 2019; Petrou et al., 2021; Schwartz et al., 2009). To be effective, educators and administrators must critically reflect on how, where, and when to integrate the MH into the medical education curriculum.

In this chapter we describe the brief history of innovation in medical education in Nepal, along with establishment of Patan Academy of Health Sciences (PAHS) and the considerations that went into the development and implementation of an MH curriculum at our institution. We also highlight the experiences and reflections of students and faculties. Finally, we provide some reflections on our experience developing an MH curriculum.

5.2 Nepalese Medical Education and Patan Academy of Health Sciences

Tribhuvan University was established in 1959 and remained the only university in Nepal until 1986. In 1978, Tribhuvan University started the country's first medical degree program to address the growing needs of doctors (Dixit, 2009). The establishment of multiparty democracy in 1990 and subsequent political transformation in Nepal coincided with a surge in the establishment of private for-profit medical colleges without a clear policy framework such that by 2020, there were 23 medical schools producing more than 1500 graduates annually (Sigdel et al., 2021). However, the rural–urban disparities in health indicators remain a formidable challenge (Ministry of Health and Population, Nepal, 2017), one of the many reasons being the unwillingness of the physicians to serve the rural population. Amid this backdrop, PAHS was established in 2008 by the Charter of the Parliament of Nepal with the mission of producing not only technically competent but compassionate health professionals who will be willing to serve the rural and marginalized population.

PAHS adopted innovative selection process with a view that the standard approach to assessing academic excellence is not sufficient to assess whether a learner is a 'good physician' (Hughes, 2002; Kaiser et al., 2007). Instead, non-cognitive attributes were tested using Personal Quality Assessment (PQA) and Multiple Mini-Interviews (MMI) and a cohort was selected after application of Social Inclusion Matrix (SIM). The SIM allowed for discrimination in favor of students from socio-economically, geographically marginalized, disadvantaged population (Upadhyay et al., 2017). PAHS continued this selection process from 2010 to 2018 (Shreshta et al., 2021) after which Medical Education Commission (MEC)[1] was tasked with conducting the admission process at the national level to improve the quality of medical education (Maskarinec et al., 2020; Sigdel et al., 2021).The initial finding indicated that PAHS approach was successful in enrolling a high proportion of candidates from rural and disadvantaged groups (Upadhyay et al., 2017; Shrestha et al., 2021).

Paralleling its concerns with the assessment of excellence, the Academy recognized early on that focus on biomedical model of health professions education was inadequate for preparing healthcare professionals to deliver effective care. Instead, PAHS wanted to develop learners' understanding of health seekers' perspectives and assess their empathic competencies in delivering compassionate care.

5.2.1 The Psychology of Empathy

Empathy reflects a core competency in the health professions, with many educational interventions focusing on its development (Adamson et al., 2018; Bas-Sarmiento et al., 2020; Hojat, 2009; Kiosses et al., 2016; Ruusuvuori, 2007; Tan et al., 2021; for a review, see Nembhard et al., 2023). Studies have revealed troubling trends associated with reduction in empathy over the course of medical training. Such trends are undoubtedly a function of objectification which is associated with reductions in prosocial behavior. Medical educators must address this critical task in a principled manner.

In psychological science, two kinds of empathy are distinguished: cognitive empathy (perspective taking) and affective empathy (feeling for another; Lamn et al., 2007). Studies of health professions have repeatedly demonstrated that high levels of empathy are positively associated with health outcomes (Nembhard et al., 2023). Despite being recognized as an important ability, the efficacy of interventions to develop empathy is contested. However, studies have revealed that empathy training can be effective. For instance, Tending van Berkhout et al. (2016) found that empathy training was more effective when (1) university students or health professionals received training (compared to other learners), (2) learners were compensated with academic credit for the training, (3) assessment examined an understanding of others' emotions, feeling the emotions, and accurate commentary of the emotions, and (4) assessment used objective measures rather than subjective measures. Similar findings have also been obtained in health professions education, although the support is not as strong (Paulus & Meinken, 2022). As it is undeniably true that healthcare professionals must develop affective skills, more work is required to design and develop educational interventions that can be implemented effectively to better serve communities given the human, material, and financial resources of an institution (Schoenherr & Hamstra, 2024).

5.2.2 A Community-Based Approach to Empathy Training

PAHS has placed considerable emphasis on community-based learning and education (CBLE), with a significant portion of the training occurring in rural communities through community health institutions. This helps learners appreciate the rural, decentralized nature of healthcare delivery and can work within the National Health System for which community postings from grassroots level to District Hospital levels are organized (Baral et al., 2016; Shreshta et al., 2021).

During their first residential rural rotation, they are required to live in the homes of villagers who act as their local guardian. In the written reflections, students express that the field experience and staying with the family has provided invaluable insights into the ground realities of the community and people, contributing significantly to their learning journey. Students' reflections highlight the important learning gained from direct engagement with diverse population, fostering a deeper appreciation for the complexities of delivering healthcare within different socio-cultural contexts (Dhital et al., 2015).

In the Basic Science years, all students complete three longitudinal patient follow-up projects in which they are allocated patients with chronic diseases (e.g., chronic obstructive pulmonary disease (COPD), renal failure, hepatic failure), patients at end of life, and children living with disability. Students must then visit these patients at home every fortnight for a period of six months each following which they have to submit a written portfolio which are evaluated in their annual exams. The objective of this activity is to get the students to internalize the reality of what happens at home when caring for such patients especially for people who come from low-income settings and the hardship experienced by the family. Home visits helped students develop unexpected insights into people's lives, a deeper understanding of patients' perspective (Solomon & Risdon, 2011), an appreciation for changes in patients' conditions over time (McWilliams et al., 2008), and approaches to caring for the chronically ill, such as individualizing care to meet patients' individual needs and improving quality of life as a goal of care (Yuen et al., 2006). Studies conducted in PAHS have shown that longitudinal visits at home or hospice help students access much deeper level of experiential learning and increase the depth of students' understanding of the challenges experienced by patients and families (Butterworth et al., 2016).

Healthcare professionals must collaborate effectively with all members of a healthcare team (Bridges et al., 2011; Havyer et al., 2016; Schot et al., 2020). One of the unique feature of PAHS is that third-year medical students work with nurses before starting clinical rotations. Healthy professional relationships are vital for effective team-based patient care for reducing medical errors and for improving patient outcomes (Martin et al., 2010; Rosenstein, 2002; Rosenstein & O'Daniel, 2005). Replicating previous studies, research conducted at PAHS found that learning in an authentic workplace during a clinical rotation engendered mutual respect between nurses and future doctors. This was an authentic way of learning interprofessional competencies around collaboration, communication, and professionalism. It enhanced respect for the nursing profession in students and engendered respect for the students by nurses. Even this brief rotation resulted in transformative learning, where students recognized nurses as independent health practitioners within the healthcare team and identified nurses as holistic patient-centered communicators (Butterworth et al., 2018).

Although interventions are included in the program to develop a human-centered approach to healthcare delivery and could be said to be part of MH, formal MH teaching as a subject was only initiated in 2018 with the inclusion of Foundation Block in the curriculum. The eight-week Foundation Block of PAHS curricula introduces students to key principles of medical ethics, communication skills, basic information technology skills, and MH.

5.3 Integrating Medical Humanities into the PAHS Curriculum

In the presence of birth and death, tragedy and loss, suffering and resilience, we can glimpse defining features of humanity (Kumagai & Wear, 2014). The MH are concerned with 'the science of human' and are designed to optimize patient care and help learners become good physicians (Kirklin, 2003; for review, see Cole et al., 2015). As an interdisciplinary field, MH includes the humanities (literature, philosophy, ethics, history, and religion), social sciences (anthropology, cultural studies, psychology, sociology, and health geography), and theaters (film and visual arts) and their application in pursuit of medical educational goals (Bleakley, 2015; Evans, 2002; Kirklin, 2003).

Conforming to these themes, the aim of integrating MH in the undergraduate medical curriculum of PAHS is for the students to develop a holistic understanding of human experience in relation to life processes like birth, aging, illness, and disability, as well as death and dying.

The objectives of the MH course are as follows:

- Understand how disease and disability affect a person, their family, and community,
- Understand the concept of suffering in relation to illness, disease, and disability,
- Understand the difference between caring and treating, curing and healing,
- Understand aging and dying as a part of life,
- Understand the role of health professionals in alleviation of suffering.

To meet these objectives, 16-hour (8-session) MH course was included in the Foundation Block, increasing its length to 20 hours distributed across 10 sessions. While we recognize the debate on the appropriate terminology like health humanities (Crawford et al., 2010, 2015), we continue to refer to this area of study as MH/humanities in medicine to simplify our discussion. PAHS has also separated MH from ethics teaching. Ethics training consists of distinct sessions in the Foundation Block and is continued during Basic Science and Clinical Science years (for a related approach, see Gago et al., 2024). The reason for this is that over time ethics session can come to dominate the MH teachings and objectives which were set out may be difficult to meet.

5.3.1 Material Included in the MH Sessions

5.3.1.1 General Overview

The MH course at PAHS covers diverse topics like death and dying, disability, social injustice, doctor–patient relationship, and aging. Various media are utilized including real patient narratives, art, movie, poetry, literature, and photography. Active learning is encouraged. After presentation of the media (e.g., story, movie, or poetry), students are divided into several groups and are asked to identify relevant issues and discuss in groups and present in plenary sessions. Reflective learning is prioritized. The details of each session are highlighted in the following sections.

5.3.1.2 Introductory Session

An hour-long introductory session is used to introduce this novel – and often unexpected – subject for the students. They are presented with the basic approach to MH, the reasons for including MH in the curriculum, and the various tasks they need to complete during this time.

In the MH course, students are required to complete:

1. Reflection Piece 1: Learners must reflect on 'What do they think life is about, what is their purpose in life? What do they want to achieve in life?'
2. Reflection Piece 2: Learners must reflect on piece on 'What do they think is death? How would they want to die?'
3. Simulated Disability Exercise: The students are asked to work in group of three. In each group, one learner adopts the role of a person with a disability (e.g., a mobility issue that requires the use of a wheelchair, or a visual impairment), a second learner adopts the role of caregiver, and third learner adopts the role of observer, noting the reaction of the other people. The three-person team must complete the task in a public area, have tea/coffee in local restaurant, and return to the campus. The activity should take approximately 2–3 hours to provide a greater sense of realism and to reduce the chances that idiosyncratic events will bias the experience. Following this, the learners must write a reflective piece on their experience.
4. Produce an Act: They are asked to work in groups of eight and produce an act (drama, dance, story, poetry, or mixture of these media) reflecting what they have experienced during the eight-week MH course. This is presented in the last session of the Foundation Block.

5. Write a final individual reflection of about 1000 words to be submitted on completion of the Foundation Block.

5.3.1.3 First Session

This session starts with a powerful letter written in Nepali language to the Health Minister by a 19-year-old girl, Sandhya Shahi, from a remote area of the country who is afflicted with metastatic bone cancer. It is about her struggle to come to terms with the disease and her death. One of the students, preferably female, is asked to read the letter in the class. After the letter we ask the students, 'How do they feel after reading the letter'? We allow three to four students to tell their feelings. The students raise various issues related to the letter like injustice, inequitable distribution of healthcare resources in the country, poverty, and the struggle of patients at end of life, their fear of death and dying, etc. We also highlight whether the health professionals are treating dying people well and the minimal expectations of the patients and their family members in such situations. The students are asked to discuss these issues in groups and present in plenary.

5.3.1.4 Second Session

In this session, an excerpt from the book *When Breath Becomes Air* by Paul Kalanithi is presented to learners. Paul is a young neurosurgeon in training who is diagnosed with metastatic lung cancer near the end of his neurosurgical residency and describes his cancer journey. His journey contrasts with the young girl's life in the first session especially in terms of acceptance of the condition. Also discussed in this session are the responsibilities of physicians to patients, doctor–patient relationship, struggle of families of patients, and our responsibilities as physicians to families.

5.3.1.5 Third Session

In this session, epilogue of *When Breath Becomes Air* written by Paul's wife is discussed which mainly revolves around Paul's last month and his end of life. The question of whether Paul's dying was good is debated and the reasons why his death could be said to be good is discussed. Students are asked how they might want to die and what is important for them at the end of life. They are also asked to write a short reflection on what is life and what is death to them and share their thoughts in plenary.

5.3.1.6 Fourth Session

Two Nepali poems are read during this session.

In the year 2017, a flood caused havoc in flat lands of Nepal. An impoverished family lost their child but as there was no land to bury him, the parents performed the last rites at the banks of flooded river and left the child to flow in the river. The poem is written in manner of a mother addressing her child. It presents an accurate representation of poverty and the social injustice, doctors' strike, and partiality of the people due to their political affiliation. We ask students how they felt after reading this poem. We then sample reactions of three to four students. Students are then asked to highlight the issue from the poem and organize them into several domains. Students are divided into eight groups to discuss various domains and present in plenary.

The second poem is about cry of the unborn child to have opportunity to live. It highlights the issues of abortion. This poem was written by one of our own students and was awarded second prize in poem contest at our Academy.

Students discuss poverty and its relation to health and our duties as physicians to the marginalized people of the society. Ethical issues concerning abortion are also discussed.

5.3.1.7 Fifth Session

In this session a movie *Awakenings* is shown. This is a movie based on a true story written by Oliver Sacks in which he describes his experience as a doctor caring for patients afflicted with 'sleeping sickness'. The movie highlights the plight of patients with chronic conditions and the families who look after them. Dr Sayer is a lovable man, who treats chronic, hopeless patients and speaks with their loved ones.

5.3.1.8 Sixth Session

Reflections from the movie are presented by the students. We ask the students to share initial response after watching movie. Some of the key points highlighted in this session are described below.

What is the impact of chronic illness on the family members of the patients? What is the hospital ward like at the start of the film? How do patients react when they realize how long they have been unconscious? How does Leonard react when the effects of the drug stop working? How does Dr Sayer care for Leonard as he starts to become more unwell again? What is the hospital ward like at the end of the film? In what ways is care on the ward different at the end?

Students are also asked to think about, for example, what does the film teach them about caring for vulnerable, persons with disability and their humanity? What does the film say about hope? What did they learn about doctor–patient relationship? What characteristics of Dr Sayer would they like to copy?

The second half of the session is focused on the presentation from the students on their disability project.

5.3.1.9 Seventh Session

Continuation of the presentation on disability project.

Second part of the session: Students are asked, "What are you proud of?" Each student has to give a short account of what they feel proud of.

5.3.1.10 Eighth Session

Extract from a Nepali novel *Jeevankanda ki phul* (Life: a thorn or a flower?) written by Jhamak Ghimire is read. The author is a lady with cerebral palsy of very poor background who is unable to speak nor use her arms. The book depicts her journey of learning to write by using her toes as pen and the dirt on the floor as her copy and how she studied without going to school and rose to the height she has attained today as literary figure winning many prestigious awards.

In this autobiography, the author has written story of suffering and struggle for freeing herself from status like animal. After much struggle, she explored the power of words, and she dares to call life a flower, and not a thorn. Whatever form it is, she says, life gives joy, and it is beautiful. She emphasizes that nothing is impossible if we are willing to pursue something and work hard for it.

5.3.1.11 Ninth Session

Photos of elderly are given to each group, and they are asked what do they see? Students are asked to write a group reflection on photographs. They are asked to highlight the following points: What is the photographer trying to show you with this photo? How do you feel about what you see? How do you think it feels to grow old? What aspects might be hard, painful, and what aspects would be good and enjoyable? How does society view the older people? How do you think health workers should care differently for older patients?

This is again presented in the plenary.

Two short movies are shown about the elderly to highlight the importance of love, care, and connections with them.

5.3.1.12 Tenth Session

This is the last session of MH class in Foundation Block. Students work in a group, prepare, and present short dramas or short films that highlight the importance of humanities in medicine. Through their creative work, they emphasize the role of empathy, compassionate care, socio-cultural understanding, and ethical consideration in healthcare practice. These presentations focus on the connection between medicine and humanity.

5.4 Students' Attitudes toward the MH Course

Feedback from the course has largely been positive, leading to the continued use of the course with only slight modifications. Here, we chart the evolution of the course from one that used elementary measures to evaluate the student's learner experience to a more robust set of measures to illustrate the construct validity of the materials (e.g., Schoenherr & Hamstra, 2024).

In 2018 we did not perform a formal evaluation but piloted a semi-structured survey tool to be formally implemented in the coming year. The survey tool consisted of 11 statement items related to student perceptions and students had to score their level of agreement to the statement using five-point Likert scale. All 65 students in the class participated in the survey. Each of them answered each item. Cronbach's alpha calculated for all 11 items was 0.74. There were also three open response questions. Participation in the survey was voluntary, and students were free to decline to participate with no adverse consequences. After the verbal consent, faculty distributed the questionnaire to each of the students and requested to submit their answers in a specific place without writing their name and roll number. The surveys were completed anonymously, and students were encouraged to give honest responses (Subedi et al., 2019) (Table 4.1).

In 2019 we performed a formal evaluation using this tool after obtaining permission from the Academy and the Institutional Review Committee of PAHS. All 65 students participated in the survey. Again, Cronbach's alpha was high (0.779) for all items (Helen et al., 2020). Most students (95%) agreed that the course was enjoyable and interesting, it was relevant to their future career, it helped them understand doctors' role in caring for patients, and it should be included in future courses. The majority (92%) also agreed that the course will help them become better doctors, and that the course materials helped them expand their perspectives and views (87%; Helen et al., 2020).

In 2020, we performed a study to see whether the MH course impacted on the students' empathy level using Jefferson Scale of Empathy (student version) among the first-year learners of 2019–2020 student cohort. Jefferson Scale of Empathy-Student Version (JSE-S), a self-administered written questionnaire, developed to measure empathetic qualities and tendencies among healthcare students and professionals. The JSE-S is a robust, 20-statement item questionnaire with participant responses scored on a seven-point Likert scale. All 65 students voluntarily participated in completing the scale. Participants were asked to complete the questionnaire prior to starting of the MH course and at completion of the course. They were also asked to indicate their choice of future specialty they were likely to pursue at the time of survey which was divided into people-orientated specialties (like internal medicine, general practice, obstetrics, pediatrics) or technology and procedure-oriented which includes surgery, neurosurgery, orthopedic surgery, and public health, and 'Undecided', for students unable to identify a future specialty they would be interested in pursuing later in their careers.

TABLE 5.1 Students' Perceptions of MH Course

Items	*Mean ±SD*	*Strongly disagree (%)*	*Disagree (%)*	*Neutral (%)*	*Agree (%)*	*Strongly agree (%)*
1 – I found the medical humanities course interesting.	4.3±0.5	0	0	4.6	63.1	32.3
2 – I enjoyed the medical humanities course.	4.2±0.6	0	0	10.8	60.0	29.2
3 – The sessions were well structured.	4.1±0.7	0	1.5	13.8	55.4	29.2
4 – The sessions were interactive and included much discussion time.	4.3±0.6	0	0	7.7	50.3	41.5
5 – I found the materials we used in the sessions (poems, books, film, art) made me think differently about disease, disability, and death	4.6±0.5	0	0	1.5	33.8	64.6
6 – The subjects discussed were relevant to my future medical career.	4.3±0.7	1.5	0	7.7	47.7	43.1
7 – The course expanded my perspective and views (for example, culturally, artistically, and intellectually) through the material discussed.	4.1±0.6	0	0	12.3	66.2	21.5
8 – The course faculty were engaging and helped to stimulate ideas and discussions.	4.4±0.6	0	0	4.6	52.3	43.1
9 – I think the medical humanities course was important and should be included in future introductory courses.	4.5±0.8	1.5	0	7.7	29.2	61.5
10 – The medical humanities course helped me to better understand a doctor's role in caring for patients.	4.5±0.6	0	0	4.6	38.5	56.9
11 – Studying medical humanities will help make me a better doctor.	4.5±0.6	0	0	7.7	35.4	56.9

There was a significant increase in mean score (M) for the entire class from pre-module to post-module: M(pre) = 105 to M(post) = 116, $p < 0.001$. Similar patterns were observed for males (M(pre) = 103 to M(post) = 116) and female students (M(pre) = 108 to M(post) = 116). Participants preferring procedure- and technology-oriented specialties showed a significant increase in mean scores: 103–117, and participants preferring people-oriented specialties demonstrated a smaller increase: 107–111 (GC et al., 2022).[2]

Reflections written by the students at the end of the course provide converging evidence for positive changes in their empathy. In developing the MH course, the PAHS has adopted the definition of reflection provided by Nguyen et al. (2014) as the process of engaging the self in attentive, critical, exploratory, and iterative interactions with one's thoughts and actions, and their underlying conceptual frame, with a view to changing them and with a view on the change itself – to be integral to learning, growing, and maturing to become a competent and compassionate professional (Gago et al., 2024). Reflective learning is prioritized from the outset of the MH course. Students are asked to write their reflections after each community visits, rural rotations, at the end of patient follow-ups as mentioned above. In the MH course, students are asked to write a short reflection after the disability project and a 1000-word reflection in a language of their comfort at the end of the MH course. The reflections, although compulsory, are not marked. This makes it more of value as feedback. Reflections written by the students are true feedback on the course and how this has impacted them.

5.5 Reflections after the Disability Project

To compliment the quantitative analysis, a qualitative analysis was conducted to identify writing themes that suggested improved development of learner empathy. The disability project has been described above in the task required to be completed by the students. This assignment is given to students with the objective that they can perceive the difficulties the persons living with disability and the caregivers have to endure in their daily lives so that when they come across such patients in their work, they are able to provide a better care. We understand that stepping in the shoes of persons living with disability for 2 hours will not get them to truly see the innumerable challenges they have to face in their life nor truly feel the pain that they have to go though – even assuming that the students can even get near to feeling such pain will be an insult to the people living with the disability. However, we feel that even if they can internalize the different aspect of how they live their lives, it can make them see life in a different dimension.

Students' reflection after this assignment provides some evidence that to a certain extent our objectives have been met. Certain themes stood out from the written reflections which included (1) respect for the persons living with disability, (2) how they had taken their own abilities for granted, (3) mixed feelings about the societies' approach toward such persons, (4) disappointment seeing the inaccessible infrastructure of the city, and (5) how the social experiment changed them.

5.5.1 Respect for the Persons Living with Disability

Most students wrote that they had never given any thought about this issue at all until this assignment which has changed their perspective about people living with disability and has developed tremendous respect for them.

One student wrote,

> *Inner me wept because at that moment I felt it is just a project work what if the person sitting on the chair was someone who I love, the one of my own family. Life is comparatively so hard and painful for them as just in an hour it broke me from inside. I promised myself that I will never disrespect the people struggling with such illness. And thanks those who take care of their loved one in such situation.*

Another student wrote,

> *One of the highlights of this course was the disability project, a memory I will never forget as long as I live. Walking with crutches for an hour or so made me understand a small portion of the true depth of feelings that disabled people may go through on a regular basis. This by far has been my strongest and most cherished experience in the foundation course. When I walked my way through the streets, I felt some strong emotions. I felt vulnerable yet empowered, pitiful yet optimistic, and saddened yet content. It was a varying mixture of emotions coming together to form a single state of mind.*

5.5.2 How They Had Taken Their Own 'Abilities' for Granted

Many students also felt that they had been taking their 'abilities' – to walk, the ability to see, ability to think – as givens and that the exercise brought them to the realization that they should not take these gifts for granted. Rather, life should be cherished. One student noted this point directly: "*So, I learnt that 'everything that we have today should not be taken for granted.' We should value the life that we have got and try our best to make the lives of the ones around us 'unchallenging.*"

Another student articulated in a similar manner,

> *Everyone has obstacles and challenges they must deal with, and disability should never be the reason to pity [oneself] and have constant focus on it. So lastly it made me realize how thankful and grateful we should be of everything that we possess and the things that are going in our life.*

Similarly, another student penned his emotions,

When we were done with the project, I got to understand my privileges a little better. In so many ways I use to victimize myself, I always complained that I don't have enough money, I am already 21 without any achievement, I have so many problems but that day I understood at least I have my hands, legs, brain and I am healthy. And how difficult would my life be without them. I thought if I didn't have my legs I would only have the desire to have legs and all of my other desires would be so insubstantial and unimportant, I have my legs so what do I have to victimize myself for? I felt like I grew as a person that day.

5.5.3 Mixed Feeling about the Societies' Approach toward Persons with Disabilities

Following the exercise, the students' perception of society was defined by complex assessments. Some students perceived people to be quite helpful, warm, and empathetic, while there were others who were harsh, cold, and unhelpful.

In this regard, one student wrote,

As we moved towards the Jawalakhel [a location approximately 1.5 kms away from the hospital where most students went to have tea]], I noticed very few people being concerned about an injured lad in a wheel chair and I felt really miserable but there were also some amazing people who advised us ways to get past every nook and cranny of the streets of Lagankhel [the location of Patan Hospital].

Another student mentioned,

"Through this project, I learned that lives of differently abled people had a lot of hurdles. First of all, people staring at me made me really uncomfortable. I felt like they were seeing not my individuality but just a person on a wheelchair. Some frowned at me, some gave me a pity look and yet some were silently judging me. People looked down at me and while I was on a wheelchair I could literally see the world through a different angle, and I was suddenly very conscious of myself.

When we reached the café to have tea there was stair through the entry way, I was very disappointed at that, but the servers there were very considerate as they set up chairs for me and my friends (care takers) right next to the entrance near the stairs. It made me feel like there are still people around me who care for others and are empathetic towards disabled."

Yet another student expressed her feelings,

On the way we met some people who helped us, some people who didn't care and some who disliked us. We found a good guy helping us with our wheelchair when it was stuck. Some helping us to cross the busy road by blocking the traffic.

5.5.4 Disappointment in the Lack of Accommodations for Disabilities in the City's Infrastructure

Many students were disappointed with the infrastructure in the city. Rather than accommodating the needs of all members of society, the city's design failed to facilitate the activities of people with disabilities and in some cases hindered their activities.

A student put in words his disappointment:

As the wheelchair rolled, I sometimes glided on the pebbles, slipped on sloppy roads, struggled at crowded places, and almost collided with a car as the driver slammed the door behind him. Witnessing so many obstacles, I realized our roads weren't constructed considering the differently abled people.

Another student echoed this sentiment:

During my journey to Jawalakhel, I realized that the roads were not friendly for the differently abled people. Moreover, the cycle lane was also converted into a parking lot. My friends were struggling hard to push me in the wheelchair in such a huge traffic jam. I felt really sad when my wheelchair was stuck in the ditch.

Similarly, another student added,

The world around is not same for everyone like walking in park. We face a lot of difficulty in every step we take. Public places were full of crowded, road was not good, there was no ramps and footways were too narrow. I think this is the worse for physically disabled people because they mostly move around in wheelchair or use crutches.

5.5.5 How the Experience Has Changed Them

Many students described this experience as having changed them as a person.

A student described his emotions,

This has rarely ever happened in my life and the emotions really stuck with me after that. Before, my feelings for the disabled were either black or white. If they couldn't walk, they must have gotten into an accident. If they were blind, they must have been born that way. But after this event, I have caught myself on several occasions thinking deeply about a disabled person when they walk by me on the streets. I think about what they might be feeling, what they might want to say, or how their day might be going. It is a trait in me that has been developed ever since that day I walked in the shoes of a man in crutches and experienced his life.

One student recounted an incidence that occurred when he was going home on a vacation after the disability experiment, what he describes as a coincidence:

It happened when I was returning to my home for the Tihar festival along with my friends. When our bus reached Naubise, there was a blind woman entering the bus with one companion. Nobody left a seat for her. When she came nearer to us [my friend,], who had been my companion during the disability role play, left his seat for the blind woman. Then I was on her side during the journey. At first, I was too shocked by this event. I used to be either afraid or discard such people previously, but that time something must be different, isn't it? I began the conversation with her. Talking with her, I felt so happy, she was very good at conversation, so the journey passed too rapidly…. I felt sad listening to her story, her difficulties in life. At that time, I felt I have not experienced even 1% during the role play that such blind people are facing daily. I even told her about my disability role play. She felt happy and told me something that I will never forget and why this medical humanity of PAHS has a significant impact on me. She told me I was different from other people because I was more compassionate. She liked how I was talking to her without hesitation that made her feel like a normal person. After building so much rapport with her finally when her departure time came, she was so sad and even cried. She was holding my hand so tight as if she was not going to leave it and told me that she would remember me all her life. Thus, after this incident I felt too grateful towards the foundation course which had given me the opportunity to bring such direct change to myself.

5.6 Final Reflections of the Students

The students' reflections over the years suggest that the MH program fulfills a need within PAHS. It has reassured us that the approach we have developed is appropriate. By exploring different issues not explicitly addressed in the traditional medical education curriculum (e.g., life and death, the meaning and experience of disease, disability, inequity and injustice, and poverty), students have come to think deeply and have challenged and shaped their views. The reflections were very powerful, to say the least.

Several themes emerged from them.

5.6.1 Changing Perception of the Course Itself

Most students had little knowledge in the MH prior to taking the course. Many initially felt that it was going to be a waste of time, expressing a preference to study anatomy or physiology for which they had come to medical school to learn. This initial impression, however, changed over time and most felt that this course was very useful, many emphasizing that this should be included in all medical schools.

A student wrote,

Recalling that day, my very first class of medical humanities, and to be honest, at that time I thought this class is not that important. But I was wrong, from the very first day of our class I felt this class is important and as more class ran I felt it more important and came to conclusion that to be a good doctor, one should have a class of medical humanities. Seriously, this class changed my mind and made me adapt a new way of vision.

Another student had a similar response:

During initial days I have wondered …why medical humanities course is included? … Why is our faculty teaching this kind of literature instead of teaching anatomy and physiology? Does this course really help me to become a good doctor? But after those lectures my perception changes…. The articles poems stories are …. gradually developed my mind to be a compassionate, believe in love and respect…. Before joining PAHS I too was a financially oriented doctor…and this course helps me change into a better person.

In a related vein, another student wrote,

Honestly speaking the first few classes held in the course felt like a waste of time. But as time passed, I noticed that the topics had left a subtle yet strong mark that is hard to describe in words, but I started feeling the joy, happiness, sadness, hopes of others became clearer by some degree.

The writing of yet another student was on the same line:

When I first started medical humanities, I was pessimistic about it, I thought it was utterly futile to teach these topics. Now that the course is over I am very grateful that medical humanities was included in foundation block. The things I learnt from medical humanities will certainly guide me to right direction in my life and also in my medical career.

Similar thought was expressed by another student who also added that the teaching method especially the group work and presentation in the plenary improved his critical thinking and communication skill.

> *At first, I felt it was unnecessary, as the lesson progressed, I felt that it was worth it and is an absolute necessity We learned about compassion and empathy toward our patient, ... critical thinking through the small groups' works assigned during our lectures, communications skills as well, as we were to present our views and ideas from our discussion and lot more of the attributes of PAHS without ever realizing that were being taught.*

Another student added how he learned to work in a group, "*As I look back on these months, I see how much I've grown. I've learned the way of group-work on how it functions and how one's contribution can make an impact on whole group's performance and learnings.*"

5.6.2 Changing Perception about Life

Many students felt that they started viewing life in a different way after the course. The dominant themes included how they should cherish every moment of life, how they had taken for granted many things in life, and how their life had become more meaningful.

One student reflected,

> *Medical humanities has taught me to look deeply into things that I usually brush off. It has taught me stories of love, pain, strength, trauma and healing. We have always taken our lives for granted. I have lived through my life in such haste that I have forgotten to appreciate the most valuable attributes like love, health, relationships etc. I have now learned to value them all and be thankful for them.*

Another student added,

> *I was convinced. I realized that in the end blessings, connections, passion and love are what really is valued. I realized that our wish for money, power, fame everything is all futile, what we really want is meaning in our life. We want it to be meaningful.*

Yet another wrote,

> *With a newfound appreciation for even the smallest things in life; warm tea on rainy days, the smell of home cooked food, being able to sleep soundly at night, the thought that my loved ones are safe and healthy. I've come to realize*

that human life is fragile, but resilient, ephemeral but meaningful. Somehow, learning about death has taught me more about life.

One student wrote,

I live the life which many people wish they had. I live the life of happiness which many people are hardly getting… I found this course strongly effective when it seriously alarmed us regarding our conducts with others…The value of little encouragement, little motivation…Life is really not about taking but it's about giving.

5.6.3 Changing Perception about Death and Dying

Many students had never thought about death or dying or had different perception of death which was changed after going through MH course. The following were some of the thoughts the students had.

One student articulated,

"*I had never quite perceived death as something that could be peaceful or liberating. It always occurred to me that "death" was a dark, desolate and terrifying thing, an ineffable reality that one can't run or hide from. Other than being born, death is the most natural, most definite thing we will experience, yet we can't quite bring ourselves to talk about it openly…*

In one of our medical humanities classes, we talked about "good" deaths and "bad" deaths. We talked about how we wanted our final moments to be like."

Another student wrote in similar line, "*Previously, death always meant darkness. It meant losing, suffering, leaving and letting go. This story taught me that death doesn't necessarily mean suffering and pain. Death can be moksha, it can be freedom and it can be beautiful.*"

Yet another student commented that death could be beautiful:

Looking at the journey of death through Paul's eyes, I knew more about life itself. I thought the perfect way to be alive was in the absence of suffering. But life isn't the absence of suffering, instead, it's learning to live with it. Paul showed me how death could also be beautiful.

A student mentioned about the need to accept the reality of death:

Life is so fragile. As everything comes with the date of expiry so does our life has. Death is part of life, and it is an unavoidable event. We need to accept this harsh reality; we will leave this world one day for forever. I think many people do not accept this reality.

Another student wrote,

To conclude, each and every topic we discussed about in medical humanities have influenced me emotionally in one or the other way. However, Paul's story was the one which went through my head and forced me to think about my death, compelled me to imagine myself in my death bed and think about the things I want to do, the things which will make me happy, the kind of doctor I should be, the things I am supposed to do as a good professional doctor, the way I should deal with every individual, the responsibilities I have towards other people and my community.

One student mentioned how death is a taboo subject:

"*Another topic that fascinated me about the course was talking about death so vividly and openly which I had never done before. Death such a stigmatized topic that whenever we speak about it, we are hushed by our parents.*

But maybe death is not the enemy after all, as it has been portrayed, it might be difficult to think about our death but, may be death is what makes us want to live all the more. Death is what brings significance to life. That certainty that I am going to cease to exist someday, makes me want to live my life to the fullest and cherish every day, every moment."

Another student penned his idea about good death:

Good death to me doesn't mean dying after having completed all my wishes and dreams but the death which I will be able to accept as and when it comes to me, raw and natural. My life is very personal to me and so should be my death.

5.6.4 Changing Perspective about Themselves as a Person

Another theme that emerged was how the students perceived a change in themselves as a person and how the course has made them a better person and will make them a better doctor in the future. The following quotes from students' reflection substantiate this thought.

One student was very frank about his intention and wrote,

"*To be honest I joined medical school thinking of being a doctor who just want to earn money and fame. But going through and learning medical humanities changed my perception. I am no more who I was few months back…*

From Medical Humanities I earned positive attitude. An attitude with vision of serving mankind.

I earned A LIFE LESSON. A lesson of love, a lesson of care."

Another had similar feelings:

> *I stepped into PAHS with a dream of becoming a successful doctor. We were introduced to a subject called medical humanities on our foundation block. Little did I know that this subject would change my whole perspective on my dream profession, and I am glad it did. After all classes on medical humanities, I can feel the change in my perspective about this profession. I have evolved a lot in terms of emotions and behaviour. I have learnt about the importance of humanity in this profession. I am paving my way towards becoming a good human and a doctor with utmost dedication, compassion, love and empathy and this course has and will play an important role in shaping me a human being I have always wanted to be.*

Another student expressed,

> "*It was something beyond my thoughts, something which could be felt but rarely could be expressed and something that influenced me to become a better human being.*
>
> *I enjoyed every class. Every week it was nourishing my soul through its different aspects of viewing life and giving me sensation of my existence.*"

Similarly, another student put down the changes he felt:

> "*I find my behavior and thought very different from the past.*
>
> *My concept about life, death, justice, doctor-patient relationship, caring and compassion has been changed….*
>
> *We the medical student or we can say we the future doctors should know the value of life and treat each and every patient with respect and love.*
>
> *Life is very precious.*"

Another student was very candid about her views about taking up medicine as career and narrated,

> "*I didn't want to study medicine for as long as I can remember. It felt too scary, too serious – I would have to be responsible for a stranger who was in pain…*
>
> *Then I slowly realized how easy I had taken my life to be, how I wasn't really grateful for being alive- for being able to breathe and 'just' exist. Reading about people with terminal diseases was sad and painful but I learnt to value life and individuals. Travelling by wheelchair looked easy, until I saw the bumpy ground so close to me, until I saw my friends' hands blistering and their wrists hurting from pushing it. Help felt insignificant, until a bus driver came*

down his seat to help pull a wheelchair into his vehicle and refused to take the bus fare…

I gradually grew to like medicine because it helped me open a path for the suffering, no matter how narrow the path may be."

5.6.5 Changing Perception about the Role of Doctors

Many students had the perception that being a doctor meant writing prescriptions, treating diseases, and earning money and possibly fame. They had not deeply reflected on the true nature of the responsibilities of a physician.

One student articulated his thoughts,

> *Previously I only used to take doctor as a profession of giving medicines and as a respectful job…Doctors' behaviour and attitude also plays in a role of healing. Doctor should value the life of patient by showing genuine empathy and love to the patients.*

Another student mentioned,

> *Introducing with medical humanities and whatever it taught me was a great turning point for my thought and perception learned that being a doctor as a profession is not all what makes our life meaningful. It's about being sincere with that duty and carrying a positive attitude with it. It let me think deep about the meaning of life and death.*

Similarly, another student commented,

> *The doctor should only not have clinical qualified but also a skillful and a good communicator. The attitude of doctor, their behaviour towards patients is not taught anywhere, it's we have to acquire, and it is given through medical humanities. Patan academy of health science is only the college which have medical humanities course, and I am very grateful to this subject as it has changed my perspective of doctors as they should not treat patient and earn money but also heal the patients.*

Another student expressed his thoughts,

> *I thought medicine is all just saving life anyway as due to following popular notion we are compared to ideal gods that saves life anyways. But there is more to it… doctors are no to save lives at any cost rather there to try to save life and if failed then to comfort human lives.*

5.6.6 Looking to Future with Positive Attitude

Many students voiced they were now ready for the future to be good doctors and better human beings, attributing this to the experiences they had during the medical humanities course.

One student articulated his notion for the future,

"*This has made me question our morality as health professionals, as human beings. Can we do anything differently? Can we be better? Can we be the glimmer of hope that people need in their darkest times? After all, it is the biggest privilege a person can get. Seeing people while they're most vulnerable. Seeing people being born and then die…*

I think the answer is definitely yes. Yes, we can do things differently, be better, and be the hopes of our patients. All we need to do is take a good, hard look at ourselves and ask ourselves, what kind of doctor do I want to be? Or more importantly, what kind of person do I want to be? Do I want to be someone who's compassionate? Empathetic? Kind?

Yes, yes and yes.

In less than 2 months, I can confidently say that this class has changed me as a person and as a future doctor."

Another voiced his view,

After this whole two month, now I think that I'm ready to start my MBBS journey. Knowing the importance of a person as a human being I can start walking toward my goal of being a humble doctor. I want to take away from these classes that each and every person is equal. I hope I would treat everyone equally with respect and compassion, be it a poor or a rich, a disabled or a healthy person. This journey from feeling sympathy to empathy to being compassionate is small but it has great effect on my life. I hope as a doctor I would ease their life a little physically, mentally and spiritually. I wish that I remember that human beings are not just physical bodies, but they have spiritual and emotional aspects as well.

Similarly, another student stated,

After all classes on medical humanities, I can feel the change in my perspective about this profession. I have evolved a lot in terms of emotions and behaviour. I have learnt about the importance of humanity in this profession. I am paving my way towards becoming a good human and a doctor with utmost dedication, compassion, love and empathy and this course has and will play an important role in shaping me a human being I have always wanted to be.

Finally, a student put forward a more global view:

On an ending note, this course, while completely new, also made me re-imagine our world. It made me question why we people are not growing sensitive to the expected degree on the real-world issues. How can we, in the capacity of doctor, contribute to make this world a better place for everyone?

5.7 Challenges and Future Directions

The positive feedback received from students provides us with evidence that the MH course has a degree of implementation validity (Schoenherr & Hamstra, 2024). Nevertheless, we encountered many challenges throughout the development of the course, both within the creation of the course and within the implementation at PAHS. Here, we briefly review a few key implementation issues.

The medical and health humanities represent extremely broad fields that are associated with their own curricula. Any program in health professions education cannot hope to capture all of the information, experiences, expertise, and perspectives. To accommodate these needs, our MH course of study attempted to sample broadly using a variety of approaches including reflection exercises and experiential learning. These approaches have been used effectively elsewhere in health professions education (Beard & Wilson, 2006; Kolb, 2015).

One of the most significant challenges in introducing subjects like MH in a health science curriculum is support from the academic leadership and the academic faculties in any institution. These are vital dimensions of the implementation validity of any educational activity (Schoenherr & Hamstra, 2024). This was not the case at PAHS. PAHS supported innovative educational activities and assessment methods and had already adopted admission entrance examinations and CBLE curriculum in MBBS program (Baral et al., 2016; Upadhyay et al., 2011). One of the key factors is that the course developers and implementers were embedded in the Academic Authority (RG as Founding Dean and Rector at the time and MS as Chair of the Department of Community Health Sciences and Coordinator of School of Public Health). This social capital helped minimize the inherent difficulties in engaging other institutional stakeholders in supporting the incorporation of the MH course into the curriculum.

Another key feature of PAHS is the socio-cultural context. The biomedical tradition has provided considerable insight into the detection, diagnosis, and treatment of pathophysiologies. Through the processes of colonization and globalization, these ideas have spread, often at the expense of holistic, traditional forms of healthcare (Schoenherr, 2027; Schoenherr & Beaudoin, 2027; Venosa et al., 2027).

Following our review of the literature and personal reflections, we realized the challenges in adding the MH course to the Foundation Block. We agreed from the outset that it would necessarily be unlike traditional 'black and white' material in the course curriculum as the subject matter required a more holistic approach. Once we began to create the objectives, it became easier to collect materials for the course. We strongly believed that the content must stir up the emotions of students, challenge them with issues related to the objectives and let them come up with answers on their own. We agreed that the MH course would not be a venue to preach to the students, but instead we will allow them to come to their own conclusions through discourse and reflection in small groups.

As in any course development, the collection and review of the literature was a time-consuming task. It took almost a year to collect the teaching materials. During the literature review process, we concluded that the inclusion of real stories was a critical element to engage learners. Once we collected the materials, we collated them and identified themes related to stories or poems and potential discussion issues. As healthcare must be practiced by, and delivered to, a local community, we prioritized the inclusion of both local and global materials.

A final challenge to ensure effective, sustainable course delivery was to train faculty members to be facilitators for the teaching sessions. Despite the experience and expertise of faculty members, the novelty of the MH course material required a different set of competencies. This was and remains the most formidable challenge, a challenge that could jeopardize the long-term continuity of the program. This is true of any educational activity (Schoenherr & Hamstra, 2024). The MH course eventually was sustained by only three permanent faculty and one foreign faculty (a general practitioner). We have not been able to add more faculties in the five years since the program started. One likely barrier is the aspect of suffering. While it features prominently in the activities of healthcare practitioners and experiences addressed by the medical and health humanities, discussions around issues related to suffering, death and dying, emotional distress can be difficult. Over time, healthcare professionals can experience empathic burnout (Brazeau et al., 2010; Paro et al., 2014; Picard et al., 2016; Von Harcher et al., 2018). Thus, the ideal of rotating faculty in and out of the course cannot yet be realized.

Challenges remain. While we believe we have demonstrated the implementation validity of the MH course, the nature of assessment, especially the long-term impact of the course, remains a problematic task. Few have attempted it. A study from Harvard showed that students who had gone through New Pathway which included weekly structured learning experiences focused on humanistic aspects of medicine, and clinical experiences designed to foster humanism and the doctor–patient relationship rated their preparation to practice humanistic medicine higher than did traditional students and expressed more confidence in their ability to manage patients with psychosocial problems 12 years after entry into medical school (Peters et al., 2000). How this translates into real-life clinical care is not known; however, such studies are imperative to answer the skeptics and ensure the place of MH into health professional curriculum long term.

5.8 Our Reflection as Faculty Members Who Developed the Course and Worked as Facilitators of the Course

When the time came to implement the course, we were likely as nervous as the students or perhaps even more as we had no idea how the students would respond to the stories we had collected. Will they reject the subject completely? Will they consider this a complete waste of time? Will they be more interested in starting their Basic Science course like anatomy, physiology? After all isn't this what they have entered medical school for? The initial assumptions the students had would seem to support these concerns.

I (RG) remember when, in the first session, after reading the letter written by a 19-year-old dying girl from a remote part of Nepal, I asked them, "How did you feel after reading this letter?" They started bringing up issues related to healthcare and health professions behavior. I asked them again, "What did you feel in your heart?" They were dumbfounded. Later, they said, we never thought we would be discussing our 'feelings' in medical school.

After the second session, 'When breath becomes air,' we had their full attention. They appeared to have embraced the rationale of the course, soaking up the emotions. Many said they cried while reading the stories. There was less hesitation in sharing personal emotional experiences as the course proceeded.

As expressed by the students (in the section Theme 1 of final reflections), the small group discussion seemed to help them think critically, work in groups as a team, and help develop their communication skill. They had not done this before during their education. They had mostly attended lectures. One person from each group had to present the general views of the group at the plenary. At first, this was very challenging as they had no prior experience. Traditionally, only the teachers speak. By the end of eight weeks, we experienced satisfaction as many of them were able to stand in front of class and speak confidently and fluently.

The reflections from the first cohort of students in 2018 were beyond what we expected. This suggested that our approach was producing the desired learning outcomes. The reflections from subsequent cohorts helped cement our feelings about the course. The success of this course is also apparent in the adoption of a humanities course in nursing curriculum from 2021 with the 2-hour sessions being spread out across three years.

The students' reflections indicate a change in their perceptions about life, aging, dying, and people living with disabilities and could be considered to be transformative learning as described by Mezirow. He describes transformative learning as the process of effecting change in a frame of reference which are the structures of assumptions through which we understand our experiences and have been acquired through a coherent body of experience – associations, concepts, values, feelings, conditioned responses – frames of reference that define their life world (Mezirow, 1993, 1997). It has been described by O'Sullivan et al. as experiencing a deep, structural shift in the basic premises of thought, feelings, and actions, a shift of consciousness that dramatically and permanently alters our way of being in the world (O'Sullivan et al., 2002). It is our belief that we have not transformed the learners, but we have challenged and encouraged them to think about issues which they had not given much thought to previously. As dedicated young professionals, they are unlikely to have much life experience, most of them brought up in very protected environments. We believe that the course has helped them delve deeper into themselves and find who they truly are. It is not a matter of transformation but a matter of self-realization.

5.9 Conclusion

Developing and implementing an MH curriculum within the undergraduate medical and nursing programs in Nepal yields several important conclusions. The research findings demonstrated that students have a positive reception to the MH course, leading to a notable shift in their attitudes toward patients and increase in empathy. For educational activities to be effective, it is crucial to assess their implementation validity by ensuring the availability of adequate resources – human, material, and financial. The MH curriculum serves as a necessary complement to the dominant biomedical model in healthcare, offering a more holistic understanding of patients, their families, communities, and even the learners themselves. This comprehensive approach challenges the often reductive and analytic frameworks used in traditional medical and nursing education, encouraging a broader perspective on health, illness, disease, disability, aging, and death.

Moreover, the MH curriculum promotes the integration of various competencies across different domains, fostering a more cohesive and enriched educational experience. However, like any curriculum element, MH courses require continuous evaluation and adaptation to maintain their relevance and effectiveness. Developing reliable methods to assess the efficacy of MH curricula remains a challenge, but it is essential for ensuring the quality and impact of the program. As MH becomes increasingly vital in medical education, particularly in the age of artificial intelligence, it provides essential insights into the human aspects of healthcare. This ensures that the focus remains on empathy, compassionate care, and ethical considerations amid rapid technological advancements.

Notes

1 The MEC was established after a civil movement against irregularities in admission process and unregulated and uncontrolled accreditation of private medical colleges.

2 Prior to analysis, the scalar data were scored or reverse scored as necessary, for the positively and negatively worded items, respectively, based on the JSE-S Professional Manual and Users Guide (2009). Statistical analysis was conducted based on simple descriptive statistics using grouped mean scores, as outlined in the JSE-S methodology. The empathy scores were compared for the whole cohort and subgroups, using independent T-test and ANOVA test, respectively. Similarly, to compare the significance

of pre-module and post-module score difference, paired t-test was applied depending on the normality of data. For non-normally distributed data, the nonparametric test Wilcoxon signed-rank test was applied. Tests were considered statistically significant at p-value of ≤ 0.05 level. All analysis was conducted using the statistical software package SPSS 20. For details https://link.springer.com/article/10.1186/s12909-022-03188-y

References

Abdo, S., Elliott, L., Micallef, J., Sivanathan, M., & Dubrowski, A. (2024). Optimizing psychomotor skills acquisition in healthcare simulation through knowledge mobilization. In *Fundamentals and Frontiers of Medical Education and Decision-Making* (pp. 186–212). Routledge.

Adamson, K., Loomis, C., Cadell, S., & Verweel, L. C. (2018). Interprofessional empathy: a four-stage model for a new understanding of teamwork. *Journal of Interprofessional Care*, *32*(6), 752–761.

Baral, K. P., Upadhyay, S. K., Bhandary, S., Gongal, R. N., & Karki, A. (2016). Development of community based learning and education system within undergraduate medical curriculum of Patan Academy of HealthSciences. *Journal of Nepal Health Research Council*, *14*(32), 58–65.

Bas-Sarmiento, P., Fernández-Gutiérrez, M., Baena-Baños, M., Correro-Bermejo, A., Soler-Martins, P. S., & de la Torre-Moyano, S. (2020). Empathy training in health sciences: a systematic review. *Nurse Education in Practice*, *44*, 102739.

Beard, C. M., & Wilson, J. P. (2006). *Experiential Learning: A Best Practice Handbook for Educators and Trainers*. Kogan Page Publishers.

Bleakley, A. (2015). *Medical Humanities and Medical Education: How the Medical Humanities Can Shape Better Doctors*. Routledge.

Brazeau, C. M., Schroeder, R., Rovi, S., & Boyd, L. (2010). Relationships between medical student burnout, empathy, and professionalism climate. *Academic Medicine*, *85*(10), S33–S36.

Bridges, D., Davidson, R. A., Soule Odegard, P., Maki, I. V., & Tomkowiak, J. (2011). Interprofessional collaboration: three best practice models of interprofessional education. *Medical Education Online*, *16*(1), 6035.

Brody, H. (2011). Defining the medical humanities: three conceptions and three narratives. *Journal of Medical Humanities*, *32*, 1–7.

Butterworth, K., Nichols, D. N., & Manca, T. A. (2016). How future doctors in Nepal are using reflective portfolios to learn compassion and empathy. *European Journal of Palliative Care*, *23*(1), 36–41.

Butterworth, K., Rajupadhya, R., Gongal, R., Manca, T., Ross, S., & Nichols, D. (2018). A clinical nursing rotation transforms medical students' interprofessional attitudes. *PloS One*, *13*(5), e0197161.

Cerceo, E., & Vasan, N. (2023). Creating alignment: How the humanities can help heal physicians and patients. *Journal of Medical Education and Curricular Development*, *10*, 23821205231203487.

Cole, T. R., Carlin, N. S., & Carson, R. A. (2015). *Medical Humanities: An Introduction*. Cambridge University Press.

Crawford, P., Brown, B., Baker, C., Tischler, V., Abrams, B., Crawford, P., ... & Abrams, B. (2015). *Health Humanities* (pp. 1–19). Palgrave Macmillan UK.

Crawford, P., Brown, B., Tischler, V., & Baker, C. (2010). Health humanities: the future of medical humanities?. *Mental Health Review Journal*, *15*(3), 4–10.

Dhital, R., Subedi, M., Prasai, N., Shrestha, K., Malla, M., & Upadhyay, S. (2015). Learning from primary health care centers in Nepal: reflective writings on experiential learning of third year Nepalese medical students. *BMC Research Notes*, *8*, 1–9.

Dixit, H. (2009). Development of medical education in Nepal. *Kathmandu University Medical Journal*, *7*(1), 8–10.

Dixon, K. M. (1999). Death and remembrance: addressing the costs of learning anatomy through the memorialization of donors. *The Journal of Clinical Ethics*, *10*(4), 300–308.

Elvins, R., & Green, J. (2008). The conceptualization and measurement of therapeutic alliance: an empirical review. *Clinical Psychology Review*, *28*(7), 1167–1187.

Evans, M. (2002). Reflections on the humanities in medical education. *Medical Education*, *36*(6), 508–513.

Ferretti, E., Schoenherr, J. R., Mattiola, A., & Daboval, T. (2023). Vulnerabilities in clinician–parent exchanges and the cascade of communication traps: a review. *Archives of Disease in Childhood*, *108*(2), 86–90.

Fitzgerald, D., & Callard, F. (2016). *Entangling the Medical Humanities* (pp. 35–49). Edinburgh University Press.

Gago, F., Echagüe, C. L., & Lázaro, M. (2024). Reflection as a core skill in bioethics education: application to the scientific and healthcare professions. In J. R Schoenherr & M. M. McConnell (Eds.), *Fundamentals and Frontiers in Medical Education and Decision-Making: Educational Theory and Psychological Practice* (pp. 245–269). Routledge.

Hallam, E. (2017). Relational anatomy: dissecting and memorialising the dead in medical education. *Medicine Anthropology Theory| An Open-Access Journal in the Anthropology of Health, Illness, and Medicine*, *4*(4), 99–124.

Havyer, R. D., Nelson, D. R., Wingo, M. T., Comfere, N. I., Halvorsen, A. J., McDonald, F. S., & Reed, D. A. (2016). Addressing the interprofessional collaboration competencies of the Association of American Medical Colleges: a systematic review of assessment instruments in undergraduate medical education. *Academic Medicine*, *91*(6), 865–888.

Helen, A. D., Subedi, M., & Gongal, R. (2020). Medical undergraduates' perceptions on medical humanities course in Nepal. *Journal of Nepal Health Research Council*, *18*(3), 436–441.

Hojat, M. (2009). Ten approaches for enhancing empathy in health and human services cultures. *Journal of Health and Human Services Administration*, *31*(4), 412–450.

Hughes, P. (2002). Can we improve on how we select medical students? *Journal of the Royal Society of Medicine*, *95*(1), 18–22.

Kaiser, F., Dewan, H. B., & Mansoor, F. (2007). Selection of medical students admission and selection policy. *RMJ*, *32*(2), 193–196.

Kim, S. C., Kim, S., & Boren, D. (2008). The quality of therapeutic alliance between patient and provider predicts general satisfaction. *Military Medicine*, *173*(1), 85–90.

Kiosses, V. N., Karathanos, V. T., & Tatsioni, A. (2016). Empathy promoting interventions for health professionals: a systematic review of RCTs. *Journal of Compassionate Health Care*, *3*, 1–22.

Kirklin, D. (2003). The centre for medical humanities, royal free and university college medical school, London, England. *Academic Medicine*, *78*(10), 1048–1053.

Kolb, D. A. (2015). *Experiential Learning: Experience as the Source of Learning and Development*. Pearson Education, Inc.

GC, K. B., Arjyal, A., Douglas, A. H., Subedi, M., & Gongal, R. (2022). A quantitative evaluation of empathy using JSE-S tool, before and after a Medical Humanities Module, amongst first-year medical students in Nepal. *BMC Medical Education, 22*(1), 159.

Kumagai, A. K., & Wear, D. (2014). "Making strange": a role for the humanities in medical education. *Academic Medicine, 89*(7), 973–977.

Lamm, C., Batson, C. D., & Decety, J. (2007). The neural substrate of human empathy: effects of perspective-taking and cognitive appraisal. *Journal of Cognitive Neuroscience, 19*(1), 42–58.

Lee, S. Y., Lee, S. H., & Shin, J. S. (2019). Evaluation of medical humanities course in college of medicine using the context, input, process, and product evaluation model. *Journal of Korean Medical Science, 34*(22), e163.

Martin, D. J., Garske, J. P., & Davis, M. K. (2000). Relation of the therapeutic alliance with outcome and other variables: a meta-analytic review. *Journal of Consulting and Clinical Psychology, 68*(3), 438.

Martin, J. S., Ummenhofer, W., Manser, T., & Spirig, R. (2010). Interprofessional collaboration among nurses and physicians: making a difference in patient outcome. *Swiss Medical Weekly, 140*(1718), 1–12.

Maskarinec, G. G., Subedi, M., Subedi, P., & Karki, A. (2020). Non-violent action to reform medical education in Nepal-the fasts-unto-death of Dr Govinda KC. *Social Medicine, 13*(1), 35–47.

McConnell, M. M. (2024). Emotions and clinical decision-making. In *Fundamentals and Frontiers of Medical Education and Decision-Making* (pp. 139–168). Routledge.

McWilliams, A., Rosemond, C., Roberts, E., Calleson, D., & Busby-Whitehead, J. (2008). An innovative home-based interdisciplinary service-learning experience. *Gerontology & Geriatrics Education, 28*(3), 89–104.

Mezirow, J. (1993). A transformation theory of adult learning. In P. Kleiber & L. Tisdell (Eds.), *Adult Education Research Annual Conference Proceedings* (Vol. *31*, pp. 141–146).

Mezirow, J. (1997). Transformative learning: theory to practice. *New Directions for Adult and Continuing Education, 1997*(74), 5–12.

Ministry of Health, Nepal, New ERA, ICF. (2017). *Nepal Demographic Health Survey 2016* (p. 581). Ministry of Health, Nepal.|

Monteiro, S., Cavanagh, A., Biswabandan, B., & Sibbald, M. (2024). Separating the noise from the signal: The role of familiarity and pattern recognition in the development of clinical expertise. In *Fundamentals and Frontiers of Medical Education and Decision-Making* (pp. 169–185). Routledge.

Nembhard, I. M., David, G., Ezzeddine, I., Betts, D., & Radin, J. (2023). A systematic review of research on empathy in health care. *Health Services Research, 58*(2), 250–263.

Nguyen, Q. D., Fernandez, N., Karsenti, T., & Charlin, B. (2014). What is reflection? A conceptual analysis of major definitions and a proposal of a five component model. *Medical Education, 48*(12), 11761189.

O'Sullivan, E., Morrell, A., & O'Connor, M. A. (2002). *Expanding the Boundaries of Transformative Learning: Essays on Theory and Praxis*. Springer.

Ousager, J., & Johannessen, H. (2010). Humanities in undergraduate medical education: a literature review. *Academic Medicine, 85*(6), 988–998.

Paro, H. B., Silveira, P. S., Perotta, B., Gannam, S., Enns, S. C., Giaxa, R. R., ... & Tempski, P. Z. (2014). Empathy among medical students: is there a relation with quality of life and burnout?. *PloS One, 9*(4), e94133.

Paulus, C. M., & Meinken, S. (2022). The effectiveness of empathy training in health care: a meta-analysis of training content and methods. *International Journal of Medical Education, 13*, 1.

Peters, A. S., Greenberger-Rosovsky, R., Crowder, C., Block, S. D., Moore, G. T. (May 2000). Long-term outcomes of the new pathway program at Harvard Medical School: a randomized controlled trial. *Academic Medicine, 75*(5), 470–479.

Petrou, L., Mittelman, E., Osibona, O., Panahi, M., Harvey, J. M., Patrick, Y. A., & Leedham-Green, K. E. (2021). The role of humanities in the medical curriculum: medical students' perspectives. *BMC Medical Education, 21*, 1–8.

Picard, J., Catu-Pinault, A., Boujut, E., Botella, M., Jaury, P., & Zenasni, F. (2016). Burnout, empathy and their relationships: a qualitative study with residents in General Medicine. *Psychology, Health & Medicine, 21*(3), 354–361.

Robbins, B. D., Tomaka, A., Innus, C., Patterson, J., & Styn, G. (2009). Lessons from the dead: the experiences of undergraduates working with cadavers. *OMEGA-Journal of Death and Dying, 58*(3), 177–192.

Rosenstein, A. H. (2002). Nurse-physician relationships: impact on nurse satisfaction and retention. *AJN The American Journal of Nursing, 102*(6), 26–34.

Rosenstein, A. H., & O'Daniel, M. (2005). Disruptive behavior and clinical outcomes: perceptions of nurses and physicians: nurses, physicians, and administrators say that clinicians' disruptive behavior has negative effects on clinical outcomes. *AJN The American Journal of Nursing, 105*(1), 54–64.

Ruusuvuori, J. (2007). Managing affect: Integration of empathy and problem-solving in health care encounters. *Discourse Studies, 9*(5), 597–622.

Schoenherr, J. R. (2022). Learning engineering is ethical. In J. Goodale & J. Kolodner (Eds.), *Learning Engineering Toolkit* (pp. 201–228). Routledge.

Schoenherr, J. R. (2027). Innovation and implementation in the health professions: Translating research in education and healthcare delivery. In J. R. Schoenherr (Ed.), *Fundamentals and Frontiers in Medical Education and Decision-Making* (pp. 1–76). Routledge.

Schoenherr, J. R., & Beaudoin, J. (2027). The evolving landscape of health professions education in East Asia: heterarchies in East Asian medicine and medical education. In J. R. Schoenherr (Ed.), *Fundamentals and Frontiers in Medical Education and Decision-Making* (pp. 462–509). Routledge.

Schoenherr, J. R., & Hamstra, S. J. (2024). Validity in health professions education: From assessment instruments to program innovation and evaluation. In *Fundamentals and Frontiers of Medical Education and Decision-Making* (pp. 80–107). Routledge.

Schot, E., Tummers, L., & Noordegraaf, M. (2020). Working on working together. A systematic review on how healthcare professionals contribute to interprofessional collaboration. *Journal of Interprofessional Care, 34*(3), 332–342.

Schwartz, A. W., Abramson, J. S., Wojnowich, I., Accordino, R., Ronan, E. J., & Rifkin, M. R. (2009). Evaluating the impact of the humanities in medical education. *Mount Sinai Journal of Medicine: A Journal of Translational and Personalized Medicine: A Journal of Translational and Personalized Medicine, 76*(4), 372–380.

Shapiro, J., Coulehan, J., Wear, D., & Montello, M. (2009). Medical humanities and their discontents: definitions, critiques, and implications. *Academic Medicine, 84*(2), 192–198.

Shrestha, S., Shrestha, A., Shah, J. N., & Gongal, R. N. (2021). Competency based post graduate residency program at Patan Academy of Health Sciences, Nepal. *Journal of Nepal Health Research Council, 19*(1), 189–195.

Sigdel, S., Ozaki, A., Dhakal, R., Pradhan, B., & Tanimoto, T. (2021). Medical education in Nepal: impact and challenges of the COVID-19 pandemic. *Academic Medicine, 96*(3), 340–342.

Solomon, P., & Risdon, C. (2011). Promoting interprofessional learning with medical students in home care settings. *Medical Teacher, 33*(5), e236–e241.

Subedi, M., Helen, A. D., Maharjan, B. R. (2019). *The Perception and Experiences of PAHS's Medical Students to a Medical Humanities Course in Foundation Block.* Rector Office, Patan Academy of Health Sciences.

Taccolini Manzoni, A. C., Bastos de Oliveira, N. T., Nunes Cabral, C. M., & Aquaroni Ricci, N. (2018). The role of the therapeutic alliance on pain relief in musculoskeletal rehabilitation: a systematic review. *Physiotherapy Theory and Practice, 34*(12), 901–915.

Tan, L., Le, M. K., Yu, C. C., Liaw, S. Y., Tierney, T., Ho, Y. Y., ... & Low, J. (2021). Defining clinical empathy: a grounded theory approach from the perspective of healthcare workers and patients in a multicultural setting. *BMJ Open, 11*(9), e045224.

Teding van Berkhout, E., & Malouff, J. M. (2016). The efficacy of empathy training: A meta-analysis of randomized controlled trials. *Journal of Counseling Psychology, 63*(1), 32–41.

Upadhyay, S. K., Bhandary, S., Bhandari, D. B., Dulal, R. K., Baral, K. P., Gongal, R. N., ... & Karki, A. (2017). Admitting deserving medical students from rural and disadvantaged: Patan Academy of Health Sciences' Approach. *Journal of Nepal Health Research Council, 15*(1), 75–80.

Upadhyay, S. K., Bhandary, S., & Ghimire, S. R. (2011). Validating a problem-based learning process assessment tool. *Medical Education, 45*(11), 1151–1152.

Vasquez, M. J. (2007). Cultural difference and the therapeutic alliance: an evidence-based analysis. *American Psychologist, 62*(8), 878.

Venosa, A. R., Baroneza, J. E., & Ferreira Fernandes, R. A. (2026). Medical education in Brazil: A history of an evolving pluralistic healthcare system. In J. R. Schoenherr (Ed.), *Fundamentals and Frontiers of Medical Education and Decision-Making*. Routledge.

Von Harscher, H., Desmarais, N., Dollinger, R., Grossman, S., & Aldana, S. (2018). The impact of empathy on burnout in medical students: new findings. *Psychology, Health & Medicine, 23*(3), 295–303.

Yuen, J. K., Breckman, R., Adelman, R. D., Capello, C. F., LoFaso, V., & Carrington Reid, M. (2006). Reflections of medical students on visiting chronically ill older patients in the home. *Journal of the American Geriatrics Society, 54*(11), 1778–1783.

6

MEDICAL EDUCATION DESPITE WAR

Innovation in the Health Professions during Armed Conflict

Inna Ivanivna Kucherenko
with Jordan Richard Schoenherr

The well-being and lifespan of Ukrainians is dependent on their healthcare system. Efficient and effective healthcare delivery is vital to ensuring the continued social and economic growth of a country. Medical education provides the foundation for healthcare professionals to develop medical expertise, interpersonal communication with patients, utilizing limited institutional and instructional resources, and work as advocates for their profession and the health of a society. In recent years, medical education in Ukraine has moved toward integration within Europe and the international healthcare systems to better achieve these goals.

As part of a large socioeconomic system, healthcare systems provide critical resources and services during a crisis (Emami et al., 2024; Wiedner et al., 2020). They can mitigate threats by providing support to citizens in times of need, providing them with mental and physical stability and acting as a symbol of a nation's continued will to support its people. In crises caused by natural disaster, devastation is typically unsystematic. In the case of armed conflict, strategic and tactical decisions systematically target specific civilian and military resources that support the lives of a country's people (Schoenherr, 2027).

Armed conflicts challenge the fabric of a society and healthcare institutions: they threaten the health and safety of citizens and deplete limited resources that are normally used to maintain the social and physical infrastructure of a country such as education and healthcare services (Gleditsch, 2018; Schoenherr, 2027a; Spiegel et al., 2010). During armed conflicts, it remains critical that educators, learners, and practitioners continue working despite war to ensure continuity and facilitate the recovery of a nation (Bdaiwi et al., 2020). The damage done to healthcare infrastructure is not always incidental. Disregarding ethics, adversarial state and nonstate actors can actively target healthcare infrastructure to destabilize, diminish,

DOI: 10.4324/9781003498155-6

and demoralize a society (Bou-Karroum et al., 2020; Briody et al., 2018; Haar et al., 2021).

Inevitably, natural and anthropogenic crises can overlap. In recent years, the Ukrainian healthcare system has faced many challenges: as the country began to recover from the global pandemic caused by COVID-19, Russia's invasion and continued attacks have placed unprecedented demands on the delivery of care (Ivats-Chabin et al., 2021; Uwishema et al., 2022). In "total wars" such as that launched by Russia on Ukraine, the distinction between civilians and soldiers, domestic and military infrastructure become progressively blurred (Schoenherr, 2023; Schoenherr, 2027c). In conflicts, some argue that this distinction is an "impossibility" (Zehfuss, 2012). Soldiers, citizens, and professionals must martial the resources of their nation together to counter foreign aggression. Practitioners in Ukraine as well as foreign volunteers responded in ways that have kept Ukraine as a functional society despite the continued attacks (Bajaj et al., 2022; Chudzicka-Czupała et al., 2023; Jain et al., 2022; Lawry et al., 2024). Examining how innovation occur during these vulnerable times can provide valuable lessons that are tragically increasingly necessary as conflicts become more prevalent globally.

Similarly, the effects of conflicts are rarely isolated to single countries (Carmignani & Kler, 2016a, 2016b; Murdoch & Sandler, 2002; Silve & Verdier, 2018; cf. Bosker & Ree, 2009). Healthcare systems represent international networks, with attacks on one nation having effects outside the original borders. For instance, the war in Ukraine has adversely impacted its neighbors and allies (e.g., Poland; Kardas et al., 2022; Lewtak et al., 2022) and continues to divert healthcare resources to respond to continued armed aggression (Schoenherr, 2027c). Assistance from state and nonstate actors has also acted as a crucial supplement to diverted resources. For instance, many governmental and nongovernmental organizations provided material, financial, and professional support, e.g., Medecins sans frontieres/Doctors Without Borders (MSF; Figure 6.1). Despite international assistance, Ukrainian medical educators and administrators must develop local solutions to meet the challenges that the country and regions cannot escape from. Geopolitical uncertainty and instability feature prominently, with private organizations (e.g., Starlink) and governments (e.g., the United States) providing intermittent and unstable support.

This chapter provides an overview of the ongoing developments in the Ukrainian healthcare system, contemporary innovations, and how it has responded to conflict. First, a historical review of the Ukrainian healthcare and medical systems is provided to establish a baseline prior to the 2022 invasion. Prior to the invasion, Ukraine was making efforts to align its healthcare infrastructure with the EU standards. Despite the conflict, Ukraine healthcare institutions continue to be restructured. Here, the experiences of one institution are described as an ongoing narrative of innovation during times of armed conflict. The chapter concludes by providing future directions for the recovery of the healthcare system in a post-conflict era.

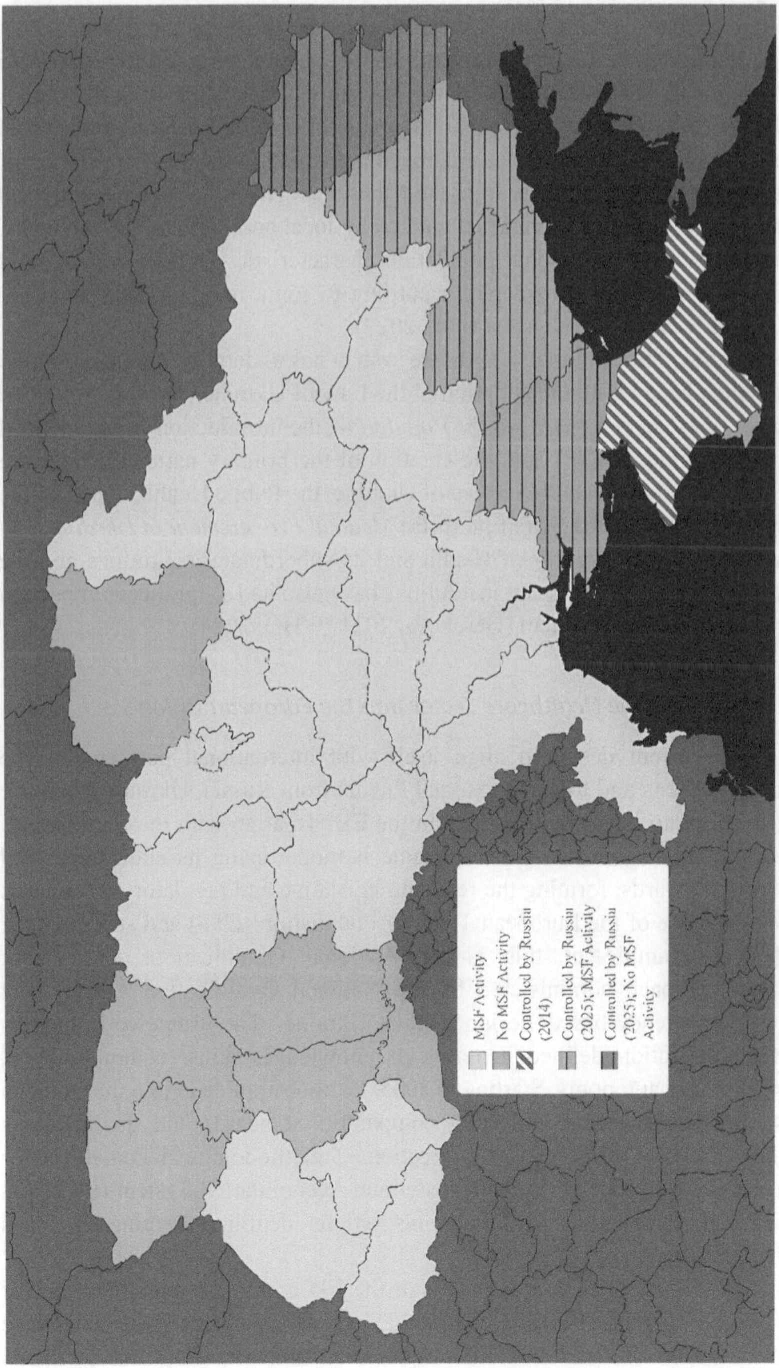

FIGURE 6.1 Map of Ukraine showing regions of MSF project delivery (light grey) and non-delivery (medium grey) in 2023.

Source: Adapted from MSF (2025) and *The New York Times* (2025). Map created with mapchat.net.

6.1 Ukrainian Healthcare and Medical Education Systems

The modern state of Ukraine gained independence in 1991 from the former Soviet Union. At that time, the Ukrainian healthcare system was based on the *Semashko Model*, a national, centralized, hierarchical system where healthcare professionals and staff were state employees. A transition period followed as the Semashko Model became untenable. The resulting reorganization resulted in the decentralization of services and devolution of power from the Ministry of Health to regional and local health authorities, which in turn are regulated by local and regional governments. Challenges remained as regional population characteristics, patient volume, and quality of care were not considered, according to some reviews (Buletsa et al., 2019; Lekhan et al., 2015; Shyshka et al., 2023).

More recently, the Ukrainian healthcare system has undergone a transformation process, which began with the adoption of the Law of Ukraine *On State Financial Guarantees of Medical Services to the Population*, the introduction of the Medical Guarantees Program (MGP), and the creation of the primary national healthcare agencies – the National Health Service of Ukraine, the Public Health Center of the Ministry of Health, and the State Enterprise *Medical Procurement of Ukraine*. The reorganization of the Ministry of Health and its subordinate institutions and the devolution of power to healthcare institutions have also had a significant impact on the Ukrainian healthcare system (Gercheva, 2021; WHO, 2024).

6.1.1 Integrating the Healthcare Sector into the European Union

Due to a concurrent desire to align itself with international partners for the health of its citizens and to resist external threats from Russia, Ukraine has made concerted efforts to integrate itself within the EU. To align with these initiatives, frameworks, and standards of care, Ukraine is modernizing its educational and professional standards, forming the relevant legislative and regulatory framework with the assistance of the European Training Foundation (ETF) and stakeholders. The clearest example of this is the National Qualifications Framework (NQF),[1] an approach administered by the National Qualification Agency that promotes competency-based design within Ukraine. The framework focuses on professionalization defined in terms of knowledge, skills, communication, responsibility, and autonomy. Starting in 2005, Ukraine applied to join the Bologna Process, directed toward establishing comparable standards and qualifications for higher education. Following the creation of methodological guidelines for implementing the European Credit Transfer and Accumulation System (ECTS) in Ukrainian higher education institutions, institutions identified learning outcomes for each course in each discipline.

Ukraine's efforts to integrate itself with the EU continued after the onset of conflict. According to the Ministry of Health, Ukraine has increased the percentage of implementation of the Association Agreement with the EU resulting in an increase from 64% (2021) to 79% (2024; Ministry of Health, 2025). Ukraine has made additional attempts to align itself with European laws by adopting the integration law "On the Public Health System" in 2022. Concurrently, the Ministry of Health has established measures to protect the workforce from the negative impacts of their work (Ministry of Health, 2025). These measures have been tested to the extreme in recent years.

In 2024, the European Commission approved the Twinning Project, developed to support institutional capacity building initiatives and improve coordination and responses to cross-border threats (European Council, 2024). Within Ukraine, these efforts also include the modernization of the blood safety system, a system that is critical to the war effort. This includes modification to the existing electronic health system (EHCS) and the eKrov (eBlood) system, with a focus on facilitating monitoring and planning by allowing for greater control and transparency in the management of blood supply. The Ministry of Health (2023) noted that changes to the EHCS focus on "maintaining primary medical records regarding the results of medical examination of donors, admission to donations, blood collection, and transfusion; accounting of recipients' blood samples; [and] recording of serious adverse reactions or serious adverse cases related to donation, etc.". In parallel, the Ministry of Health updated the requirements for the blood safety system authorities with the strategy for the development of blood donation until 2028 and licensing conditions for blood collection and testing (Ministry of Health, 2025).

Since 2023, updates have also been made to the medical care standards and clinical protocols. Strengthening international ties with the European Union and involvement in EU institutions is an important part of the daily work of the Ministry of Health team. In response to the demands placed on healthcare systems in Europe during the COVID-19 pandemic, the EU proposed an ambitious €5.1 billion ($5.54 US) health program, EU4 Health. EU4 Health creates a strategic reserve of healthcare staff and medical supplies for prevention, preparedness, and response to health crises.

In addition to Ukraine's continued participation in the EU4Health program, it has also entered an administrative arrangement on access of Ukrainian healthcare institutions to the European Reference Networks (ERNs) IT system. ERNs facilitate the collaboration of European hospital centers of expertise and reference across borders, especially those that are complex or uncommon to augment the efforts of healthcare professions to address these issues. As of 2024, these networks span 382 hospitals and their 1,619 specialized healthcare units in 27 EU Member States (and Norway). They facilitate communication and foster virtual expert discussions, provide educational and training activities, develop registries of rare diseases, and develop and maintain clinical practice guidelines (European Commission, 2024). ERNs must be assessed, appraised, and evaluated as defined by a legal framework and supported by monitoring and assessment systems.

Ukraine has also joined the Critical Medicines Alliance (CMA). Established in January 2024, the CMA was created as a consultative mechanism to facilitate interactions between key stakeholders from EU Member States, scientific communities, industry, and civil society. It currently has two working groups directed toward strengthening EU manufacturing capacities of critical pharmaceutical ingredients and medicines, creating a strategic stockpile of medicines, and fostering cooperation and partnerships (Ministry of Health of Ukraine, 2025).

6.2 Adaptation to Continuing Challenges

An overemphasis on recent challenges faced by the Ukrainian healthcare system can obscure the continuous innovation that is a feature of health professions education and delivery. Here, we describe developments leading to the armed conflict to provide a point of comparison.

Since 2017, Ukraine has made a concerted effort to reform its healthcare system. The main objectives of the reform focus on changing approaches to financing the healthcare system, digitalization and creation of digital services for patients, formation of a patient-centered healthcare model, which will lead to an increase in the quality and accessibility of medical care, creation of conditions for effective resource management, minimization and complete elimination of informal payments and other corruption, and formation of a fair and manageable healthcare system (e.g., Terentyuk et al., 2024).

More recently, Ukraine has made significant progress toward European integration in the healthcare sector, including improving legislation, bringing medical standards closer to those of Europe, and actively cooperating with EU countries. This will create new opportunities for patients and facilitate Ukraine's integration into the European medical space, including the development of medical tourism (Ministry of Health, 2025). However, war has fundamentally altered the conditions in which healthcare is taught and practiced. Medical education has undergone a rapid, unplanned transformation: classes have shifted format, simulation training and evidence-based medicine are more widely used, digitalization has accelerated across the health sector, and mental health support for veterans and civilians has become a priority.

The state's top priorities have become lifelong learning, developing and strengthening human potential, and implementing European principles, approaches, practices, and tools in education and science. Previously, the Ministry of Education and Science of Ukraine has defined strategic priorities and directions for activities until 2030:

- Preschool, school, extracurricular, special, and inclusive education.
- Vocational pre-higher, higher, and adult education.
- Professional (vocational) education.
- Science and innovation.
- Digital transformation of education and science.
- European integration of education and science.

Additionally, the "Strategic Plan of the Ministry of Education and Science of Ukraine until 2027" defines the strategies for Ukraine's development and its integration into the European Union (Ministry of Education and Science, 2024). The plan outlines nine ministerial priorities until 2027, covering key areas of the ministry's work including early childhood and preschool education, support for persons with special education needs, a new model for Ukrainian schools, extracurricular education and transformation of vocational education, the development and integration of science and education with Europe, and recognition of the need to engage in digital transformation.

Despite these interruptions, medical education persists. Educators acknowledge that efforts must be directed to achieve international standards, integrate modern technologies into instructional and assessment practices, continue the process of digitalization, and meet the needs of the military (Kuchyn et al., 2023). New specialties and specializations have been introduced, such as "Therapy and Rehabilitation", which includes physical therapy, ergotherapy, as well as speech and language therapy. An important new direction in Technologies of Medical Diagnostics and Treatment that has taken on an even greater importance due to the ongoing war is prosthetics and orthotics. In the first year of this program students were enrolled in many institutions including Kharkiv National Medical University, Danylo Halytsky Lviv National Medical University, Shupyk National University of Healthcare of Ukraine, and Ternopil National Medical University.

6.3 Medical Education in Ukraine

Beyond the development of international health networks to share knowledge and resources, Ukraine has also responded to changing pedagogical models from healthcare professions (Holomb et al., 2022; Kalyniuk et al., 2024; Radziievska et al., 2022; Yelahina, 2023). Here, we review developments in the medical education system of Ukraine.

6.3.1 Principles of the Medical Education in Ukraine

Medical education in the region currently referred to as Ukraine has a lengthy history, with the Collegium Medicum established in 1773 in Lviv and incorporated into the medical faculty of Lviv University 44 years later. In 1894, a full medical faculty provided a comprehensive set of courses. By the early twentieth century, medical education was offered at Kharkiv University (1805), Kyiv University (1840), Lviv University (1894), Odesa University (1900), and Katerynoslav University (1918; Encyclopedia of Ukraine, 1993).

During the Soviet Era (1922–1991), the *Semashko Model* "generated innovations, models, and examples to be emulated or avoided, but certainly not ignored, around the world" (Krementsov, 2017, p. 1693). Rather than a principled adoption due to its comparative advantages, the model was forced onto nations such as Ukraine in Central and Eastern Europe, which had largely adopted social health insurance system prior to World War II due to the influence of the Austro-Hungarian and Prussian Empires (Kaminska, 2022).[2] Healthcare professionals worked in clinics and hospitals as employees of the state, subordinate to other industrial sectors. The system was defined by limited autonomy of healthcare professionals, low quality of care, and inefficient distribution of limited healthcare resources (Kaminska, 2022; Kornai & Eggleston, 2001).

At the onset of the Russian invasion, Ukraine had 23 medical institutions with medical degrees recognized by the European Council and World Health Organization. These institutions served over 18,000 learners from within and outside of Ukraine's borders, including those who could not obtain degrees due to prohibitive costs or political exclusion in their own countries (Jain et al., 2022; Srichawla et al., 2022).

Broad recognition of the value of competency-based medical education (CBME) has led many nations to adopt these basic principles (Schoenherr, 2027a;

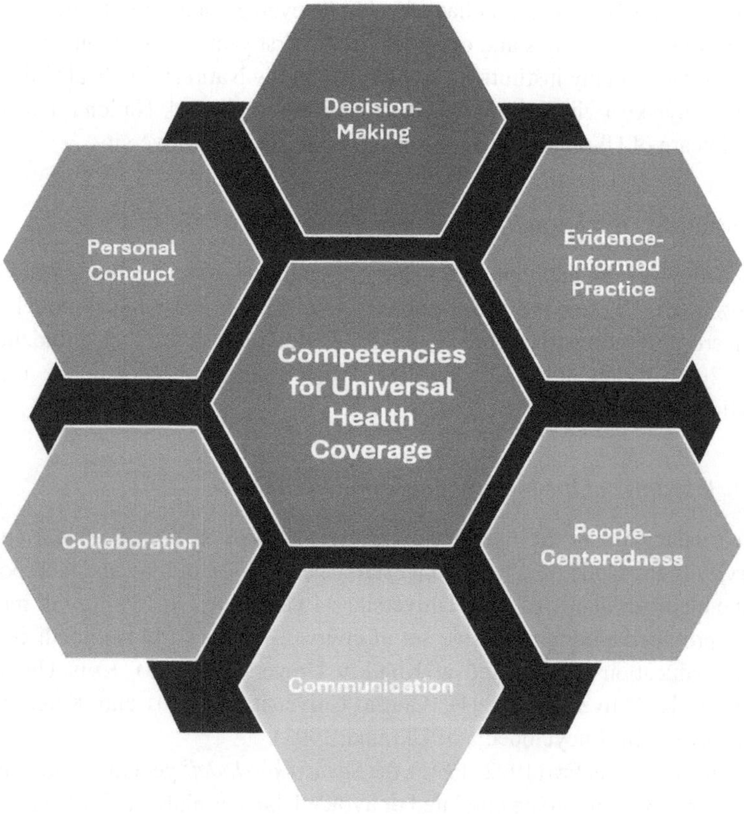

FIGURE 6.2 Six competencies defined in the WHO Competencies for Universal Health Coverage Framework.

Schoenherr & McConnell, 2024). In their review of the medical education system in Ukraine, Radziievska et al. (2022) note,

> Ukraine, one of the former republics of the Soviet Union, is still at the beginning of reform. Ukraine's educational system (including medicine) is still dominated by the Soviet educational system, which is already morally and intellectually obsolete. Students are most often offered textbooks that are 40 years old.
>
> *(p. 115)*

To address these needs, Ukraine's Ministry of Health has adopted international standards for medical education such as the *Global Competency Framework for Universal Health Coverage* (World Health Organization (WHO), 2022), as the basis of general, special, and professional competencies. This framework focuses on creating a curriculum on the outcomes of educational practices rather than content-delivery. Instead of prioritizing acquisition of knowledge in a hierarchical relationship from teacher to learner, it prioritizes a non-hierarchical model wherein direct observations are made of how learners apply their knowledge, using multiple measures of assessment. While the generality of the WHO approach would appear to be ideal in that it could be applicable to any country, the lack of specificity introduces the need for more interpretation and concomitant variability (Schoenherr & McConnell, 2024; Schoenherr, 2027a).

As a novel approach, CBME has not yet been implemented within Ukraine. For instance, commentators have noted that "[a]t the current stage, there is a need to reconsider the content of activities for educators in medical education institutions in accordance with new requirements" (Yelahina, 2023, p. 85). However, the limited evidence of implementation of CBME would seem to be no different from other institutions outside of Ukraine, such that the CBME paradigm is more aspirational than apparent in practice (Schoenherr, 2027a).

6.3.2 Structure of Medical Education in Ukraine

The structure of higher medical education in Ukraine has been influenced by other education systems of other developed countries and is in accordance with the recommendations of the EU, UNESCO, UN, and other international organizations (Ministry of Education and Science of Ukraine, 2021). Higher medical education in Ukraine is regulated by the law "On Higher Education" and the regulation "On Internship". Here, we provide an overview of the basic structure of the medical education curriculum in the Ukrainian system.

Training of specialists in Ukraine in the field healthcare has been classified into several primary areas of care: Dentistry, Medicine, Nursing, Technologies of Medical Diagnostics and Treatment, Medical Psychology, Pharmacy, Industrial Pharmacy, Therapy and Rehabilitation, Pediatrics, and Public Health (see Table 6.1). Enrollment in these primary areas will determine the course of training for learners. For instance, the length of training students receive is dependent on their specialty, varying from five years (e.g., Dentistry and Pharmacy) to six years (e.g., Medicine, Medical Psychology, and Pediatrics). In some specialties, training requires the completion of a Bachelor's and Master's, i.e., Nursing, Technologies of Medical Diagnostics and Treatment, Therapy and Rehabilitation (Figure 6.2).

The educational and professional programs of each specialty are defined by both compulsory and optional components. The compulsory components of educational and professional programs include training activities focused on social and humanitarian issues in addition to fundamental and professional training and practice. Optional components contain original courses that make up at least 25% of the total number of European Credit Transfer and Accumulation System (ECTS)[3] credits of the educational and professional program.

6.3.2.1 International Standards in Ukrainian Medical Education

Ukrainian healthcare system is integrated with global standards of care and education. External exams such as the KROK (Integrated License exam under ECTS) and ESP (English for professional purposes) are important for students. These examinations are conducted by the Testing Board for Assessment of Professional Competence of Higher Education Applicants in the fields of Medicine and Pharmacy at the Ministry of Health of Ukraine (abbreviated as Testing Board).

Consisting of three assessments, the KROK was established as the primary means to assess learners' performance in 1998. The KROK 1 is an exam that is used to assess knowledge and general scientific disciplines in their third year of study. If a learner fails the KROK 1, they have one additional attempt. If they fail to meet this standard a second time, they are expelled. In their final year of study, the KROK 2 assesses their clinical competencies and is part of the state certification of applicants. The minimal passing score is 64.0%[4] for both the KROK 1 and KROK 2 tests (Table 6.1). The KROK 3 is provided to interns to assess their competency. Without completing an internship, learners cannot become a medical specialist or pharmacist/chemist in Ukraine. Specific variants of KROK have been developed for areas of specialization.[5]

Since 2014, Ukraine's higher education systems have undergone significant changes. The law "On Higher Education" outlines three priorities for this transformation. In general, it was introduced to align Ukraine with European standards, increase the autonomy and competitiveness of Ukrainian universities by decentralizing the management and implementation of educational programs and financing, increase the research and scientific capacities and capabilities of Ukraine, establishing clear standard and rules for admission, and increase the skill of the workforce. Learners are placed at the center of this approach, ensuring the students are aware of how they will be assessed in advance of a course, as well

TABLE 6.1 List of Specialties and Duration of Training in Internship in Accordance with the Specialty Obtained in Higher Education

№	*Specialty in the higher education establishment*	*Internship specialty*	*Duration of internship training*
1.	**Medicine, Pediatrics**	Obstetrics and gynecology	3 years
2.	**Medicine, Pediatrics**	Anesthesiology and intensive care	3 years
3.	**Medicine, Pediatrics**	Internal medicine	2 years
4.	**Medicine, Pediatrics**	General practice – family medicine	2 years
5.	**Medicine, Pediatrics**	Epidemiology	1 year
6.	**Medicine, Pediatrics**	Infectious diseases	2 years
7.	**Medicine, Technologies of medical diagnostics and treatment, Pediatrics**	Laboratory diagnostics, virology, microbiology	1.5 years
8.	**Medicine, Pediatrics**	Emergency medicine	2 years
9.	**Medical psychology**	Medical psychology	1 year
10.	**Medicine**	Neurology	2 years
11.	**Medicine, Pediatrics**	Orthopedics and traumatology	2 years
12.	**Medicine, Pediatrics**	Otolaryngology	2 years
13.	**Medicine, Pediatrics**	Ophthalmology	2 years
14.	**Medicine, Pediatrics**	Radiology	1.5 years
15.	**Medicine, Pediatrics**	Pathological anatomy	1.5 years
16.	**Medicine, Pediatrics**	Psychiatry	2 years
17.	**Medicine**	Surgery	3 years
18.	**Medicine, Pediatrics**	Physical and rehabilitation medicine	2 years 3 years – for those, who enter internship from 2024
19.	**Medicine, Pediatrics**	Dermatovenereology	2 years
20.	**Pediatrics, Medicine**	Pediatric surgery	3 years

(*Continued*)

TABLE 6.1 (Continued)

№	*Specialty in the higher education establishment*	*Internship specialty*	*Duration of internship training*
21.	**Pediatrics, Medicine**	Pediatrics	2 years
22.	**Dentistry**	Dentistry	1 year
23.	**Pharmacy, industrial pharmacy**	Pharmacy	1 year
24.	**Medicine, Pediatrics**	Forensic medical examination	2 year

Note: In accordance with the Orders of the Ministry of Health of Ukraine dated May 6, 2024 No. 788 "On Amendments to Certain Regulatory Legal Acts of the Ministry of Health of Ukraine" and dated May 11, 2024 No. 820 "On Amendments to the Order of the Ministry of Health of Ukraine dated May 6, 2024 No. 788".

as giving students the right to strike and self-governance, with students having administrative access to 0.5% of university income. Learners can also choose the pace of their study, with Bachelor's degrees being available for three- or five-year durations, aligning Ukrainian institutions with European and other international systems.

6.3.2.2 Institutional Context: Bogomolets National Medical University

An exclusive focus on national policies and institutions within Ukrainian healthcare ignores the specific innovations and implementation experiences that ultimately determine the successes and failures of an innovation. Here, we consider Bogomolets National Medical University and how it has adapted historically and presently to the Russian invasion.

Founded in 1840, Kyiv University was reorganized into the Kyiv Medical Institute in 1920, later to be renamed after Bogomolets in 1946 and given the status of the National Medical University in 1995. Despite being scheduled to open in 1842, a dire need for clinicians due to an epidemic lead to the admission of the first medical students in 1841 for anatomy lectures. In addition to housing departments including anatomy, medical chemistry, therapy, ophthalmology, and surgery, state medical studies additionally included a focus on forensic medicine, "medical police hygiene", medical law, and veterinary police. Degrees were conferred three years later to the first three graduates (Bogomolets National Medical University (BNMU), 2025).

Like other medical institutions, Bogomolets National Medical University provides quality education. All PhD programs launched at the university are accredited. As for the Master's degree, Medicine, Medical Psychology, and Pediatrics are accredited. Dentistry and Public Health are accredited by the

National Agency for Quality Assurance in Education. As of 2024, other programs will be accredited in Medical Diagnostics and Treatment Technologies (Master's Program) and Pharmacy and Industrial Pharmacy. Programs have been developed to support mental health, and trainings are held for everyone on mental support, inclusiveness, etc. There are training programs for veterans.

6.4 Medical Education during Conflict: Institutional Experiences

The ongoing efforts to establish improvement to the Ukrainian healthcare system and implementation of these innovations have been stunted by externalities. For instance, the COVID-19 pandemic presented significant challenges, forcing higher medical education institutions to adapt to new learning conditions at short notice. The Russian invasions of 2014 and 2022 have also drained considerable economic and human resources that would otherwise have been dedicated to the improvement of community and national health and medical education (Schoenherr, 2027c). Prior to discussing the specific adaptations and changes made by educators, healthcare institutions, and Ukrainian society to armed conflict, we review factors that affect healthcare delivery and health professions education.

6.4.1 Armed Conflict and Healthcare

Armed conflicts are a ubiquitous feature of human history. Conflicts act as a catalyst for innovation in healthcare delivery and health professions education (Schoenherr, 2027a). Responses can either be directed toward prospective or preventative measures or reactive to the realities of conflict. In his discussion of prospective medical education delivery during total war (nuclear conflict), Casberg (1958) notes that medical educators (administrators) should consider potential targets, coordination mechanisms with relevant authorities, availability and vulnerability of faculty and learner resources, peripheral support and facilities, as well as the available relevant basic and clinical translational research. Civil wars present another area of research. For instance, a study of 58 Sudanese medical schools found that most institutions experienced multiple attacks (64.7%), looting (73.5%), and were converted into military bases (67.6%). Resumption of educational programs was also observed in most institutions (60.3%). Studies suggesting the medical students experience adverse effects ranging from distractions (65.2%) to anxiety and depression (51% and 49%, respectively; Omer et al., 2024).

More generally, Bou-Karroum et al. (2020) identified over 470 studies examining the impact of armed conflict of violence against healthcare workers during conflicts and workforce performance after the conflict in the Middle East, focusing on Syria, Iraq, Israel, and Palestine with other areas including Africa, the Americas and South Asia. Sixty-seven of these papers focused on impacts on education (e.g., Balalian et al., 2014; Barnett-Vanes, 2016; Barnett-Vanes et al., 2016; Challoner & Forget, 2011; Donaldson et al., 2011; Hexom et al., 2012; Penfold & Ali, 2014). With studies primarily focusing on the impact on medical students and residents with nursing students' experiences examined to a lesser extent (Dobiesz et al., 2022). Some results were counterintuitive. For instance, Batley et al. (2008) found that despite the stress resulting from working in conflict, both medical students and residences indicated that they reported positive effects, such as novel challenges, pride in their professions, and increased motivation. Such results stand in contrast to widespread findings of posttraumatic stress in soldiers and healthcare workers exposed to armed conflict (e.g., Ahmead et al., 2024; Engelhard et al., 2015; Gibbons et al., 2012; Veronese et al., 2022) but are consistent with the phenomenon of post-traumatic stress disorder (PTSD) growth, i.e., the self-reported positive states that contrast with actual mental health (Frazier et al., 2009). Healthcare professionals and medical educators must therefore not take such reported outcome measures at face value.

Following a decade of conflict, the experiences of Syrian healthcare professions provide critical insight into the impacts of long-term conflict on the delivery of health professions education. One basic distinction is that between government-controlled areas (GCAs) and non-GCAs (NGCAs), with GCAs associated with more human resources and institutional capacities relative to NGCAs. Summarizing the research on Syria, Bdaiwi et al. (2023) identified multiple factors across studies (Table 6.2). For instance, due to the demands on healthcare professionals, efforts have also focused on "accelerated medical education" (Cangiarella et al., 2017; Drees & Omurtag, 2012; Leong et al., 2017), with such efforts existing since World War II (Johnson et al., 1943). [6] Due to the limits on internal capacity, they note that "International and regional academic institutes collaboration and coordination efforts are needed to formulate educational platforms using innovative approaches (such as online/blended/ store-and-forward/ peer-training/ online tutoring) to strengthen and build the capacity of the health workforce in conflict-affected area" (p. 8).

6.4.2 Health Professional Education during Armed Conflict: Ukrainian Experiences

As the bombs began to fall, Ukrainians perished indiscriminately. By August 2024, 11,743 civilians were killed and 24,614 were injured in the conflict, predominantly in areas controlled by the Ukrainian government (United Nations (UN), 2024). The attacks also threatened the healthcare infrastructure in the country, impacting healthcare facilities daily. By August 2024, the World Health Organization confirmed more than 1,940 attacks on healthcare by Russian force, noting that 86% of these attacks have affected healthcare facilities, with 42% of the attacks affecting primary care facilities. They additionally note that approximately 200 ambulances are damaged or destroyed per year in shelling

TABLE 6.2 Features of Health Professions Education during Conflict

Factor	*Government-Controlled Areas*	*Nongovernment Controlled Areas*
Attacks and security	- Arresting, bombing, and missiles	- Violation of international humanitarian laws - Weaponization of healthcare, restricting access to care as a weapon - Healthcare assets are attacked (facilities) - Reprisal, detention, and torture of students and healthcare professionals
Personal experiences and quality of training/ education	- Training interruptions - Exposure to war-related medical conditions - Shortages of water and electricity - Overcrowded transportation	- Training interruptions - Sieges and forced evacuation - Permanent physical disabilities - Junior staff required to perform outside of the professional activities they have been trained to perform - Limited number of educators - Low HCP:population ratio
Mobility and human resources	- Departure of 70% of healthcare professionals - Low HCP:population ratio - 40% of medical students planned to study abroad	- Departure of 70% of healthcare professionals - Low HCP:population ratio
Innovation	- Remote training - Peer-led teaching/"training the trainers" - Student-led initiatives - Calls for community-based learning - Calls for conflict-focused curriculum - Testing bilingual teaching approaches	- Creation of field hospitals and fortification against attacks - Creation of new universities, institutes, and postgraduate training programs - Homemade and locally manufactured training facilities and devices - Task shifting - Remote training - Peer teaching/"training the trainers" - Conflict-focused curriculum and training - Equal partnerships with stakeholders (academic and humanitarian orgs.) - Courses in supporting resilience

Source: Adapted from Bdaiwi et al. (2023).

attacks (WHO, 2024). While many medical facilities were either damaged (28) or destroyed (2), more educational facilities were damaged (38) or destroyed (13; UN, 2024). These attacks continue to disrupt medical education. In March 2023, an estimated 76,000 students including students from Africa and Asia returned to take their KROK 2 exam. As one student recounted about the incident, "We had to interrupt the exam seven times because of missile alarms. The room was cold and there was almost no light. The exam lasted from 9:00 to 16:00 because of different interruptions" (quoted in Di Stasi, 2023). To address the realities and stress of the conflict, the Ministry of Health temporarily reduced the passing grade for KROK 1 from 60.5% to 55.5%.

Beyond ruined cities, rockets, and drones, and the lives that have been lost, the effects of conflict on medical education can be illustrated by examining changes in the enrollment numbers for foreign students in Ukrainian institutions (Jain et al., 2022). Due to its location in the capital (Kyiv) and status as one of Ukraine's oldest institutions, we review the experiences of Bogomolets National Medical University. Over a five-year period, the contingent of foreign applicants to the Bogomolets National Medical University sharply decreased. Between 2020 and 2021, foreign enrollment remained largely unchanged. However, between 2021 and 2022, enrollment decreased by 142 foreign students. This trend accelerated between 2022 and 2023, with 1669 fewer students enrolling, and 625 between 2023 and 2024. Based on changes in prior years, war is clearly the primary factor leading to this change. While statistics convey the general nature of the educational environment, I (IIK) have presented a firsthand account of how Ukrainian medical education has continued despite war, and how practitioners and institutions have adapted to the demands (Figure 6.3 and Table 6.3).

From February 24, 2022, to October 1, 2024, 1,275 air raid alarms were sounded in Kyiv, and the danger lasted more than 1,395 hrs (https://kyiv.digital/storage/air-alert/stats.html). Martial law was declared shortly after. During the first week of the

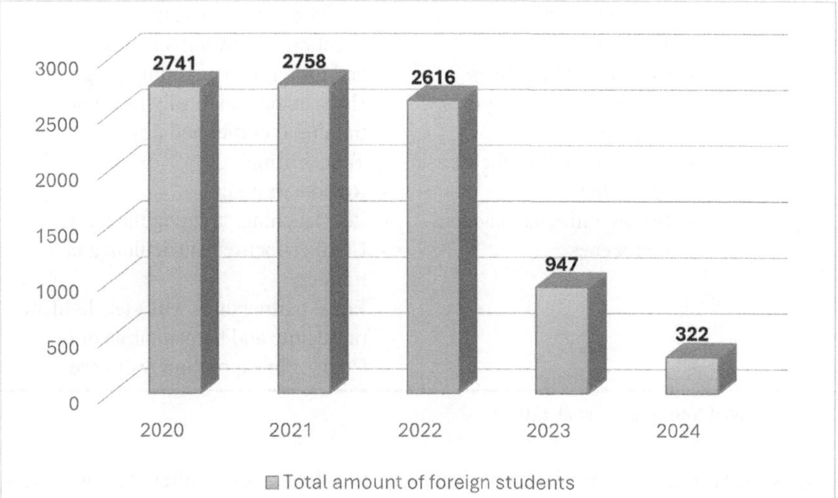

FIGURE 6.3 International student enrollment in Ukrainian medical education institutions.

full-scale invasion, emergency care was provided by Bogomolets National Medical University – in the University Clinic and Outpatient Clinic in 24/7 mode. Students and teachers of the Faculty of Dentistry were at the Dental Center of the National Medical University. Orthopedists and traumatologists of the surgical department from the Faculty of Medicine No. 1 provided surgical care. The faculty's therapeutic departments were in contact with the clinics and provided consultations. Students and teachers of the Faculty of Medicine No. 4 were involved in volunteering and territorial defense. Employees of the Department of Obstetrics and Gynecology No. 2 performed their duties at the clinical base, carried out duty, and provided consultations.

Following the wave of attacks, some medical services and institutions need to halt their activities. However, as communities continue to require both primary and critical care, the demands of practice remain. For instance, faculty in the Department of Surgical Dentistry and Maxillofacial Surgery continued to operate during the attacks, with the Stomatology Center resuming its work on March 2, 2022. Amid shelling and hostilities, dental services were provided to military and civilians (Figure 6.4). Currently, education at the Bogomolets National Medical University is conducted in a mixed format. Lectures are held online, and practical classes are held in classrooms. The university has its own distance learning platform, LIKAR_NMU, which is filled with educational and methodological complexes for students (13; Kuchyn et al., 2021, 2022). As critical infrastructure is intentionally and incidentally damaged, power shortages and blackouts are frequent occurrences. The university uses back-up power sources that allow it to provide students with lighting.

Full-time employees of the Department of Clinical Immunology and Allergology with the Section of Medical Genetics of the Medical Faculty No. 4 provided medical care to victims of the emergency that arose during the martial law in Ukraine. They also consulted remotely with patients who had previously contacted the university clinical bases.

Students enrolled in a variety of courses worked in different hospitals in Kyiv and other cities of Ukraine, with sixth-year students providing a variety of medical care throughout Ukraine. Teachers of the clinical departments of the faculties of the Bogomolets National Medical University provided medical care in medical institutions in urban and rural environments.

Many Ukrainian students of the faculty left Kyiv and joined local territorial defense units and volunteer movement and donated blood for the needs of the country's medical service. Local students and those in occupied territory work as volunteers in both medical institutions and public works to defend the city. The demands of conflict placed considerable strain on faculty as they attempted to develop and maintain human resources as well as act as advocates for Ukrainian healthcare professionals. For instances, the Faculty of Dentistry sent letters to many professional dental organizations of the world with an appeal to condemn

TABLE 6.3 Enrollment in Medical Programs by Year, Year of Study, and Discipline

Year	*Year of Studying*	*Medicine*	*Dentistry*	*Pharmacy, Industrial Pharmacy*	*Total Amount of Students*
2024	1	4	1		5
	2	6	4	2	12
	3	28	14	3	45
	4	53	15	1	69
	5	22	31	13	66
	6	125			125
Total for the year:		**238**	**65**	**19**	**322**
2023	1	2	2	1	5
	2	19	6	1	26
	3	113	20	3	136
	4	48	22	4	74
	5	115	68	11	194
	6	512			512
Total for the year		809	118	20	947
2022	1	70	6	3	79
	2	360	86	17	463
	3	137	46	4	187
	4	408	84	19	511
	5	686	178	22	886
	6	490			490
Total for the year:		**2,151**	**400**	**65**	**2,616**
2021	1	94	49	11	154
	2	185	60	4	249
	3	478	74	17	569
	4	764	206	23	993
	5	497	94	18	609
	6	184			184
Total for the year		**2,202**	**483**	**73**	**2,758**
2020	1	45	25	3	73
	2	501	79	7	587
	3	752	218	33	1003
	4	553	118	27	698
	5	156	38	13	207
	6	173			173
Total for the year		**2,180**	**478**	**83**	**2,741**

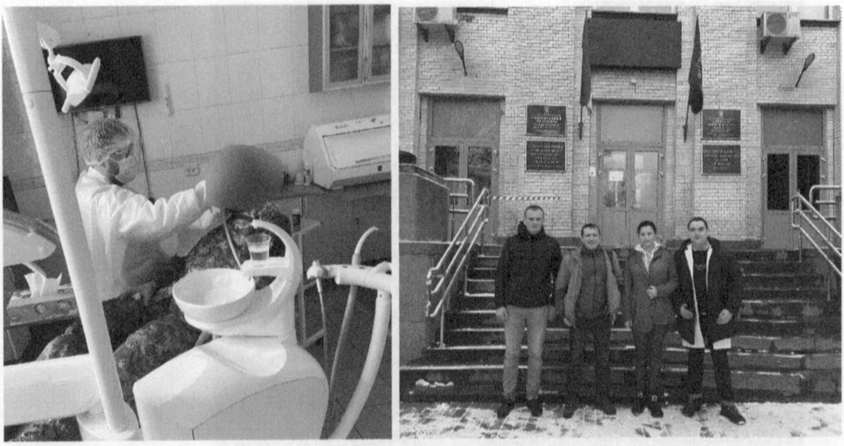

FIGURE 6.4 Dental services provided during shelling.

the Russian aggressors who started the war and to support Ukraine's aspiration for peace and independence.

The staff of the Faculty of Medicine and Psychology provide online consultations to people who experience panic attacks, are stressed, depressed, or experienced other acute stress conditions. During the first four days of the war, more than 100 consultations were provided. Technological innovations were also developed to supplement practitioners, providing health seekers with continuous care during the crisis. In addition, a Telegram bot (https://t.me/friend_first_aid_bot.) and a Telegram channel (www.mvk.if.ua/cssm/29453) were created to broaden access to anyone who needed clear instructions for self-help: what to do and what not to do during a threat to life and health and after a traumatic experience.

As stewards of the students in their charge, educational institutions also sought to protect their students. Over a thousand students were in the dormitories in the universities of Vinnytsia and Zaporizhzhia. These students were transported to Kyiv to increase their safety (Figure 6.5).

Teachers and students of the Faculty for the Training of Doctors for the Armed Forces of Ukraine joined the territorial defense, volunteering in clinics. The Department of General Surgery No. 2 deployed approximately 20 reserve operating rooms. The demands of conflict also required a greater focus on specific competencies, with the educational activities adapted to ensure that these skills were developed in a timely manner, consistent with an accelerated medical education model. To meet the demands of conflict, consulting work and training on the topic of "Sorting the Wounded" (triage) were carried out to teach civilian doctors tactical medicine and work with the wounded.

On February 28, 2022, the first lecture on military medical training was held online, and on March 1, 2022. A second lecture on "Application of tactical

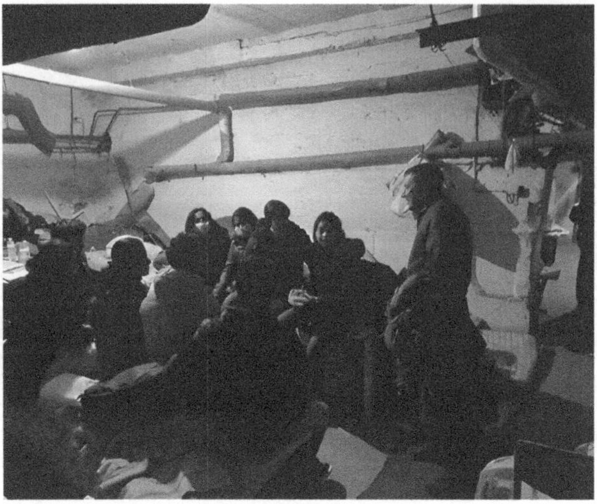

FIGURE 6.5 Sheltered foreign students in the basement.

medicine standards in modern conditions" was then offered. Generally accessible online lectures were also delivered on tactical medicine, a practically oriented training course of the professional school "Trauma and its consequences" on the topic "Combat injuries to the musculoskeletal system", "Protection of the population and medical personnel from chemical weapons, actions of medical personnel upon admission to the ZOZ of patients after a chemical attack".

The first week of the full-scale invasion was the ultimate test of the Ukrainian medical education system and the resolve of its practitioners. A significant number of teachers did not leave the operating rooms or basements that they worked in, helping colleagues and maintaining contact with their students (Bogomolets National Medical University, 2022).

The need to resume formal instruction was outlined in the letter of the Ministry of Education and Science of Ukraine dated March 10, 2022 No. 1/3417-22 "On the completion of the academic year", the specifics of the work of teachers during the martial law regime were explained in the letter of the Ministry of Education and Science of Ukraine dated March 15, 2022 No. 1/3463-22 "On the provision of information", and the specifics of the completion of the academic year were approved by the order of the Ministry of Education and Science of Ukraine dated April 1, 2022 No. 290 "On approval of Methodological recommendations on certain issues of completion of the 2021/2022 academic year".

Therefore, Bogomolets University returned to distance learning, to ensure the safety situation of learners, educators, and administrators and deliver consistent education and training experience. For over a month, staff of surgical departments

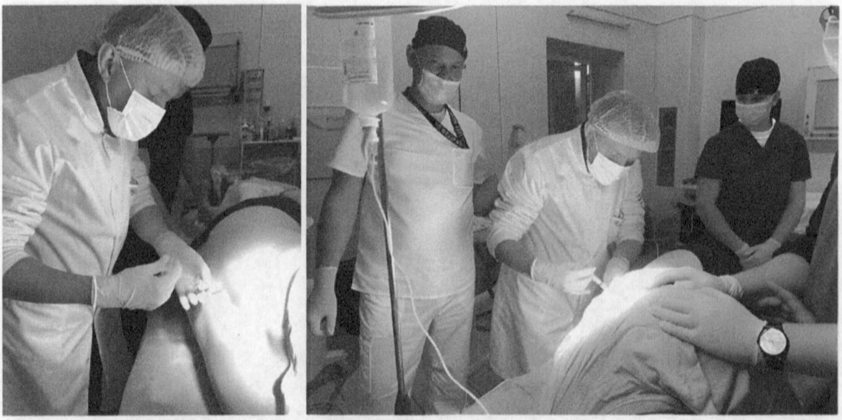

FIGURE 6.6 Images from two operating rooms. Dr. Yuri Kuchin supervises.

continuously operated to save lives, with the rector of the university, Dr. Yuri Kuchin, often joined them (Figure 6.6).

The demands of total war require that civilians and professionals engage in many other activities other than those for which they have training (Casberg, 1958). Students and teachers also volunteered their time in other activities, including weaving camouflage nets, purchasing ammunition for the military, delivering food and medicine and humanitarian aid, providing first aid to evacuees from the war zone, and helping people evacuated from the war (Figure 6.7).

On May 9, 2022, the first public defense of Vasyl Romanovych Horoshko's dissertation for the degree of Doctor of Philosophy in the field of knowledge "Health Care" in the specialty "Medicine" took place in the conference hall of the university's administrative building in a mixed format. It is symbolic that the defense took place on the Day of Victory over Nazism in World War II. On November 28, 2022, Valentyn Rohozynskyi a young scientist, a postgraduate student of the Department of Pediatric Surgery, who was voluntarily mobilized into the Armed Forces of Ukraine, defended the dissertation and got the degree Doctor of Philosophy (BNMU, 2022a).

In May 2022 Kyiv region was de-occupied and training was restored for applicants who had the opportunity to attend classes. Schedules for practical skills training in the simulation center were created. Consequently, the educational process was organized according to mixed (classroom-distance) or distance learning forms. As opposed to 2022, when KROK 2 was canceled, in the 2022/2023 and 2023/2024 academic years, higher education applicants in the specialties "Dentistry", "Medicine", "Medical Psychology", "Pharmacy", "Industrial pharmacy", "Therapy and Rehabilitation" (Master's degree), "Therapy and Rehabilitation" (Bachelor's), "Pediatrics", "Public Health" (Bachelor's degree) took the Unified State Qualification Exam (USQE)-2: the integrated test exam

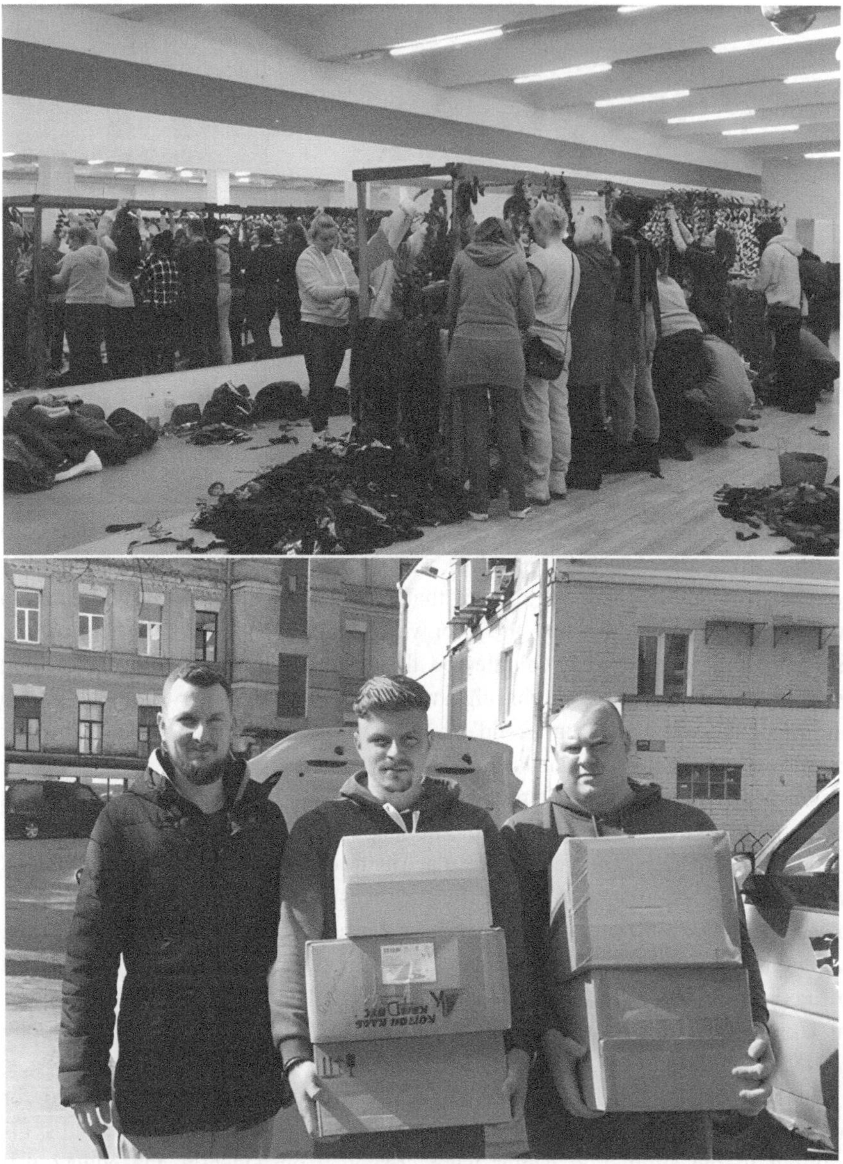

FIGURE 6.7A Students and teachers volunteer weaving camouflaged netting.

KROK, the English language exam for specific purposes, conducted by the Testing Center at the Ministry of Health of Ukraine, and the objective structured practical (clinical) exam (OSCE), conducted at the Bogomolets National Medical University (Figure 6.8).

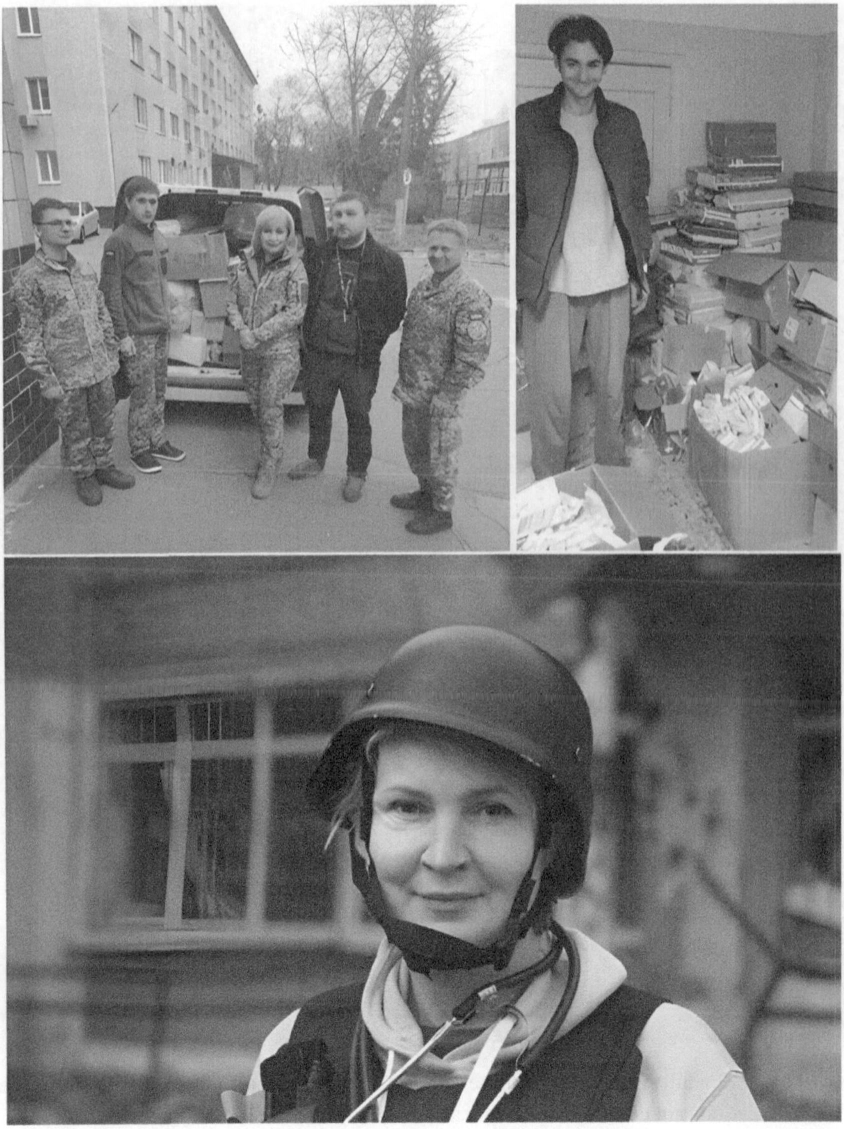

FIGURE 6.7B Delivering food, medicine, and humanitarian aid.

Higher education applicants and the academic staff were provided with routes to shelters, guidelines for organization and conduct classes during air raid alerts. During this difficult period, our international colleagues provided significant assistance. The university signed memorandums of cooperation with multiple European universities, and colleagues were happy to invite applicants and teachers

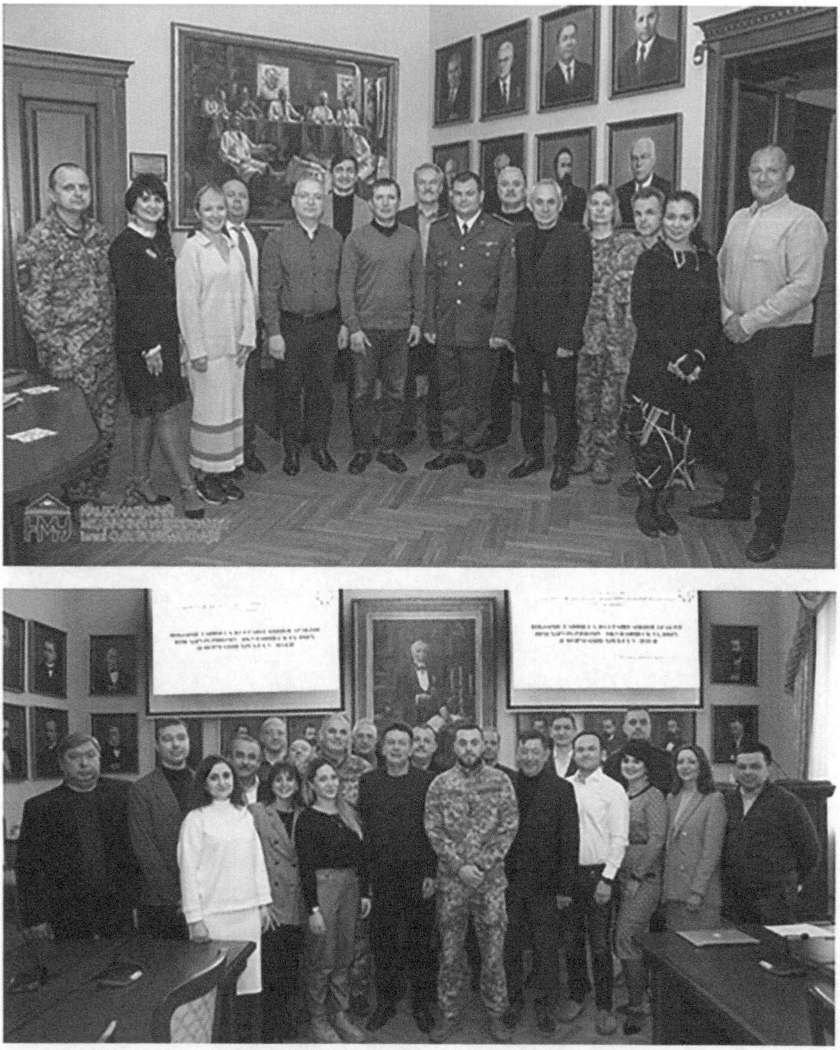

FIGURE 6.8 Faculty members – some in fatigues – stand around to demonstrate the continued delivery of education.

to join their staff, starting with temporary free training and ending with offers of exchanges of scientists and teachers and the possibility of employment (Figure 6.9).

For assistance to our university in a difficult period, the following were awarded the title of honorary professors (Figure 6.10). For example, on October 17–20, 2022, at the invitation of Polish colleagues, a meeting was held between the delegation of the Bogomolets National Medical University and the administration of the Medical University of Warsaw, where they discussed a significant expansion

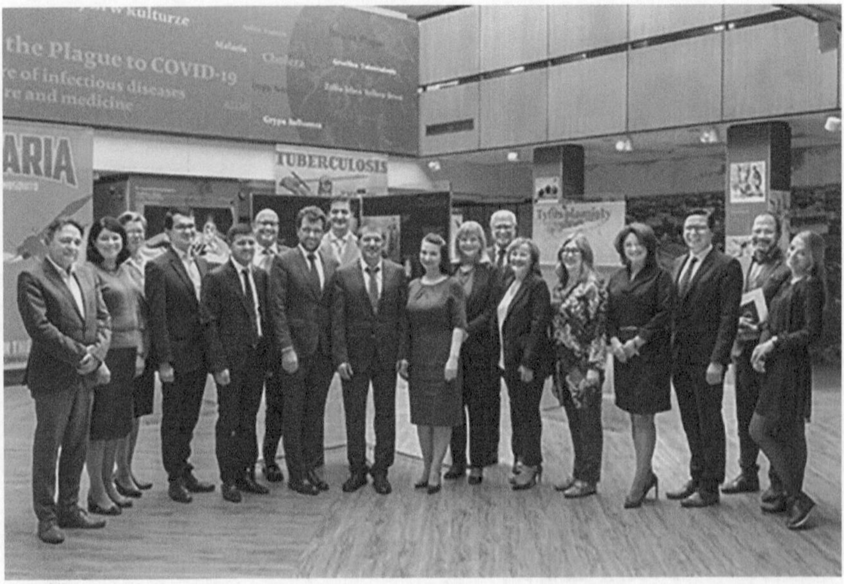

FIGURE 6.9 Attendees at a meeting between Ukrainian Bogomolets National Medical University) and Polish delegates (Medical University of Warsaw).

of the horizons of cooperation, in particular, joint research projects, simulation training, and academic mobility for both students and teachers (BNMU, 2022b).

Teachers of the Crisis Rescue Foundation (UK) also provided online lectures to students of the Bogomolets National Medical University. The Crisis Rescue Foundation has more than 250 experienced British medical teachers. Most of them are faculty and staff members of hospitals or primary care facilities.

Teachers and students on the front lines, returning for rotation, share the experience gained in real military field conditions with students, police, and others, conducting training and simulation training. From February 24, 2022, to October 1, 2024, 58 employees from Bogomolets National Medical University were mobilized. As of October 1, 2024, 44 remain mobilized, 7 people were demobilized, 6 people are discharged, 1 person is missing in action, 14 have the status of combatant. Among BNMU students as of October 1, 2024, 35 people are mobilized into the Armed Forces of Ukraine, National Guard of Ukraine, Territorial defense, volunteer battalions; 15 students have the status of combatant; 37 have the status of volunteer. In total, 17 BNMU students, teachers, and graduates have died since 2014.

WiderImpact and Response in Ukrainian MedEd Community. The experiences of a single institution serve as an important reminder of the innovation that occur on a small- to medium-scale. On a larger scale, Ukraine healthcare education and services have undergone significant attacks and responses during early stages of

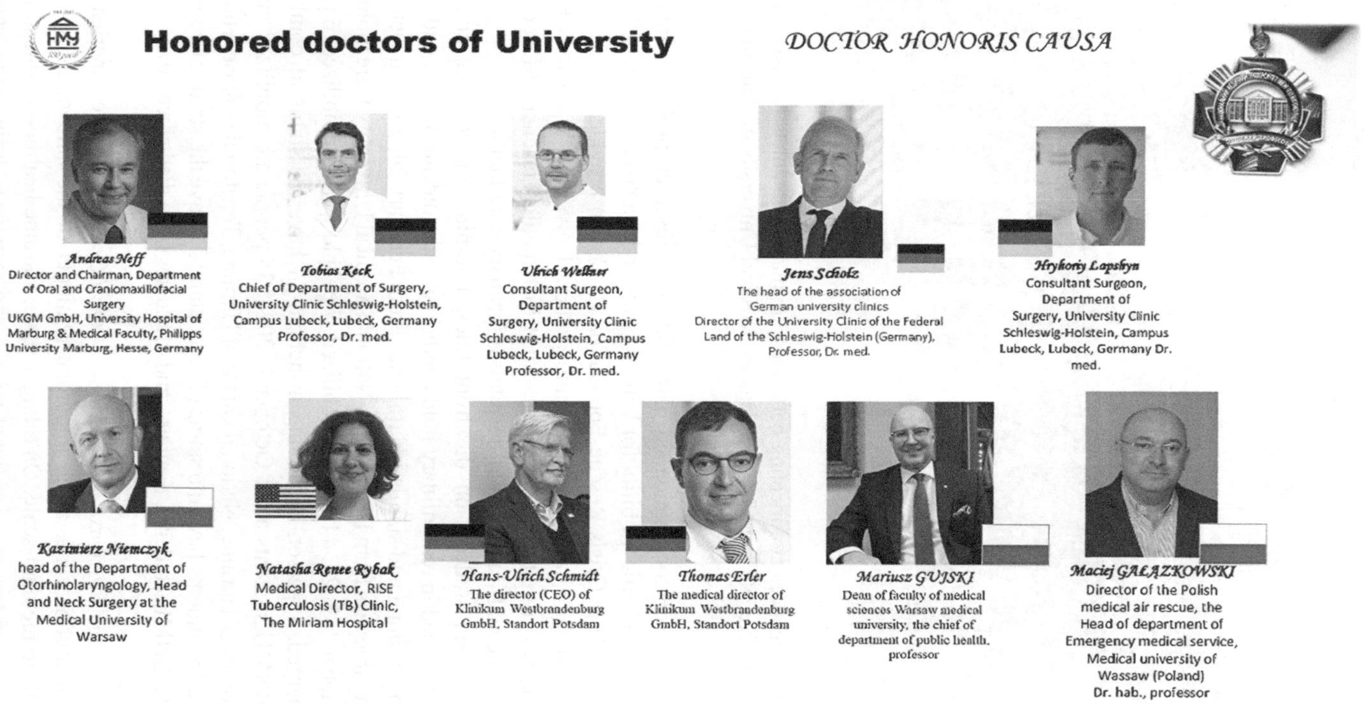

FIGURE 6.10 Images of honored doctors of the university. Honorees were awarded the title of honorary professor.

the conflict. While a comprehensive review is premature due to the ongoing nature of the conflict, we review available peer-reviewed studies to provide a (snapshot) of Ukrainian experiences.

Empirical studies have also shed light on general pattern of adaptation in Ukraine. Between October and November 2022, Mayer et al. (2023) conducted a survey of nearly 50 faculty and 200 students. Unsurprisingly, the majority of faculty (86%) and students (69%) respondents experienced significant changes to their work or study that were attributable to the war. Similarly, Goncharuk-Khomyn et al. (2023) found that foreign students' satisfaction with their safety and comfort and collaborative learning in medical education decreased, caused by the need for migration and the conflict itself. Mayer et al. (2023) also conducted more extensive interviews with nine respondents. Their thematic analysis identified multiple themes including "disruption of teaching, increased workload, mental stress, financial restrictions, non-war related needs, international cooperation, quality of education, and prospects of future professionals". While providing insight into higher education institutions within Ukraine, it is critical to note that the experience of conflict differs by regions and institution based on the features of the learners and educators, specialities, the proximity to conflict, and the available resources.

Despite the adaptation to conditions in which practitioners and students were deprived of the stability and resources necessary to ensure effective implementation (for general discussions, see Debarre, 2022; Schoenherr & Hamstra, 2024), areas for improvement have also been noted. For instance, semi-structured interviews were conducted with 24 Ukrainian informants (program leaders, surgeons, and residents) during April and September 2023 by Dzhemiliev et al. (2024). They identified multiple areas that continued to challenge the delivery of medical education. Some of these themes were unique relative to the circumstances of conflict while others were more deeply rooted. Informants indicated that learning objectives, assessments criteria, and guidelines were not clear. This placed considerable emphasis on self-directed learning and the initiative of the learner in obtaining experience. Neither research opportunities nor simulation experiences were available, with one respondent noting that they had to rely on "a self-made lap simulator, but it was of poor quality, and there was always a queue for it, so its utility was almost nonexistent" (p. 1816). Moreover, few clinical opportunities were available due to surgeons being engaged in critical duties. However, the conflict itself presented new training opportunities (e.g., bullet extraction, treatment of combined injuries) but was also seen as more emotionally difficult due to the stress experienced by learners, colleagues, and patients. However, these circumstances also created opportunities for independence and collaboration with foreign colleagues through workshops and online conferences.

6.5 Conclusions

Healthcare systems are powerful symbols of a society. They represent the knowledge and competency of its experts, the care and concern it has for its people, and resilience of the institutions that are created by, and support, the members of its communities. Focusing solely on its scientific, medical, and education basis can obscure the influence of geopolitical factors and incidents as well as the social and natural environment, often considered as externalities. The most effective training and educational programs must be mindful of the historical and current social context in which they are delivered. Crises such as armed conflicts represent a critical test of the resiliency of a society and its institutions. Along with other forms of critical infrastructure, healthcare provides an undeniable pillar that fulfills the practical needs of a people that are must defend themselves and reestablish a new equilibrium.

This chapter has provided a snapshot of current state of the healthcare system in Ukraine before and during an ongoing conflict with the Russian Federation, focusing on the experiences of one institution, Bogomolets National Medical University.

Innovation and Implementation in Armed Conflict. Necessity is often the primary driver for innovation. Most healthcare professionals are faced with daunting tasks of de-implementation such as shifting from apprenticeship models to CBME. In the years leading up to the Russian invasions of 2014 and 2022, Ukraine has made concerted efforts to align itself with international and European standards of education and healthcare. Ukraine has faced four factors that critically impact program implementation: de-implementation of an existing education system, integration into an international body (European Union), recovery from a global pandemic that depleted its institutional capacities, and an ongoing armed conflict. These four elements are intertwined. Reforms designed to move away from the Semashko Model and healthcare reforms illustrate Ukraine's shift away from the Russian Federation and toward the European Union. With looming EU membership and its weakened state from the COVID-19 pandemic, a hostile Russian government found an opportunity, framing it as a "special operation". During this time, Ukraine has received considerable support from its allies. However, this support has not always been stable nor unconditional, making Ukrainian innovations the most reliable source of the nation's survival, with NGOs providing additional support.

Shared Experience of Conflict. Many features and dimensions can be used to define cultures. Cultural variation should be accounted for the delivery of educational programs and healthcare (Schoenherr, 2027a, 2027d; Schoenherr & Beaudoin, 2027). However, the narrative account of Bogomolets National Medical University demonstrates that regardless of the theatre of war, healthcare professions education and healthcare professionals face the same challenges. When comparing the experiences of Bogomolets National Medical University to other studies, we find very similar patterns. For instance, Bdaiwi et al.'s (2023) division of GCAs and NGCAs have many parallels in Russia–Ukraine conflict. The Russia Federation's attacks on Ukraine's water supply, power grids, and other critical infrastructure, the need for Ukrainian learners and educators to decentralize education, shift the focus of curriculum delivery, and adapt to resource constraints reflect typical patterns of healthcare adapting to armed conflict. Indirect impacts are also observed such as the disproportional effect of conflict on women (e.g., Shalak et al., 2023). As UN Women (2025) reported, gender-based violence has increased, women and girls are reporting higher levels of depression, women have taken on additional burdens in childcare (from 49 hrs/week to 56 hrs/week), income gaps have increased, and displaced women are more likely to be unemployed (50.6%) than men (29%). Equally critical, the next generation of Ukraine's doctors have also been impacted. At a time when clinicians are most needed, their lives and profession are being targeted and attacked. Learners must adapt to the interruptions, constrained resources, and assaults that armed conflict introduce, with issues in curriculum delivery.

Toward a Post-Conflict Era. Building resilient health professions education not only requires a focus on preparing for crises such as natural disasters and armed conflict, it additionally requires that we consider how best to re-build social institutions like healthcare and education systems. Recovery plans must also consider the psychological toll of war on healthcare professionals. Whether in terms of PTSD, secondary PTSD, or moral injury incurred from observed combat or practicing and learning in a time when the foundations of a society have been destabilized, we cannot neglect the health of those that deliver care. Narratives of "growth" that might stem from individual and group adaptation to armed conflict are not supported by evidence (Frazier et al., 2009).

As Ukraine moves into a post-conflict era, it will need to consider how to address the needs not only of its citizens, but of healthcare workers. Intense armed conflict is associated with trauma for combatants and noncombatants that have long-lasting effects. During conflict, Healthcare Professionals (HCPs) might be able to motivate themselves by focusing on the need to care for others, support their nation, and maintain quality of life for those within their community. They are unlikely to have time for self-care. The recovery of Ukraine and other nations subjected to conflict requires ensuring that healthcare workers' needs are prioritized. If we do not care for the carers, the impact of conflict will affect a society's ability to recover and reclaim its health.

Notes

1 NQS the framework was developed to address all levels of education and training.
2 The Socialist Federal Republic of Yugoslavia maintained its own system.

3 The ECTS provides a comparison standard for all European nations.
4 Center of Education Quality of the Ministry of Health of Ukraine (2025). *Minimum Passing Score*. Retrieved November 17, 2025 from: www.testcentr.org.ua/en/exams/minimum-passing-score
5 Krok M is an exam in professionally oriented disciplines such as the educational and professional program for junior bachelors. Krok M is part of the state certification of applicants and is taken in the final year of study. Krok B is an exam in professionally oriented disciplines that correspond in content to the bachelor's degree program. Krok B is part of the state certification of applicants and is taken in the final year of study.
6 Consistent with CBME, AME focuses on ensuring that essential competencies are established, this can be conceived of as a form of satisficing wherein minimal standards are met to ensure an adequate quality of care. Despite differences in performance between typical and accelerated students, evidence suggests that such accelerated programs (e.g., Santen et al., 2024; Satyamoorthi et al., 2024).

References

Ahmead, M., Abu Turki, M., & Fawadleh, L. (2024). The prevalence of PTSD and coping strategies among Palestinian mental health professionals during political violence and wartime. *Frontiers in Psychiatry*, *15*, 1396228.

Bajaj, S. S., Mandell, S., Epstein, A., & Lim, R. (2022). The hidden surgical humanitarian response in Ukraine–Correspondence. International Journal of Surgery, *105*, 106865.

Balalian, A. A., Simonyan, H., Hekimian, K., & Crape, B. (2014). Adapting continuing medical education for post-conflict areas: assessment in Nagorno Karabagh-a qualitative study. Human Resources for Health, *12*, 1–6.

Barnett-Vanes, A. (2016). Armed conflict, medical training and health systems. *Medicine, Conflict and Survival*, *32*(1), 30–39.

Barnett-Vanes, A., Hassounah, S., Shawki, M., Ismail, O. A., Fung, C., Kedia, T., ... & Majeed, A. (2016). Impact of conflict on medical education: a cross-sectional survey of students and institutions in Iraq. BMJ open, *6*(2), e010460.

Batley, N. J., Makhoul, J., & Latif, S. A. (2008). War as a positive medical educational experience. Medical education, *42*(12), 1166–1171.

Bdaiwi, Y., Rayes, D., Sabouni, A., Murad, L., Fouad, F., Zakaria, W., ... & Abbara, A. (2020). Challenges of providing healthcare worker education and training in protracted conflict: a focus on non-government controlled areas in north west Syria. *Conflict and Health*, *14*, 1–13.

Bdaiwi, Y., Sabouni, A., Patel, P., Ekzayez, A., Alchalati, S., Abdrabbuh, O., ... & Glogowska, M. (2023). Impact of armed conflict on health professionals' education and training in Syria: a systematic review. *BMJ Open*, *13*(7), e064851.

Bogomolets National Medical University (BNMU) (2022b). *НМУ імені О.О. Богомольця та Варшавський медичний університет розширюють горизонти співпраці / Bogomolets National Medical University and Warsaw Medical University are expanding the horizons of cooperation.* Retrieved March 9, 2025, from https://nmuofficial.com/news/nmu-imeni-o-o-bogomoltsya-ta-varshavskyj-medychnyj-universytet-rozshyryuyut-goryzonty-spivpratsi/

Bogomolets National Medical University (BNMU) (2022c). Звернення ректора Ю.Л.Кучина до студентів НМУ імені О.О.Богомольця https://nmuofficial.com/news/zvernennya-rektora-yu-l-kuchyna-do-studentiv-nmu-imeni-o-o-bogomoltsya/

Bogomolets National Medical University (BNMU) (2022a). *Ступінь доктора філософії здобув Валентин Рогозинський: науковець, практикуючий лікар, військовий хірург / Valentyn Rogozinskyi: scientist, practicing physician, military surgeon received the degree of Doctor of Philosophy*. Retrieved March 9, 2025, from https://nmuofficial.com/news/stupin-doktora-filosofiyi-zdobuv-valentyn-rogozyskyj-naukovets-praktykuyuchyj-likar-vijskovyj-hirurg/

Bogomolets National Medical University (BNMU) (2025). *About University*. Retrieved February 21, 2025, from https://nmuofficial.com/en/pro-universytet/

Bosker, M., & de Ree, J. (2009). *Localizing conflict spillovers: introducing regional heterogeneity in conflict studies*. Groningen: University of Groningen.

Bou-Karroum, L., El-Harakeh, A., Kassamany, I., Ismail, H., El Arnaout, N., Charide, R., ... & Akl, E. A. (2020). Health care workers in conflict and post-conflict settings: systematic mapping of the evidence. *PloS Oone*, *15*(5), e0233757.

Briody, C., Rubenstein, L., Roberts, L., Penney, E., Keenan, W., & Horbar, J. (2018). Review of attacks on health care facilities in six conflicts of the past three decades. *Conflict and Health*, *12*, 1–7.

Buletsa, S., Deshko, L., & Zaborovskyy, V. (2019). The peculiarities of changing health care system in Ukraine. *Medicine & Law*, *38*, 427.

Cangiarella, J., Fancher, T., Jones, B., Dodson, L., Leong, S. L., Hunsaker, M., ... & Abramson, S. B. (2017). Three-year MD programs: perspectives from the consortium of accelerated medical pathway programs (CAMPP). *Academic Medicine*, *92*(4), 483–490.

Carmignani, F., & Kler, P. (2016a). Surrounded by wars: Quantifying the role of spatial conflict spillovers. *Economic Analysis and Policy*, *49*, 7–16.

Carmignani, F., & Kler, P. (2016b). The geographical spillover of armed conflict in Sub-Saharan Africa. *Economic Systems*, *40*(1), 109–119.

Casberg, M. A. (1958). Medical education in total war. *The American Journal of Surgery*, *95*(4), 493–500.

Challoner, K. R., & Forget, N. (2011). Effect of civil war on medical education in Liberia. *International Journal of Emergency Medicine*, *4*, 1–4.

Chudzicka-Czupała, A., Chiang, S. K., Tan, C. M., Hapon, N., Żywiołek-Szeja, M., Karamushka, L., ... & Ho, R. (2023). Association between mental health, psychological characteristics, and motivational functions of volunteerism among Polish and Ukrainian volunteers during the Russo-Ukrainian War. *Scientific Reports*, *13*(1), 20725.

Debarre, A. (2022). *Hard to Reach: Providing Healthcare in Armed Conflict*. International Peace Institute.

Di Stasi, L. (2023). *'The exam was stopped 7 times': Foreign students angry at being forced to return to Ukraine for test*. Retrieved January 1, 2024 from https://www.euronews.com/my-europe/2023/04/09/the-exam-was-stopped-7-times-foreign-students-angry-at-being-forced-to-return-to-ukraine-f

Dobiesz, V. A., Schwid, M., Dias, R. D., Aiwonodagbon, B., Tayeb, B., Fricke, A., ... & Erickson, T. B. (2022). Maintaining health professional education during war: A scoping review. *Medical Education*, *56*(8), 793–804.

Donaldson, R. I., Mulligan, D. A., Nugent, K., Cabral, M., Saleeby, E. R., Ansari, W., ... & Gausche-Hill, M. (2011). Using tele-education to train civilian physicians in an area of active conflict: certifying Iraqi physicians in Pediatric Advanced Life Support from the United States. *The Journal of Pediatrics*, *159*(3), 507–509.

Drees, B. M., & Omurtag, K. (2012). Accelerated medical education: past, present and future. *Missouri Medicine*, *109*(5), 352.

Dzhemiliev, A., Antoniv, M., Huivaniuk, I., Kizub, D., Reich, A. J., Kochis, M., ... & Melnitchouk, N. (2024). Strengths and opportunities for improvement in surgical education in Ukraine: a qualitative study. *World Journal of Surgery*, 48(8), 1811–1819.

Emami, S. G., Lorenzoni, V., & Turchetti, G. (2024). Towards resilient healthcare systems: a framework for crisis management. *International Journal of Environmental Research and Public Health*, *21*(3), 286.

Encyclopedia of Ukraine (1993). Medical education. Retrieved February 1, 2025. https://www.encyclopediaofukraine.com/display.asp?linkpath=pages%5CM%5CE%5CMedicaleducation.htm

Engelhard, I. M., Lommen, M. J., & Sijbrandij, M. (2015). Changing for better or worse? Posttraumatic growth reported by soldiers deployed to Iraq. *Clinical Psychological Science*, *3*(5), 789–796.

European Commission (2024). European Reference Networks. Retrieved February 19, 2025 from https://health.ec.europa.eu/rare-diseases-and-european-reference-networks/european-reference-networks_en

European Council (2024). European Health Union: protecting Europeans against cross-border health threats. Retrieved February 2, 2025, from https://www.consilium.europa.eu/en/policies/protecting-against-cross-border-health-threats/

Frazier, P., Tennen, H., Gavian, M., Park, C., Tomich, P., & Tashiro, T. (2009). Does self-reported posttraumatic growth reflect genuine positive change? *Psychological Science*, *20*(7), 912–919.

Gercheva, D. (2021). Building a more effective, efficient and equitable healthcare system in Ukraine. *Interfax Ukraine Information Agency.* Retrieved November 1, 2025 from: www.undp.org/ukraine/blog/building-more-effective-efficient-and-equitable-healthcare-system-ukraine

Gibbons, S. W., Hickling, E. J., & Watts, D. D. (2012). Combat stressors and post-traumatic stress in deployed military healthcare professionals: an integrative review. *Journal of Advanced Nursing*, *68*(1), 3–21.

Gleditsch, N. P. (2018). Armed conflict and the environment. In *Environmental Conflict* (pp. 251–272). Routledge.

Goncharuk-Khomyn, M., Kaliy, V., Pohorilyak, R., Cavalcanti, A., Keniuk, A., Yavuz, Y., & Olena, B. (2023). Impact of war on foreign students' satisfaction with quality of dental and medical education in Ukraine. *Brazilian Oral Research*, *37*, e026.

Haar, R. J., Read, R., Fast, L., Blanchet, K., Rinaldi, S., Taithe, B., ... & Rubenstein, L. S. (2021). Violence against healthcare in conflict: a systematic review of the literature and agenda for future research. *Conflict and Health*, *15*(1), 37.

Hexom, B., Calvello, E. J., Babcock, C. A., Fowler, R., Theodosis, C., Sirleaf, J. A., ... & Tupesis, J. P. (2012). A model for emergency medicine education in post-conflict Liberia. *African Journal of Emergency Medicine*, *2*(4), 143–150.

Holomb, L., Rogachevskyi, O., Karbovanets, O., Senkevych, O., & Vivsyannuk, V. (2022). Modernization of theoretical and practical aspects of the development of higher medical education in Ukraine. *Amazonia Investiga*, *11*(55), 163–171.

Ivats-Chabin, A. R., Korolchuk, O. L., Kachur, A. Y., & Smiianov, V. A. (2021). Healthcare in Ukraine during the epidemic: difficulties, challenges and solutions. *Wiadomosci lekarskie*, *74*(5), 1256–1261.

Jain, N., Panag, D. S., Srivastava, M., Mohan, S., Chodnekar, S. Y., Akbari, A. R., ... & Pilmane, M. (2022). Fate and future of the medical students in Ukraine: A silently bubbling educational crisis. *Medical Education, 56*(8), 779–782.

Jain, N., Prasad, S., Bordeniuc, A., Tanasov, A., Shirinskaya, A. V., Béla, B., ... & Reinis, A. (2022). European countries step-up humanitarian and medical assistance to Ukraine as the conflict continues. *Journal of Primary Care & Community Health, 13*.

Johnson, V., Swett, F. H., & Green, J. (1943). The accelerated program of medical education. *Academic Medicine, 18*(2), 73–79.

Lawry, L. L., Korona-Bailey, J., Juman, L., Janvrin, M., Donici, V., Kychyn, I., ... & Koehlmoos, T. P. (2024). A qualitative assessment of Ukraine's trauma system during the Russian conflict: experiences of volunteer healthcare providers. *Conflict and Health, 18*(1), 10.

Kalyniuk, N. M., Franchuk, V. V., Selskyy, P. R., Humenna, N. V., & Hladii, O. I. (2024). Blended form of education as an innovative approach in the training of medical students: The experience of Ukraine. *Educación Médica, 25*(6), 100965.

Kaminska, M. E. (2022). Variations on Bismarck: Translations of Social Health Insurance in Post-Communist Healthcare Reforms in Central and Eastern Europe—The Role of Vertical and Horizontal Interdependencies. In F. Nullmeier, D. González de Reufels, & H. Obinger (Eds.), *International Impacts on Social Policy: Short Histories in Global Perspective* (pp. 449–462). Cham: Springer International Publishing.

Kardas, P., Babicki, M., Krawczyk, J., & Mastalerz-Migas, A. (2022). War in Ukraine and the challenges it brings to the Polish healthcare system. *The Lancet Regional Health–Europe, 15, 1.*

Kornai, J., & Eggleston, K. (2001). Choice and solidarity: the health sector in Eastern Europe and proposals for reform. *International Journal of Health Care Finance and Economics, 1*, 59–84.

Krementsov, N. (2017). The promises, realities, and legacies of the Bolshevik Revolution, 1917–2017. *American Journal of Public Health, 107* (11), 1693–1694.

Kuchyn, I., Vlasenko, O., Gashenko, I., Mykytenko, P., & Kucherenko, I. (2021). Creating the informational and educational environment of the University based on the distance learning platform LIKAR_NMU. *Archives of Pharmacy Practice*, 12(2), 66–74.

Kuchyn, Y., Naumenko, O., Vlasenko, O., Lytvynova, S., Burov, O., Kucherenko, I., & Mykytenko, P. (2022). The experience of designing a single information and educational environment of the university "NMU Digital". *Educational Technology Quarterly, 2022*(1), 73–87.

Kuchyn Y., Vlasenko O., Kucherenko I., Mykytenko P. (2023). Individual educational trajectory of higher medical education students: methodological and technical aspects of implementation. In *General Pedagogy and History of Pedagogy*. (pp. 163–169).

Lekhan, V., Rudiy, V., Shevchenko, M., Nitzan-Kaluski, D., & Richardson, E. (2015). Ukraine: Health system review. Health systems in transition, 1–154. World Health Organization.

Leong, S. L., Cangiarella, J., Fancher, T., Dodson, L., Grochowski, C., Harnik, V., ... & Pusic, M. (2017). Roadmap for creating an accelerated three-year medical education program. *Medical Education Online, 22*(1), 1396172.

Lewtak, K., Kanecki, K., Tyszko, P., Goryński, P., Bogdan, M., & Nitsch-Osuch, A. (2022). Ukraine war refugees-threats and new challenges for healthcare in Poland. *Journal of Hospital Infection, 125*, 37–43.

Mayer, A., Yaremko, O., Shchudrova, T., Korotun, O., Dospil, K., & Hege, I. (2023). Medical education in times of war: A mixed-methods needs analysis at Ukrainian medical schools. *BMC Medical Education*, 23(1), 804.

Ministry of Education and Science of Ukraine (2021). Diagram of the Structure of Higher Education in Ukraine. URL: https://mon.gov.ua/static-objects/mon/sites/1/nrk/2021/11.10/Zvit.pro.samosertyfikatsiyu.NRK-dodatok.2-10.11.pdf

Ministry of Education and Science of Ukraine (2024). Strategy for the Development of the Health Care System until 2030. URL: https://moz.gov.ua/uploads/ckeditor/%D0%A1%D1%82%D1%80%D0%B0%D1%82%D0%B5%D0%B3%D1%96%D1%8F/UKR%20Health%20Strategy%20Feb%2024.2022.pdf

Ministry of Health of Ukraine (2023). A European integration government decree on the introduction of the information and communication complex of the blood system was adopted. Retrieved February 16, 2025 from https://moz.gov.ua/en/a-european-integration-government-decree-on-the-introduction-of-the-information-and-communication-complex-of-the-blood-system-was-adopted

Ministry of Health of Ukraine (2025). *Ukraine on the way to the EU: achievements in health care during two years of European integration.* Retrieved February 16, 2025 from https://moz.gov.ua/uk/ukrayina-na-shlyahu-do-yes-dosyagnennya-v-ohoroni-zdorov-ya-za-dva-roki-yevrointegraciyi

Murdoch, J. C., & Sandler, T. (2002). Economic growth, civil wars, and spatial spillovers. *Journal of Conflict Resolution, 46*(1), 91–110.

Omer, A. T., Ali, E. M., Elhassan, M. E., Ibrahim, S. A., & Ahmed, Y. S. (2024). Medical education challenges during the war crisis in Sudan: a cross-sectional study, 2023–2024. *BMC Medical Education, 24*(1), 1354.

Penfold, R., & Ali, M. (2014). Building medical education and research capacity in areas of conflict and instability: experiences of the OxPal Medlink in the occupied Palestinian territories. *Medicine, Conflict and Survival, 30*(3), 166–174.

Radziievska, I., Trepet, G., Radzikhovska, N., Sukhostavets, N., Yuryk, O., & Saienko, V. (2022). Modern achievements and prospects for the development of higher medical education: Ukrainian realities. *Amazonia Investiga, 11*(55), 114–123.

Santen, S. A., Yingling, S., Hogan, S. O., Vitto, C. M., Traba, C. M., Strano-Paul, L., ... & Park, Y. S. (2023). Are they prepared? Comparing intern milestone performance of accelerated 3-year and 4-year medical graduates. *Academic Medicine, 99*, 1267–1277.

Satyamoorthi, N., Marin, M., Ludlow, P., Triola, M. M., Gillespie, C., Cohen, E., ... & Cangiarella, J. (2024). Outcomes of accelerated 3-year MD graduates at NYU Grossman School of Medicine during medical school and early residency. *Academic Medicine, 100*, 184–190.

Schoenherr, J. R. (2023). The first total war and the sociotechnical systems of warfare. IEEE Technology and Society Magazine, *42*(3), 42–56.

Schoenherr, J. R. (2027a). Innovation and implementation in the health professions: Education and healthcare delivery. In J. R. Schoenherr & M. M. McConnell (Eds.), *Fundamentals and Frontiers of Medical Education and Decision-Making: Innovation, Implementation, and Translational Research* (pp.77–131). Routledge.

Schoenherr, J. R. (2027b). Human-centered artificial intelligence in health professions education and decision-making: A sociotechnical systems perspective. In Schoenherr, J. R. (Ed.), *Fundamentals and Frontiers of Medical Education and Decision-Making: Innovation, Implementation, and Translational Research* (pp. 132–190). Routledge.

Schoenherr, J. R. (2026c). The development and dynamics of heterarchical structure in Mayan medical education and healthcare ecosystems. In Schoenherr, J. R. (Ed.), *Fundamentals and Frontiers of Medical Education and Decision-Making: Innovation, Implementation, and Translational Research* (pp. 359–411). Routledge.

Schoenherr, J. R. (2027c). War Against Systems: Healthcare Infrastructure and Irregular Warfare during the Total War in Ukraine. In *Ukraine, Competitive Statecraft, and Irregular Warfare*.

Schoenherr, J. R. & Beaudoin, J. (2027). The evolving landscape of health professions education in East Asia. In Schoenherr, J. R. (Ed.), *Fundamentals and Frontiers of Medical Education and Decision-Making: Innovation, Implementation, and Translational Research* (pp. 462–509). Routledge.

Schoenherr, J. R., & Hamstra, S. J. (2024). Validity in health professions education: From assessment instruments to program innovation and evaluation. In J. R. Schoenherr & M. M McConnell (Eds.), *Fundamentals and Frontiers of Medical Education and Decision-Making* (pp. 80–107). Routledge.

Schoenherr, J. R., & McConnell, M. M. (2024). Human-centered design in health professions education: Informing competency-based education with psychological science. In *Fundamentals and Frontiers of Medical Education and Decision-Making* (pp. 3–36). Routledge.

Shalak, M., Markson, F., & Nepal, M. (2023). Gender-based violence and women reproductive health in war affected area. *Korean Journal of Family Medicine*, *45*(1), 12.

Shyshka, I., Mashchenko, O., & Tomareva, V. (2023). Theoretical And Methodological Foundations of The Healthcare System of Ukraine. Baltic Journal of Economic Studies, *9*(4), 253–261.

Silve, A., & Verdier, T. (2018). A theory of regional conflict complexes. *Journal of Development Economics*, *133*, 434–447.

Spiegel, P. B., Checchi, F., Colombo, S., & Paik, E. (2010). Health-care needs of people affected by conflict: future trends and changing frameworks. *The Lancet*, *375*(9711), 341–345

Srichawla, B. S., Tabari, M. A. K., Găman, M. A., Munoz-Valencia, A., & Bonilla-Escobar, F. J. (2022). War on Ukraine: Impact on Ukrainian medical students. *International Journal of Medical Students*, *10*(1), 15.

Terentyuk, V. G., Matukova-Yaryga, D. G., & Kucherenko, I. I. (2024). Digital education as an integral part of the digital transformation of healthcare. In *The Impact of Digitization on Higher Medical Education*. (pp. 67–71). Scientific and Pedagogical Internship. Republic of Poland.

United Nations (UN) (2024). *Ukraine – Protection of Civilians in Armed Conflict*. Retrieved October 20, 2024 from https://ukraine.ohchr.org/en/Protection-of-Civilians-in-Armed-Conflict-October-2025

United Nations Women (2025). Three years of full-scale war in Ukraine roll back decades of progress for women's rights, safety and economic opportunities. Retrieved February 21. 2025 from www.unwomen.org/en/news-stories/press-release/2025/02/three-years-of-full-scale-war-in-ukraine-roll-back-decades-of-progress-for-womens-rights-safety-and-economic-opportunities

Uwishema, O., Sujanamulk, B., Abbass, M., Fawaz, R., Javed, A., Aboudib, K., ... & Onyeaka, H. (2022). Russia-Ukraine conflict and COVID-19: a double burden for

Ukraine's healthcare system and a concern for global citizens. *Postgraduate Medical Journal, 98*(1162), 569–571.

Veronese, G., & Pepe, A. (2022). Psychological distress, professional burnout, and trauma in Palestinian health care helpers: A two-wave quantitative longitudinal study. *Psychological Trauma: Theory, Research, Practice, and Policy, 14*(4), 523.

WHO (2024). *Health financing in Ukraine: Reform, resilience and recovery*. World Health Organization. Retrieved November 3, 2025 from: www.who.int/europe/publications/i/item/WHO-EURO-2024-10570-50342-75964

World Health Organization (WHO) (2022). *Global Competency Framework for Universal Health Coverage*. URL: www.who.int/publications/i/item/9789240034686

World Health Organization (WHO) (August 19, 2024). *Grim milestone on World Humanitarian Day: WHO Records 1940 Attacks on Health Care in Ukraine Since Start of Full-Scale War*. Retrieved on October 20, 2204 from www.who.int/europe/news/item/19-08-2024-grim-milestone-on-world-humanitarian-day--who-records-1940-attacks-on-health-care-in-ukraine-since-start-of-full-scale-war

Wiedner, R., Croft, C., & McGivern, G. (2020). Improvisation during a crisis: hidden innovation in healthcare systems. *BMJ Leader*, 1–40.

Yelahina, H. I. (2023). Teacher's professional competence development as an integral part of higher medical education in the United States and Ukraine. *Медична Освіта*, 4, 84–89.

Zehfuss, M. (2012). Killing civilians: thinking the practice of war. *The British Journal of Politics and International Relations, 14*(3), 423–440.

7

INNOVATIONS IN HEALTH PROFESSIONS EDUCATION IN CANADA TO ADDRESS THE TRUTH AND RECONCILIATION COMMISSION OF CANADA'S CALLS TO ACTION AND THE HEALTH INEQUITIES EXPERIENCED BY INDIGENOUS PEOPLES

Catherine B. Chan, Leah Gramlich, Lisa M. Littlechild, Rick Lightning, Jenna Ganske, and Jessica Thorlakson

7.1

Health disparities suffered by Indigenous peoples stemming from colonialism, past and present, and its associated practices in Canada have been well-documented. These inequities occur to this day despite the Canada Health Act's goal of creating one of the healthiest populations in the world, and access to healthcare without barriers, in respectful environments (Government of Canada, 2019; Health Canada, 1985). Health inequities result in lower life expectancy (First Nations Information Governance Centre, 2016; Government of Canada, 2017; Statistics Canada, 2005), higher chronic and infectious disease burden, and worse self-reported health (Wylie & McConkey, 2018). Poorer quality of life or wellbeing is assumed, but its measurement is hindered by a lack of tools that measure themes considered important by Indigenous peoples (Gall et al., 2021). During the COVID-19 pandemic, Indigenous people had 60% higher odds of being infected, experiencing severe illness or dying based on 29 studies from the USA and Canada (Williams, Alberton, & Gorey, 2022). The authors reported that although they had an insufficient number of studies to test differences between countries, the overall rate appeared similar (Williams et al., 2022). These outcomes occurred despite many communities using their sovereign authority to enact protective measures, such as quarantine and lockdown strategies, limiting access to outsiders, banning ceremonial gatherings, promoting traditional ways of knowing, spending time in outdoor activities on their traditional lands, providing meals to elders, and

DOI: 10.4324/9781003498155-7

maintaining the health of elders by getting vaccinated (Mashford-Pringle, Skura, Stutz, & Yohathasan, 2021; Williams et al., 2022). Indeed, underlying inequities in access to housing and safe water exacerbated COVID-19 infection rates (Brant-Birioukov, 2021), as did loss of social supports such as school nutrition programs (Cranston & Whitford, 2022).

The barriers to equitable healthcare access have been reported using the Structural and Social Determinants of Indigenous People's Health Framework, which include proximal, intermediate, and distal barriers (Reading & Wien, 2009). Under intermediate barriers, health education systems were prominent, while under distal barriers the interconnected impacts of colonialism, racism, and social exclusion were identified (Nguyen, Subhan, Williams, & Chan, 2020).

Health education systems hierarchies perpetuate colonial attitudes. Decolonization, or removal of colonial elements of such systems, must acknowledge that the Eurocentric lens and processes upon which these hierarchies were built are not the only way of seeing and doing. Health education systems and their attempts to decolonize education can be examined through at least two lenses: the experience of Indigenous students or that of non-Indigenous students. While programs for health professionals usually attempt strategies that address both, in this review we focus on the interventions directed at non-Indigenous students because it is highly likely that providers encountered by Indigenous people seeking healthcare will be overwhelmingly non-Indigenous. Therefore, providing efficacious means of reducing healthcare inequities through the education of non-Indigenous students is of great importance. Introduction of concepts including cultural competence and cultural safety, serious consideration of traditional medicine and holistic practices within the curriculum, and partnering with Indigenous communities (Nguyen et al., 2020) are some of the strategies discussed in greater detail below.

7.1.1 Canada, Colonization, and Its Legacy

Canada is often perceived as a progressive society but like many others, it has a dark colonial past, which has been judged the most potent distal determinant of existing health inequities. Colonial policies were created to exert political control over Indigenous nations, in part through occupying their territories (with or without treaty agreements), forced resettlement, economic marginalization through denial of rights to resources, creation of the concept of "status", and forbidding traditional cultural practices and language (McGann, 2013). For over 100 years, ending only in the 1990s, the residential school system was used to isolate Indigenous children from their families and culture while promulgating Western religious and education with the goal of assimilation (Hanson, Gamez, & Manuel, 2020). Within living memory, the "Sixties Scoop" refers to forcible removal of Indigenous children from their families without consent, often placing them with White foster parents far from their homes. In addition, the creation of Indian Reserves under the Indian Act often resulted in dispossession of their traditional lands with forced relocation, often to remote territories with poor economic prospects (Hanson, 2009). These actions have created lasting, intergenerational physical and mental traumas that may manifest in self-destructive behaviors, lack of trust in White institutions, negative bias of White people towards Indigenous people, and continued marginalization, all of which contribute to health inequities (Nguyen et al., 2020). In 2007, the Truth and Reconciliation Commission (TRC) of Canada was established as part of a class action lawsuit (the Indian Residential Schools Settlement Agreement) brought against the Federal Government (Crown-Indigenous Relations and Northern Affairs Canada, 2024). Its purpose was to reveal the history of the residential school system from an Indigenous perspective and to educate Canadians about it.

In 2015, the TRC concluded its work with the publication of the Calls to Action, 94 important steps towards redressing colonialism, the residential school system, and the systemic racism continuing to this day. Action #18 calls for all levels of government to "acknowledge that the current state of Aboriginal health in Canada is a direct result of previous Canadian government policies…" and Action #19 calls for the federal government to "…close the gaps in health outcomes between Aboriginal and non-Aboriginal communities". Action #22 calls on "those who can effect change within the Canadian healthcare system to recognize the value of Aboriginal healing practices and use them in the treatment of Aboriginal patients in collaboration with Aboriginal healers and elders where requested by Aboriginal patients." While not specifically targeting health professional education programs, the successful execution of these calls will depend upon the wholehearted participation of the healthcare system, including appropriate, culturally relevant training for all existing and future staff. Specifically, regarding education, Action #23.iii. is to "provide cultural competency training for all healthcare professionals" and Action #24 calls upon

> medical and nursing schools to take a course dealing with Aboriginal health issues, including the history and legacy of residential schools, the United Nations Declaration on the Rights of Indigenous Peoples, Treaties and Aboriginal rights, and Indigenous teachings and practices. This will require skills-based training in intercultural competency, conflict resolution, human rights, and anti-racism.

Implementing the Calls to Action in educational programming for healthcare professionals requires the universities and colleges offering these programs to act both collectively and individually. We acknowledge that many activities have occurred in boardrooms and classrooms that have not found their way to the published literature. The literature review presented in this chapter provides a snapshot of the peer-reviewed literature on innovations and interventions meant to increase cultural awareness, safety, and competency in newly graduated healthcare professionals from Canadian institutions.

7.1.2 Indigenous Perspectives in Health Professional Education

In this review, perspectives from Indigenous authors, medical professionals, and students are respectfully identified and considered to recognize their insights on decolonizing education programs. Only 2.9% of Canadian registered nurses and less than 1% of physicians identify as Indigenous (Canadian Medical Association; Canadian Indigenous Nurses Association, 2016). There is a growing appreciation that the incorporation of Indigenous knowledge (Van Bewer, Woodgate, Martin, & Deer, 2020) and a strength-based approach (Kennedy et al., 2022), which focuses on solutions rather than problems, into health professional education programs provides an important counterpoint to the Eurocentric model of education focused on the biomedical model (Van Bewer et al., 2020). Acknowledging and building on inherent strengths empowers individuals and communities to identify health promotion activities that embrace positive determinants of health and effect social change (Jardine & Lines, 2018). Relationality (to help each other in a collective sense) and holistic care (embracing a broad definition of caring and healing) are Indigenous perspectives that could be applied in all nursing education and practice for the betterment of the profession (Stansfield & Browne, 2013; Van Bewer et al., 2020).

Providing Indigenous perspectives in health professional education can play a pivotal role in understanding the complexities that are faced by Indigenous peoples and emphasize the importance of hearing their perspectives. Presently, the lack of documentation of perspectives shared by Indigenous nurses creates a sense of invisibility among them (Thurston & Mashford-Pringle, 2015). Many barriers still exist within traditional education systems with a lack of accountability for curriculum revision. However, multiple examples of incorporating Indigenous knowledge into nursing (and other healthcare professional) curricula exist as evidence of progress as reviewed by Van Bewer et al. (2020). Sharing principles and traditions practiced by Indigenous healthcare students contributes to reconciliation within an education

Diabetes in Canada

Non-indigenous adult (aged 18+) population 7.4%
First Nations adults living on reserve 17.2%
First Nations adults off-reserve 12.2%
Métis adults 8.9%
Inuit adults 9.0%

Incidence of childhood-onset type 2 diabetes (per 100,000 per year)
Indigenous peoples 23.2
White 0.54

FIGURE 7.1 Diabetes in Canada information (Public Health Agency of Canada, 2022).

system. Opportunities for Indigenous nurses or nursing students to role-model and provide mentorship for their non-Indigenous peers have been highlighted within the literature (Rohatinsky, Exner-Pirot, Parent-Bergeron, Bosevski, & Pratt, 2018; Thurston & Mashford-Pringle, 2015; Van Bewer & Sawchyn, 2024; Van Bewer et al., 2020).

Following similar observations of indigenous healthcare traditions (Schoenherr, 2027), collaboration with Indigenous leaders and community-based engagement is recommended in addressing educational inequities, as well as incorporating local Indigenous knowledge and guidance (Thurston & Mashford-Pringle, 2015; Van Bewer et al., 2020). Lastly, increasing accountability to understand the historical impacts on Indigenous peoples and engaging in self-reflection is a crucial step by non-Indigenous healthcare professionals towards developing cultural competency and demonstrating their willingness to engage in culturally safe practices (Rohatinsky et al., 2018) (Box 7.1).

BOX 7.1 CASE STUDY

Conrad's Story as Told by Dr. Leah Gramlich

Narratives are an important tool that can be used to illustrate authentic human experiences through storytelling. This is the story of the late Conrad Bull, a young Cree with diabetes and a resident of Maskwacîs, in the province of Alberta. It is about 70 km south of Edmonton – Canada's fifth largest city – and about 20 km from the nearest hospital. The story is told here by Dr. Leah Gramlich, to whom Conrad gifted his story. It is presented with the permission and participation of Lisa Littlechild, Conrad's mother, and all rights to his story, including in this telling, remain with her.

Conrad Bull gifted us his story – that of an Indigenous youth, living and struggling with diabetes. He faced challenges because of the disease itself and at the hands of the health system and its healthcare providers. He succumbed to his disease too early, his life cut short. In sharing his story, Conrad and his mother Lisa allow us to critically examine our knowledge and beliefs as healthcare professionals working with Indigenous peoples. Our work includes service (providing culturally sensitive and safe care), education of future health professionals, ongoing education of our existing healthcare workforce and research and evaluation to address health inequity and systemic racism that impact Indigenous peoples.

I met Conrad a year before he passed, 11 years after being diagnosed with diabetes.

Conrad was 11 when he initially became ill in 2012. Although he was a robust boy, he had lost a lot of weight and had nausea and vomiting. Lisa noticed "sticky pee" on the toilet seat at home and knew from her experiences with her father-in-law that this was a symptom of diabetes (related to glucosuria). When she first took Conrad to the emergency department, the staff did not want to test Conrad for diabetes, because they felt it was unlikely that a child that young would develop diabetes, despite a family history. It was only when she threatened to leave and come back to see a different provider that they agreed to test his blood sugar and when it registered "high" on the glucometer, she was whisked out of the room so that, in her words, "the healthcare team could provide the right care". In the early days following his diagnosis, there were the usual challenges and a lot of trial and error as Conrad and Lisa worked to learn to live with diabetes and deal with the impact it had on the entire family, including employment and the cost of living. Conrad's diabetes was well-managed when living at home, but he struggled when he sought to be an independent adult. Mental health challenges, including depression and suicide concerns during his teenage years, were not addressed, acknowledged, or treated as part of the diabetes care that Conrad received.

Conrad was "transitioned" to adult care at 16 years of age, deemed capable of making his own decisions and without communication with his family. No one seemed to really "get" Conrad during his difficult teenage years, including Alberta Health Services and Maskwacîs care, programs, and services. Lisa noted that it seemed like the diabetes affected Conrad's brain and behavior, but this was not addressed or acknowledged even when he was too sick to make his own decisions. It was during this time that Conrad became a "baby dad" to Kinsley, his daughter. Kinsley was ultimately a strong motivator for life as Conrad's disease progressed.

Conrad had stomach problems for many years including poor appetite, nausea, vomiting, and diarrhea that did not seem to be taken seriously or addressed. These symptoms were a source of distress and embarrassment for Conrad as he was at risk of having "accidents" and soiling himself or having to throw up into the kitchen sink. These symptoms had a great impact, contributing to distress for the entire extended family at Lisa's home.

Conrad was referred to see me in the Malnutrition Clinic in Edmonton in 2022. At the time he was 6 ft tall and weighed 110 lbs (body mass index 14.9 kg/m^2 (normal is considered 18–24.9 kg/m^2)). He had a chronically low weight and prominent, persistent gastrointestinal symptoms. At this time he already had evidence of complications of diabetes including nephropathy (proteinuria on urinalysis) and neuropathy (diabetic gastroparesis). He was willing to be admitted for investigations, assessment of his diabetes skills and nutrition support, even though it kept him far from his family. That was when I got my first glimpse of his inner strength and resolve. During this admission, it was evident that he had insight into diabetes management including an understanding of the role of food and insulin. Conrad was scared of low blood sugars – he had had episodes of profound hypoglycemia and also had an ongoing fear of vomiting after meals and was worried about taking too much insulin for meals. During that admission, it became evident that he felt he was a burden at home to Lisa and that he needed support for living independently. Conrad and I agreed to use the admission to get the right social supports in place as well as to optimize his diabetes and nutrition care. Unfortunately, Conrad was not "sick enough" to warrant ongoing admission to acute care and he was discharged home.

Over the next month, Conrad continued to struggle with medical and social issues, so we re-admitted him to the acute care hospital in the city, knowing it was not ideal. Once again, he was discharged without a solid plan to ensure support in his local community.

Conrad re-presented to his local hospital within one week with pain in his right wrist and arm, noting that it was swollen, red, and hot. He waited in the emergency department for many hours before he was seen. He was diagnosed with "flesh-eating disease" – necrotizing fasciitis. He was rushed to the regional hospital where he required urgent surgery to amputate his right arm. He had a cardiac arrest during surgery but came back to life. His kidneys failed following this, and he required dialysis. The necrotizing fasciitis extended to his right leg and although there were concerns because of his heart stopping during his first surgery, he survived a right leg amputation. Lisa felt that the arm infection and leg pain were not taken seriously. After the surgeries, there were a lot of delays and Conrad was in a lot of pain, and the wound was starting to smell.

During this hospital stay, Conrad and Lisa noted many challenges with their care. Nurses were often rough and unhelpful with getting Conrad out of his wheelchair, and not being helped up when he fell. In addition, Conrad felt shamed by the staff when he had accidents and soiled himself. He felt like they were grossed out by him and made him feel like **** about himself. Conrad's room was often messy, with full garbage bins and dirty sheets, as though he was to fend for himself while in hospital. He overheard nurses in the hallway providing personal and sensitive information about him where everyone could hear it, which made him very upset. He was wrongly accused of accessing his intravenous line. Being in care was a constant battle for his dignity and human rights, in addition to basic care.

Conrad was discharged after his arm and leg amputations with painkillers but no antibiotics. When the homecare nurse came to change the dressing, she asked if she could take a picture of the open wound and it felt like he was discharged too soon. Lisa did not agree with the discharge plan but felt that the hospital just wanted to get rid of Conrad.

By this time, Conrad's weight was down to 100 lbs (with edema and anasarca) and his BMI was estimated to be around 11. Eating was a challenge, especially given his right arm amputation. The burden of mobilization given his

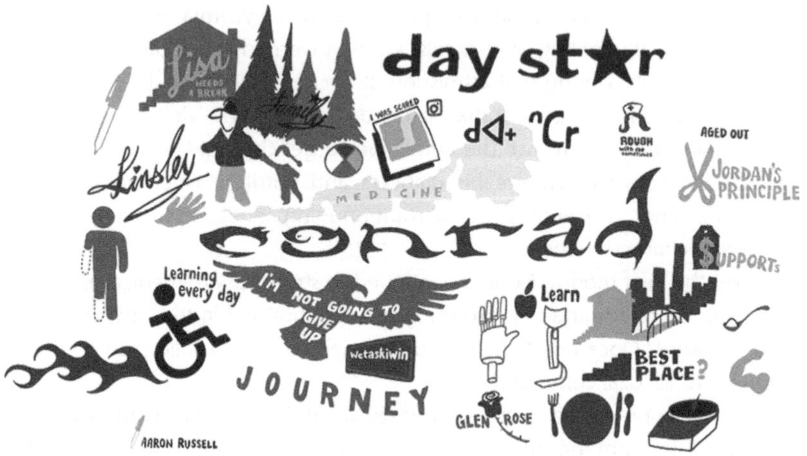

FIGURE 7.2 Graphic artist Aaron Russell's representation of Conrad's Story.

right leg amputation was new for Conrad, but he quickly adapted to using a wheelchair. The need for ongoing dialysis was a challenge.

Around this time, I spoke with Conrad – by this time, he had earned my total respect and support and I had earned Conrad's trust. I was impressed by his equanimity and composure in the face of a life-threatening and debilitating disease. I developed a deep appreciation for how important Conrad's family, particularly Lisa and Kinsley, were to his wellness and healing. The physician in me knew the odds of survival were low in a 21-year-old double amputee with profound malnutrition, kidney failure, diabetes, and all of the complications. I was frank in my discussions with Conrad and encouraged him to focus on what he truly wanted. We talked about what it would take to "get better" and what "getting better" might look like, including consideration of prostheses, ongoing dialysis and support for nutrition with tube feeding. We discussed the fact that this work would need to take place in the city, away from his family home and community. It was around this time that Conrad shared his story with us, told through graphic artist Aaron Russell (Figure 7.2).

Despite the odds, Conrad managed to get home for Christmas and after thinking about it, decided upon transfer to the city for feeding and a mobility plan. Once again, the hospital environment, its rigidity, and the expectations of the healthcare providers were too much and Conrad decided to leave, to be closer to home, with his people, on his terms.

Conrad developed pneumonia and died in early 2023, leaving his loving mom Lisa, his daughter Kinsley, and a lot of family. He left us his story so that we can learn and do better.

7.2 Addressing Inequity and Inequality in Indigenous Healthcare through Education of Health Professions Students

Improving the knowledge, beliefs, and attitudes of healthcare professionals is incumbent upon educators, so that Conrad's gift to us – and the experiences of countless others – is not in vain. His story is painful to hear, an exemplar of the many factors that contribute to health inequalities and inequities in Indigenous peoples (Nguyen et al., 2020) and a reminder that there is a long way to go towards achieving social accountability and health equity (Markham et al., 2021). Within the last few decades, there has been increasing global recognition of the disparate accessibility of healthcare services, health outcomes, and participation in the healthcare workforce experienced by indigenous communities (King, Smith, & Gracey, 2009; Reid & Robson, 2007) as well as initiatives to address these challenges (Lavoie et al., 2016; Tiwari et al., 2018).

One approach to addressing inequities is to explicitly teach about concepts recommended by the TRC, such as cultural competency during the training of medical and nursing students. The purpose of this literature review is to summarize institutional attempts to adopt philosophies, leadership, and organizational initiatives as well as specific course materials with a focus on schools of medicine and nursing in Canada. Although the initial intent of this review chapter was to highlight initiatives that have been evaluated, scarcity of data precludes this limitation. Hence, programs lacking a formal evaluation are also included to illustrate a broader perspective. Details of the literature search are provided in Appendix A.

7.2.1 Foundational Institutional Shifts

Prior to the publication of the TRC Calls to Action in 2015, several medical and nursing schools reported increased emphasis on teaching concepts such as social justice, cultural safety and self-efficacy, racism, and prejudice in their curricula. Since 2015, these efforts have intensified. An international Consensus Statement, developed over a decade by leaders in Indigenous medical education in Canada, Australia, New Zealand, and the United States, provides guidance to medical educators regarding principles for action to address key themes of colonization, racism, and privilege (Jones et al., 2019). These include anti-racism training, embedding Indigenous health as a formal discipline in medical education and alignment of the whole curriculum. The Consensus Statement authors acknowledge that taking action involves more than addressing overt and obvious instances of colonization, racism, and privilege, as these practices are built into the fabric of our society (Jones et al., 2019). Thus, educators in the health professions must be wary of complicity in these hidden obstacles to equity for Indigenous peoples (for a case study in Indigenous healthcare, see Schoenherr, 2027; for another discussion of reconciling pluralistic traditions within the Americas see Venosa et al., 2027, and Africa, see Oluwabunmi Olapade-Olaopa et al., 2027).

Frameworks have been developed to help Canadian educators in medical and other health professional programs implement these principles. Indigenous leadership provided important input into the development of these frameworks. While not covered by the framework developed by the Royal College of Physician and Surgeons Canada (i.e., CanMeds; see, Schoenherr & McConnell, 2024), this approach is consistent with competency-based medical education which assumes that core competencies can be identified, measured, assessed, and used to determine whether healthcare professionals can be entrusted to engage in practice (e.g., Ma, 2024).

Indigenous communities have developed unique adaptations to the socioecology (Schoenherr & Beaudoin, 2027; Venosa et al., 2027). Capturing specific competencies is critical for effective care. The Core Competencies of graduating students articulated by the Indigenous Physicians Association of Canada include demonstration of (1) "compassionate, culturally safe, relationship-centred care for First Nations, Inuit, Métis patients, their families or communities"; (2) "effective and culturally safe communications…"; (3) "skills of effective collaboration with both Aboriginal and non-Aboriginal health care professionals, traditional/medicine peoples/healers in the provision of effective health care for First Nations, Inuit, Métis patients/populations"; (4) describe approaches to optimizing First Nations, Inuit, Métis health through a just allocation of healthcare resources, balancing effectiveness, efficiency, and access, employing evidence based and Indigenous best practices; (5) "identify the determinants of health of Aboriginal populations and use this knowledge to promote the health of individual First Nations, Inuit, Métis patients and their communities" and (6) "contribute to the development, dissemination, critical assessment of knowledge/practices and dissemination related to the improvement of First Nations, Inuit, Métis health in Canada" (Indigenous Physicians Association of Canada–Association of Faculties of Medicine, 2008). While these competencies predate the TRC Calls to Action, they are consistent with and extend the responsibilities of medical professionals to address Indigenous health inequities.

The Association of Faculties of Medicine in Canada has published a Joint Commitment to Action on Indigenous Health to assist the schools of medicine in developing innovations that address the TRC Calls to Action. Key themes identified included the building of Indigenous community relationships, actions related to the learning environment and curriculum, and supporting admissions of Indigenous students. Importantly, several quantifiable indicators were developed for each theme/action, which in theory allows the medical schools to self-evaluate their progress. At the time, there was no accreditation standard related to the adoption of these actions against which the medical schools could be held accountable (Anderson et al., 2019). After releasing the Joint Commitment to Action, the progress of medical schools across Canada was surveyed relative to the recommendations and whether they self-identified as being at various stages of implementation (Association of Faculties of Medicine of Canada, 2020). Moreover, the accreditation document released in 2021 now includes standard 7.6, which states:

> The faculty of a medical school ensures that the medical curriculum provides opportunities for medical students to learn to recognize and appropriately address the unique needs of people of diverse cultures, genders, races and belief systems, in particular the Indigenous peoples of Canada. The medical curriculum prepares medical students to:
>
> a) recognize and appropriately address the manner in which people of diverse cultures, genders, races and belief systems perceive health and illness and respond to various symptoms, diseases, and treatments;
> b) recognize and appropriately address personal biases (cultural, gender, racial, belief) and how these biases influence clinical decision-making and the care provided to patients;
> c) develop the basic skills needed to provide culturally competent health care;
> d) identify health care disparities and participate in developing solutions to address them.
>
> *(Committee on Accreditation of Canadian Medical Schools, 2021)*

Likewise, the Canadian Association of Schools of Nursing's most recent accreditation standards section on curriculum explicitly specifies the inclusion of Action 24 of the TRC. Specifically, Standard 4 Program Framework and Curriculum, Key Element 14 states:

> The curriculum implements Action 24 of the Truth and Reconciliation Commission's call to programs of nursing to integrate the United Nations Declaration on the Rights of Indigenous Peoples, human rights, the history of Indigenous peoples in Canada, Indigenous teachings and practice, intercultural competency, and anti-racism.
>
> *(Canadian Association of Schools of Nursing, 2020)*

Any change in competency requires specific resources to successfully implement it within a curriculum (Schoenherr & Hamstra, 2024). Addressing colonialism, racism, and privilege requires effort and funding by the program's leadership team to ensure that educators can address these topics authentically and appropriately (Schoenherr, 2027b; Venosa et al., 2027). While these actions will now be spurred by the necessity of meeting accreditation standards, some medical and nursing schools have been addressing the need to confront health inequities in Indigenous populations over the past two decades. The remainder of this chapter reviews these efforts and the lessons learned by these institutions as they implemented these changes.

7.2.2 Structural Shifts in the Delivery of Medical and Nursing Curricula

Implementation of the key principles described above is contextual (Jones et al., 2019) and therefore needs to be addressed individually by each institution and program to ensure the validity of implementation by considering the available institutional resources, the role educational activities play in a curriculum, and their relationship to existing activities (Schoenherr & Hamstra, 2024). Some examples of such educational and training activities have been published.

The University of Manitoba reimagined a longstanding entity, the Northern Medical Unit, to address the issue of colonial power structures as a barrier to achieving healthcare transformation for Indigenous peoples. Originally founded in 1970, the Northern Medical Unit was based in Churchill, Manitoba, as a tertiary referral center for First Nations communities in the north as well as in the Kivalliq region of Nunavut. It was also engaged in research and educational activities, evolving through the years to include some Indigenous input to its activities and governance (Cook, MacKinnon, Anderson, & Whetter, 2019). As described by Cook et al. (Cook et al., 2019), Ongomiizwin, the Indigenous Institute of Health and Healing at the University of Manitoba launched in 2017, currently spans education, research, and health services. Its development was led by Indigenous–non-Indigenous pairs of faculty or staff, whose working groups addressed six identified priorities: relationship building, recognition of rights, reconciliation and respect, reflective programs and practice, recruitment and retention, and anti-racism (Cook et al., 2019). Examples of activities addressing health professional education include two-week visits by interdisciplinary groups of students to partnering First Nations communities and the development of a longitudinal course in Indigenous health delivered throughout the four years of the medical curriculum, beginning in 2010. A tangible benefit of these initiatives has been increased recruitment and retention of healthcare professionals to Ongomiizwin Health Services (Cook et al., 2019). However, evaluation of the program on outcomes such as racism, reconciliation, and respect for Indigenous peoples has not been published.

The most ambitious initiative in Canada was the creation of the Northern Ontario School of Medicine (NOSM) in 2005, with a specific purpose of advancing social accountability by graduating medical doctors whose training enhances their likelihood of practicing in rural and Indigenous communities (Jacklin, Strasser, & Peltier, 2014).

In northern Ontario, Indigenous people comprise 17% of the population (OECD, 2020). Health inequities are clearly evidenced in northern Canadian populations. They can be attributed to the remoteness of Indigenous communities, low educational attainment, and difficulty in recruiting and retaining personnel in addition to the issues rooted in colonialism (Nguyen et al., 2020). The NOSM has physical campuses in both Sudbury and Thunder Bay, two cities approximately 1000 km apart in central and western sectors of northern Ontario, but considers the entire north as their campus (Strasser et al., 2018). Ongoing meaningful involvement of Indigenous partners shapes the overall program and curriculum (Jacklin et al., 2014) including specific community engagement activities (see below). The evolution of the program structure, process of curriculum delivery, and interactions with Indigenous communities and program content highlight the necessity of embedding review and renewal processes to adapt to changing environments and build upon previous learnings (Jacklin et al., 2014).

Sustainability requires institutional buy-in and development of a supportive culture, provision of financial and time resources, and ongoing trust of the many Indigenous partners involved in the initiative (Jacklin et al., 2014). Despite having a unique opportunity to build the Aboriginal Health Program into an entirely new curriculum and hire faculty who support the ideals of social justice and other advantages, authors note continuing challenges with ensuring equal billing for Indigenous content and learning objectives, low participation of faculty in Indigenous health continuing education, and developing content that, while accurately portraying Indigenous health issues may also perpetuate stereotypes. Underlying these challenges is the continuing tension between Indigenous and non-Indigenous knowledge systems and the ongoing need to address the power imbalance that exists (Jacklin et al., 2014).

7.2.3 Community Partnerships and Immersion

Underlying many initiatives to address the TRC recommendations in medical and nursing schools is the development of partnerships with Indigenous communities. Partnership is a component of a framework guiding the placement of equity and social justice concepts within health professional curricula (Blanchet Garneau, Belisle, Lavoie, & Laurent Sedillot, 2021). These authors argue that such efforts must go beyond short experiences rooted in traditional colonial structures. Partnerships should be built upon the 4Rs: respect, relevance, reciprocity, and responsibility. The products (i.e., curricular elements) should provide benefits to both the learners and the communities (Blanchet Garneau et al., 2021). When developing content and teaching strategies, Indigenous partners, including Indigenous instructors, should be involved as critical partners (Beavis et al., 2015), imparting their own "wise practices" (Blanchet Garneau et al., 2021).

The NOSM focused on community partnerships, including Indigenous communities, as part of its ethos. They call their education model Distributed Community Engaged Learning (DCEL; (Strasser et al., 2018)). By placing medical students in Indigenous communities, NOSM strives to capitalize on evidence that positive experiences will increase their likelihood of subsequently seeking postgraduate training and practicing in such communities. To lay the foundation for community placements, planners incorporated Indigenous perspectives provided by the Nishnawbe Aski Nation into the proposal for building a new medical school. Community workshops emphasized that true learning could not occur without authentic experiences. This defines a unique pillar of NOSM's curriculum that all students – not just those with expressed interest – would have a placement in an Indigenous community (Hudson & Maar, 2022). Hudson and Maar have outlined a detailed chronology of the development of the community placement for NOSM (Hudson & Maar, 2022). Some of the recommendations developed through community consultation include integrating traditional medicine throughout the curriculum, involving non-academic Indigenous healers in teaching, expanding opportunities for students to immerse themselves in Indigenous communities, and ensuring that NOSM staff, faculty, and learners all participate in gaining cultural safety training. The fifth Indigenous Community Partnership Gathering celebrated successes but also outlined many areas for continuous refinement and improvement of the partnership (Northern Ontario School of Medicine, 2018), which included more research into the long-term impacts of the cultural placements.

Another long-term partnership between the Stó:lō First Nation's Fraser Valley Aboriginal Children and Family Services Society (Xyolhemeylh) and the University of British Columbia (UBC) known as the Community as Teacher program was initiated in 2006. The Xyolhemeylh had offered cultural camps for youth and families, and then, building on prior relationships with UBC researchers, invited a partnership with UBC's Division of Health Care Communication (DHCC), which encompasses the health disciplines (Bain, 2014). The students participate in the Community as Teacher program and experience a three-day cultural immersion, the outcomes of which are described under curricular interventions. Similarly, some outcomes of NOSM and Ongomiizwin initiatives mentioned above are noted below in the sections on curricular interventions.

While the benefits of community partnerships have been repeatedly articulated in Canada and elsewhere (Brock, Fowler, Freeman, Richardson, & Barnes, 2019), such relationships require ongoing effort, particularly to ensure value-added outcomes for both parties. Challenges include geographic separation of the universities from many of the communities and ensuring authentic shared decision-making and mutual benefits. At NOSM, regular face-to-face meetings, the creation of local steering committees, and an advisory Reference Group have been created (Strasser et al., 2018). Similarly, the Ongomiizwin program relies on close communications within working groups (Cook et al., 2019) and the Xyolhemeylh initiative emphasizes a shared purpose in education, incorporating the patient (or community) voice, and partnership in relevant research (Bain, 2014).

7.2.4 Curricular Interventions

For this discussion, "interventions" refers to distinct curricular elements (e.g., a course, community placement, workshop, or lecture) aimed at reducing colonialism, racism, and privilege and increasing learners' empathy for Indigenous peoples and, often, an underlying goal of having more graduates practice in communities with a high proportion of Indigenous peoples.

7.2.5 Cultural Immersion Experiences

Cultural immersion is a method within experiential learning practices that is intended to increase the participants' knowledge of self and the host community (de Leeuw et al., 2021). Cultural immersion experiences may increase cultural sensitivity and awareness (Brock et al., 2019; Buchanan, Velandia, Weckend, & Bayes, 2021) and evidence is accumulating regarding their efficacy to improve learners' attitudes and knowledge of Indigenous health inequities and other outcomes (Burgess & Cavanagh, 2015; de Leeuw et al., 2021). There is an emerging consensus that self-reflection is a critical component of cultural immersion, to allow students to understand their unfamiliar environment and come to terms with their experience (Burgess, 2017; Matthews, Clune, Luhanga, & Loewen, 2021). There are ways to maximize cultural immersion benefits, such as including pre-immersion preparation for students to enable them to better appreciate the nuances of their learnings into a cultural framework (Matthews et al., 2021).

7.2.5.1 Northern Ontario School of Medicine Distributed Community Engaged Learning

The NOSM DCEL occurs in year one of the medical curriculum (preceded by extensive orientation) when pairs of students spend four weeks in one of 36 partner communities (Strasser et al., 2009). The structure builds on Indigenous preference for independent learning as participants in the community (Hudson & Maar, 2022). Students learn beside elders, community members, and healthcare professionals situated in each community (which are rarely physicians). Since the pilot placement in 2005, the program has evolved, including the provision of more resources to the communities to organize and prepare to receive students. In keeping with Indigenous self-determination, NOSM does not vet or approve the cultural and clinical activities planned for the students by each community although guidelines for the number of hours spent in cultural versus clinical activities are provided (Hudson & Maar, 2022). Notably, the emphases have changed over the years, from cultural "competence" to "safety" and fewer clinical and more cultural experiences.

The acceptance and success of this initiative can be inferred from its continued existence with formalized agreements between 32 Indigenous communities and NOSM. After 20+ years of experience, the publication of outcomes is still scanty. Coke et al. (Coke, Kuper, Richardson, & Cameron, 2016) interviewed residents of Kenora, a northwestern Ontario town with many Indigenous residents and a service center for remote First Nations. While not specifically undertaken to evaluate NOSM's program, several respondents singled out NOSM students, for example,

"...since NOSM University has been around, they are way more prepared than the other universities". Another individual said,

> it's an immersion in the culture and they are sent to different First Nations communities for 4 weeks. So their awareness and knowledge really develops very early in the program. As far as living conditions, social economic conditions, health challenges.

Students who have participated in the program report greater cultural awareness and empathy (Strasser et al., 2018). Another NOSM program matches mentors and medical student researchers with communities wishing to conduct health research on questions of importance to them. Such activities provide a limited number of trainees with the opportunity to increase their awareness of health-related priorities of First Nations people and build trust in those communities (Maar, Boesch, & Tobe, 2018).

7.2.5.2 First Nations Community Education Partnership

The Northern Medical Program of the University of Northern British Columbia, situated in Prince George, developed a cultural immersion in partnership with the First Nations Health Authority (FNHA; Northern Region), which saw an opportunity for place-based, shared learning in northern rural and remote First Nations communities to improve medical students' understanding of First Nations health issues and increase their social accountability and encourage graduates to consider practicing in these communities (de Leeuw et al., 2021).

The program called the First Nations Community Education Partnership (FNCEP) was piloted and then introduced as a regular elective offering in 2015. Small groups of students spend two to four nights with a host family, participating in the host's lives and community events to acquire a realistic perspective, gain empathy, and build relationships (de Leeuw et al., 2021). It is emphasized that students are not there to "help" the community. Before attending FNCEP, students have completed a mandatory course in Indigenous Cultural Safety, which is part of the University of British Columbia medical curriculum but, unlike the NOSM immersion experience, little other orientation is provided.

An important foundation of the FNCEP course is humanities-based education, including a guided critical reflection process that was evaluated for the de Leeuw et al. publication to understand post-FNCEP shifts in attitudes and beliefs, what students observed during their placement and how this compared to pre-FNCEP reflections. The authors reported that most learners experienced transformative learning, beginning with little understanding but demonstrating increased cultural sensitivity post-FNCEP. However, the possibility of entrenching stereotypes in some individuals was observed. The authors also noted that the course in Indigenous Cultural Safety, if the only background students possess, may be insufficient to prepare them for clinical placements in Indigenous communities, as revealed by pre-FNCEP reflections (de Leeuw et al., 2021).

UBC health professional students self-select to participate in camps developed by the Stó:lō First Nation to experience the community-as-teacher model, engaging with the camp leaders, elders and youth to learn about aspects of Indigenous culture over three to four days. The community in return creates opportunities for the students to participate in the event organization or to lead group discussions on specific health topics. Researchers interviewed camp leaders, youth, and students for their perspectives and conducted a thematic analysis. Some benefits to students were increased cultural awareness, negation of stereotypes, and overall increased cultural sensitivity and appreciation of culturally safe practices. Community members concurred that students were enthusiastic and appreciative of the opportunities to interact with and learn from the community, while the youth also found them approachable and helpful. A long-lasting impact of this short immersion experience was the resilience and strengths within the community (Kline et al., 2013), which is consistent with current thinking on utilizing strength-based approaches when partnering with Indigenous communities to address health equity (Kennedy et al., 2022).

7.2.5.3 *Intraprofessional Practice Education*

Nursing programs have also introduced community placements into their curricula. In Saskatchewan, the Institute of Applied Science and Technology entered a three-way partnership between community advisors, the Division of Nursing faculty advisors, and students to create community placements in rural/remote areas. The primary driver of this initiative was the expansion of nursing programs increasing the need for placements (Hoffart, Kuster-Orban, Spooner, & Neudorf, 2013). Specific learning objectives related to clinical care were developed by the faculty advisors to be relevant to nursing students in three programs (licensed practical, registered, and registered psychiatric), including holistic health and cultural safety. The students worked alongside a variety of healthcare providers in the community and also participated in culturally relevant health promotion activities, a powwow and other activities provided by community members (Hoffart et al., 2013). Evaluation of the pilot (involving three students from each program) highlighted strains on the capacity of the community to host nine students as well as other pedagogical issues. Students reported an enhanced appreciation of cultural diversity, holistic practices, and the determinants of health (Hoffart et al., 2013).

7.2.6 *Didactic and Short Experiential Learning Experiences*

The University of Victoria nursing program developed a 13-week course called Understanding Indigenous Health and Wellness, which uses "storytelling, self-reflection and experiential learning methods and engages a critical social lens that explores power, white privilege, racism and culture" (University of Victoria, 2024).

The strengths and gifts of Indigenous knowledge and teachings are interwoven. Evaluation of this course was provided by 16 students responding to a survey. Despite the students having awareness of the historical reasons for Indigenous peoples' mistrust of the healthcare system and the need to provide trauma-informed care, they nonetheless felt poorly equipped to navigate cultural tensions and unjust policies or deal with racist comments or power differentials exhibited by coworkers (Braithwaite, Kelly, & Chakanyuka, 2022). These results indicate that knowledge is important but insufficient for entry-level nurses to confront the reality of the system in which they practice and point to the need for multi-level education across the health system, implementation of policies that promote health equity and encourage culturally sensitive practices. Some respondents indicated that earlier provision of the course material along with toolkits could help them in practice (Braithwaite et al., 2022).

Based on research suggesting that teaching about the impact of colonialism on Indigenous health inequities could improve the causal beliefs of health professional students, the Western University medical school introduced a four-week mandatory course called Introduction to Culturally Safe Care for Indigenous Peoples for first-year students in 2019. In 2022, the course was extended to six weeks. Topics included modules addressing historical contexts, Indigenous perspectives on health issues, and clinical strategies. Course developers partnered with elders, knowledge keepers, and community members and focused on culturally safe care. Learners from the 2019, 2020, and 2022 cohorts volunteered to complete pre- and three-month post-course surveys. An Indigenous Advisory Council provided advice on survey questions interrogating beliefs and attitudes (Melro, Matheson, & Bombay, 2023). Differences in the outcomes between cohorts make the overall results difficult to interpret and most changes were non-significant. The authors highlighted that the course had unintended consequences in some outcomes, particularly in one cohort, that might relate to a weaker pre-course belief that ongoing colonialism contributes to health inequities. They recommend that the implementation of Indigenous educational interventions be rigorously evaluated to ensure that outcomes are as intended (Melro et al., 2023).

Several Canadian schools of medicine have also implemented shorter, less resource-intensive experiences but most of those published focused on medical residents. For example, similar to a poverty simulation model used to teach interns about sociodemographic factors impacting health (Hsieh & Coates, 2018), medical students in Ontario developed a series of 14 scenarios in which the learner role-played an Indigenous person. The scenarios were co-developed by a team involving members of four Indigenous communities (urban, rural, and remote) using a sharing circle to capture experiences involving health system encounters and addressing various social determinants of health. The program was called Stand Up for Indigenous Health and was piloted in two Ontario residency programs with 29 non-Indigenous volunteers. The intervention consisted of 2-hour facilitated modules, and the facilitators included a local Indigenous community member.

As learners worked through the modules, they were provided a running monetary and stress balance, to reflect the difficulties they encountered and the choices they made to overcome obstacles. The session concluded with a group discussion/debrief. Residents reported higher empathy scores, self-perceived knowledge of social determinants of health in Indigenous communities, and higher motivation to use culturally safe practices when interacting with Indigenous clients (Sauve, Cappelletti, & Murji, 2022).

Although longer courses with experiential components might be desirable, they must be effectively integrated within curricula (Schoenherr & Hamstra, 2024). Before introducing the four-week course described above, Western University trialled a 3-hour seminar for first and second-year medical students. The learning objectives focused on Indigenous health issues, socioeconomic influences on their health, communicating with people with different cultures and languages, and addressing stereotypes. The material was presented by two professors with Indigenous ancestry. Students completed pre–post surveys. In the short term, students had increased knowledge and a better understanding of socioeconomic impacts on health and felt more confident about providing care for Indigenous people after the seminar. However, longer-term impacts have not been reported (Zhou et al., 2012).

The University of Toronto used the KAIROS Blanket Exercise (KBE) to raise the critical consciousness of medical students. Critical consciousness is defined as an awareness of the views of individuals, others, and the world to appreciate embedded social inequities and to challenge existing power dynamics thereby increasing the practice of cultural safety (Herzog, Wright, Pennington, & Richardson, 2021). The KBE is a short, immersive role-playing experience followed by a reflective debriefing led by Indigenous facilitators that was developed by Indigenous elders and teachers and the Aboriginal Rights Coalition (KAIROS Canada, 2019). Most KBE participants appreciated the opportunity to reflect on their experience and enhance their knowledge. They reported perspective shifts on issues like health inequity, privilege, and bias and acknowledged the need to be active participants in reconciliation (Herzog et al., 2021).

7.3 The Elder-in-Residence Program at the University of Alberta

As described by Mosom (Cree "Grandfather") Rick Lightning, the Elder-in-Residence program has evolved over approximately the last six years to include providing his perspective on University and Faculty of Medicine and Dentistry policies, increase awareness of Indigenous issues amongst the faculty ("None of them had met an Indian at the beginning"), advocacy and support Indigenous and non-Indigenous students in their medical school journey. The position is part of Wâpanachakos ("Morningstar", Indigenous Health Program) at the University of Alberta, whose mandate is to increase the number of Indigenous students pursuing medical degrees and to provide those students with the resources and support they need to be successful. Working with Alberta First Nations, Wâpanachakos has created cultural safety in admission processes and coursework, increased culturally relevant program content, and provided training on-reserve and in other northern, rural, and remote communities.

As Mosom, Mr. Lightning's perspective is to embrace all ancestries and cultures. When he invites individuals to participate in traditional Cree ceremonies, such as a sweat, he encourages everyone to bring their families and reflect upon their place in their family, to pray in their language, and to better understand themselves ("White people have ancestors, too"). Over the years, he has invited the entire medical and dental undergraduate cohort, Indigenous and non-Indigenous to his community of Maskwacîs, to participate in ceremonies at the community powwow grounds, share a potluck meal featuring foods from all participants' cultures, pray in each person's language, and meet with Cree elders. He notes that "…this is a human thing, not an Indian thing". Confronting misconceptions arising from ignorance is important for building trusting relationships. In recent years, he has partnered with Métis communities to provide similar experiences and is working to identify opportunities with Inuit peoples. Through these encounters, he seeks to build lasting partnerships because "partners will stand with you" and promote coming together as nations.

The Elder-in-Residence has many opportunities to use his position and vast life experience at the policy level. He has promoted the concept of tenured elders across the university, to ensure the longevity of their association so that enduring relationships can be built with students. He serves on many committees and is usually the only voice for Indigenous concerns or perspectives. He consults across the College of Health Sciences (which includes nursing, pharmacy, kinesiology, public health, and rehabilitation medicine). Having had a 25-year career with the United Nations, he is unafraid to exercise his policy expertise, confront colonialism, and racism within the University and advocate for change. When asked if he felt University initiatives such as creating an Indigenous strategic plan make a difference, he replied that even moving an inch is progress and that we must continue to ask uncomfortable questions and be motivated to change by the uncomfortable answers to those questions.

7.4 Discussion

The purpose of this chapter was to highlight innovations in health professions education that were designed to reduce health inequities experienced by Indigenous peoples in Canada through decolonizing practices. Unfortunately, despite clear Calls to Action of the TRC and, in many instances much goodwill on all sides, many challenges still exist. Conrad's story illustrates many of the issues prevalent in our current healthcare systems across Canada:

- Lack of knowledge of healthcare professionals of the burden of chronic diseases such as diabetes in Indigenous populations, including children and youth,
- Poor access to healthcare facilities, including distance and lack of transportation,
- Isolation from family and friends while receiving care; no one to advocate for the patient or help interpret and implement the care plan,

- Unprofessional conduct of healthcare staff, including overt and covert racism, prejudice, lack of consultation with the patient and family,
- Difficulty in navigating the system, including community supports.

The literature documents many advances towards decolonizing curricula of nursing and medical schools in Canada, yet faces ongoing challenges such as the "hidden curriculum" – lingering colonial, institutional, and structural processes that obstruct learning goals, difficulty in prioritizing cultural safety and competency education amongst all the other demands of the curriculum and being mindful of unintended consequences, such as entrenching rather than reducing stereotypes (de Leeuw et al., 2021; Jacklin et al., 2014). A review of material published online by Canadian nursing and midwifery programs, found that only about 20% had fully implemented the TRC recommendations up to June 2020 (Metheny & Dion Fletcher, 2021). Moreover, teaching cultural safety appropriately means exposing students to Indigenous perspectives that are locally relevant (Thurston & Mashford-Pringle, 2015). Indigenous nursing students from one Canadian program identified persistent gaps or practices that made them feel culturally unsafe, the need for ongoing training of faculty, and opportunities for them to create relationships with their peers using traditional Indigenous methodologies such as sharing circles (Van Bewer & Sawchyn, 2024).

The examples provided in this review all involve input from Indigenous partners or consultants to a varying degree, including course development, community involvement, and/or Indigenous teachers in the classroom. Clearly, partnerships are at the core of many sustained interventions but this raises the issue of knowledge ownership and the potential for misappropriation (Stansfield & Browne, 2013). Interestingly, trainees are driving some of the change, as exemplified by the publications from (Sauve et al., 2022; Zhou et al., 2012) but sustainability is likely to be low without institutional backing. It also appears that many of the programs have not published their innovations. Consequently, there is a gap in the full understanding of curricular innovation, and explicit assessment of their successes and failures. Explicit attempts must be made to assess the implementation validity of these programs and ensure that the curriculum addresses the community of learners and health seekers that they serve (Schoenherr & Hamstra, 2024).

Some authors express pessimism that settler-educators can overcome their backgrounds rooted in our racial-colonial hierarchy and lack of a deep understanding of racism, despite their empathy for the health inequities faced by Indigenous peoples (Sylvestre, Castleden, Denis, Martin, & Bombay, 2019). Moreover, even after training using Indigenous instructors and epistemologies, students entering their profession encounter entrenched attitudes and behaviors that they find difficult to counter (Braithwaite et al., 2022); thus it could take a generation to adequately change the work environment. Still, others argue that in our post-COVID educational environment, "Indigenuity" or resilience, innovation, and adaptation delivered using traditional Indigenous methods are needed more than ever to counter the upheaval (Brant-Birioukov, 2021).

7.5 Land Acknowledgement

The University of Alberta in Edmonton, Alberta, is situated in Treaty 6 Territory. The City of Edmonton (Amiskwaciwâskahikan in Cree) is home to more than 76,000 Indigenous people. The authors respectfully acknowledge the peoples who have inhabited these lands since time immemorial: the Cree, Blackfoot, Métis, Nakota Sioux, Iroquois, Dene, Ojibway/Saulteaux/Anishinaabe, Inuit, and many others. We thank them for their stewardship of these lands, for enriching our lives with their histories, languages, and cultures and for their willingness to engage with us on a journey of reconciliation.

References

Anderson, M. A., Crowshoe, L., Diffey, L., Green, M., Kitty, D., Lavallee, B., … Richardson, L. (2019). *Joint Commitment to Action on Indigenous Health*. Retrieved from www.afmc.ca/wp-content/uploads/2022/10/AFMC_Position_Paper_JCAIH_EN.pdf.

Association of Faculties of Medicine of Canada. (2020). *Joint Commitment to Action on Indigenous Health (JCAIH) Update Report*. Retrieved from www.afmc.ca/wp-content/uploads/2022/10/JCAIH_School-Survey-Responses_FINAL-REPORT_v4.pdf.

Bain, M. (2014). *Community-University Engagement: Case Study of a Partnership on Coast Salish Territory in British Columbia*. (Master of Arts Thesis). Vancouver, BC: University of British Columbia.

Beavis, A. S., Hojjati, A., Kassam, A., Choudhury, D., Fraser, M., Masching, R., & Nixon, S. A. (2015). What all students in healthcare training programs should learn to increase health equity: Perspectives on postcolonialism and the health of aboriginal peoples in Canada. *BMC Medical Education, 15*, 155. doi: 10.1186/s12909-015-0442-y.

Blanchet Garneau, A., Belisle, M., Lavoie, P., & Laurent Sedillot, C. (2021). Integrating equity and social justice for indigenous peoples in undergraduate health professions education in Canada: A framework from a critical review of literature. *International Journal for Equity in Health, 20*(1), 123. doi: 10.1186/s12939-021-01475-6.

Braithwaite, T. J., Kelly, L. P., & Chakanyuka, C. (2022). File of uncertainties: Exploring student experience of applying decolonizing knowledge in practice. *Quality Advancement in Nursing Education – Avancées en Formation Infirmière, 8*(3), 1–37. doi: 10.17483/2368-6669.1351.

Brant-Birioukov, K. (2021). Covid-19 and In(di)genuity: Lessons from indigenous resilience, adaptation, and innovation in times of crisis. *Prospects (Paris), 51*(1–3), 247–259. doi: 10.1007/s11125-021-09557-7.

Brock, M. B., Fowler, L. B., Freeman, J. G., Richardson, D. C., & Barnes, L. J. (2019). Cultural immersion in the education of healthcare professionals: A systematic review. *Journal of Educational Evaluation for Health Professions, 16*, 4. doi: 10.3352/jeehp.2019.16.4.

Buchanan, K., Velandia, M., Weckend, M., & Bayes, S. (2021). Learning objectives of cultural immersion programs: A scoping review. *Nurse Education Today, 100*, 104832. doi: 10.1016/j.nedt.2021.104832.

Burgess, C. (2017). Beyond cultural competence: Transforming teacher professional learning through aboriginal community-controlled cultural immersion. *Critical Studies in Education, 60*(4), 477–495. doi: 10.1080/17508487.2017.1306576.

Burgess, C., & Cavanagh, P. (2015). Cultural immersion: Developing a community of practice of teachers and aboriginal community members. *The Australian Journal of Indigenous Education, 45*(1), 48–55. doi: 10.1017/jie.2015.33.

Canadian Association of Schools of Nursing. (2020). *CASN Accreditation Standards and Framework.* Retrieved from https://accred.casn.ca/content/user_files/2023/10/EN-CASN-Accreditation-Standards-Aug-30-2022-plus-TRC.pdf.

Coke, S., Kuper, A., Richardson, L., & Cameron, A. (2016). Northern perspectives on medical elective tourism: A qualitative study. *CMAJ Open, 4*(2), E277–E283. doi: 10.9778/cmajo.20160001.

Committee on Accreditation of Canadian Medical Schools. (2021). *CACMS Standards and Elements*. Retrieved from https://cacms-cafmc.ca/wp-content/uploads/2022/12/CACMS_Standards_and_Elements_AY_2022-2023.pdf.

Cook, C., MacKinnon, M., Anderson, M., & Whetter, I. (2019). Structures last longer than intentions: Creation of ongomiizwin – Indigenous Institute of Health and Healing at the University of Manitoba. *International Journal of Circumpolar Health, 78*(2), 1571381. doi: 10.1080/22423982.2019.1571381.

Cranston, J., & Whitford, R. (2022). Still thriving: A case illustrating how COVID-19 affected indigenous health and wellness. *Canadian Journal of Educational Administration and Policy, 200*, 96–103.

Crown-Indigenous Relations and Northern Affairs Canada. (2024). Truth and Reconciliation Commission of Canada. Retrieved from www.rcaanc-cirnac.gc.ca/eng/1450124405592/1529106060525.

de Leeuw, S., Larstone, R., Fell, B., Cross, N., Greenwood, M., Auerbach, K., & Sutherland, J. (2021). Educating medical students' "hearts and minds": A humanities- informed cultural immersion program in indigenous experiential community learning. *International Journal of Indigenous Health, 16*(1), 87–107. doi: 10.32799/ijih.v16i1.33078.

First Nations Information Governance Centre. (2016). Our Data, Our Stories, Our Future: The National Report of the First Nations Regional Early Childhood, Education and Employment Survey. Retrieved from https://fnigc.ca/sites/default/files/docs/fnigc_fnreees_national_report_2016_en_final.pdf.

Gall, A., Anderson, K., Howard, K., Diaz, A., King, A., Willing, E., … Garvey, G. (2021). Wellbeing of indigenous peoples in Canada, Aotearoa (New Zealand) and the United States: A systematic review. *International Journal of Environmental Research and Public Health, 18*, 5832. doi: 10.3390/ijerph18115832.

Government of Canada. (2017). Indigenous Peoples and Communities. Retrieved from www.rcaanc-cirnac.gc.ca/eng/1100100013785/1529102490303.

Government of Canada. (2019). Canada Health Act. *Justice Laws Website.* Retrieved from https://laws-lois.justice.gc.ca/eng/acts/c-6/fulltext.html.

Hanson, E. (2009). Reserves – Indian Reserves. *Indigenous Foundations.* Retrieved from https://indigenousfoundations.arts.ubc.ca/reserves/#:~:text=Colonial%20authorities%20and%20some%20Aboriginal,so%20practices%20varied%20between%20regions.

Hanson, E., Gamez, D., & Manuel, A. (2020). The residential school system. *Indigenous Foundations.* Retrieved from indigenousfoundations.arts.ubc.ca/residential-school-system-2020/.

Health Canada. (1985). About Mission, Values, Activities. Retrieved from www.canada.ca/en/health-canada/corporate/about-health-canada/activities-responsibilities/mission-values-activities.html.

Herzog, L. S., Wright, S. R., Pennington, J. J., & Richardson, L. (2021). The KAIROS blanket exercise: Engaging indigenous ways of knowing to foster critical consciousness in medical education. *Medical Teacher, 43*(12), 1437–1443. doi: 10.1080/0142159X.2021.1956679.

Hoffart, C., Kuster-Orban, C., Spooner, C., & Neudorf, K. (2013). Intraprofessional practice education using a community partnership model. *Journal of Nursing Education, 52*(2), 104–107. doi: 10.3928/01484834-20130121-01.

Hsieh, D. T., & Coates, W. C. (2018). Poverty simulation: An experiential learning tool for teaching social determinants of health. *AEM Education and Training, 2*(1), 51–54. doi: 10.1002/aet2.10076.

Hudson, G. L., & Maar, M. (2022). *The Making of the World's Only Medical School Mandatory Placement in Indigenous Communities: Northern Ontario School of Medicine (NOSM)*. In D. Gavrus, & S. Lamb (Eds.), *Transforming Medical Education: Historical Case Studies of Teaching, Learning, and Belonging in Medicine* (pp. 252–277). McGill-Queen's University Press

Indigenous Physicians Association of Canada–Association of Faculties of Medicine. (2008). *First Nations, Inuit, Métis Health Core Competencies: A Curriculum Framework for Undergraduate Medical Education*. Retrieved from www.nccih.ca/634/First_Nations,_Inuit_and_Métis_Health_Core_Competencies__A_Curriculum_Framework_for_Undergraduate_Me....nccih?id=984&col=3.

Jacklin, K., Strasser, R., & Peltier, I. (2014). From the community to the classroom: The aboriginal health curriculum at the Northern Ontario School of Medicine. *Canadian Journal of Rural Medicine: The Official Journal of the Society of Rural Physicians of Canada = Journal canadien de la medecine rurale: le journal officiel de la Societe de medecine rurale du Canada, 19*(4), 143–150.

Jardine, C., & Lines, L.-A. (2018). Social and structural determinants of indigenous health. In H. Exner-Pirot, B. Norbye, & L. Butler (Eds.) *Northern and Indigenous Health and Healthcare*. Saskatoon, Canada: University of Saskatchewan.

Jones, R., Crowshoe, L., Reid, P., Calam, B., Curtis, E., Green, M., … Ewen, S. (2019). Educating for indigenous health equity: An international consensus statement. *Academic Medicine: Journal of the Association of American Medical Colleges, 94*(4), 512–519. doi:10.1097/ACM.0000000000002476.

KAIROS Canada. (2019). History of the blanket exercise. Retrieved from www.kairoscanada.org

Kennedy, A., Sehgal, A., Szabo, J., McGowan, K., Lindstrom, G., Roach, P., … Barnabe, C. (2022). Indigenous strengths-based approaches to healthcare and health professions education – Recognising the value of elders' teachings. *Health Education Journal, 81*(4), 423–438. doi: 10.1177/00178969221088921.

King, M., Smith, A., & Gracey, M. (2009). Indigenous health part 2: The underlying causes of the health gap. *The Lancet, 374*, 76–85.

Kline, C. C., Godolphin, W. J., Chhina, G. S., & Towle, A. (2013). Community as teacher model: Health profession students learn cultural safety from an Aboriginal community. *Michigan Journal of Community Service Learning, 20*(1), 5–17.

Lavoie, J. G., Kornelsen, D., Wylie, L., Mignone, J., Dwyer, J., Boyer, Y., … O'Donnell, K. (2016). Responding to health inequities: Indigenous health system innovations. *Global Health, Epidemiology, and Genomics, 1*, e14. doi: 10.1017/gheg.2016.12.

Ma, T. P. (2024). Considerations for implementation of a competency-based education program for preclerkship courses. In J. R. Schoenherr, & M. M. McConnell (Eds.), *Fundamentals and Frontiers of Medical Education and Decision-Making* (pp. 37–79). Routledge.

Maar, M., Boesch, L., & Tobe, S. (2018). Enhancing indigenous health research capacity in Northern Ontario through distributed community engaged medical education at

NOSM: A qualitative evaluation of the community engagement through research pilot program. *Canadian Medical Education Journal*, *9*(1, Special Issue), e21–e32.

Markham, R., Hunt, M., Woollard, R., Oelke, N., Snadden, D., Strasser, R., … Graham, S. (2021). Addressing rural and Indigenous health inequities in Canada through socially accountable health partnerships. *BMJ Open*, *11*(11), e048053. doi: 10.1136/bmjopen-2020-048053.

Mashford-Pringle, A., Skura, C., Stutz, S., & Yohathasan, T. (2021). *What We Heard: Indigenous Peoples and COVID-19*. Retrieved from www.canada.ca/content/dam/phac-aspc/documents/corporate/publications/chief-public-health-officer-reports-state-public-health-canada/from-risk-resilience-equity-approach-covid-19/indigenous-peoples-covid-19-report/cpho-wwh-report-en.pdf.

Matthews, E. J., Clune, L., Luhanga, F., & Loewen, R. (2021). The impact of cultural immersion international learning experiences on cultural competence of nursing students: A critical integrative review. *Journal of Professional Nursing*, *37*(5), 875–884. doi: 10.1016/j.profnurs.2021.07.002.

McGann, S. (2013). *Manifestations of Colonialism in Canada.* (MSc). Toronto, Canada: Metropolitan University, (Paper 2088).

Melro, C. M., Matheson, K., & Bombay, A. (2023). Beliefs around the causes of inequities and intergroup attitudes among health professional students before and after a course related to indigenous peoples and colonialism. *BMC Medical Education*, *23*(1), 277. doi: 10.1186/s12909-023-04248-7.

Metheny, N., & Dion Fletcher, C. (2021). An environmental scan of indigenous cultural safety in Canadian baccalaureate nursing and midwifery programs. *Canadian Journal of Nursing Research*, *53*(4), 417–425. doi: 10.1177/08445621211016143.

Nguyen, N. H., Subhan, F. B., Williams, K., & Chan, C. B. (2020). Barriers and mitigating strategies to healthcare access in indigenous communities of Canada: A narrative review. *Healthcare (Basel, Switzerland)*, *8*(2). doi: 10.3390/healthcare8020112.

Northern Ontario School of Medicine. (2018). *Gathering Together for Life and Wellbeing. Gididaa Bimaadiziwin Wenji-Maamoobiidin*. Retrieved from www.nosm.ca/wp-content/uploads/2019/02/Gathering-Report-Gididaa-Bimaadiziwin-Wenji-Maamoobiiding.pdf.

OECD. (2020). Linking indigenous communities with regional development in Canada. *OECD iLibrary*. Retrieved from www.oecd-ilibrary.org/sites/e6cc8722-en/index.html?itemId=/content/component/e6cc8722-en.

Olapade-Olaopa, E. O, Adisa, A. O., Olopade, F. E., Lawal, T., A., Hammad, N., Iputo, J. E. & Scott-Emuakpor, A. B. (2027). Medical Education in Sub-Saharan Africa. In J. R. Schoenherr (Ed.), *Fundamentals and Frontiers of Medical Education and Decision-Making: Innovation, Implementation, and Translational Research* (pp. 412–461). Routledge.

Public Health Agency of Canada. (2022). *Framework for Diabetes in Canada*. Retrieved from www.canada.ca/en/public-health/services/publications/diseases-conditions/framework-diabetes-canada.html.

Reading, C. L., & Wien, F. (2009). *Health Inequalities and Social Determinants of Aboriginal Peoples' Health*. Prince George, Canada: National Collaborating Cengtre for Aboriginal Health.

Reid, P., & Robson, B. (2007). Understanding health inequities. In B. Robson & R. Harris (Eds.), *Hauora: Māori Standards of Health IV. A Study of the Years 2000-2005.* (pp. 3–10). Wellington, New Zealand: Te Rōpū Rangahau Hauora a Eru Pōmare.

Rohatinsky, N., Exner-Pirot, H., Parent-Bergeron, M., Bosevski, K., & Pratt, C. (2018). Indigenous nursing students' readiness for practice perceptions - Les perceptions d'étudiantes autochtones en sciences infirmières quant à leur préparation à la pratique.

Quality Advancement in Nursing Education - Avancées En Formation Infirmière, *4*(2). doi: 10.17483/2368-6669.1133

Sauve, A., Cappelletti, A., & Murji, L. (2022). Stand up for indigenous health: A simulation to educate residents about the social determinants of health faced by indigenous peoples in Canada. *Academic Medicine: Journal of the Association of American Medical Colleges*, *97*(4), 518–523. doi: 10.1097/ACM.0000000000004570.

Schoenherr, J. R. (2027a). The development and dynamics of heterarchical structure in Mayan medical education and healthcare ecosystems. In Schoenherr, J. R. (Ed.), *Fundamentals and Frontiers of Medical Education and Decision-Making: Innovation, Implementation, and Translational Research* (pp. 359-411). Routledge.

Schoenherr, J. R. (2027b). Innovation and implementation in the health professions: Translating research in education and healthcare delivery. In Schoenherr, J. R. (Ed.), *Fundamentals and Frontiers of Medical Education and Decision-Making: Innovation, Implementation, and Translational Research* (pp. 359–411). Routledge.

Schoenherr, J. R. & Beaudoin, J. (2027). Medical heterarchies in East Asian medical education: The evolving landscape of health professions education in East Asia. In Schoenherr, J. R. (Ed.), *Fundamentals and Frontiers of Medical Education and Decision- Making: Innovation, Implementation, and Translational Research* (pp. 462–509). Routledge.

Schoenherr, J. R. & McConnell, M. (Eds.) (2024). Human-centered design in health professions education: Informing competency-based education with psychological science. In Schoenherr, J. R. & McConnell, M. (Eds.), *Fundamentals and Frontiers of Medical Education and Decision-Making Educational Theory and Psychological Practice*, Routledge.

Schoenherr, R. J. & Hamstra, S. J. (2024) Validity in health professions education. From assessment instruments to program innovation and evaluation. In Schoenherr, R. J. & McConnell, M. M. (Eds.), *Fundamentals and Frontiers of Medical Education and Decision-Making* (p. 28). 1st Edition. Routledge.

Stansfield, D., & Browne, A. J. (2013). The relevance of indigenous knowledge for nursing curriculum. *International Journal of Nursing Education Scholarship*, *10*(1), 143–151.

Statistics Canada. (2005). Projections of the Aboriginal Populations, Canada, Provinces and Territories 91-547-X. Retrieved from www150.statcan.gc.ca/n1/en/catalogue/91-547-X.

Strasser, R., Hogenbirk, J., Jacklin, K., Maar, M., Hudson, G., Warry, W., … Carson, D. (2018). Community engagement: A central feature of NOSM's socially accountable distributed medical education. *Canadian Medical Education Journal*, *9*(1), e33–e43. Retrieved from www.ncbi.nlm.nih.gov/pmc/articles/PMC6104326/pdf/CMEJ-9-e033.pdf.

Strasser, R. P., Lanphear, J. H., McCready, W. G., Topps, M. H., Hunt, D. D., & Matte, M. C. (2009). Canada's new medical school: The Northern Ontario School of Medicine: Social accountability through distributed community engaged learning. *Academic Medicine: Journal of the Association of American Medical Colleges*, *84*(10), 1459–1464. doi: 10.1097/ACM.0b013e3181b6c5d7.

Sylvestre, P., Castleden, H., Denis, J., Martin, D., & Bombay, A. (2019). The tools at their fingertips: How settler colonial geographies shape medical educators' strategies for grappling with anti-indigenous racism. *Social Science and Medicine*, *237*, 112363. doi: 10.1016/j.socscimed.2019.112363.

Thurston, J. M., & Mashford-Pringle, A. (2015). Nursing & indigenous education integration. *Journal of Nursing Educaion and Practice*, *5*(10), 9. doi: 10.5430/jnep.vXnXpXX.

Tiwari, T., Jamieson, L., Broughton, J., Lawrence, H. P., Batliner, T. S., Arantes, R., & Albino, J. (2018). Reducing indigenous oral health inequalities: A review from 5 nations. *Journal of Dental Research*, *97*(8), 869–877.

University of Victoria. (2024). Undergraduate calendar – September 2024: NURS484 – Understanding indigenous health and wellness. In U. O. Victoria (Ed.): University of Victoria.

Van Bewer, V., & Sawchyn, M. (2024). Enhancing nursing education for indigenous students: Indigenous nursing students' insights and strategies. *Nurse Educaion Today*, *137*, 106157. doi: 10.1016/j.nedt.2024.106157.

Van Bewer, R., Woodgate, R., Martin, D., & Deer, F. (2020). The importance and promise of integrating indigenous perspectives in nursing education. *Witness: The Canadian Journal of Critical Nursing Discourse*, *2*(1), 11–24. doi: 10.25071/2201-5796.46

Venosa, A. R., Baroneza, J. E., & Fernandes, R. A. F. (2027). Medical Education in Brazil: A History of An Evolving Pluralistic Health Care System. In J. R. Schoenherr (Ed.), *Fundamentals and Frontiers of Medical Education and Decision-Making: Innovation, Implementation, and Translational Research* (pp. 310–335). Routledge.

Williams, N. G., Alberton, A. M., & Gorey, K. M. (2022). Morbid and mortal inequities among indigenous people in Canada and the United States during the COVID-19 pandemic critical review of relative risks and protections. *Journal of Indigenous Social Development*, *11*(1), 3–32.

Wylie, L., & McConkey, S. (2018). Insiders' insight: Discrimination against indigenous peoples through the eyes of health care professionals. *Journal of Racial and Ethnic Health Disparities*, *6*(1), 37–45. doi: 10.1007/s40615-018-0495-9.

Zhou, A. W., Boshart, S., Seelisch, J., Eshaghian, R., McLeod, R., Nisker, J., … Howard, J. M. (2012). Efficacy of a 3-hour aboriginal health teaching in the medical curriculum: Are we changing student knowledge and attitudes? *Health Education Journal*, *71*(2), 180–188. doi: 10.1177/0017896910394544.

8

MEDICAL EDUCATION IN BRAZIL

A History of an Evolving Pluralistic Healthcare System

Alessandra Ramos Venosa, José Eduardo Baroneza, and Rachel Aparecida Ferreira Fernandes

8.1 Introduction

Brazilian medical education turns 218 years old in 2026. Before the first medical educational course was created in 1808, in the city of Salvador, Bahia, the teaching and exercise of healing practices were already widespread in Brazilian territory defined by the eclectic cultural influences of indigenous, African, and European practitioners (Zank et al., 2017; Miliken & Albert, 1996; Alves, 2009). Like many other healthcare systems in the world, these traditions have both complimented and conflicted with one another in terms of health beliefs, the authority of practitioners, and how knowledge is transmitted (Baer et al., 2013; Hanh, 1995; for examples in this volume, see Schoenherr, 2027; Schoenherr & Beaudoin, 2027) (Figure 8.1).

With the arrival of the Portuguese on the east coast of South America in 1500 AD, the indigenous peoples already had extensive knowledge of the medicinal properties of plants and many ancestral healing practices (de Mello, 1980; Monteiro & Brandelli, 2017). Reports from the first explorers describe that the indigenous peoples of Brazil enjoyed exceptional health conditions, had plenty of food, and had many developed social norms and conventions (Botelho & Costa, 2006).

In the Brazilian pre-colonial period (1500–1530), there were no formal medical institutions in the territory and both the indigenous people and most explorers resorted to the ancestral practices and indigenous knowledge when they needed treatment for illnesses (Johnson & Silva, 1992). Predominantly Jewish and Christian surgeons, barbers, and apothecaries were among those who left Europe fleeing the Inquisition and landed in Brazil in the 1530s with the approval of the Portuguese court (Rodrigues & Fiolhais, 2013).

From 1530 to the present, Brazil went from being a Portuguese colony (1530–1822) to an independent nation and, as such, changed its government regime from

DOI: 10.4324/9781003498155-8

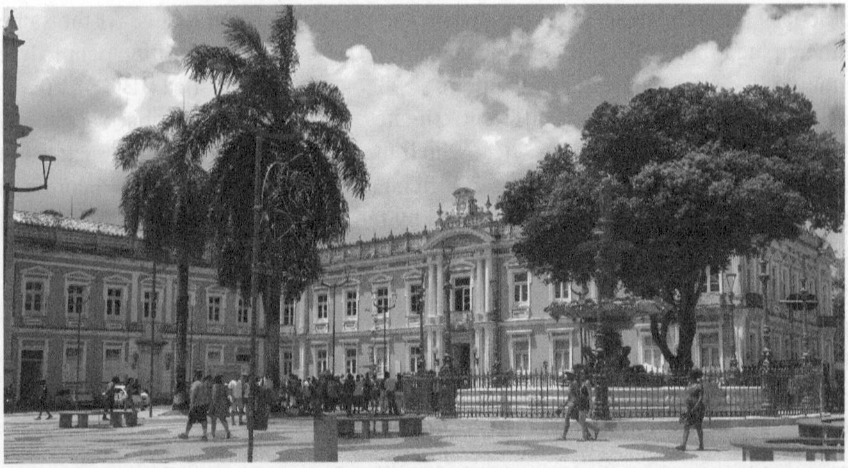

FIGURE 8.1 Building of the Bahia School of Surgery, the first medical school in Brazil.
Source: Gomes (2020).

a monarchy (1822–1889) to a Republic (1889 to the present). During those years, immigrants from different parts of the world arrived in Brazil; many of these people were Africans and their descendants, brought by European colonizers. They constituted more than two thirds of the Brazilian population between the 17th and 19th centuries (Mussa, 1991) and remain in the majority today.

In the 500 years that have passed, healing practices and the knowledge associated with them have developed and transformed in Brazil, due to the relationships between its indigenous peoples, colonizers, and immigrants. Traditional knowledge remains a persistent influence on medical practice (Alves, 2009), while scientific, technological, and humanistic developments outside of Brazil have also revolutionized both the practice and teaching of Medicine (Batista et al., 2015). For instance, as Barbosa et al. (2016) have noted:

> it can be said that this set of knowledge, although modified, reinvented and resignified in the current reality of the current social context in Brazil, coexists with the medical knowledge instituted by scientism, constitutes a rich heritage of human history and of the human sciences and of health, still representing a vast field for research today.
>
> *(p. 75)*

Currently, Brazil is the fifth largest country in the world, with approximately half of its territory covered by forests (Serviço Florestal Brasileiro (SFA), 2013). These forests are home to approximately 500,000 indigenous people (Instituto Brasileiro de Geografia e Estatística (IBGE), 2012), who continue to use ancestral healing practices through rituals invoking spirits and using medicinal plants. At the same time, in the urban and agrarian regions of Brazil, more than 200 million people live today, 85% in cities (Instituto Brasileiro de Geografia e Estatística (IBGE), 2015), in a complex territory with different climates, demographic distributions, social and epidemiological characteristics, which makes the unique healing practices in each region, although the teaching of official medicine is conducted by a common national curriculum guideline, supported by the most modern concepts of medical education.

8.2 Teaching Healing Practices in Colonial Brazil: From 1530 to 1889

8.2.1 Prehistory of Medical Practice and Education in Brazil

The prehistory of medical practice in Brazil reflects three parallel systems, one European, one indigenous, and one African, with little interaction between the three due to social, cultural, and linguistic barriers. In 1500 when the Portuguese navigators arrived in the region now known as Brazil, there were thousands of indigenous ethnic groups living a semi-nomadic lifestyle. Due to the pre-literate nature of these First Nations, the little we know about the culture and traditions comes from the descriptions left by the explorers (Holanda, 2003) (Figure 8.2).

The indigenous people were guided by the *Pajés*,[1] who were healers, religious and political leaders of the natives. The Pajés transmitted their knowledge orally to their people and to the European explorers (Batista et al., 2015). They had significant status in their societies. In addition to their leadership roles, Pajés treated the sick and wounded in wars through medicinal plants and begged the deities for help in rituals. These practices were very different from those practiced in European medicine and were typically misinterpreted by Christian colonizers, who believed that they were sorcerers guided by evil spirits (Botelho & Costa, 2006).

Because of their differences with the colonizers, the Pajés encouraged the native peoples to resist the deep changes represented by the arrival of the Europeans (Clastres, 1978). However, as they dominated the territory and saw the possibility of using the natives as a labor force (e.g., to collect medicinal plants; Soublin, 2000, p. 65), the colonizers passed laws and regulations that authorized them to

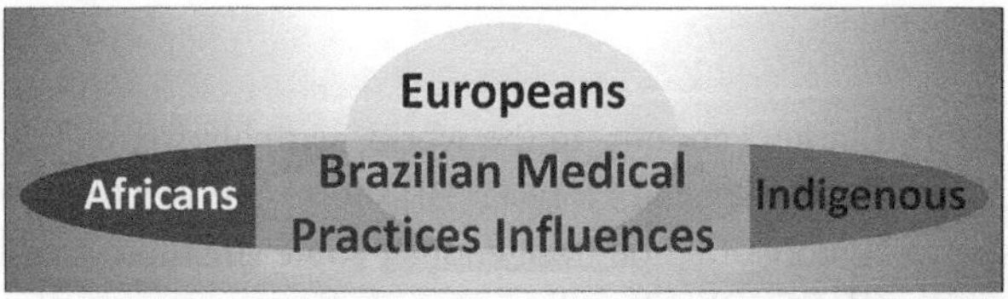

FIGURE 8.2 Source of influence in early Brazilian medical practices.

enslave the natives and eliminate the power of the *Pajés* (Freire, 1991, pp. 41–53; Porro, 2002, pp. 175–96). The enslavement of the natives led to genocide, as stated in the testimony of Manoel Teixeira, a priest who lived in the city of Belém, in the Amazon region, who said on his deathbed in 1654, “In the space of thirty-two years during which this region was conquered, more than 2 million Indians were extinguished, belonging to more than 400 villages” (Freire, 1991, p. 16).

Despite the conflicts with the explorers and their effort to eliminate Pajés’ influence to conquer and maintain the territory, the contact with the South American native people introduced European doctors to important knowledge about the healing properties of local plants and herbs. Over time, they adopted and adapted these indigenous practices to the European traditions that they brought with them, disseminating their newfound knowledge of Brazilian medicinal plants when they returned to Europe (Botelho & Costa, 2006; Walker, 2013, 2016). The exchange of knowledge between the indigenous peoples and the explorers happened since the 16th century, since the ships that docked in Brazil brought, among other professionals, doctors trained in European schools (Rodrigues & Fiolhais, 2013; Peard, 1999).

In addition to the native indigenous, African immigrants have also been part of Brazilian society. Nearly 5 million enslaved Africans were transported to Brazil by the Portuguese (Voeks, 2012) and they brought their own distinct knowledge and healing practices.

Africans made a distinction between what they called "body diseases", such as sores and worms, and “spirit diseases”, which they understood to be caused by witchcraft. Their healing practices involved prayers, and magic rituals (Edler, 2010). Many practices were categorized as “witchcraft” and were condemned in Europe and Brazil due to inquisitorial visits from the Tribunal of the Holy Office, in search of the so-called heretics (Ribeiro, 1997). However, there was greater tolerance of these in the colony, so that many Europeans used the practices of traditional African medicine, in a hidden way, inside their homes (Schwartz, 1988).

The first wave of European practitioners to land in Brazil between the 16th and 18th centuries received their training in Portuguese and Spanish medical schools, where teaching was predominantly based on the theoretical Greek (Hippocrates and Galen) and Arabic texts (Avicenna and Averróis; Batista et al., 2015). Such doctors limited themselves to caring for the colonizers and teaching healing practices to Catholic missionary priests, with the priest being responsible for the healthcare of the indigenous populations at the beginning of the colonial period, who accepted European therapeutic techniques when they converted to Christianity (Torres-Londono, 2000).

To treat the sick, priests used European knowledge about healing practices and indigenous peoples’ knowledge about the properties of medicinal plants, knowledge that is transmitted across generations, through cultural transmission about the relations between health, diseases, and the curative properties of plants (Pezzuti & Chaves, 2009). In addition, Europeans worked as apothecaries who were responsible for planting and harvesting medicinal herbs – of native and of European origin – from which they prepared medicines. The missionaries remained in Brazil from 1549 to 1759, writing therapeutic compendiums that achieved great reputation both in Brazil and in Europe, combining the knowledge of European and indigenous curative practices (Calainho, 2005).

Written by Fernão Cardim between 1548 and 1625, "*Tratados da terra e gente do Brasil*" (Treatises on the land and people of Brazil) described trees and herbs that were useful for medicine. One of the chapters, entitled "Trees that serve as medicine", described plants that could be used to treat diseases, among them the description of herbs used to treat dysentery, sores, headaches, and stomachaches (Cardim, 1925). Similarly, in the 18th century, the publication entitled "*Coleção de várias receitas e segredos particulares da nossa companhia de Portugal, da Índia, de Macau e do Brasil*" (Collection of various recipes and private secrets of our company from Portugal, India, Macau, and Brazil) was a guide for the production of pharmaceuticals from medicinal plants that projected Portuguese America internationally due to the property of its medicinal herbs (França, 2019).

Despite the Portuguese monarchy restricting the practice of medicine to missionaries, healthcare professionals began to become more common after the mid-18th sanctuary. Doctors, barber-surgeons, and apothecaries trained in Portugal began to practice their professions in Brazil (Gurgel, 2011). Often, apothecaries had the greatest knowledge of medical practices and many of them also worked as barbers, surgeons, doctors, and teachers, teaching their skills to citizens. Professions began to form. The Chief Physicist and Chief Surgeon appointed by the Portuguese monarchy to coordinate health services in the colony were at the top of this hierarchy (Romera et al., 2020).

From a decree published in 1800, every year four Brazilian students[2] had to go to the Portuguese city of Coimbra to study Medicine and Surgery (Batista et al., 2015). When they returned to Brazil, they worked as physicians and taught their skills to apprentices who accompanied them in daily practices. Once they were considered suitable by their masters, they took exams in local chambers to obtain a kind of consent for medical practice (Botti, 2009).

In addition to the professionals authorized to work, there were many *curandeiros*, who treated the sick without official medical qualification. The presence of the curandeiros addressed the lack of qualified professionals for health practices, in a workplace where medicine, religion, and magic became inseparable, due the convergence of different origins of the Brazilian people (Lima, 2020).

In indigenous populations who had yet to have contact with the colonizers, their traditional healing practices endured for many centuries. In these traditions, Pajés used rituals that included the interpretation of dreams, the invocation of spirits, and the ingestion of potions prepared with medicinal plants and animal products. Paralleling the European tradition, the pajés also received training using an apprenticeship model between master and learner, focusing on oral transmission of knowledge (Gurgel, 2011). Even today there are similar cultures in indigenous communities in Brazil, in which the pajés are sought both by the natives and people who live outside the native villages as an alternative in the search for a cure for diseases (Silva, 2016).

8.2.2 Formalizing Medical Education in Brazil

In 1808, the Portuguese royal family left Lisbon and moved to Brazil, fleeing the invasion of Portugal by French troops led by Napoleon Bonaparte. Thereafter, the Brazilian territory became the seat of the Portuguese Empire. In the same year, the first official educational courses in medicine were created with the Bahia School of Surgery, founded on February 18 in Salvador, and with the Anatomy and Surgery Course, founded on March 8 in Rio de Janeiro. These three-year courses aimed at training doctors for the Navy and the Army, used military hospitals as a practical teaching setting, and prioritized the teaching of anatomy and surgery, emphasizing the training of surgeons instead of clinicians, since pharmaco-clinical disciplines were absent (Prata, 2010; Flores, 2017).

In 1813, the Director of Medical-Surgical Studies of the Court decided to reform the course located in Rio de Janeiro, transforming it into a medical-surgical academy, which was repeated in 1815 in Salvador. As a result, both medicine courses lasted five years, including the disciplines of Chemistry, Botany, Pharmacology, Hygiene, Internal Medicine, and Etiology of Diseases, beginning the training of clinicians in Brazil and ending the period in which those who worked in the country were only those trained in Europe (Batista et al., 2015).

Following its independence from Portugal, Brazil briefly entered the Imperial Period from 1822 to 1889, ending with the Proclamation of the Republic which resulted in a shift from a monarchy to a presidency. During the Imperial Period, higher education was maintained as centralized under the Crown's monopoly (Flores, 2017). Although advances were made, medical education courses in Brazil were part-time and consisted of multidisciplinary curricula in which each discipline was taught separately without worrying about the integration of knowledge. Theoretical content was provided through lectures and practical activities provided in hospitals (Teixeira, 1989).

Major changes began to emerge in Brazilian medical education in 1829 with the creation of the Medicine Society of Rio de Janeiro. Debates frequently focused on the need for reforms and decision-making in the teaching models adopted in medical education courses (Edler, 2000). In 1832, the two medical-surgical academies were transformed into Faculties of Medicine, with the course of study lasting six years. The curriculum consisted of physics, botany, zoology, mineralogy, general and descriptive anatomy, medical chemistry, pharmacy, physiology, pathology, surgery, internal medicine, clinical surgery, obstetrics and gynecology, pediatrics and childcare, legal medicine, history of medicine and hygiene (Prata, 2010).

Before reforms in the early 1800s, the French anatomical-clinical teaching model dominated. This approach had students attend theoretical classes in conventional classrooms and observed patients in hospital beds. In the hospital, the focus on practical healthcare strategies included auscultation, percussion, pathological analysis of histological sections, clinical instrumentation, autopsy, and statistical analysis (Edler & Fonseca, 2006). Following the French approach that separated theoretical and practical science, the model did not consider the importance of experimental research in teaching, nor the knowledge arising from the use of model organisms to understand human diseases (Bonner, 1995).

Pressured by the dissatisfaction of professors and students in relation to medical education in Brazil, which was considered conservative and obsolete, reforms in 1882 led to changes in the pedagogical projects of the courses. At the core of this approach was the development of a hybrid teaching model that combined the French model and a German model (Santos Filho, 1991). The German model placed emphasis on the use of evidence-based education and decision-making along with humanistic training (Kemp & Edler, 2004). The reform, however, did not change the conservatism that defined medical education in Brazil, which, associated with the foundations of the Roman Catholic Apostolic Church, denied modern materialist, Darwinist, and positivist conceptions (Santos Filho, 1991).

In 1889 Brazil became a Republic, and the Brazilian Constitution of 1891 allowed the provision of higher education by private institutions. In 1898, the third Brazilian medical school was created in Porto Alegre, in southern Brazil. Thus, as the 19th century ended, Brazil now had three medical schools distributed throughout its territories in the northeast, southeast, and south regions (Batista et al., 2015).

8.3 Influences, Reforms, and Expansion of Medical Education from the 20th Century to the Present Day

Although there were some modifications to the curriculum and pedagogical practices of medical education in Brazil during the 19th century, it took over a century after the establishment of the first national school for significant structural, epistemological, and methodological transformations to commence. Following the Republic proclamation, both internal factors (economic, educational, and health policies) and external factors (the Flexner report in the United States, scientific advances in patient care, and new teaching methodologies) directly and indirectly influenced the changes in Brazilian medical education during the 20th century and into the first 20 years of this millennium (Oliveira et al., 2019).

8.3.1 The Evolution of Medical Education in Modern Brazil

The number of medical education courses in Brazil continues to grow. From its three original medical schools, Brazil now has 389 medical schools (Scheffer et al., 2023), second only to India, which has 421 schools in 2016 (Supe, 2016; see Khan,

2024). Although this growth process was continuous, it was not linear but marked by booms in specific periods reflecting their respective political and socioeconomic scenarios (Lopes, 2018).

From 1967 to 1971, Brazil experienced substantial economic growth, known as the "economic miracle" (Bueno & Pieruccini, 2005). The youth population grew quickly, and education quality improved. As a result, there were five times as many students meeting university admission requirements as available spots, leading to pressure to expand the university network, particularly for medical programs. This expansion has been attributed to (a) a national shortage of doctors (Haddad et al., 2010) and (b) the government's concern for the health of workers to ensure the nation's economic progress. This led to a significant increase in medical schools from 40 to 72 in just five years (Braghini, 2014; Nassif, 2022).

Although the opening of these schools was legally authorized by the Ministry of Education and Culture of Brazil (MEC), the government agency responsible for accrediting higher education courses in our country, the abrupt expansion of medical courses raised concerns about the quality and homogeneity of training among medical schools. For this reason, the MEC limited the opening of new courses so that existing courses could be evaluated on-site and checked for compliance with the legal norms for their operation. Only ten new programs were added over the next 25 years (Bueno & Pieruccini, 2005).

In 1988, the enactment of the new Brazilian Constitution, enshrining health as a right of the population and duty of the State (Brazil, 1988), paved the way for the implementation of the current national health system, called the "Sistema Único de Saúde" (SUS; Amaral, 2016). With the principles of universality, equity, and completeness of health for the population, provided for by the SUS (Paim, 2009), a larger number of physicians were required, leading to the second period of expansion of courses in the country. From 1997 to 2008, 93 new courses were created (Sampaio de Carvalho & de Sousa, 2013).

Despite this expansion of medical schools, in 2013, the ratio of physicians to inhabitants was 1.9/1000, below the government target of 2.7/1000 (Saúde, 2015) (see endnote 2)[3] and the World Health Organization recommendation of 2.5/1000 (World Health Organization, 2006). To address this deficit, the More Doctors Program (Programa Mais Médicos) was created that defined three pillars of action: (a) emergency provision of professionals, (b) infrastructure, and (c) medical training (Pinto et al., 2014). The "emergency provision" axis selected professionals who had graduated in Brazil and abroad, to provide care to areas that traditionally did not have sufficient access (Oliveira et al., 2015). The "infrastructure" axis increased funding for the construction of new basic care units and the expansion of existing ones (Saúde, 2015). Finally, the "medical training" axis authorized the creation of new medical schools and additional vacancies in ongoing courses. From 2013 to the present, the greatest expansion of national medical education has been observed, with the creation of 145 new schools and more than 20,000 vacancies for new entrants (Scheffer et al., 2023).

Accompanying the growth of Brazilian medical education courses, there were also trends toward the privatization and the internalization of teaching. Since the founding of the first private school in 1951, the expansion of the private network has been encouraged by various measures that include the following: government tax incentives (at the federal, state, and municipal levels); financing and scholarships for underprivileged students; loans from the National Bank for Economic and Social Development (BNDES) for adapting physical structures; and recommendation for partnerships with existing health establishments, without the need for the costly construction of teaching hospitals by teaching institutions. In the 1980s, the proportion of private medical schools surpassed that of public schools and has continued to rise since then. Currently, there are 268 private and 121 public medical schools.

8.3.2 The Influences of International Context, Public Education, and Health on Curricular Guidelines in Medical Education

The pedagogical model of medical education in Brazil that was marked by French academicism and research by the German school (Gonçalves & Benevides-Pereira, 2009) was replaced in the 20th century by the hegemonic American model molded by the postulates of the Flexner report (Flexner, 1910). The Flexnerian paradigm was defined by the need for creation of medical schools based on university structures, the implementation of a selection process for the admission of students, the construction of equipped laboratories, the replacement of chairs by departments, the segmentation of the course into a basic cycle and a professional cycle, the creation of teaching hospitals, the integration of teaching with research, and the implementation of medical residency. This model came to dominate Brazilian medical education after the 1940s (Boelen, 2002; Kemp & Edler, 2004; González & Almeida, 2010).

Despite its strengths, the Flexnerian paradigm has important limitations. Its emphasis on the regulation and scientific standardization of medical schools, grounded in mechanistic thinking, biologicism, the assumption of disease unicausality, early specialization, and a hospital-centered, curative, and individual approach to care, has contributed to the neglect of biopsychosocial dimensions of the health–disease process. (Singer & Clair, 2003; Singer et al., 2017). It additionally failed to address the need for primary care with the incorporation of collective practices of prevention and health promotion, in addition to purely curative and individual approaches (Boelen et al., 1995; González & Almeida, 2010).

Starting in the 1960s, and intensifying after the creation of SUS, the Ministries of Health and Education took multiple actions that greatly shaped the structure of medical education in Brazil. The Ministries began to place a greater emphasis on interdisciplinarity, basic healthcare in an outpatient setting, and generalist and humanist training (Amoretti, 2005; Lampert et al., 2009). This new direction for national medical education was consolidated with the publication of the first

National Curriculum Guidelines for Medical Education (DCN) in 2001 (Brasil, 2001), which added to the previous guidelines the focus on training reflective professionals, committed to the real needs of the population, willing to work in health planning activities and with the ability to continuously "learn to learn" (Brasil, 2014). Ten years later, in 2025, new guidelines were published, reaffirming the main points of the 2014 version while introducing innovations in the methods used for student and institutional assessment and placing greater emphasis on mental health during the internship period (Brasil, 2025a, 2025b). Also in 2025, ENAMED, the National Examination for the Evaluation of Medical Training, was introduced, led by the Ministry of Education and applied to students in the final year of medical school.

Presently, around 85% of Brazilian medical schools follow the new DCN, although the syllabus may vary (Zanolli et al., 2014). The programs include a minimum of 7200 hours of training, over six years, at least two of which are in-service training (called Internships), under the supervision of professors. Internships require at least 30% of their total workload, which is dedicated to primary care as well as intensive and emergency care. Basic science teaching is contextualized to practice (real or simulated), and practical skills training takes place in clinics and hospitals. Theoretical-practical knowledge must be centered on active methodologies and follow a "spiral" trajectory, from the first years of graduation. This process requires that students coexist with professionals and users of health services, having opportunities to associate the theoretical contents with those absorbed in the practice, building autonomy, capacity for reflection, and meaningful learning. Throughout their training, medical students learn about the importance of social, cultural, behavioral, psychological, ecological, ethical, and legal determinants on both individual and collective levels of the health-disease process (Brasil, 2014). In this holistic context of education, it is noteworthy to highlight that the teaching of "spirituality and health" in Brazilian medical schools has significantly expanded in the last decade, following the example of what has occurred in other parts of the world (Lima, 2020).

The current emphasis in Brazil on training general practitioners who are capable of swiftly entering the job market after graduation, in conjunction with substantial public investment in specialization through medical residency programs (87% funded by public resources), has led to a decline in the ratio of available residency positions to the number of recently graduated physicians (Scheffer et al., 2023). Exclusively within the field of Family Health, there has been a modest rise in the quantity of medical residency vacancies, undertaken as a measure to address the dearth of physicians operating in primary care within remote regions. Consequently, for physicians who choose to pursue specialization and face challenges in obtaining a position within medical residency programs that adhere to the American model (Dezee et al., 2012) regulated by the Ministry of Education, there are two alternative avenues available: (a) specialization following the Taiwanese model (Chow et al., 2012), with criteria approved by the Scientific Council of the Brazilian Medical

Association (AMB), and (b) exams administered by the AMB to obtain the title of specialist, similar to the German model (Nikendei et al., 2009).

While residency and specialization time varies from two to six years, depending on the specialty, a minimum of five years of previous training, supervised by specialists, is necessary for the professional to be able to take the exams to obtain the title. The selection process for admission to residency or medical specialization comprises a written test covering basic areas of practice (Internal Medicine, Pediatrics, Surgery, Gynecology and Obstetrics, Family Medicine, and Public Health), curriculum analysis, and interview. The use of oral or performance tests is still uncommon.

8.3.3 Democratization of Access to Medical Education in Brazil

The educational system in Brazil is composed of both public and private schools, which offer education from early childhood through higher education. Public education is free of charge and government-managed, and it is often the main option for lower social classes with fewer financial resources until the end of high school, while higher social classes tend to attend private schools. When it comes to higher education, the situation is different; access to the public education system is highly competitive. Students who attend private high schools have twice the chance of being accepted into public higher education courses and, in terms of medical schools, the impact of socioeconomic status is significant. In a nationwide study conducted in 2004, it was found that only 9% of graduates from public medical programs had attended public high schools, 79.4% were white and 67% were from families with an income above ten minimum wage salaries (Figueiredo et al., 2022).

The public debate regarding access to higher education has gained importance in Brazil and has encouraged the adoption of inclusion policies based on affirmative action that includes governmental or institutional resolutions. Such policies aim to benefit historically discriminated minorities, mainly blacks, natives, low-income people, and people with disabilities.

In 2012, Law No. 12,711/2012 introduced the requirement that 50% of vacancies at public Universities and Federal Institutes of Education must be allocated to students who attended public high schools and have the objective of minimizing the inequality of access to university education in the country. The distribution of vacancies is assigned based on criteria such as low-income, self-declaration of black or brown skin, indigenous people, and candidates with disabilities. Predating the so-called Law of Quotas, admission policies were already implemented in several institutions, which, supported by state laws, adopted the reservation of a percentage of vacancies for students who attended public schools. The University of Brasília, in 2004, was the first federal university to establish similar affirmative action. The approval of the quota law at the federal level had an impact on many educational institutions that were not obliged, by law, to offer quotas, but which began to implement affirmative admission policies, thus expanding the offer of vacancies for quota holders (Guimarães & Zelaya, 2022).

The implementation of bonus and reservation systems has had a significant impact on the profile of Brazilian university students. As Figure 8.3a demonstrates, there has been a progressive increase in the number of medical students who are self-declared as black or brown with a concomitant decrease in white students between 2013 and 2019. As Figure 8.3b demonstrates, this trend is particularly pronounced in public institutions relative to private institutions (Scheffer et al., 2020).

Affirmative actions have also been adopted to meet the needs of Brazilian indigenous people in terms of their patterns of movement and to ensure access for this population to medical schools. Currently, 43 courses at public institutions have indigenous students enrolled in their programs. This experience brings several positive factors, including contributing to changes in medical education and opening space for protagonism in the academic, scientific, and political environment (Luna et al., 2021).

In addition to democratizing access to places in higher education, it is also essential to adopt measures that help the permanence and conclusion of the course. Assessments of dropout rates show that dropout rates among quota holders were lower or similar to rates among non-quota holders, showing the success of these actions. At the University of Brasilia, for example, the dropout rate among quota and non-quota students was 3.4% and 3.1%, respectively. At the State University of Rio de Janeiro, 26% of quota students dropped out before completing their course, a lower number than the 37% of non-quota students who left before completing their undergraduate degree (Guimarães & Zelaya, 2022).

Another concern is to ensure that the quality of professional training is equal among quota holders and non-quota holders. This information can be accessed by the National Student Performance Exams (ENADE), which evaluates students at the end of the undergraduate course in Brazil. The results obtained in recent years show that the average grades vary between quota holders and non-quota holders, between 5% and 10%, a statistically close value (Guimarães & Zelaya, 2022).

Currently, 73.8% of the vacancies available in Brazilian medical courses are in the private sector and the financial cost of monthly fees is high. Government programs have also been developed to help keep students in private courses such as FIES, a student finance-funding program, and PROUNI (University for All Program) that grants partial and full scholarships, encouraging institutional participation through tax exemption. Both programs positively impact access to private education; in 2014, 35% of higher education vacancies in the private sector were occupied through this type of financing (Nassar et al., 2021).

8.3.4 The Growing Role of Women in Brazilian Medical Education?

Women were initially absent in medical education in the 19th century due to the belief that they were incapable of formally exercising professions in scientific

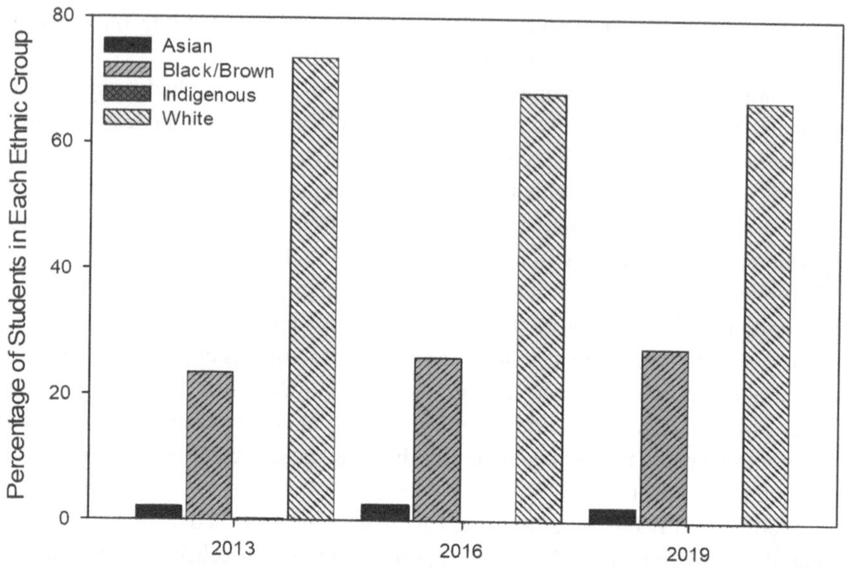

FIGURE 8.3A Self-declared color or race of students completing medical education programs.

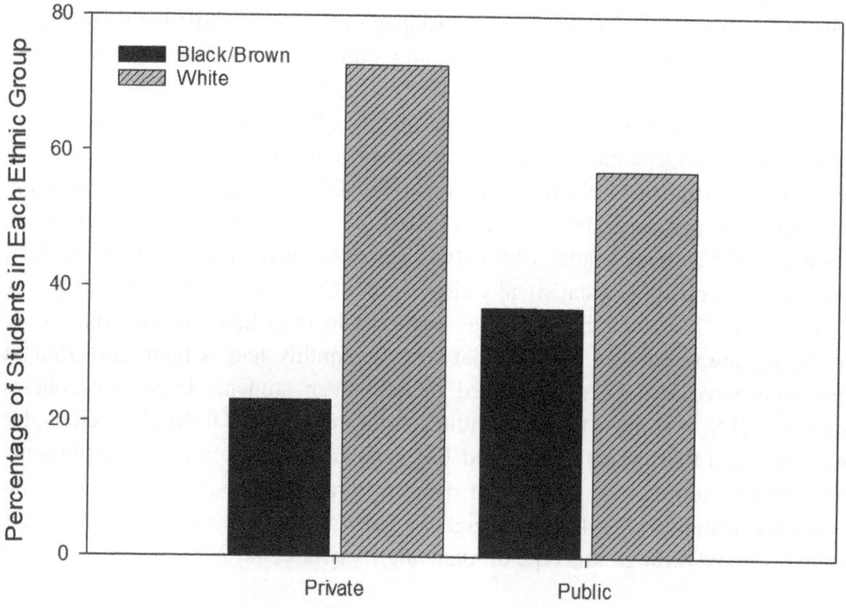

FIGURE 8.3B Self-declared color or race of students completing the medical course distributed by type of institution – public or private – in 2013 and 2019.

areas. This combined with a lack of access to university courses, were obstacles overcome by the first female clinicians: Maria Augusta Generoso Estrela, Rita Lobato Velho Homem, and Maria Odília Teixeira. Maria Augusta Estrela graduated in 1879 from New York Medical College and Hospital for Women. The year of her graduation was a historic milestone in the conquest of space by women in universities, as it marks the moment when women began to have the right to attend higher education courses. Her impact was such that she is honored as the Patroness of the Academia de Medicina de São Paulo (Begliomini, 2022). Rita Lobato has the distinction of becoming the first Brazilian to study medicine in Brazil. She graduated in 1887 from the Faculty of Medicine of Bahia, the first medical school in Brazil. Daring and ahead of her time, she faced strong criticisms for her choice of thesis topic, which was considered offensive at the time for addressing a modest and reserved subject, "Parallel between Methods Commended in Cesarean". Thanks to her strong will and determination, she was also the first woman in Brazil, and second in Latin America, to get the doctorate. Always supported by her family, she continued to practice medicine until the age of 74. Maria Odília Teixeira is also notable in that she was the first black woman to graduate, in medicine in Brazil in 1909. In addition to being a pioneer for an unprecedented achievement for her race, Maria Odília became the first black professor at the Faculty of Medicine of Bahia (Santos, 2019).

These pioneers, examples of courage and persistence, have opened space for Brazilian women who over the decades have been gaining space in the profession.

According to a demographic survey conducted by the Federal Council of Medicine, although men are still the majority among professionals working in the country, the number of women who enroll in medical courses has progressively increased. In the year 2000, women constituted the minority (44%) relative to men (56%). However, by 2009, the number of women enrolled in medical education (50.4%) exceeded that of men for the first time (49.6%). From then on, the number of women has continued to increase. For instance, in 2019, of the 21,941 new doctors in Brazil, 57.5% were women (Scheffer et al., 2020).

Despite the ongoing feminization of medicine, barriers still affect women's professional progress. The structure of medical training requires a great dedication of time and effort, from entering undergraduate courses to medical residency and postgraduate courses. It is in this context that women who choose medicine as a profession are faced with dilemmas common to their gender, such as the option for motherhood and dedication to the family and the career. In the case of a medical student, the challenges will be many and the need for a support network that includes family, friends, and institutional participation stands out (Ávila, 2014).

The rigorous selection criteria for medical residency programs and other postgraduate modalities can present a significant challenge for female candidates, particularly those who are, or plan to be, mothers. Although not an explicit or legal criterion, the responsibilities of motherhood can often disadvantage female candidates in the selection process for residency programs and scholarships, as they may face additional challenges in balancing the demands of their personal and professional lives. A possible consequence is the discrepancy in the presence of women in certain specialties, notably male-dominated fields such as surgery. The limited female representation in the faculty of specialties considered "masculine" aggravates this situation, since female doctors are unlikely to find a tutor or advisor to encourage them. This fact marks the relevance of the presence of women in academic positions, both teaching and administrative, providing a break from gender stereotypes rooted in medical culture (Ávila, 2014).

Brazilian society is experiencing a significant transition in medical history with medical schools playing a fundamental role. The creation of opportunities for discussion between the students, administrators, and professors, as well as affirmative policies that support women in their student careers, can contribute significantly to achieving gender equity in medical education in Brazil (Reigada et al., 2021).

8.4 Challenges of the 21st Century: An Analysis of the Present with Eyes on the Future

8.4.1 Adaptations of Brazilian Medical Schools to Pedagogical and Technological Innovations in the 21st Century

Medical education has been facing the great challenge of adapting to the transformations in the first decades of the 21st century. Changes in individual and collective health needs, technological advances, the growing amount of scientific information, and the changes in scenarios of action in health require institutions, professors, and students to have all contributed to a dynamic healthcare system in a constant state of evolution, such as the COVID-19 pandemic (Rocha et al., 2021; cf. Litewka et al., 2020). The Brazilian medical education system has adopted measures that have greatly facilitated adaptation, both on the initiative of medical schools and ABEM – Brazilian Association of Medical Education, and by government directives. All medical education courses in Brazil, whether public or private, have their syllabi guided by the National Curriculum Guidelines and the structure of the undergraduate medical school should contain the following features (Brasil, 2014):

- From a didactic standpoint, it is a requirement to utilize teaching methods that promote active student participation in knowledge construction, integrating content and engaging students in practical activities relevant to their future professional life at an early stage.
- To incorporate ethical and humanistic dimensions, developing citizenship-oriented attitudes and values in the student.
- To utilize diverse teaching and learning scenarios, enabling the student to explore and experience various life situations, the organization of practice, and multidisciplinary teamwork.

- To provide active interaction opportunities for students with healthcare users and professionals right from the beginning of their education, allowing them to engage with real-world problems and gradually assume increasing responsibilities as care providers. This process aligns with their level of autonomy, which culminates during the internship phase in undergraduate studies.

Currently, a student-centered approach, including their active participation in the teaching and learning process, is fundamental for their proper formation. The application of active learning methods satisfies these requirements, and the guidance contained in the curricular guidelines, listed above, encourages courses to adopt this type of practice. Education courses offered in Brazil include a variety of methods, with courses with traditional, mixed, and problem-based learning (PBL).

Along with the use of active methods, Brazilian guidelines require that medical education courses have continuing professional development activities. Teaching professional medical education has always been a challenge, as it requires a professional who combines knowledge in the medical field with didactic and pedagogical skills. To meet these expectations, professors must be able to transmit knowledge in a clear and objective way, create a stimulating learning environment, and be prepared to guide students in practical activities, both in laboratories and in different teaching scenarios in the area of health. Oliveira et al. (2019) in a descriptive integrative review of the literature highlight that the professionalization of the professor becomes an essential strategy to rethink the medical education and medical schools are responsible for creating spaces for professor's training and improvement.

ABEM – Brazilian Association of Medical Education – is a national organization whose mission is to promote the development of medical education. It plays an important role in the development of medical education in Brazil, organizing courses and conferences, like COBEM (Brazilian Congress of Medical Education), encourages the training of tutors, maintains publications and information repositories, and promotes student and institutional evaluation processes.

Both in Brazil and in the world, the role of the educational system has been questioned, requiring a reorganization around the pillars of knowledge and it is up to medical courses to adapt to this new reality. An analysis of Brazilian medical schools reveals that most of the evaluated courses (80.7%) are at advanced or innovative levels of curricular structure (Aguilar-da-Silva et al., 2009). These results point to a tendency for medical education courses in Brazil to adapt to the current moment, a fundamental factor for the country to be ready to face the coming decades, absorb the use of technologies, adapt to the acceleration of the digital age, and train professionals with adequate skills, both from a humanistic and technical point of view to the 21st century.

Studies have also suggested that the teaching of traditional approaches to healthcare is alive and well. For instance, in 2021 Lucchetti et al. (2023) surveyed the practices that they categorize as related to "spirituality and health" (S/H) in Brazilian medical schools. In their study, they found that over a decade (from 2011 to 2021), there was a marked increase in medical school provided S/H, from 40% to 65.5%. As Figure 8.4 illustrates, they also identified multiple barriers to integrating S/H teaching into the curriculum. For instance, while they found that few respondents (representatives of officially licensed Brazilian medical schools) believed that the topic should not be addressed, most indicated that there was a lack of professional knowledge (53.3%) or a lack of time (43.3%). However, many respondents also indicated that they did not see any barriers (26.7%).

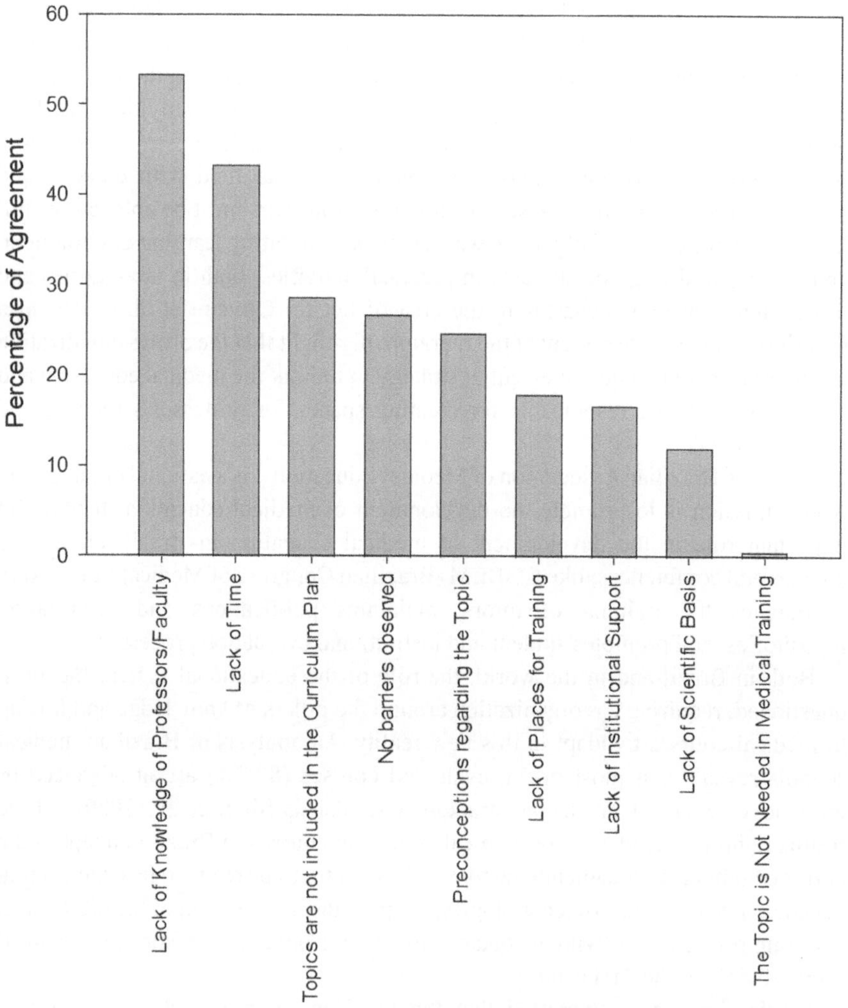

FIGURE 8.4 Barriers to integrating spirituality and health teaching into the curriculum.

8.4.2 The Impact of Educational Policies on Access to Health Services in Brazil

An important global obstacle to universal health coverage is undoubtedly the inequality in the geographic distribution of doctors, with a greater concentration in urban centers, to the detriment of rural communities (Dussalt & Franceschini, 2006). Brazil is no exception to this rule; however, this issue is particularly pronounced given its large territory and larger regional differences in socioeconomic, cultural, and epidemiological features (Figueiredo et al., 2019; Scheffer et al., 2023).

Following the example of other countries (Rourke, 2010; Mathers et al., 2011; Garces & Mickey-Pabello, 2015), several measures have been advocated nationally to favor equal access to health services for all citizens. These measures include expanding the number of undergraduate vacancies and opening schools outside the capitals, prioritizing municipalities with 50,000–100,000 inhabitants (Saúde, 2015). Furthermore, proposals for the democratization of education by implementing policies aimed at including historically discriminated minorities have been put forward and achieved through the implementation of the "Law of Quotas". Finally, there has been a push to adopt educational policies that aim to train generalist and humanist professionals who are equipped to work in primary and emergency care immediately upon graduation (Brasil, 2014).

Although the effects of these measures may take time to manifest themselves and only in the future will more robust studies be possible to assess their real results for society, preliminary analyses point to positive impacts. Recently, there has been a 65% increase in the density of physicians per population in municipalities in the interior of the country (Scheffer et al., 2023), in addition to the finding that approximately 60% of physicians who work in poorer regions are graduates who, in some way, benefited from public policies for the democratization of education. It is also important to emphasize the association between training in medical schools located in smaller cities and the performance of graduates in primary healthcare in remote areas and in municipalities with less than 20,000 inhabitants (Figueiredo et al., 2022).

8.4.3 What to Expect from the Future of Medical Education in Brazil

At the beginning of the third decade of the 21st century, the global pandemic of COVID-19 changed teaching dynamics around the world due to the need for social isolation, re-signifying the use of simulators and resources associated with information and communication technologies, which were disseminated as teaching and learning optimizing instruments (Coelho et al., 2021). Medical education was also faced with these challenges: teachers and students were required to use virtual learning environments to discuss theoretical contents and to carry out assessments, accelerating the inclusion of these technologies in their pedagogical practices. While many positive lessons can be learned from these experiences, there were also many negative outcomes. For instance, the need to limit contagion negatively impacted the acquisition of procedural skills desired for the practice of medicine (Papapanou et al., 2022).

The hybrid teaching model, in which virtual learning environments are used in parallel with face-to-face activities, is currently a trend and should be consolidated in the future, as well as the use of resources arising from the popularization of technologies and the internet, such as virtual libraries and laboratories, online evaluation forms and the use of simulators and applications associated with artificial intelligence (Lobo, 2018). In addition, medical schools in Brazil, in which the lecture method still predominates, have been encouraged to diversify their dynamics and value the adoption of active student-centered methods, such as learning by problems, by teams and peers, design thinking, flipped classes, among others (Moura et al., 2022).

Breaking with the Flexnerian model, based on isolated disciplines and on the fragmentation of the teaching process, the future points to a flexible medical education course curriculum, which emphasizes inter- and transdisciplinary activities, the integration of the contents of multiple disciplines and indigenous knowledge, extension actions in the community, the expansion of practice scenarios, and the inclusion of disciplines that discuss ethics and humanities (Gomes et al., 2014, Machado et al., 2018).

The current curriculum guidelines (Leis de Diretrizes e Bases) for undergraduate courses in Medicine in Brazil establish that graduates in Medicine must have:

> general, humanistic, critical, reflective and ethical training, with the capacity to act at different levels of health care, with actions for the promotion, prevention, recovery and rehabilitation of health, in the individual and collective spheres, with social responsibility and commitment to the defense of citizenship, human dignity, integral health of the human being and always having as a transversality in its practice, the social determination of the health and disease process.
>
> *(Brasil, 2014)*

To meet those guidelines, modernize pedagogical practices, and prepare teaching spaces to accommodate both new technologies and active teaching methods, Brazilian medical schools need continuing education programs for teachers and managers, which update and allow them to reflect on the pedagogical practice, in addition to policies for investment in infrastructure and the enhancement of the teaching career that make it stimulating to retain good professionals, whether doctors or professionals in the basic areas of health sciences.

Currently, however, most Brazilian courses do not efficiently stimulate entry and maintenance in the teaching career, offering unattractive salaries when compared to the gains obtained from exercising the medical profession outside academia, and with few initiatives of investments in new technologies and in the continuing education of teachers. In this way, in view of the technological, digital, and educational revolution that the whole world has been going through, although the trend for the future of medical teaching in Brazil is promising, its success is conditioned to changes that need to be made from the present time.

Notes

1 This term roughly corresponds to the idea of "Shaman"; however, see Langdon (2013).
2 The specifics of the selection process are unknown.
3 This ratio can be compared to those of Mexico (2.2), Japan (2.3), Canada (2.5), Germany (4.3), and Portugal (4.4; World Health Organization, 2023).

References

Aguilar-da-Silva, R. H., Perim, G. L., Abdalla, I. G., Costa, N. M. D. S. C., Lampert, J. B., & Stella, R. C. D. R. (2009). Abordagens pedagógicas e tendências de mudanças nas escolas médicas. *Revista Brasileira de Educação Médica*, *33*(suppl 1), 53–62. http://educa.fcc.org.br/scielo.php?script=sci_abstract&pid=S1981-52712009000500006&lng=pt&nrm=iso

Alves, R. (2009). Fauna used in popular medicine in Northeast Brazil. *Journal of Ethnobiology and Ethnomedicine*, *5*(1), 1–11. https://pubmed.ncbi.nlm.nih.gov/19128461/

Amaral, J. L. (2016). O exame terminal salvaguarda a medicina. *Revista da Associação Paulista de Medicina*, *682*(1), 16–17.

Amoretti, R. (2005). A Educação Médica diante das Necessidades Sociais em Saúde. *Revista Brasileira de Educação Médica*, *29*(2), 136–146. https://doi.org/10.1590/1981-5271v29.2-020

Ávila, R. C. (2014). Formação das mulheres nas escolas de medicina. *Revista Brasileira de Educação Médica*, *38*, 142–149. https://doi.org/10.1590/S0100-55022014000100019

Baer, H. A., Singer, M., & Susser, I. (2013). *Medical Anthropology and the World System: Critical Perspectives*. Santa Bárbara: Praeger.

Barbosa, M. O., Lemos, I. C. S., Kemtopf, M. R., & Fernandes, G. P. (2016). A prática da medicina tradicional no Brasil: Um resgate histórico dos tempos coloniais. *Revista Interdisciplinar de Estudos em Saúde*, *5*(1), 65–77. https://periodicos.uniarp.edu.br/index.php/ries/article/view/832

Batista, N. A., Vilela, R. Q. B., & Batista, S. H. S. S. (2015). *Educação Médica no Brasil*. São Paulo, SP: Cortez. https://doi.org/10.17566/ciads.v5i3.321

Begliomini, H. (2022). Biografias de Acadêmicos. www.academiamedicinasaopaulo.org.br/?pg=download&acao=1&id=91&biografia=Maria%20Augusta%20Generoso%20Estrela#gsc.tab=0

Boelen, C. (2002). A new paradigm for medical schools a century after Flexner's report. *Bulletin of the World Health Organization*, *80*, 592–593. www.ncbi.nlm.nih.gov/pmc/articles/PMC2567557/pdf/12163925.pdf

Boelen, C., Heck, J. E., & World Health Organization. (1995). *Defining and Measuring the Social Accountability of Medical Schools* (No. WHO/HRH/95.7. Unpublished). World Health Organization. https://apps.who.int/iris/handle/10665/5944

Bonner, T. N. (1995). *Becoming a Physician: Medical Education in Britain, France, Germany, and the United States, 1750-1945*. Baltimore: The Johns Hopkins University Press.

Botelho, J. B., & Costa, H. L. (2006). Pajé: reconstrução e sobrevivência. *História, Ciências, Sáude-Manguinhos*, *13*(4), 927–956. https://doi.org/10.1590/S0104-59702006000400009

Botti, S. H. O. (2009). *O papel do preceptor na formação de médicos residentes: um estudo de residências em especialidades clínicas de um hospital de ensino (Tese de Doutorado)*. Rio de Janeiro, RJ, Brasil: Escola Nacional de Saúde Pública Sérgio Arouca da Fundação Oswaldo Cruz. www.arca.fiocruz.br/handle/icict/2582

Braghini, K. M. Z. (2014). A história dos estudantes "excedentes" nos anos 1960: a superlotação das universidades e um torvelinho de situações improvisadas. *Educar em Revista*, *51*, 123–144. https://doi.org/10.1590/S0104-40602014000100009

Brasil. (1988). Constituição da República Federativa do Brasil, de 1988. Diário Oficial da República Federativa do Brasil, Poder Executivo, Brasília, DF, 05 de outubro. 1988. Seção I, p. 1. www.planalto.gov.br/ccivil_03/constituicao/constituicao.htm

Brasil. (2001). Conselho Nacional de Educação, Câmara de Educação Superior. Resolução CNE/CES no. 4/2001 – Institui Diretrizes Curriculares Nacionais do Curso de Graduação em Medicina. Diário Oficial da União. Brasília (Brasil). https://portal.mec.gov.br/index.php?option=com_docman&view=download&alias=15864-rces004-01&category_slug=junho-2014-pdf&Itemid=30192

Brasil. (2014). Resolução CNE/CES n. 3, de 20 de junho de 2014. Institui as Diretrizes Curriculares Nacionais do Curso de Graduação em Medicina e dá outras providências. Diário Oficial da União. https://portal.mec.gov.br/index.php?option=com_docman&view=download&alias=14957-rces001-14&category_slug=janeiro-2014-pdf&Itemid=30192

Brasil. (2025a) Instituto Nacional de Estudos e Pesquisas Educacionais Anísio Teixeira – INEP. Portaria no 413, de 18 de junho de 2025. Regulamenta o Exame Nacional de Avaliação da Formação Médica – Enamed. Diário Oficial da União: Seção 1, pp. 28–29, 23 june 2025. Disponível em: www.in.gov.br/en/web/dou/-/portaria-n-413-de-18-de-junho-de-2025-*-638296809.

Brasil. (2025b). Ministério da Educação. Conselho Nacional de Educação. Câmara de Educação Superior. Resolução CNE/CES nº 3, de 30 de setembro de 2025. Institui Diretrizes Curriculares Nacionais do Curso de Graduação em Medicina. Brasília: MEC/CNE, 2025. Disponível em: http://www.abmes.org.br/arquivos/legislacoes/Resolucao-cne-ces-003-2025-09.

Bueno, R. D. R. L., & Pieruccini, M. C. (2005). Abertura de escolas de medicina no Brasil: Relatório de um cenário sombrio tório de um cenário sombrio. 2 ed. https://portal.cfm.org.br/images/stories/biblioteca/abertura%20de%20escolas%20de%20medicina%20no%20brasil%20-%20relatrio%20de%20um%20cenrio%20sombrio%202%20edio.pdf

Calainho, D. B. (2005). Jesuítas e medicina no Brasil colonial. *História e Saúde*, *10*(19), 61–75. https://doi.org/10.1590/S1413-77042005000200005

Cardim, F. (1925). *Tratados da terra e gente do Brasil*. Rio de Janeiro: J. Leite & Cia. https://digital.bbm.usp.br/handle/bbm/4788

Chou J. Y., Chiu C. H., Lai E., Tsai D., & Tzeng C. R. (2012). Medical education in Taiwan. *Medical Teacher, 34*, 187–191. https://doi.org/10.3109/0142159x.2012.652238

Clastres, H. (1978). *Terra sem mal: o profetismo tupi-guarani*. São Paulo: Brasiliense.

Coelho, B. M., Meira, E. B., Araújo, L. S., Araújo, P. T. F., Tenisi, S. S., Santos, A. C., Dourado, D. N., ... & Silva, R. B. (2021). O impacto da pandêmica da COVID-19 na formação médica: uma revisão integrativa. *Revista Ibero-Americana de Humanidades, ciência e Educação, 7*(12), 522–545. https://periodicorease.pro.br/rease/article/view/3363/1351

De Mello, J. F. (1980). Plants in traditional medicine in Brazil. *Journal of Ethnopharmacology, 2*(1), 49–55. www.sciencedirect.com/science/article/abs/pii/0378874180900306

DeZee, K. J., Artino, A. R., Elnicki, D. M., Hemmer, P. A., & Durning, S. J. (2012). Medical education in the United States of America. *Medical Teacher, 34*(7), 521–525. https://doi.org/10.3109/0142159x.2012.668248

Dussault, G., & Franceschini, M. C. (2006). Not enough there, too many here: understanding geographical imbalances in the distribution of the health workforce. *Human Resources for Health, 4*, 12. https://doi.org/10.1186/1478-4491-4-12

Edler, F. C. (2010). Saber médico e poder profissional: do contexto luso-brasileiro ao Brasil Imperial. In: Ponte, C. F. (org) *Na corda bamba de sombrinha: a saúde no fio da história*. Rio de Janeiro: Fiocruz.

Edler, F. C., & Fonseca, M. R. F. (2006). A formação médica e o nascimento da anátomo-clínica. *Cadernos ABEM, 2*, 14. https://website.abem-educmed.org.br/wp-content/uploads/2019/09/CadernosABEM__Vol02.pdf

Figueiredo, A. M., de Lima, K. C., McKinley, D. W., del Carmen Junco Goméz, M., & Azevedo, G. D. (2022). Impacto of educational policies on access to health care in Brazil. A cross-sectional study. *Medical Education. 57*(6), 587–594. https://doi.org/10.1111/medu.15012

Figueiredo, A. M., McKinley, D. W., Lima, K. C., & Azevedo, G. D. (2019). Medical scholl expansion policies: educational access and physician distribuition. *Medical Education, 53*(11), 1121–1131. http://doi.org/10.1111/medu.13041

Figueiredo, A. M. D., Lima, K. C. D., Massuda, A., & Azevedo, G. D. D. (2022). Políticas de ampliação do acesso ao ensino superior e mudança no perfil de egressos de medicina no Brasil: um estudo transversal. *Ciência & Saúde Coletiva, 27*, 3751–3762. https://doi.org/10.1590/1413-81232022279.07092022.

Flexner, A. (1910). Medical education in the United States and Canada: a report to the carnegie foundation for the advancement of teaching. Bulletin No. 4. Updyke. www.ncbi.nlm.nih.gov/pmc/articles/PMC2567554/pdf/12163926.pdf

Flores, S. R. (2017). Democratização do ensino superior no Brasil, uma breve história: da colônia a República. *Revista Internacional de Educação Superior, 3*(2), 401–416. www.researchgate.net/publication/318845398_A_democratizacao_do_ensino_superior_no_Brasil_uma_breve_historia_da_Colonia_a_Republica

França, J. M. C. (2019). *Coleção de várias receitas e segredos particulares das principais boticas da nossa Companhia de Portugal, da Índia, de Macau e do Brasil*. São Paulo: Loyola.

Freire, J. R. B. (1991). *A Amazônia no período colonial (1616–1798)*. Manaus: Metro Cúbico.

Garces, L. M., & Mickey-Pabello, D. (2015). Racial diversity in the medical profession: the impact of affirmative action bans on underrepresented student of color matriculation in medical schools. *The Journal of Higher Education, 86*(2), 264–294. https://doi.org/10.1353/jhe.2015.0009

Gomes, A. P., & Rego, S. (2014). Paulo Freire: contribuindo para pensar mudanças de estratégias no ensino de Medicina. *Revista Brasileira de Educação Médica, 38*(3), 299–307. https://doi.org/10.1590/S0100-55022014000300003

Gomes, W. C. (2020). Prédio da Antiga Faculdade de Medicina da Bahia. Public Domain, by Wikimedia Commons. Photo: Salvador, Bahia, 2020. https://commons.wikimedia.org/wiki/File:Faculdade_de_Medicina_da_Bahia_Salvador_2019-8603.jpg#metadata

Gonçalves, M. B., & Benevides-Pereira, A. M. T. (2009). Considerações sobre o ensino médico no Brasil: consequências afetivo-emocionais nos estudantes. *Revista Brasileira de Educação Médica, 33*(3), 482–493. https://doi.org/10.1590/s0100-5502200900 0300020

González, A. D., & Almeida, M. J. D. (2010). Integralidade da saúde: norteando mudanças na graduação dos novos profissionais. *Ciência & Saúde Coletiva, 15*(3), 757–762. https:// doi.org/10.1590/s1413-81232010000300018

Guimarães, E. D. F., & Zelaya, M. (2022). Política de cotas raciais nas universidades públicas do brasil duas décadas depois. *Trabalho & Educação, 30*(3), 133–148. https:// periodicos.ufmg.br/index.php/trabedu/article/view/26556/29733

Gurgel, C. (2011). *Doenças e curas: o Brasil nos primeiros séculos.* São Paulo: Contexto.

Haddad, A. E., Morita, M. C., Pierantoni, C. R., Brenelli, S. L., Passarella, T., & Campos, F. E. (2010). Formação de profissionais de saúde no Brasil: uma análise no período de 1991 a 2008. *Revista de Saúde Pública, 44*, 383–393. https://doi.org/10.1590/S0034-891020 10005000015

Hahn, R. A. (1995). *Sickness and Healing: An Anthropological Perspective*. New Haven: Yale University Press.

Holanda, S. B. (2003). *História Geral da Civilização Brasileira: A Época Colonial.* Lisboa: Bertrand Editora. https://doi.org/10.11606/issn.2316-9141.rh.1961.120204

Instituto Brasileiro de Geografia e Estatística (IBGE). (2012). *Censo Demográfico 2010: Características Gerais dos Indígenas – Resultado do Universo.* Rio de Janeiro: IBGE. www.ibge.gov.br/indigenas/indigena_censo2010.pdf

Instituto Brasileiro de Geografia e Estatística (IBGE). (2015). *Pesquisa Nacional por Amostra de Domicílios: Síntese de Indicadores 2014.* Rio de Janeiro: IBGE. www.ibge. gov.br/estatisticas/sociais/populacao/9127-pesquisa-nacional-por-amostra-de-domicil ios.html

Johnson, H., & Silva, M. B. (1992). *O império luso-brasileiro, 1500–1620.* Lisboa: Estampa.

Kemp, A., & Edler, F. C. (2004). A reforma médica no Brasil e nos Estados Unidos: uma comparação entre duas retóricas. *História, Ciências, Saúde-Manguinhos, 11*, 569–585. https://doi.org/10.1590/s0104-59702004000300003

Lampert, J. B., Costa, N. M. D S. C., Perim, G. L., Abdalla, I. G., Aguilar-da-Silva, R. H., & Stella, R. C. D R. (2009). Tendências de mudanças em um grupo de escolas médicas brasileiras. *Revista Brasileira de Educação Médica, 33*(suppl 1), 19–34. https://doi.org/ 10.1590/s0100-55022009000500003

Langdon E. J. (2013). New perspectives of shamanism in Brazil *civilisations* [Online], 61–62. http://journals.openedition.org/civilisations/3227

Lima, I. S. (2020). *Benzedeiras – fé e cura no sertão: relações entre ciência, espiritualidade e saúde.* Belo Horizonte: Dialética.

Litewka, S. G., & Heitman, E. (2020). Latin American healthcare systems in times of pandemic. *Developing World Bioethics, 20*(2), 69–73. www.ncbi.nlm.nih.gov/pmc/artic les/PMC7262025/

Lobo, L. C. (2018). Inteligência artificial, o Futuro da Medicina e a Educação Médica. *Revista Brasileira de Educação Médica, 42*(3), 3–8. https://doi.org/10.1590/1981-52712015v42n3RB20180115EDITORIAL1

Lopes, A. C. (2018). A explosão numérica das escolas médicas brasileiras. *Educación Médica, 19*, 19–24. https://doi.org/10.1016/j.edumed.2018.03.004

Lucchetti, G., Almeida, P.O.A., Martin, E.Z., Góes, A.G., Cotta, K.C.G., Lima, A.C., Ezequiel, O.S. & Lucchetti, A.L.G. (2023). The current status of "spiritualitu and health" teaching in Brazilian medical schools: a nationwide survey. *BMC Medical Education, 23*(1), 172. https://doi:10.1186/s12909-023-04153-z

Luna, W. F., Teixeira, K. C., & Lima, G. K. D. (2021). Mapeamento e experiências de indígenas nas escolas médicas federais brasileiras: acesso e políticas de permanência. *Interface – Comunicação, Saúde, Educação, 25*, e200621. https://doi.org/10.1590/interface.200621

Machado, C. D. B., Wuo, A., & Heinzle, M. (2018). Educação médica no Brasil: uma análise histórica sobre a formação acadêmica e pedagógica. *Revista Brasileira de Educação Médica, 42*(2), 66–73. https://doi.org/10.1590/1981-52712015v42n4RB20180065

Mathers, J., Sitch, A., Marsh, J. L., & Parry, J. (2011). Widening access to medical education for under-represented socioeconomic groups: population based cross sectional analysis of UK data, 2002-6. *BMJ, 342*, d918. https://doi.org/10.1136/bmj.d918Milliken, W., & Albert, B. (1996). The use of medicinal plants by the Yanomami Indians of Brazil. *Economic Botany, 50*(1), 10–25. www.jstor.org/stable/4255967

Monteiro, S. C., & Brandelli, C. L. (2017). *Farmacobotânica: Aspectos Teóricos e Aplicação*. Porto Alegre: Artmed.

Moura, H. F. N., Oliveira, L. A. B., Venosa, A. R., Lourenço, L. H. M., & Baroneza, J. E. (2022). Uma estratégia para avaliação da percepção de docentes e discentes acerca dos métodos de ensino. *Revista Brasileira de Educação Médica, 46*(2), e088. https://doi.org/10.1590/1981-5271v46.2-20210327

Mussa, A. B. N. (1991). *O papel das línguas africanas na história do português do Brasil* (Dissertação de Mestrado). Rio de Janeiro, RJ, Brasil: Universidade Federal do Rio de Janeiro. https://periodicos.uff.br/gragoata/article/view/33165

Nassar, l. M., Couto, M. H. D. C., & Pereira Júnior, G. A. (2021). Financiamento público (fies e prouni) para o ensino de medicina no brasil: uma revisão da literatura e as distorções criadas. *Educação Em Revista, 37*, e25246. https://doi.org/10.1590/0102-469825246

Nassif, A. C. N. (2022). *Placar de criação das Escolas Médicas no Brasil*. www.escolasmedicas.com.br/index.php.

Nikendei, C., Weyrich, P., Jünger, J., & Schrauth, M. (2009). Medical education in Germany. *Medical Teacher, 31*(7), 591–600. https://doi.org/10.1080/01421590902833010

Oliveira, B. L. C. A. de, Lima, S. F., Pereira, M. U. L., & Pereira Júnior, G. A. (2019). Evolução, distribuição e expansão dos cursos de medicina no Brasil (1808–2018). *Trabalho, Educação E Saúde, 17*(1), e0018317. https://doi.org/10.1590/1981-7746-sol00183

Oliveira, F. P. de., Vanni, T., Pinto, H. A., Santos, J. T. R. D., Figueiredo, A. M. D., Araújo, S. Q. D., ... & Cyrino, E. G. (2015). Mais Médicos: um programa brasileiro em uma perspectiva internacional. *Interface-Comunicação, Saúde, Educação, 19*(54), 623–634. https://doi.org/10.1590/1807-57622014.1142

Paim, J. (2009). *O que é o SUS*. Rio de Janeiro: Editora FIOCRUZ. https://doi.org/10.1590/S0102-311X2010000600019

Papapanou, M., Routsi, E., Tsamakis, K., Fotis, L., Marinos, G., Lidoriki, I., ... & Schizar, D. (2022). Medical education challenges and innovations during COVID-19 pandemic. *Postgraduate Medical Journal, 98*(1159), 321–327. https://doi.org/10.1136/postgradmedj-2021-140032

Peard, J. G. (1999). *Race, Place, and Medicine: The Idea of the Tropics in Nineteenth-Century Brazil*. Durham: Duke University Press.

Pezzuti, J., & Chaves, R. P. (2009). Etnografia e manejo de recursos naturais pelos índios Deni, Amazonas, Brasil. *Acta Amazônica, 39*(1), 121–138,

Pinto, H. A., Sales, M. J. T., Oliveira, F. P. D., Brizolara, R., Figueiredo, A. M. D., & Santos, J. T. D. (2014). O Programa Mais Médicos e o fortalecimento da atenção básica. *Divulg. saúde debate*, 51, 105–120. https://pesquisa.bvsalud.org/portal/resource/pt/lil-771502

Porro, A. (2002). *História dos índios no Brasil*. São Paulo: Companhia das Letras.

Prata, P. R. (2010). Duzentos anos de formação médica no Brasil: onde e quando devem ser comemorados? *Interface (Botucatu)*, *14*(33), 471–473. https://doi.org/10.1590/S1414-32832010000200020

Reigada, C. L. D. L., Oliveira, D. O. P. S. D., Carrijo, A. P. B., Chueiri, P. S., Moherdaui, J. H., & Albuquerque, N. P. D. (2021). Liderança feminina: relato do primeiro encontro de mulheres Médicas de Família e Comunidade do Brasil. *Saúde Em Debate*, *45*, 212–223. https://saudeemdebate.emnuvens.com.br/sed/article/view/4599

Ribeiro, M. M. (1997). *A ciência dos trópicos:* a arte médica no Brasil do século XVII. São Paulo: Hucitec.

Rocha, R., Atun, R., Massuda, A., Rache, B., Spinola, P., Nunes, L., ... & Castro, M. C. (2021). Effect of socioeconomic inequalities and vulnerabilities on health-system preparedness and response to COVID-19 in Brazil: a comprehensive analysis. *The Lancet Global Health*, *9*(6), e782–e792. www.thelancet.com/journals/langlo/article/PIIS2214-109X(21)00081-4/fulltext

Rodrigues, I. T., & Fiolhais, C. (2013). O ensino da medicina na Universidade de Coimbra no século XVI. *História, Ciências, Saúde-Manguinhos*, *20*(2), 435–456. www.scielo.br/j/hcsm/a/BGSDRxTWx7XJcxqBfBfBZht/?format=pdf&lang=pt

Romero, F. R., Boeira, A. S., & Oliveira, L. P. O. (2020) A regulamentação legal e a prática da Medicina no Brasil Colonial. *Diálogo e Interfaces do Direito*, *3*(2), 1–28. https://dir.fag.edu.br/index.php/direito/article/view/68

Rourke, J. (2010). How can medical schools contribute to the education recruitment and retention of rural physicians in their region? *Bulletin of the World Health Organization*, *88*(5), 395–396. http://doi.org?10.2471/blt.09.073072

Sampaio de Carvalho, M., & de Sousa, M. F. (2013). Como o Brasil tem enfrentado o tema provimento de médicos? *Interface-Comunicação, Saúde, Educação*, *17*(47), 913–926. https://doi.org/10.1590/1807-57622013.0403

Santos Filho, L. (1991). *História geral da Medicina brasileira.* São Paulo: Hucitec/Edusp.

Santos, M. P. de J. dos. (2019). Maria Odília Teixeira: a primeira médica negra da Faculdade de Medicina da Bahia (1884–1937). https://repositorio.ufba.br/handle/ri/33196?mode=full

Saúde, B-Md. (2015). *Mais médicos para o Brasil*. Brasília (Brazil): Ministério da Saúde – Governo Federal. https://www.gov.br/saude/pt-br/composicao/sgtes/mais-medicos

Scheffer, M., Cassenote, A., Guerra, A., Guilloux, A., Brandão, A., Miotto, B., ... & Miotto, R. (2020). *Demografia Médica no Brasil 2020.* São Paulo, SP: FMUSP, CFM. p. 312. www.fm.usp.br/fmusp/conteudo/DemografiaMedica2020_9DEZ.pdf

Scheffer, M., Guilloux, A. G. A., Miotto, B. A., Almeida, C., Guerra, A., Cassenote, A., Matijasevich., A., Brandão, A. P. D., Castilho, E. A., Russo, G., Moreira, J. P. L. Bahia, L., Andrietta, L. S., Dal Poz, M. R., Vilela, P.R.C., Miotto, R. A., Duatre, V. C., & Araújo, W. (2023). *Demografia Médica no Brasil 2023.* São Paulo, SP: FMUSP, AMB. p. 344. https://amb.org.br/wp-content/uploads/2023/02/DemografiaMedica2023_8fev-1.pdf

Schwartz, S. (1988). *Segredos internos. Engenhos e escravos no Brasil colonial.* São Paulo: Companhia das Letras.

Schoenherr, J. R. (2027). Innovation and implementation in the health professions: Translating research in education and healthcare delivery. In Schoenherr, J. R. (Ed.), *Fundamentals and Frontiers of Medical Education and Decision-Making: Innovation, Implementation, and Translational Research* (pp. 1–76). Routledge.

Schoenherr, J. R. & Beaudoin, J. (2026). Medical heterarchies in East Asian medical education: The evolving landscape of health professions education in East Asia.

In Schoenherr, J. R. (Ed.), *Fundamentals and Frontiers of Medical Education and Decision-Making: Innovation, Implementation, and Translational Research* (pp. 462–509). Routledge.

Serviço Florestal Brasileiro (SFA). (2013). *Florestas do Brasil em resumo – 2013.* Brasília: SFB. www.gov.br/florestal/pt-br/centrais-de-conteudo/publicacoes/publicacoes-diversas/florestas_do_brasil_em_resumo_2013_atualizado.pdf

Singer, M., Bulled, N., Ostrach, B., & Mendenhall, E. (2017). Syndemics and the biosocial conception of health. *The Lancet, 389*(10072), 941–950. www.researchgate.net/publication/314200704_Syndemics_and_the_biosocial_conception_of_health

Singer, M., & Clair, S. (2003). Syndemics and public health: reconceptualizing disease in bio-social context. *Medical Anthropology Quarterly*, *17*(4), 423–441. www.researchgate.net/publication/8924026_Syndemics_and_Public_Health_Reconceptualizing_Disease_in_Bio-Social_Context/link/0fcfd50605dd70e8c3000000/download

Silva, K. L. (2016). *O ser Pajé: histórias de pajelança e encantaria em Curupuru no tempo presente (Monografia)*. São Luiz, MA, Brasil: Universidade Estadual do Maranhão.

Soublin, J. (2000). *Histoire de l'Amazonie*. Paris: Payot.

Supe, A. (2016). NEET: India's single exam for admission to medical school promises transparency and quality. *BMJ, 354*, i405. https://doi.org/10.1136/bmj.i4051

Teixeira, A. (1989). *Ensino superior no Brasil: análise e interpretação de sua evolução até 1969.* Rio de Janeiro: Editora da Fundação Getúlio Vargas. www.bvanisioteixeira.ufba.br/livros/chama_introducao.htm

Torres-Londono, F. (2000). O Índio como Selvagem: "O diálogo da conversão dos gentios" e a memória. *Projeto História: Revista do Programa de Estudos Pós-Graduados de História, 20*, 269–279. https://revistas.pucsp.br/revph/article/download/10818/8036

Voeks. R. (2012). *Ethnobotany of Brazil's African diaspora: the role of floristic homogenization.* New York: Springer. https://link.springer.com/chapter/10.1007/978-1-4614-0836-9_14#citeas.

Walker, T. D. (2013). The medicines trade in the Portuguese atlantic world: acquisition and dissemination of healing knowledge from Brazil (c. 1580–1800). *Social History of Medicine*, *26*(3), 403–431. https://academic.oup.com/shm/article-abstract/26/3/403/1619698?redirectedFrom=fulltext

Walker, T. D. (2016). Global cross-cultural dissemination of indigenous medical practices through the Portuguese colonial system: evidence from sixteenth to eighteenth-century ethno-botanical manuscripts. In: Wendt, H. (ed.) *The Globalization of Knowledge in the Iberian Colonial World* (pp. 161–192). Berlin: Editon Open Access.

World Health Organization. (2023). World health organization's global health workforce statistics, OECD, supplemented by country data [Statistical data]. Geneva: WHO Publications. https://databank.worldbank.org/source/health-nutrition-and-population-statistics/Series/SH.MED.PHYS.ZS

Zank, S., & Hanazaki, N. (2017). The coexistence of traditional medicine and biomedicine: a study with local health experts in two Brazilian regions. *PloS One*, *12*(4), e0174731. www.ncbi.nlm.nih.gov/pmc/articles/PMC5393556/

Zanolli, M. B., Maciel, D. T., Streit, D. S., Muraguchi, E. B. O. (2014). Internato Médico: Diretrizes Nacionais da ABEM para o internato no curso de graduação em Medicina, de acordo com as Diretrizes Curriculares Nacionais. In: Lampert, J. P., & Bicudo, A. M. (eds.) *10 anos das Diretrizes Curriculares Nacionais do Curso de Graduação em Medicina* (pp. 57–87). Rio de Janeiro: Associação Brasileira de Educação Médica.

9

INEQUALITY AND SOCIAL MOBILITY IN THE MEDICAL PROFESSIONS IN INDIA

Career Availability and Vulnerabilities

Khalid Khan

Introduction

Health professions education involves the socialisation of learners into healthcare professionals (HCPs) that can deliver effective and efficient care to a population. Yet, education cannot be denatured from the society in which the learners, patients, and public are situated. The governance of the healthcare system requires understanding the needs of a population and developing a workforce that can not only serve these communities but is representative of these communities. While all cultures have indigenous medical traditions, the legacy of colonialism and globalisation has resulted in blending – often forcefully – of educational and treatment practices in the health professions.

Medical education and practice occur within sociocultural traditions. Workforce development is necessarily influenced by existing social categories, identities, and structures (Schoenherr, 2027; Schoenherr & Beaudoin, 2024). Crucially, the healthcare professions are often defined by social stratification, with hierarchical relationships between healthcare professionals and between the healthcare professionals and society. Ideally, all members of society should have access to quality care and HCPs should be representative of the populations they serve to facilitate the development of the therapeutic alliance and shared understanding of socioeconomic conditions thereby facilitating communication (Schoenherr & LeBour, 2024). However, the ability for an individual from one group to 'move' up or down within a society (social mobility) can create barriers which might limit the number of HCPs from any given group. Entering the health professions in countries with high social mobility (e.g., Denmark, Norway, and Finland) might therefore be easier than countries with limited social mobility (e.g., Cameroon, India, and Pakistan; World Economic Forum, 2020). However,

DOI: 10.4324/9781003498155-9

studies conducted in Australia, Canada, the UK, and the US suggested that social mobility in medical education is generally limited (Association of Faculties of Medicine of Canada, 2012; Cleland et al., 2012; Department of Education, 2014; Fenton et al., 2016).

This chapter examines the availability of health professionals in India with a focus on the status of the underprivileged groups. It examines how the existing social inequality gets reproduced in access to a career in medicine. Following a brief background of healthcare practices and policy in India, this chapter estimates the availability of health professionals in India, their concentration in different types of jobs, and the quality of employment they are engaged in (Chikersal, 2015; Khan, 2022). This chapter investigates the broad inequities in the availability of health professionals recognising that the underrepresentation of underprivileged groups is not random but systematically connects to their group identity. It fills the gap in literature in the wake of the paucity of research focused on the availability of health professionals and their job characteristics in India. This chapter shows how inequalities existing in society may entail significant social injustices with regard to access to a career in medicine. The empirical analysis of the study is based on data from the Periodic Labour Force (PLF) Survey, 2019–20.

Social Organisation of Indian Society

Indian society is quite diverse which very often creates barriers in social mobility for the underprivileged groups (Jodhka, 2017; Srinivas, 2017; Vaid, 2014). The caste system is one of the most pervasive forms of division within India. Hindu society in India is divided into various cohesive groups, or Jatis, thereby leading to a highly fragmented social structure defined by a graded hierarchy consisting of Brahmins, Kshatriyas, Vaishyas, and Shudras.

The untouchables are other groups outside the domain of ritual hierarchy considered the lowest in social hierarchy. Due to their disadvantaged status throughout much of history, Scheduled Castes (SC) are eligible for affirmative action policies following independence. SC comprise nearly 17% of India's population. The Other Backward Class (OBC) are relatively better placed but lag behind the Hindu Higher Caste. They are also the subject of affirmative action in jobs and educational institutions based on their disadvantaged socioeconomic status. Tribal represent other ethnic groups comprising nearly 8% of the total population of India.

India has many religious practitioners, including Hindus, Muslims, Christians, Sikhs, Jains, Buddhists, and Zoroastrians. Muslims are the largest minority (14.2% of the population) and are the most disadvantaged group among the religious groups (Sachar Committee Report (2006). Different groups of Muslims have historically occupied heterogeneous positions in India; some Muslims are descendants of India's 15th to 18th century ruling classes,[1] while others descend from lower-caste groups who converted to Islam to escape their low social status. As a result, class disparity is very high with a minuscule elite coexisting with a very high share of the deprived section.

Occupational segregation is another important factor which likely influenced the choice of a profession among socio-religious groups. Muslims are largely confined to self-employment particularly in urban areas while SC are concentrated into casual employment. As per the author's calculation based on the PLF survey data, 2019–20, 45% of the total Muslim workers are concentrated into self-employment in comparison to 37% of Hindus. The SC and ST are concentrated in casual employment. In urban areas, nearly 23% of the casual employment workers are from these groups while the corresponding figures are 15% and 7% among OBC and HC, respectively. In rural areas 43% of SC and 30% ST workers are casually employment while this figure is 24% and 17% among OBC and HC, respectively.

The Healthcare System: Practice and Education/Policy in India

India has a rich tradition of six prominent systems of health, with Ayurveda and Siddha rooted in Indian traditions. Ayurveda is the oldest system in India, dated to the 2nd century BCE. The other allied systems of medicine in India are Unani, Siddha, Homoeopathy, Yoga, and Naturopathy. Ayurveda is based on the ancient philosophical teachings of *Vaisheshika* and the *Nyaya* School of logic. The *Vaisheshika* School advocated for practitioners to make inferences and perceptions obtained about a patient's pathological condition for treatment and *Nyaya* school teaches on knowledge of patient's condition, and the disease condition before proceeding for treatment (Jaiswal & Williams, 2016).

The Siddha system considers that the human body is constituted of the five elements of the universe with 96 systems that govern the physical, moral, and physiological well-being of an individual. The treatment in this system is based on the preparations from plant and mineral origin. ***Unani*** system of medicine, originated in Greece during the 460–366 BCE period, was introduced in India by the Arabs and Persians in the medieval period. This system of medicine is also recognised by the Indian government for clinical practice. In this system, plant-based compounds such as oils, tinctures, powders, and ointments are used in treatment (Mukherjee, 2001). ***Homoeopathy*** was originated in Germany in the mid-17th and 18th centuries (Jaiswal & Williams, 2016). Due to cultural exchanges, this system has been in practice in India for more than a century. It is recognised by the government of India as a system of medicine (Campbell, 1999). ***Yoga*** is another system of health originating in ancient times. It is based on meditative exercises and lifestyle management to improve health (Gina et al., 2013; Hoyez, 2007; Posadzki et al., 2011). Finally, ***Naturopathy*** is also practised in India for a long time. It originated in Germany in the 19th century and today it is practised in several countries (NIH, 2012).

The policy for the provision of the healthcare services predates independence. Multiple committees were established to examine the requirement for the health provisioning to the common people. The most comprehensive plan for health policy was prepared by the Bhore Committee popularly known as Health Survey and Development Committee Report (1946). The Report outlines comprehensive guidelines to develop the structure of the health system in India.

Once India regained independence, features of the British systems persisted. In 1959, another committee known as 'Health Survey and Planning Committee' and popularly known as Mudaliar Committee was appointed to survey the progress made in the health sector since submission of the Bhore Committee report and to make recommendations for the development and expansion of health services in future. The committee submitted its report in 1962, concluding that the quality of the healthcare services provided by the primary health centres was unsatisfactory. It suggested strengthening the existing primary health centres, sub-divisional and district hospitals, and to consolidate the progress made in the first decade and strengthen the district hospitals with specialists. A special committee was established in 1963 to study the requirements related to primary healthcare planning and priority according to need and utilisation of staff to eradicate Malaria.

By the mid-1970s, there was a growing recognition that a uniquely Indian approach to medical education was required. In 1975, the Shrivastav Committee advocated reorientation of medical education by national priorities and needs. In 1986, the Bajaj Committee called for the establishment of an educational commission for health sciences. It also noted that medical school faculty, though efficient in their clinical specialties, were deficient as educators. This resulted in the creation of numerous government and private medical colleges to meet the needs of India society.

The prevalent disparities in human resources in the health sector can be found as early as the 1960s. The Mukherjee Committee which was set up in 1965 observed a huge shortage of staff for the family planning programme. The prevention of private practice was a major issue raised by the Jungalwalla Committee (1967). They found that non-allowance should be reasonable to prevent private practice. The interstate disparities in staffing and pay scale were observed by the Kartar Singh Committee (1973).

Following independence, there have been three national health policies to guide health programmes.

The first national policy on health began to emerge in 1983. It emphasised the preventive, promotive, and rehabilitation aspects of health care and public health. It sought to establish a distributed network of comprehensive primary healthcare services. In addition to clinicians, these decentralised healthcare services would be supported by volunteers, paramedics, and community participation. Unfortunately, the goals of health could not be realised by the year 2000. The need for a new strategy was felt then.

Regional imbalance in healthcare services was also observed. In 2002, a revised health policy was adopted to address these issues. This policy also continued the goal of a decentralised health system. Further, convergence of all health programmes under a single umbrella was also targeted. The focus was on strengthening and expanding the public health services. So, the increasing contribution of the private sector was envisaged in this policy document. This policy also targeted enhancing the contribution of the private and NGO sector.

The National Health Policy (2017) identified seven priority areas for improvement in the health environment. It envisaged that these priority areas need coordinated action. Programmes and schemes were announced to achieve this goal. The interventions are the Swachh Bharat Abhiyan, balanced, healthy diets, and regular exercises, addressing tobacco, alcohol, and substance abuse, preventing deaths due to rail and road traffic accidents for achieving Yatri Suraksha, Nirbhaya Nari through action against gender violence, reduced stress and improved safety in the workplace, reducing indoor and outdoor air pollution.

Contemporary Issues with the Indian Healthcare Workforce

In India, the shortage of health workforce has been a persistent challenge, limiting the realisation of Universal Health Care. *The National Health Policy* (2017) (Government of India (GOI), 2017) envisaged attaining the highest possible level of health and well-being for all members of society across the lifespan, by adopting both a promotive and preventative healthcare orientation in all developmental policies, and universal access to good quality healthcare services without patients experiencing financial hardship. Challenges remain in achieving these goals.

The out-of-pocket expenditure by the households constitutes more than 95% of all health expenses in India (Ministry of Health and Family Welfare (MOHFW), 2014). This has been cited as a major factor pushing many members of the populations below the poverty line (Kolasa & Weychart, 2023). The government has made reducing out-of-pocket expenditure on health a priority and created the National Health Assurance Mission (2013). With this objective, the availability of adequate health workforce in the public sector becomes far more important. Thus, it is critical to examine the shortage of doctors in general and in the public sector to support developing a roadmap towards affordable access to Universal Health Care services. The government of India has developed multiple initiatives to address the needs of the healthcare sector. For instance, the flagship initiative Ayushman Bharat seeks to comprehensively strengthen the health system from the primary level to the tertiary level (NITI Ayog, 2021). The most attractive feature of this scheme is its emphasis on improving the performance of public facilities and leveraging the potential of the private sector in delivering health care to the poor. The scheme provides 500 million beneficiaries with annual hospitalisation coverage of up to INR 500,000 per family thereby improving public delivery (NITI Ayog, 2021).

Though attempts have been made to cover the deficit in health services for the underprivileged groups and backward regions, the uneven distribution of opportunities for medical education continues to be a major hurdle in this direction. Despite being one of the largest medical systems in the world, medical colleges in India are skewed towards urban locations. Further, the seats available at undergraduate and post-graduate levels are not sufficient with regard to the demand (The Hindu, 2024). The low levels of enrolment and limited supply of trained professionals is greatly impacted by the limited expenditure on medical education and the considerable cost of attending medical school. In the absence of a large number of places in medical education programmes, students frequently venture to countries like Russia, Ukraine, China, and the Philippines to obtain their medical degrees. The comparatively low cost in these countries is a major factor for students' outmigration from India. For instance, private colleges in India charge over USD 18,200 per annum while it costs from USD 24,266 to USD 36,399 for getting a medical degree for six years from Ukrainian institutions (Times of India (TOI), 2022).

The existing literature suggests a severe shortage of healthcare workers in India (Kasthuri, 2018). India is categorised among the most severe crisis-facing countries in terms of human resources in health care (Karan et al., 2019). Though there are claims that the country has enough doctors, the existing evidence raises concerns. In India there are 0.9 doctors per thousand population (OECD, 2021) against the required one doctor per thousand population as per the criteria set by the World Health Organisation (WHO) with India ranking among the lowest (106th) of the developed (112) countries (OECD, 2021).

There is no single reason for the limited number of healthcare professionals in India (Hazarika, 2013). For instance, studies of nurses have suggested multiple barriers, including long working hours, lack of recognition, poor teamwork, and workplace violence (Chhugani & James, 2017). In the case of physicians, studies suggest that the low availability of doctors in rural areas can be attributed to competition from the private sector, lower salaries, and poor working and living environment. However, research conducted by Rao et al. (2010) based on interviews found that financial and educational incentives can attract doctors and nurses to rural postings. The lack of infrastructure, support staff, and drugs, local political interference and lack of security are the major factors behind low retention of doctors and nurses. The inadequate facilities of basic amenities like water, electricity, and education facilities for children also lead to low retention. Job satisfaction as measured by autonomy at work and job responsibility has also been identified as a critical factor in determining the availability of a healthy workforce in rural settings (Sharma et al., 2014). These issues create problems of retention that must be addressed to create a sustainable workforce (Goel et al., 2016).

Workforce Analysis in India

In this section, I extended my previous work on the Indian workforce (Khan, 2022). This analysis examines the availability of health professionals, the inter-group inequality in their distribution, and quality of jobs in the medical profession in India. The analysis is based on the data from PLF Survey, 2019–20 (National Statistical Organisation, 2020). The number of health professionals is used as a proxy of medical doctors. The occupational classification of workers provides information about the health professionals engaged as physicians and surgeons (Allopathic, Ayurvedic, Homoeopathic, Unani system), dental specialists, veterinarians, and other health professionals (excluding nurses). This group of occupations largely covers doctors and, hence, can be used to measure the number of healthcare professionals in India.

The result of an analysis using the industrial classification system must proceed with caution. This alternative measure does not directly measure the number of doctors as it does not identify the medical profession directly. Rather, it shows the distribution of these workers by industrial groups. This classification has been used in the analysis to investigate the nature of jobs among health professionals. It provides details about the institutional and non-institutional classification of the medical profession. The industrial groups are analysed by gender, social, and religious groups, and across rural and urban areas. This analysis examines the availability of healthcare professionals per thousand population, their percentage distribution by types of employment namely regular employed and self-employed, and their distribution by industrial categories. The average earning per month per worker is also calculated for the analysis.

Health Professionals in India

There are two ways of estimating the number of health professionals in India from the secondary data. One by examining the industrial concentration and second by examining the occupational concentration of the workers. The figure based on the occupational concentration is close to the figure from other sources (Press Information Bureau, 2022). The total number of health professionals is 13.1 million (Table 9.1). This is close to the figures provided by the National Medical Commission reporting 13,08,009 Allopathic doctors (Press Information Bureau, 2022). As Table 9.1 demonstrates, the share of Hindu High Castes (HHCs) is highest followed by Hindu Other Backward Castes (HOBCs) and SCs. Tribals and Muslims are seriously underrepresented. Most of the health professionals are concentrated in urban areas though the population is highly concentrated in rural areas.

There is a very high disparity in availability of healthcare workers in rural and urban areas. As Table 9.1 demonstrates, there are 4.2 million healthcare workers in rural areas while the figure is nearly 8.9 million in urban areas. The rural areas comprise 32% of the total health professional while the remaining are concentrated in urban areas. This is concerning as nearly 68% of the population resides in rural areas as against 32% in urban areas.

To address the existing disparities in health services programmes such as National Rural Health Mission (NRHM) have been adopted by the government with a focus on rural areas. As a result, the country has well-established primary healthcare services and community healthcare service. However, human resources increased commensurately, particularly in rural areas and remote areas. Studies (NHM, 2011) show that during the period of NRHM, the shortfall of nurses and ANMs has decreased, though the availability of doctors did not increase at a similar pace (Motkuri & Mishra, 2018; Nair, 2019). For instance, Shahrawat and Joon (2010) have suggested that the shortage of health workforce in rural areas might be attributed to the migration of doctors, better income prospects in the private sector, unfavourable working environment and living conditions in rural areas.

The low supply of doctors due to the expensive nature of medical courses also works as a bottleneck in addressing the shortage of doctors.

Data from the PLF Survey clearly demonstrate that females are also seriously underrepresented among health professionals even though the medical profession is considered women-friendly due to the conventional social norms in India. As Table 9.1 demonstrates, women comprise 28% of the total health professionals in India while their share in population is close to half.

While India comes close to the WHO recommended minimum of one doctor for 1000 population, rural areas appear to be underserved. The OECD (2021) data noted above show how India is poorly positioned in terms of availability of healthcare professionals. When examined by region, the number of doctors in rural areas is 0.5 per thousand (half of the minimum requirement) while the number is 2.2 in urban areas, more than double of the minimum requirement. Thus, regional inequality is clearly evidenced when disaggregated figures are examined (Table 9.2).

Similar observations can also be made when considering other demographic factors that define India's healthcare workforce. There are only 0.6 female doctors per 1000 population while the corresponding figure is 1.4 for male doctors. The availability of doctors slightly falls short of the minimum requirement among SC and HOBC while it is higher among HHC. The majority of Hindus also meet the minimum requirement; Christians also have slightly higher availability than the minimum requirement while Sikhs are the best performer among the religious groups. There are 3.4 doctors per thousand population among Sikhs. In sharp contrast, tribal populations and Muslims are the most poorly served groups in this regard: there are 0.4 and 0.5 doctors per thousand population among these two groups, respectively.

Only 11 out of 25 major states satisfy the standard requirement of doctors as stipulated by WHO. The states of Punjab, Maharashtra, Karnataka, and Manipur are among the best served while states like West Bengal, Odisha, Rajasthan, and Bihar are the worst served. Almost all the states that are well-served have high socioeconomic status whereas those states which suffer from serious shortages have a comparatively low socioeconomic status.

In trying to understand where differences in the number of healthcare professions arise, a useful point of comparison is the monthly per capita consumption expenditure (MPCE). When comparing the MPCE with the healthcare workforce

TABLE 9.1 Number of Health Professionals, 2019–20

	Number (in thousand)					*Share (%)*	*Share (in %)*	
	Rural	*Urban*	*Male*	*Female*	*Total*		*Rural*	*Female*
Scheduled Tribes	12.5	33.6	32.3	13.7	46.1	3.5	27.1	29.8
Scheduled Castes	170.4	70.1	190.9	49.6	240.6	18.4	70.8	20.6
Hindu Other Backward Castes	166.2	217.9	296.7	87.5	384.1	29.3	43.3	22.8
Hindu Higher Castes	50.1	410.5	305.8	149.2	460.6	35.1	10.9	32.4
Muslims	12.8	73.6	59.2	27.3	86.5	6.6	14.8	31.6
Total	421.6	888.8	933.6	371.2	1310.3	100	32.2	28.3

Source: Periodic Labour Force Survey (PLFS), 2019–20.

TABLE 9.2 Availability of Health Workers, 2019–20

Demographic groups	*Number (per thousand)*
Rural	0.5
Urban	2.2
Male	1.4
Female	0.6
Scheduled Tribes	0.4
Scheduled Castes	0.9
Other Backward Castes	0.8
Higher Castes	1.7
Hindus	1.0
Muslims	0.5
Christians	1.3
Sikhs	3.4

Source: Periodic Labour Force Survey (PLFS), 2019–20.

(per thousand), a clear correlation is obtained, $r(25) = 0.69, p = 0.01$. Thus, the availability of healthcare professionals is linked to overall economic conditions.

Healthcare Workforce Categories

Most of the health workers are engaged as regular/salaried (RS) workers, though this varies widely across different groups (Figure 9.1). Nearly 61% of the total healthcare workers are engaged in salaried jobs. This share is slightly higher among females than male. This result reflects gender-based norms as the majority of women – particularly from middle-class families – are only allowed to work in secure, high-paying jobs (Sudarshan, 2017). The number of salaried jobs is lower in rural areas. This result stems from the lower concentration of hospitals in rural areas relative to urban areas. Similarly, lower share of salaried workers is observed among tribals and Muslims reinforcing that these communities are underserved. The health professionals among SC are highly confined to salaried employment: nearly 72% of these workers among them are salaried workers. This might be attributable to the caste-based reservation in government jobs improving their presence. One may ponder about the contrasting pattern among ST and SC, though both come under the ambit of job reservation. The geographical isolation among the former might be an important factor constraining their participation in regular employment particularly in urban areas. Muslims excluded from any affirmative action in job struggle to get into white-collar salaried jobs. The pattern among HOBC is comparable to the all-India level. In general, HHC remain overrepresented in salaried jobs. The medical profession is a departure from this pattern as the share of self-employment is higher in this case. This might be possible due to their better presence among the independent practitioners with a better earning potential. The share of casual employment is negligible among every group except Muslims.

TABLE 9.3 Number of Health Professionals per Thousand Population, 2019–20

State	*Health Professionals*	*Average monthly per capita consumption expenditure (USD)*	*Earnings: RS (USD)*	*Earnings: SE (USD)*
Delhi	3.2	45.3	722.5	NA
Punjab	3.1	35.7	568.1	229.9
Manipur	2.3	29.1	362.4	36.4
Maharashtra	2.3	26.7	183.5	521.8
Karnataka	1.8	24.5	485.0	958.9
Gujarat	1.2	28.1	341.3	182.5
Telangana	1.2	29.0	531.3	392.3
Tripura	1.2	24.4	188.9	606.6
Mizoram	1.1	33.4	374.9	NA
Uttarakhand	1.0	25.6	655.4	182.0
Kerala	1.0	35.8	751.2	766.8
Haryana	0.9	30.1	537.1	242.7
Jharkhand	0.9	19.2	384.5	118.4
Andhra Pradesh	0.9	30.0	163.8	150.8
Nagaland	0.9	22.9	232.3	84.9
Chhattisgarh	0.8	18.1	505.5	366.3
Madhya Pradesh	0.8	19.3	217.8	128.1
Jammu and Kashmir	0.7	28.0	670.8	388.9
Himachal Pradesh	0.7	28.0	270.2	266.9
Assam	0.6	23.7	397.4	48.9
West Bengal	0.6	26.0	629.5	189.2
Odisha	0.5	18.4	283.7	121.3
Rajasthan	0.3	23.1	664.5	190.9
Uttar Pradesh	0.3	18.9	187.8	334.9
Bihar	0.2	16.9	556.5	277.7

Source: Periodic Labour Force Survey (PLFS), 2019–20.

However, the higher presence of self-employed workers among Muslims cannot be regarded as an advantage. This rather follows the conventional pattern where Muslims are highly concentrated into self-employment.

Labour force issues are also evidenced in filling positions. The government jobs are the more preferred option due to the job security and social security benefits associated with it. In general, underprivileged groups are less represented in regular employment while their representation remains high in casual employment (Mamgain & Khan, 2020). However, the medical profession does not always confirm this pattern. In fact, the privileged professionals with high levels of expertise would find enough demand in the market to earn a dignified livelihood as self-employment rather than being tied to regular employment. This is why low turn-out against job advertisement in the government sector is not surprising in this profession. For example, in the state of Punjab recently, 58% of

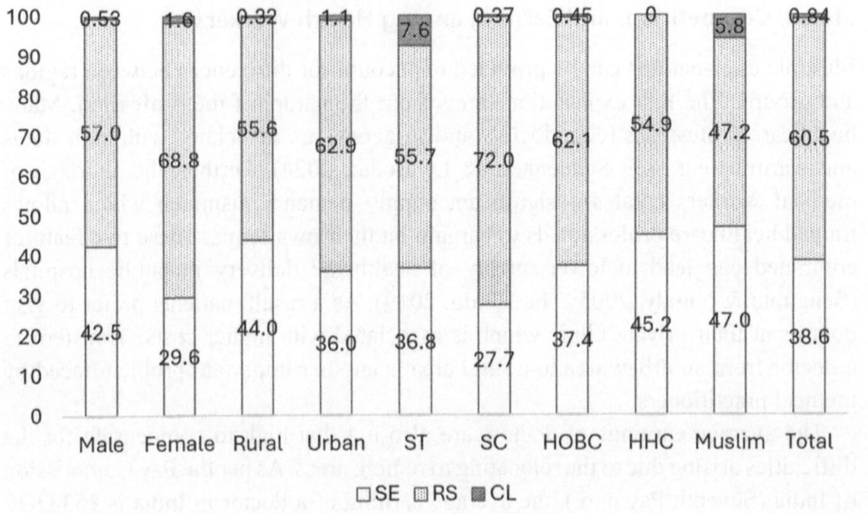

FIGURE 9.1 Health professionals by type of work, 2019–20.

Source: Based on Periodic Labour Force Survey (PLFS), 2019–20.

TABLE 9.4 Requirement and Working Specialists in Haryana State of India

	Requirement	*Working*
MD (Medicine)	241	50
Gynaecologists	193	95
Anaesthetists	231	100
Paediatrics	146	65
Surgeons	143	75

Source: Tribune India, (2023).

the advertised posts of the Medical Specialist remained vacant after the first round of interview. Of the 513 advertised posts, only 215 doctors were successfully hired, leaving 297 posts vacant. The authorities decided to hold another round of interviews to fill the posts. The shortage is higher for specialists and super specialists. Branches of medicine, paediatrics, and radiology have the highest vacancies. Of the 46 advertised posts in the radiology branch, only three were filled while 23 paediatricians joined against 121 vacant posts. In medicine, only 21 out of the 69 posts were filled. No vacancy of specialist was left in the ENT and pathology branches (Tribune India, 2019). A similar scenario is observed in Haryana which is a neighbouring state of Punjab. There is a shortage of nearly 800 doctors out of the total cadre strength of 3500. There is an emerging trend of doctors consistently quitting their job due to high pressure and low salary in the government sector (Tribune India, 2023, Table 9.4).

Status, Competition, and Earning among Health Workers

Multiple explanations can be provided to account for differences between regions and groups. The first explanation stems from the nature of the profession. Many healthcare professions (e.g., doctors and surgeons) are associated with high status and warmth (e.g., see Schoenherr & Le Bouar, 2024). Further, the shortage of medical workers creates a significant supply–demand mismatch which allows trained healthcare professionals to bargain on their own terms. These two features combined can lead to lower quality of healthcare delivery in public hospitals (Sengupta & Nundy, 2005; The Hindu, 2019). As a result, patients prefer to visit doctors at their private clinic which is associated with higher costs. Transferring a doctor from an urban area to a rural area is another important problem faced by medical practitioners.

The average earnings of doctors are also not that high to compensate for the difficulties arising due to the relocating to remote areas. As per the Pay Commission of India (Seventh Pay, n.d.), the average earning of a doctor in India is ₹533,932 per year (6478 USD) with an average monthly salary of ₹44,494 (540 USD). The earnings of an MBBS doctor with at least 5.5 years of experience vary from ₹20,000 (243 USD) to ₹60,000 (728 USD) per month. The earnings of medical professionals with a specialisation in Doctor of Medicine (MD) vary from ₹45, 000 (546 USD) to ₹2,00,000 (2427 USD) per month (Table 9.5).

Further, the earnings of doctors in private hospitals are also higher than that in government hospitals particularly for the highly specialised ones. Thus, the private sector attracts the better-skilled doctors by crowding out the skilled doctors from the government sector. Table 9.6 shows the average monthly earnings, minimum and maximum monthly salary of a doctor in different types of hospitals in India. This is to note that the average earnings of a doctor are higher in the government

TABLE 9.5 Salary Range of Doctors as per the Pay Commission

	Min[a]	*Max*[a]
MBBS doctors	35,000 (424 USD)	65,000 (789 USD)
Ophthalmologist	80,000 (97 USD)	175,000 (2123 USD)
General surgery	100,000 (121 USD)	175,000 (2123 USD)
Paediatrician	100,000 (121 USD)	200,000 (2427 USD)
Orthopaedician	100,000 (121 USD)	200,000 (2427 USD)
Anaesthesia	100,000 (121 USD)	200,000 (2427 USD)
General physician	100,000 (121 USD)	200,000 (2427 USD)
Gynaecologist	100,000 (121 USD)	250,000 (3033 USD)
Radiologists	150,000 (1820 USD)	350,000 (4247 USD)

Source: Based on Pay Commission of India.

Note:

[a] Rupee (₹) has been converted into USD by dividing by 82.42, i.e., exchange rate on 12.06.2023.

TABLE 9.6 Average Monthly Salary of Doctors in Different Hospitals (in USD)

	Hospitals	*Avg.*	*Min.*	*Max.*
1	Apollo Hospitals	834.1	218.4	764.4
2	All India Institute of Medical Sciences (AIIMS)	1069.5	752.2	10,106.8
3	Government of India	1947.3	473.2	3494.3
4	Thermaco	6341.0	1747.1	19,679.7
5	Fortis Healthcare	610.8	388.3	5156.5
6	Yashoda Hospital	521.7	388.3	812.9
7	Sahyadri Speciality Hospital	328.6	279.1	946.4

Source: Accessed from https://doctorsreview.in/health/doctor-salary-in-india/.

Note: Rupee (₹) has been converted dollar by dividing by 82.42, i.e., exchange rate on 12.06.2023.

TABLE 9.7 Earnings among Health Professionals, Salaried

	Rural	*Urban*	*Male*	*Female*	*All-India average*
Scheduled Tribes (ST)	400.4	661.5	588.8	387.9	533.6
Scheduled Castes (SC)	158.1	351.9	203.5	257.6	213.0
Hindu Other Backward Castes (HOBC)	412.2	393.8	388.0	427.3	400.2
Hindu High Castes (HHC)	534.6	548.1	509.6	560.4	547.1
Muslims	177.3	248.1	214.5	312.3	251.8
Total	285.5	488.9	401.8	459.1	426.5

Source: Periodic Labour Force Survey, 2019–20.

Note: Rupee (₹) has been converted dollar by dividing by 82.42, i.e., exchange rate on 12.06.2023.

sector than the private sector. However, the range is higher in most of the private hospitals. Only the earnings in AIIMS are higher than the private sector.

The earnings vary by socio-religious background of the health professionals also. The PLFS data show that the average earning of a health professional is USD 426.5 per month. It is the highest among HHCs. They earn USD 547.1 per month. The earning among tribals is also better than all-India average, USD 533.6. All the remaining groups earn less than the all-India average, the lowest being among SCs followed by Muslims and HOBCs. This is to note that SCs are highly concentrated into the salaried jobs, but their earnings are the lowest which shows that they are largely confined to jobs with low earning potentials. Like SCs, the quality of jobs is low among Muslims also (Table 9.7).

It is generally believed that earnings for health professionals in the private sector (especially, doctors) are higher in comparison to those within the government sector. This would seem to be a reasonable conclusion if we consider the small proportion of doctors that have a high degree of specialisation. In these cases, they might be engaged with multiple hospitals as a consultant, leading to incomes that are higher

TABLE 9.8 Earning from Government and Private Sector, 2019–20

Groups	*Non gov*	*Gov PSE*	*Total salaried*	*SE*
Male	332.2	500.0	426.0	365.5
Female	400.3	512.9	467.8	347.1
ST	96.0	583.4	535.8	294.2
SC	151.9	239.8	218.2	227.6
HOBC	201.1	660.8	436.0	221.2
HHC	532.0	610.8	569.9	488.5
Muslim	132.8	484.2	263.9	390.1
Total	353.8	514.9	446.7	361.9

Source: Periodic Labour Force Survey, 2019–20.

Note: Rupee (₹) has been converted dollar by dividing by 82.42, i.e., exchange rate on 12.06.2023.

than the average. However, as Table 9.6 suggests, the earnings of an average doctor are higher for government salaried jobs (USD 514.9 per month) in comparison to those of private salaried jobs (USD 353.8 per month). Notably, earning from self-employment is higher than that of earning from regular jobs in the private sector. They earn USD 361.9 on an average (Table 9.9). This pattern itself shows the peculiar inequality existing in medical profession based on one's specialisation. As discussed already, the privileged professionals with high levels of expertise would find enough demand in the market to earn a dignified livelihood as self-employment rather than being tied to regular employment. As a result, the turn-out against job employment in the government sector remains low at a higher level of specialisation. The highly specialised professionals prefer and would choose the private sector as an independent consultant with a high return to their services. The high pressure in the government jobs and location of such jobs in remote areas are also important reasons for the shift of the specialised professionals towards the private sector (Table 9.8).

An analysis of geographic differences in salary is also revealing. As Table 9.3 indicates, salaried doctors earned higher income in states like Arunachal, Kerala, Delhi, and Jammu and Kashmir while it is lowest in Madhya Pradesh, Tripura, Uttar Pradesh, Maharashtra, and Andhra Pradesh. Self-employed doctors earn higher income in Karnataka, Kerala, Tripura, and Maharashtra while it is lowest in Odisha, Jharkhand, Nagaland, Assam, and Manipur. Unlike availability of doctors, the earnings do not appear to follow any pattern relative to the developmental position of the state. Supporting this observation, the correlation between earnings from regular employment and number of healthcare professionals (reported above) was small and not significant, $r(25) = 0.126, p = 0.550$. The absence of a relationship is likely due to the wide arrays of multiple factors. For instance, doctors from poor states might also earn high income due to the low supply of medical services. The correlation between earnings from self-employment and the availability of health professionals is relatively higher but still is not significant, $r(25) = 0.211$.

Industrial Categories

As mentioned earlier, the information on workers from the available secondary data by industrial categories does not specifically provide information on doctors. So, the estimated workforce might not truly reflect the actual state of affairs. However, the patterns of earnings provide an important insight into the variations in different categories of industry under the broader umbrella of the healthcare sector. Table 9.9 depicts the earnings of HCPs in different industrial roles. Given that it covers a wide array of occupations, the average earnings are underestimated. However, the variation shown by this data is worth examining. At aggregate level the average earning of self-employed professionals is higher than salaried workers. This is to note that this finding contradicts with the estimates obtained from the occupational categories wherein earnings from regular employment are higher than that from self-employment (see Table 9.3). Given that the occupational classification better represents the medical sector, I will prefer to go with the earlier explanations.

In regular employment the highest earning is observed in practices outside hospital activities. However, earning in hospital activities is the next highest. The earnings from the remaining activities fall drastically. The pattern remains the same in SE jobs. It is highest in hospital activities followed by medical and dental practice activities and so on (Tables 9.9 and 9.10).

The earning in every industrial activity follows the conventional identity-based patterns. In human health, the earning of HHCs from SE is highest followed by ST, HOBC, and SC. Muslims earn slightly higher than SC but lower than all other groups. In residential care, the earning is far lower among SC/ST than HOBC/HHC. HOBC and HHC continue to occupy top positions. The earning among

TABLE 9.9 Earning among Self-Employed and RS by Type of Industry (in USD)

	RS	*SE*
Hospital activities	253.5	408.8
Medical and dental practice activities	310.0	316.3
Other human health activities Ayurveda, Unani, Homoeopath, independent laboratory, and blood banks	175.8	237.2
Nursing care for elderly, convalescent homes, rest homes	178.8	86.5
Residential care facilities for mental retardation, Mental, and substance abuse	227.0	0.0
Residential care activities for the elderly and disabled	174.3	0.0
Other residential care activities	126.3	261.7
Social work activities without accommodation for the elderly and disabled	146.6	119.0
Other social work activities without accommodation	101.3	135.5
Total	219.1	304.5

Source: Periodic Labour Force Survey, 2019–20.

Note: Rupee (₹) has been converted dollar by dividing by 82.42, i.e., exchange rate on 12.06.2023.

TABLE 9.10 Earnings, SE (in USD)

	Human health	*Residential care (87)*	*Social work activities without accommodation*	*Total*
Self-employment				
ST	386.8	36.4	96.8	336.3
SC	202.3	12.1	120.9	193.4
HOBC	221.4	198.2	59.9	215.1
HHC	400.5	225.5	284.3	395.5
Muslim	206.2	182.0	32.3	196.7
Total	312.5	252.1	133.3	304.5
Regular/salaried employment				
ST	217.6	123.5	112.8	188.7
SC	164.0	121.3	79.1	153.9
HOBC	242.5	200.8	95.9	219.4
HHC	300.8	136.9	131.5	277.0
Muslim	168.1	254.7	137.8	167.8
Total	240.4	154.7	109.0	219.1

Source: Periodic Labour Force Survey, 2019–20.

Note: Rupee (₹) has been converted dollar by dividing by 82.42, i.e., exchange rate on 12.06.2023.

Muslims is lower than HOBC/HHC and higher than SC/ST. However, the earning of Muslims in social activities without accommodation is lowest while it continues to be highest among HHC. The earning among SC/ST is higher than Muslims and HOBC but lower than HHC (Table 9.9).

In regular employment also the earning from human health is highest among HHCs and HOBCs. Muslims and SCs are the lowest earning groups. The earning of tribals is higher than them. However, earning from residential care and social work departs from the conventional patterns. In residential care the earning is highest among Muslims followed by HOBC, HHC, and ST and SC. In social works also the earning is highest among Muslims followed by HHC, ST, HOBC, and SC, respectively. This is to note that the earning from human health is higher than that of other two industrial groups which indicates that jobs under this category are of better quality (Table 9.9).

Conclusion

This study examines the availability of healthcare professionals in India with a focus on the status of the underprivileged groups. It shows that social injustice that exists in a society might limit access to a career in medicine. It is observed that the availability of health professionals satisfies the criterion set by the WHO. However, less-developed countries continue to face a serious shortage of healthcare professionals. Further, the distribution of health professionals by socio-religious groups, location and gender is uneven. The underprivileged groups particularly people from tribal communities, Muslims, and women face a serious underrepresentation of health professionals vis-à-vis their population share. All workers are either regular employed or self-employed while casual workers are completely absent reflecting the elite nature of this profession. The result of this study indicates that salaried workers earn more than the self-employed professional despite the popular perception of the contrary. This is indicative of the fact that only a minuscule elite section of these professionals manages to establish a well-developed clinic while the majority struggle. This disparity indicates that merely a choice of medical profession does not ensure one's success in the job market. A graduate belonging to the privileged background having a degree from prestigious institutions with sufficient social networks may be more successful than the others. In such a scenario, the choice of self-employment as an independent consultant might be a more attractive choice than the regular employment. In fact, a relatively better performance of reserved groups such as SC/ST in regular employment is an indication of the success of affirmative action.

There are indications of a better share of RS health professionals among underprivileged caste/ethnic groups, probably due to the presence of affirmative action, but inequality prevails in self-employment and high-quality occupations, thus reflecting the inequality prevalent in society. However, the pattern among Muslims is different from the caste/ethnic groups as the share of RS workers is lower and while the level of self-employment is higher among Muslims. Such policies would also improve the availability of health professionals from the underprivileged socio-religious background which in turn would play an instrumental role in ensuring better access to healthcare services for patients from underprivileged communities.

The findings of this study also suggest that improving the availability of the healthcare workforce demands intervention towards how recruitment and training is conducted in medical education in India. Ensuring equal access for students from underprivileged groups is critical for addressing the existing inequality in the availability of health professionals. For this, affirmative action for students from poor families and first-generation learners might be worthwhile to address the problem of inequality of access to medicine courses. Such policies would also improve the availability of healthcare professionals from varied socio-religious backgrounds which would play an instrumental role in ensuring better access to healthcare services for patients from underprivileged communities.

Note

1 This group is often referred to as the Mughals in English, derived from the term 'Mongol'.

References

Association of Faculties of Medicine of Canada. (2012). *The Future of Medical Education in Canada*. Ottawa: AMFC.

Bajaj Committee. (1986) National Health Portal. Accessed from https://web.archive.org/web/20170119150205/; www.nhp.gov.in/sites/default/files/pdf/Bajaj_Committee_report.pdf.

Bhore Committee. (1946). National Health Portal. Accessed from https://web.archive.org/web/20151009034256/; www.nhp.gov.in/directory-services-and-regulations/committees-and-commissions/bhore-committee1946.

Campbell, A. (1999). The origins of classical homoeopathy? *Complementary Therapies in Medicine*, *7*, 76–82.

Chhugani, M., & James, M. M. (2017). Challenges faced by nurses in India-the major workforce of the healthcare system. *Nurse Care Open Access Journal*, *2*(4), 112–114.

Chikersal, A. (2015). *Physician Shortages in the Indian Public Sector.* Health Policy Brief. New Delhi: Centre for Policy Research.

Cleland, J., Dowell, J., McLachlan, J., Nicholson, S., & Petterson, F. (2012). *Identifying Best Practice in the Selection of Medical Student*. London: General Medical Council.

Department of Education. (2014). *Undergraduate Applications, Offers and Acceptances: 2014 Report and Appendices*. Canberra: Department of Education.

Fenton, J. J., Fiscella, K., Jerant, A. F., Sousa, F., Henderson, M., Fancher, T., & Franks, P. (2016). Reducing medical school admissions disparities in an era of legal restrictions: Adjusting for applicant socioeconomic disadvantage. *Journal of Health Care for the Poor and Underserved*, *27*(1), 22–34.

Gina, K., Kim, E., Terry, K., & Cynthia, J. (2013). More than I expected: Perceived benefits of yoga practice among older adults at risk for cardiovascular disease. *Complementary Therapies in Medicine*, *21*, 14–28.

Goel, S., Angeli, F., Bhatnagar, N., Singla, N., Grover, M., & Maarse, H. (2016). Retaining health workforce in rural and underserved areas of India: What works and what doesn't? A critical interpretative synthesis. *The National Medical Journal of India*, *29*(4), 212.

Government of India (GOI). (2017). National Health Policy, Ministry of Health and Family Welfare. Accessed from https://main.mohfw.gov.in/sites/default/files/9147562941489753121.pdf.

Hazarika, I. (2013). Health workforce in India: Assessment of availability, production and distribution. *WHO South-East Asia Journal of Public Health*, *2*(2), 106–112.

Hoyez, A. (2007). The 'world of yoga': The production and reproduction of therapeutic landscapes. *Social Science & Medicine*, *65*, 112–124.

Jaiswal, Y. S., & Williams, L. L. (2016). A glimpse of Ayurveda – The forgotten history and principles of Indian traditional medicine. *Journal of Traditional and Complementary Medicine*, *7*(1), 50–53.

Jodhka, S. (2017). *Caste in Contemporary India*. New Delhi: Routledge India.

Jungalwalla Committee. (1967). National Health Portal. Accessed from https://web.archive.org/web/20200923142137/; www.nhp.gov.in/sites/default/files/pdf/Jungalwal_Committee_Report.pdf.

Karan, A., Negandhi, H., Nair, R., Sharma, A., Tiwari, R., & Zodpey, S. (2019). Size, composition and distribution of human resource for health in India: New estimates using National Sample Survey and Registry data. *BMJ Open*, *9*, e025979. https://doi.org/10.1136/bmjopen-2018-025979.

Kartar Singh Committee. (1973) National Health Portal. Accessed from https://web.archive.org/web/20200923115004/; www.nhp.gov.in/sites/default/files/pdf/Kartar_Singh_Committee_Report.pdf.

Kasthuri, A. (2018). Challenges to healthcare in India: The five A's. *Indian Journal of Community Medicine: Official Publication of Indian Association of Preventive & Social Medicine*, *43*(3), 141–143. https://doi.org/10.4103/ijcm.IJCM_194_18.

Khan, K. (2022). Inequality in access to medical education in India: Implications for the availability of health professionals. *Caste: A Global Journal on Social Exclusion*, *3*(2), 319–334.

Kolasa, A., & Weychert, E. (2023). The causal effect of catastrophic health expenditure on poverty in Poland. *European Journal of Health Economics*. https://doi.org/10.1007/s10198-023-01579-6.

Mamgain, R. P., & Khan, K. (2020). Trends in employment and unemployment in India: Dimensions of gender, caste and education. In N. V. Varghese, & M. Khare (Eds.), *India Higher Education Report 2020: Employment and Employability of Higher Education Graduates in India*. India: Routledge.

Ministry of Health and Family Welfare (MOHFW, 2013–14). Household Health Expenditures in India. https://main.mohfw.gov.in/sites/default/files/38300411751489562625.pdf.

Motkuri, V., & Mishra, U. S. (2018). Human Resources in Healthcare and Health Outcomes in India MPRA Paper No. 85217. Accessed from https://mpra.ub.uni-muenchen.de/85217/.

Mukherjee, P. (2001). Evaluation of Indian traditional medicine. *Drug Information Journal*, *2*, 623.

Nair, K. S. (2019). Health workforce in India: Opportunities and challenges. *International Journal of Community Medicine and Public Health*, *6*(10), 4596–4604.

National Health Policy. (2017). *Ministry of Health and Family Welfare*. Government of India. Accessed from https://main.mohfw.gov.in/sites/default/files/9147562941489753121.pdf.

National Statistical Organisation. (2020). *Periodic Labour Force Survey*. Ministry of Statistics Programme and Implementation, Government of India.

NHM. (2011). *Evaluation Study of National Rural Health Mission (NRHM) in 7 States*. Government of India. Accessed from https://nhm.gov.in/images/pdf/publication/Evaluation_study_of_NHM_in_7_States.pdf.

NIH U.S. Department of Health and Human Services; USA. (2012). *Naturopathy: An Introduction*. National Institutes of Health. http://nccam.nih.gov/health/naturopathy/naturopathyintro.htm.

NITI Ayog. (2021). *Investment opportunities in India's healthcare sector*. Government of India. Accessed from www.niti.gov.in/sites/default/files/2021-03/InvestmentOpportunities_HealthcareSector_0.pdf.

OECD. (2021). *Health at a Glance 2021*. Paris: OECD Indicators, OECD. https://doi.org/10.1787/ae3016b9-en.

Posadzki, P., Edzard, E., Rohini, T., & Myeong, S. (2011). Is yoga effective for pain? A systematic review of randomized clinical trials. *Complementary Therapies in Medicine*, *19*, 281–287.

Press Information Bureau. (2022). Government has taken multiple steps to further increase availability of doctors in the country. Accessed from https://pib.gov.in/PressReleseDetailm.aspx?PRID=1845081#:~:text=As%20per%20information%20provided%20by,)%20as%20on%20June%2C%202022.

Rao, K. D., Sundaramana, T., Bhatnagar, A., Gupta, G., & Jain, K. (2010). *Health Workers Attitudes Toward Rural Service in India: Results from Qualitative Research*. HNP Discussion Paper. Washington DC: World Bank.

Sachar Committee Report. (2006). *Sachar Committee Report: Social, Economic and Educational Status of the Muslim Community of India; A Rreport, Prime Minister's High Level Committee*. Cabinet Secretariat, Government of India.

Schoenherr, J. R. (2027). Innovation and implementation in the health professions: Translating Research in Education and Healthcare Delivery. In J. R. Schoenherr (Ed.),

Fundamentals and Frontiers of Medical Education and Decision-Making: Innovation, Implementation, and Translational Research (pp. 1–76). Routledge.

Schoenherr, J. R., & Le-Bouar, C. (2024). Representing and communicating health information: Fundamentals of persuasive health communication. In *Fundamentals and Frontiers of Medical Education and Decision-Making: Educational Theory and Psychological Practice* (pp. 270–312). Routledge.

Schoenherr, J. R., & Hamstra, S. J. (2024). Validity in health professions education: From assessment instruments to program innovation and evaluation. In *Fundamentals and Frontiers of Medical Education and Decision-Making: Educational Theory and Psychological Practice* (pp. 80–107). Routledge.

Sengupta, A., & Nundy, S. (Nov 19, 2005). The private health sector in India. *BMJ*, *331*(7526), 1157–11578. https://doi.org/10.1136/bmj.331.7526.1157. PMID: 16293815; PMCID: PMC1285083.

Seventh pay. (n.d.). Doctor Pay Scale Grade Matrix. Accessed from https://7thpaycommissioninfo.in/doctor-pay-scale-grade-matrix-allowances/.

Sharma, M. et al. (2014). Determinants of Indian physicians' satisfaction & dissatisfaction from their Job. *Indian Journal of Medical Research*, *139*, 409–417.

Shehrawat, R., & Joon, V. (2010). Rural health care system in India and the challenges of retention of health manpower in rural India. *Health and Population: Perspectives and Issues*, *33*(4), 217–225.

Srinivas, M. N. (2017). Mobility in the caste system. In J. C. Singer & B. S. Cohn (Eds), *Structure and Change in Indian Society* (pp. 189–200). Routledge.

Sudarshan, R. M. (2017). Higher education and gendered norms: Enabling the 'use' of women's education. In N. V. Varghese, N. S. Sabharwal & C. M. Malish (Eds.), *India Higher Education Report 2016*: Equity. New Delhi: SAGE Publications India Pvt. Ltd.

The Hindu. (Feb, 2019) Corruption blamed for healthcare sector woes. Accessed from www.thehindu.com/news/cities/ozhikode/corruption-blamed-for-healthcare-sector-woes/article26361494.ece.

The Hindu. (Feb 11, 2024). Comprehensive India-specific approach needed for growth of medical education: Parliamentary panel. www.thehindu.com/education/comprehensive-india-specific-approach-needed-for-growth-of-medical-education-parliamentary-panel/article67834932.ece.

Times of India (TOI). (Nov 20, 2022). How limiting student migration for medical school will benefit India and advance its educational leadership. https://timesofindia.indiatimes.com/blogs/voices/how-limiting-student-migration-for-medical-school-will-benefit-india-and-advance-its-educational-leadership/.

Tribune India. (Feb 17, 2019). Doctors stay away from government sector. www.tribuneindia.com/news/archive/chandigarh/doctors-stay-away-from-government-sector-730035.

Tribune India. (May 28, 2023). www.tribuneindia.com/news/features/why-doctors-are-quitting-haryana-government-jobs-511967.

Vaid, D. (2014). Caste in contemporary India: Flexibility and persistence. *Annual Review of Sociology*, *40*, 391–410.

World Economic Forum. (2020). *Global social mobility report 2020: Equality, opportunity and a new economic imperative*. Geneva: World Economic Forum. www3.weforum.org/docs/Global_Social_Mobility_Report.pdf

SECTION 3

International and Transnational Systems

Evolution and Adaptation

10

THE DEVELOPMENT AND DYNAMICS OF HETERARCHICAL STRUCTURE IN MAYAN MEDICAL EDUCATION AND HEALTHCARE ECOSYSTEMS

Jordan Richard Schoenherr

Spread across parts of modern-day Mexico, Guatemala, Belize, Honduras, and El Salvador, the Maya live in diverse landscapes, with over 30 documented dialects (Aissen et al., 2017; Brown & Witschey, 2001; Law, 2020; Reyes-Foster, 2014; Wichmann, 2006). Rather than focusing on their successful innovations in continuously adapting to changes in their physical and social environment, research has tended to focus on health disparities between ladinos and mestizos (people of 'mixed' heritage), and the comparatively worse health outcomes for the Maya and other indigenous groups (Bhatt, 2012; Bogin et al., 1992; Lee et al., 2012; Melville & Lykes, 1992). This pattern is consistent with other colonized populations (Asamoah et al., 2023; Lewis & Myhra, 2018; Marrone, 2007; Smallwood et al., 2021; Valeggia & Snodgrass, 2015; for specific studies, see Bramley et al., 2005; Chan et al., 2026). In North America and elsewhere, these efforts were often framed paternalistically, 'to "save the Indians" from disease' (Few, 2015, pp. 9–10), often ignoring indigenous knowledge or medical traditions arriving with enslaved Africans.

Historically, studies of Mesoamerican medical knowledge have largely been motivated by bioprospecting, with the goal of decontextualizing therapeutic knowledge (e.g., plants, animals), and incorporate it into Biomedical Western Medicine (BWM; Anderson, 2002; Berlin & Berlin, 2004a, 2004b; Berlin et al., 1999; Greene, 2004; Leonti et al., 2013; Nigh, 2002; Pushpangadan et al., 2018; Shiva, 2007; Soejarto et al., 2005). While such processes might qualify the efficacy of pharmacologically active compounds and validate them in Western science, they do not override the agency and generations of cumulative experimentation of indigenous populations as the originators of the innovation. Nor does validation and assimilation of knowledge with BWM necessarily affect adoption rates by health seekers.

DOI: 10.4324/9781003498155-10

Restricting what constitutes healthcare using BWM medicalization can also severely misrepresent the healthcare ecosystem. By limiting who can practice as a healer and what treatment alternatives are legitimated, inequalities can be created in access to training, assessment, and healthcare services (Broom et al., 2009). For instance, healthcare services tend to be found in urban communities with clinicians largely absent in remote locations, use diagnostics and pharmaceuticals that are difficult to produce, and might not incorporate the attitudes, values, and conventions of the communities they serve (Dussault & Franceschini, 2006; Gall et al., 2019; Gilliland et al., 2019; Nigenda, 2013; Thomas et al., 2014; Wilson et al., 2009). The interactions between the Maya, their neighbors, and BWM practitioners have frequently been defined in these terms. The observation that traditional medicine plays a vital role in health ecosystem further underscores the need to situate healthcare education and delivery practices in their implementation context (Schoenherr, 2027). By understanding the practices of healers, the lifeways and epistemologies of communities, and the adaptations of communities to available resources, healthcare professionals (HCPs) can foster an environment of mutual respect and understanding that improves the quality of care, develops a strong therapeutic alliance with health seekers, and makes them more effective advocates for the communities that they serve (Allen et al., 2020; Chary et al., 2022; Green & Colucci, 2020; Little et al., 2019; Nyembezi et al., 2024; Schoenherr et al., 2026).

In this chapter, I assume that medical decision-making and health-seeking behavior is dependent on belief systems about the material and immaterial world that are created, maintained, and modified in social networks of practitioners and patients (e.g., Coreil et al., 1994; Feyisetan et al., 1997; Kleinman, 1980). The chapter surveys the sensemaking processes of rejection, adoption, and adaptation of diagnostics and therapeutic products and techniques, and relational models of healers and health seekers which creates medical pluralism. In addition to processes internal to these social networks, the influence of externalities such as colonialism are also reviewed (Griffiths et al., 2016).

Making 'Medicine'. Healthcare beliefs and practices are typically defined by the overlapping processes of medicalization and scientification. Medicalization and scientification concern the identification and classification of features of the world as parts of paradigms (e.g., methods and instruments, concepts, and sources of evidence) of medicine and science, respectively. In BWM, medicine and science are intimately bound, often defined by 'evidence-based' approaches to healthcare. In other health traditions, paradigm*s* for the maintenance and treatment of health can take a variety of forms, varying the role and authority of the healer, health seekers, and community, the evidence used to diagnose, the criterion used for therapy adoption, and creation of formal and informal healthcare social organizations. Thus, while diagnostics and treatment methods, products, and services might not align with BWM, they can constitute a coherent medical paradigm (Bunniss & Kelly, 2010; Hill, 2009; McKivett & Paul, 2024; Tataryn, 2002).

Due to passive and active cultural exchanges, multiple medical paradigms can exist within the same healthcare ecosystem. *Medical pluralism* is defined by cooperation, coexistence, competition, and cooptation of health beliefs, diagnostic, and therapeutic practices between more than one healthcare tradition (Amzat et al., 2014; Baer, 2011; Berry, 2008; Broom et al., 2009; Fort et al., 2022; Goldstein, 2004; Kroeger, 1983; Leslie, 1980; Minocha, 1980; Shih et al., 2010; cf. Han, 2002). Given that a variety of treatment and illness models that are available within the healthcare ecosystem, a health seeker's agency is a critical determinant of why, how, when, and where they seek health information, what information is accepted, and whether they adopted the product or services offered.

Framed in these terms, the apparent dominance of BWM cannot be taken at face value. In some cases, BWM might appear to be preferable, with indigenous healers frequently recommending – and indigenous health seekers frequently selecting – solutions provided by BWM. However, critiques of the efficacy, adequacy, and safety of BWM are also prevalent (Berry, 2008; Harvey, 2011; Lehman et al., 2017). Instead, health seekers' behavior is likely best defined as *satisficing syncretism*, drawing from the products, services, and practices that are most accessible and effective (e.g., Young & Garro, 1982). Provided the maintenance or restoration of a state of health (defined by the health seeker) is sufficient, health seeker will continue to rely on these methods. To provide the best care, indigenous healers and HCPs will need to understand the historical and social dynamics of the healthcare ecosystem they practice within.

The Socioecology of Healthcare. Healthcare systems represent adaptations to the local physical and social environment including resources, climate, pathogens, population density, and the structure of the social networks. Concepts of health and illness are attempts to organize and disseminate knowledge, to provide explanations of the association and causal connections between factors (e.g., genetics, diet, social interaction) and outcomes (e.g., maintenance or changes in well-being) to reduce the uncertainty about the possible courses of action available to healers and health seekers, whereas they can be organized into coherent paradigms, they can also be created through trial-and-error.

Unlike many other beliefs,[1] health beliefs are critical determinants for the survival and success of a group. From an evolutionary perspective, norms and conventions will increase or decrease the likelihood of individual or group survival (Goodnight & Stevens, 1997; O'Gorman et al., 2008; Simon et al., 2013; Williams, 1966). A socioecology approach emphasizes how cognitive, affective, and behavioral processes, along with the structure and function of social networks, influence, and are influenced by, the physical environment communities inhabit (Oishi, 2014; Oishi & Graham, 2010; Schaller, 2020; Uskul & Oishi, 2020). By adopting a socioecological approach, the indigenous medical practices of communities such as the Maya can be placed in context.

Overview. This chapter reviews innovations within the healthcare system created, used, and imposed on indigenous people in Mesoamerica, primarily focusing on Mayan groups in Guatemala while also considering practices and groups outside these immediate geopolitical and ethnic boundaries. Section 10.1 briefly defines historical features of the Mayan world to provide a foundation for an understanding of the concepts, resources, practices, and social organization of Mayan society. Starting with an overview of pre-contact Mayan civilization and intellectual tradition from available archaeological and ethnographic sources, Mayan ontology, epistemology, and social organization are described. The influence of colonization is reviewed, emphasizing the origins of the contemporary pluralistic society of Guatemala along with the civil war. Section 10.2 reviews the indigenous Mayan approach to medicine. It focuses on conceptual models of illness, diagnostic methods, diagnoses, and treatment, and kinds of healers. Section 10.3 provides a contemporary view of medical pluralism in Mesoamerica. Here, the concept of heterarchy can be used to understand how healthcare is organized in multiethnic, multiregional societies. By adopting a socioecological perspective to healthcare, more efficient and effective care can be provided to communities.

10.1 Social and Ecological Features of the Mayan World

Colonization of the Americas has occurred in multiple waves, starting with paleolithic hunter-gatherers migrating from Northern East Asia via Beringia and continuing today as non-native populations migrate to these regions. By 2000 BCE,[2] complex sedentary societies had established themselves in Mesoamerica. Cities that grew out of these settlements would come to be defined by public plazas, monuments, ball courts, and palaces that were connected by vast networks of paved roadways (*sak b'eh*; 'white road'), the arteries for the transport of information and physical resources. Roads also linked vital local resources such as gardens, fields, fishponds, orchards, reservoirs as well as farmsteads, forests, wetlands, and cenotes (collapsed sinkholes). Cenotes were particularly important as they connected the people to sources of water and the Mayan sacred underworld (Canuto et al., 2018; Dunning et al., 1998; Farahani et al., 2017; Graham & Isendahl, 2018; Krause et al., 2021; Scarborough, 1998; Sheets et al., 2015).

As the Maya emerged as a distinct society, their interaction with neighboring groups proved critical. Knowledge of medicinal plants, practices, and deities helped shape approaches to health and illness (e.g., Teotihuacan; Braswell, 2004; Foley, 2017; Miller, 2013; Reilly, 1986; Spence, 1996; Sugiyama & Sugiyama, 2020). Like many other civilizations, the Maya people persisted, while classical Mayan society declined (Douglas et al., 2016; Medina-Elizalder & Rohling, 2012). Losses in the social organization would have altered the distribution of labor, undoubtedly resulted in concomitant loss of knowledge. Here, I briefly review the basic features of Mayan society that provide greater context for healthcare practices.

10.1.1 *Social Organization of Pre-Columbian Mayan Society*

Mayan communities were largely divided between the commoners[3] who were believed to be born of earth and grass and the elites (i.e., nobility, kings/lords, and priests) who had a celestial origin. Most community members engaged in labor such as farming, art, and construction. Monumental architecture built by commoners depicted the cosmovision of the Maya, creating social representations[4] that acted as mutual reference points for all members of a society. Rather than a simple dichotomous social hierarchy, evidence suggests the existence of an intermediate group (e.g., *açmen winik*): commoners who increased their status through appointment or achievement (Marcus, 2004; Martínez, 1929). Some of these individuals were healers.

In Mayan society, broad distinctions are found between healers serving commoners (*ahicon*) and nobles (*ah cut*; Miles, 1957; Orellana, 1987). Insight into the training and practice of these healers can be found in Aztec society (Guerra, 1966; Ortiz de Montellano, 1975). Rather than high status, 'the male physician [was] on a par with the carpenter, mason and scribe, and classed the female physician with the cook, the seamstress and the spinner' (Guerra, 1966, p. 321). This suggests that traditional healers might occupy an intermediate social position within Aztec and Mayan communities, perhaps implying a degree of social mobility. In contrast, nobles completed an apprenticeship at the *calmecac*, an institution of higher learning where they learned health ceremonies and preparation of medicinal compounds. The efficacy of their methods is demonstrated by the fact that Spanish conquistadors recognized them as doctors, using their services in the early colonial period (Treviño, 1984, 2001).[5]

10.1.1.1 *Heterarchical Structure*

While hierarchical relations can define social organizations, multiple relational models present alternatives (Fiske, 1991, 1993, 2012). When more than one principle of social organization exists within a group, it reflects a *heterarchy* (Crumley, 1995, 2015).[6] In this way, community members can be organized concurrently into multiple social groups. This framework has also been used to describe social organization of learners and professionals (Schoenherr & Dopko, 2019) and provides help to qualify medical pluralism (see also Schoenherr & Beaudoin, 2027).

Like other societies, Mayan civilization has been defined as a heterarchical structure (Cook, 2007; Lohse & Valdez, 2010; Potter & King, 1995). For instance, evidence of heterarchical structures can be found in religious and secular roles within communities (Cancian, 1965), as well as indigenous forms of justice that operate in parallel with those of the government (Bybee et al., 2013; Girón, 2007).[7] Gender has often been presented as a canonical case for studies of social organization (e.g., Grauer, 2021; Hutson et al., 2012; Joyce & Hendon, 2012; Stanton, 2000; Ortner

& Whitehead, 1981; Weiner, 1976; cf. DeMarrais, 2013). For instance, Hendon (1999) identifies the existence of 'multiple prestige structures, underwritten by different forms of social evaluation' (p. 257). Specifically, whereas men tended to occupy dominant sociopolitical positions in society (e.g., kings, priests), women dominated textile production (weaving) and trade which endowed men with the symbols of leadership. Such claims are also supported by the inclusion of weaving artifacts as prestige goods in the burials of high-status women (Chase et al., 2008).

The observation of multiple prestige structures does not imply that individuals necessarily have or had an equal or equivalent status. Focusing on relationships between women and men in Zapotec society, Kellogg (2005) notes that

> [w]omen are powerful because of their important economic activities and because … women function in parallel, semiautonomous female domains through which they hold socially recognized roles of authority… *[however, we must conclude] that women's power, real as it is, is lesser than Zapotec men's.*
>
> *(p. 105; italics added)*

Relational models can also change over time, such as a communal relationship in guerilla units during the Guatemala Civil War. Thus, even though Mesoamerican societies are defined by heterarchical structure, relational models contain distinction based on occupational and social groups and associated status.

Contemporary healthcare delivery in Latin America can be understood in similar terms (Gellego-Pérez et al., 2023; Hill et al., 2022; Koss-Chioino et al., 2003). The process of colonization was directed toward reducing, removing, and replacing indigenous cultural traditions in favor of those of the colonizers (Cooper & Stoler, 1989; Dirlik, 2002; Fryberg et al., 2018). However, in Guatemala, early attempts to maintain a divided society of two republics – one Spanish (*repúblicas de los españoles*) and one indigenous (*repúblicas de los indios*) – were thwarted by the interactions between indigenous, Spanish, and African slaves (Lutz, 1994). The intermingling of genes and ideas and rich societies that they create continues to be a defining feature of Latin American societies such as Guatemala.

Indigenous practices have adapted and remain vital in many communities. For instance, the practices of *empiricos*[8] (e.g., bonesetters, healers (*curanderos*), and midwives (*comadronas*)), along with practitioners of BWM, define a heterarchical healthcare ecosystem. Supporting this, despite discriminatory practices, traditional healers were often regarded as exceedingly competent, and often preferred (Few, 2015). Midwives continue to play a critical role in healthcare delivery in rural areas although their role and attitudes toward them differ across social groups (Cominsky, 2001; Van Dijk et al., 2013; Summer et al., 2017). Moreover, while BWM might be valued in some communities, its limited accessibility (geographic and financial), compatibility with indigenous attitudes and beliefs, and reductive analytic focus on biology and physiology do not necessarily make it the preferred choice (Glei & Goldman, 2000, 2003; Schoenherr & Hamstra, 2024).

10.1.1.2 Health, Homes, and Habits

Concepts of 'health' cannot be understood in isolation. Perceptions of health and illness are integrated with the physical, social, and the immaterial world. Traditional Maya society is intimately associated with the forest, with some referring to traditional healing practices as 'forest medicine'. Agroforestry practices of the Maya include the cultivation of upwards of 400 plant species, including *milpa* polyculture which includes 20 plant species that are used for food, improvement of soil quality, and medicine (Diemont et al., 2006). Such practices represent an evolutionary sustainable strategy that promotes biodiversity and has led to functional plant groups (Argens et al., 2023). Cultivation practices that support polyculture can include extensive irrigation systems (employing multiple terraces) and crop rotation. The effects of these ancient practices remain apparent today (Ross & Rangel, 2011).

Alone, horticultural knowledge is insufficient to guarantee the health of a population. Nutrients within plants and animals are not necessarily accessible to human, requiring specific preparation methods. In the Americas, this is exemplified by maize preparation techniques, allowing for the extraction of calcium and niacin (Béhar, 1968; Katz et al., 1974; Kodicek et al., 1959) to be used in food staples such as tortilla (Bressani, 1990; Serna-Saldivar et al., 2015). Without these adaptations, nutrient-deficient diets can result in diseases, such as pellagra which plagued colonial settler communities (Berdanier, 2019).

Sweat/steam lodges are another widespread cultural adaptation supporting health in the Americas (Struthers et al., 2004). In Mesoamerica, evidence of these practices can be dated to the Classic period in Mayan civilization (Clarke, 2022). The use of sweat lodges is often seen as a spiritual practice for cleansing, however, there are multiple mental and physical health benefits including the elimination of microbes and participation in these communal practices (Colmant et al., 2005). Unsurprisingly, indigenous healers, midwives, and bonesetters make use of these sites. Healing practices such as these undoubtedly contributed to the physical and social stability of Mesoamerican societies.

Spirits and their ecology (e.g., mountains, cenotes) are prominent features of the traditional Mayan worldview and must be accounted for in a socioecological approach to healthcare delivery (Bassie-Sweet, 2014). As I will note below, some practitioners believe that it is through their communion with spirits that insight can be gained about the causes of illness and appropriate course of treatment.

10.1.2 Discontinuities

Despite cultural achievements including writing system, astronomical knowledge, architecture, archaeologists estimate that pre-contact Mayan communities went into decline between 850 and 1000 CE. This decline has largely been attributed to an inability of traditional Mayan society to cope with repeated, sustained droughts (Haug et al., 2003; Hodell et al., 1995; Kennett et al., 2012; for a review, see Douglas et al., 2016). The later arrival of European explorers and colonists led to the further catastrophic reductions in indigenous populations with the incidental and intentional introduction of pathogens (for a review, see Mann, 2005). Concurrently, colonial powers sought to eliminate the belief systems of indigenous groups. For instance, perception, representation, and treatment of female healers appear to have markedly declined during the colonial period (Giralt, 2012; Klein, 1995). Similarly, the colonial powers' destruction of sweat lodges and other traditional practices during epidemics due to fear of contagion likely contributed to the spread of diseases (e.g., Guatemala; Carey, 2023; Grandin & Oglesby, 2011).

Despite these challenges, certain knowledge survived including the medicinal properties of plants and use of sweat baths (Ferrier et al., 2020; Watson et al., 2023). This suggests that while institutional healthcare systems that are based on complex social organizations are vulnerable to social, ecological, and biological threats, folk medicine offers a comparatively resilient resource to communities.

As cultural exchanges occurred across Mesoamerica, insight into healing practices of Mayan healers can also be gained from the practice of neighboring groups. In a comparison of the practices of the conquistadors and Aztec healers, Ortiz de Montellano (1976) argued that 'the ideal Aztec healer was one who tested his remedies, [...] the Aztec distinguished between healers whose cures were effective and healers whose cures were not'. As I will note below, empiricism also informs contemporary Mayan healing practices. While this might be an illusory correlation between diagnoses and treatment outcomes, it nevertheless represents a clear demonstration of an emphasis on empirical analysis and abductive reasoning that defines most healthcare traditions, including BWM.

10.1.2.1 Guatemalan Civil War

While Mayan communities were geographically dispersed, the borders imposed by colonial powers impacted the evolution of the practices of indigenous groups (Carey, 2023; García Ortega, 2021; Hamilton & Chinchilla, 1991; Nolan-Ferrell, 2012). The population density of the Mayan population varies throughout the departments in Guatemala due to migration, resettlement, and seasonal work (Figure 10.1).

Internal conflicts across the regions have been a persistent influence on indigenous communities (e.g., Cleary et al., 2000; Reed, 2001). The Guatemalan Civil War (1960–1996) had a uniquely devastating effect on the Maya. Despite a series of democratic reforms in the 1940s and 1950s, a CIA-backed coup in 1954 led to a military dictatorship (Immerman, 1982; Schlesinger & Kinzer, 2005). Early tensions between the ruling ladino elite who had discriminated against the larger rural Mayan population came to a head (Carmack, 1988). Guerilla forces emerged

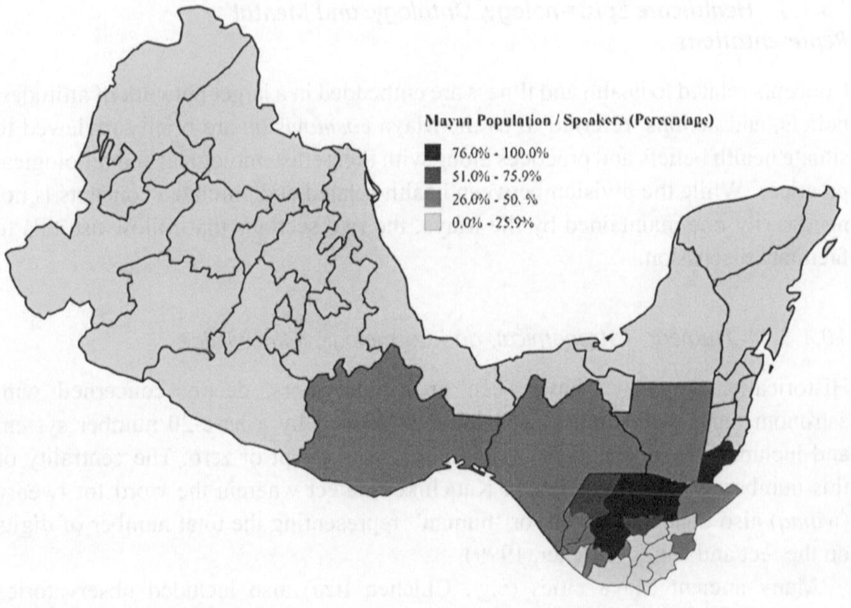

FIGURE 10.1 Mayan population density within Guatemalan departments, and density of indigenous and Mayan language speakers in Mexican states and Belizean districts.

to challenge the government (Schirmer, 1998), with government forces committing vicious acts of reprisal, displacing over 1 million, and killing or 'disappearing' more than 200,000 more people (Commission for Historical Clarification, 1999; Sanford, 2003). In addition to the destruction of local ecology that threatened traditional medicines (Cosminsky, 2001), the deaths of healers and healthcare workers created critical shortages (Cosminsky, 1977; Médecins Sans Frontières, 1999). Unsurprisingly, the prevalence of disease, child mortality, and malnutrition increased during this time (Metz, 1999).

Collective memory of these events has led to deep-seated distrust in state-based organizations and silence (Copeland, 2014; Greem, 1999; Maupin, 2009). Among other behaviors, this is evidenced in the high rates of lynchings, which have been framed as a form of legal pluralism ('Mayan Justice'), due to the perception of an ineffective government (Bybee et al., 2013; Girón, 2007), paralleling colonial attempts at creating 'two republics' and the use of double-naming conventions.[7] Beyond the psychological impact of war and concomitant distrust (Kirmayer et al., 2010), the contemporary healthcare system faces challenges stemming from misalignment between indigenous beliefs and modes of healthcare delivery (Maupin, 2009). Consequently, when healthcare resources are available, they might be underutilized.

10.1.3 Healthcare Epistemology, Ontology, and Mental Representations

Concepts related to health and illness are embedded in a larger network of attitudes, beliefs, and actions, referred to as the Maya *cosmovision* are briefly reviewed to situate health beliefs and practices along with their epistemological and ontological practices. While the division between health-related and unrelated concepts is not necessarily one maintained by the Maya, the two sections that follow use this to facilitate discussion.

10.1.3.1 Numeric, Astronomical, and Cosmological Knowledge

Historically, the Maya have been great innovators, deeply concerned with astronomy and mathematics. The latter is defined by a base-20 number system and includes the independent invention of the concept of zero. The centrality of this number system is evident in Kaqchikel dialect wherein the word for twenty (*winaq*) also denotes 'person' or 'human', representing the total number of digits on the feet and hands (Fischer, 1999).

Many ancient Maya cities (e.g., Chichen Itza) also included observatories to record, study, and predict events. Time (*kin*) is integral to Mayan thinking (Edmonson, 1988). The Mayan calendrical systems represent time using an interlocking set of three cycles: the *Tzolk'in*[9] (a 260-day sacred calendar), the *Haab* (a 365-day civil calendar defined by the solar year), and the Long Count (a system based on ~5,000 years; Figure 6.2).[10] The Tzolk'in continues to be used today by Mayan priests (Tedlock, 1982, p. 89; Earle, 2008, p. 69) (Figure 10.2).

Beyond agriculture and gestation, the calendar has an important meaning for individuals as it concerns *maatan*, translated variously as destiny/fate, favor, or luck (Fischer, 1999; Waldram & Hatala, 2015). Each day is represented by a different lord, each with their own power (Lincoln, 1942; Roys, 1933), phase of the moon (Nash, 1970) as well as their co-essences (Bunzel, 1952; Tedlock, 1982; Vogt, 1976). As Waldram (2020) notes, 'the day someone was born is crucial information; two people with the same set of signs and symptoms but different birth dates may have different sicknesses' (p. 102).[11,12] Similarly, the time of day that a therapeutic is administered is also believed to be an important determinant of its efficacy (pp. 190–191).

10.1.3.2 Biological Knowledge and Ontologies

To navigate the world, we must identify objects, forces, and entities. Mayan ontologies do not follow the (Western) taxonomic approach (e.g., Atran, 1999). Moreover, there are many kinds of nonhuman agents which are believed to interact with and influence the Maya people. For instance, minor spirits (*chiichi'*) have comparable knowledge to that of human agents. Masters of the forest (*yumil*

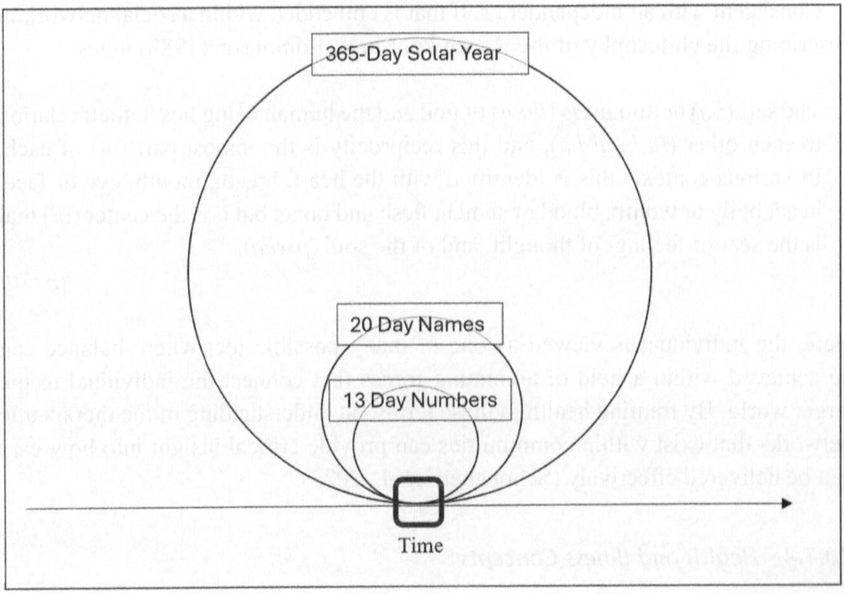

FIGURE 10.2 Mayan calendrical system. Dates are understood in terms of the permutations of day numbers and day names, defining the 260 days of the Tzolk'in (sacred calendar), along with the days in the Haab (solar year). Combinations repeat after 52 years. Each calendar cycle consists of 5128 years (ending December 12, 2012). Spheres are not to scale.

k'axob') and the sun (*k'in*) have greater knowledge, with the greatest knowledge being assigned to God (*diyoos*; Knight et al., 2004). These results suggest the realism of nonhuman agents to the Maya such that they can be solicited for reliable knowledge and health interventions.

10.1.3.3 Self and Social Network

In Western society, individual autonomy and self-identity is typically prioritized (Hofstede, 1980). This approach tends to ignore the influence of other agents in a social network. In contrast, societies in the Americas are often defined by a focus on collective action, ethics, and identities. Recent studies have demonstrated the complexity of social interdependency and individual values. For instance, Guatemalan society is comparatively low in individualism, with higher levels of communal embeddedness (rather than autonomy; Krys et al., 2022). Yet, these societies also prioritize an *independent* self rather than a collective self (Ashdown & Gibbons, 2012; Krys et al., 2019; Minkov et al., 2017; Vignoles et al., 2016). Supporting the socioecological approach, these findings have been attributed to historical pathogen prevalence (relative interdependence), modes of subsistence (relative independence), and intercultural exchanges resulting from colonization.

Consistent with an independent self that is embedded within a social network in describing the philosophy of the Kaqchikel Maya, Edmonson (1988) notes:

> The self (*ba*) or thingness (*baal*) of god and the human being lies in their relation to each other (*tu baal ba*), and this reciprocity is the inmost part (*ol*) of each. In various contexts this is identified with the heart, breath, mouth, eye or face, head, belly or womb, blood or semen, flesh and bone, but it is the center (*ol*) that is the seat of feeling, of thought, and of the soul (*pixan*).
>
> *(p. 70)*

Here, the individual is viewed as one of many possible loci where balance can be achieved within a field of animating forces that connect the individual to the larger world. By framing health in these terms, an understanding of the therapeutic networks that exist within communities can provide critical insight into how care can be delivered effectively (Schoenherr et al., 2027).

10.1.4 Health and Illness Concepts

Like Western scientists and medical practitioners (Magnani, 1992, 1997; Martini, 2023; Mirza et al., 2014), Mayan healers rely on abductive reasoning to understand health and illness (Moriarty, 1970). Abductive reasoning consists of a broad range of inferential techniques that use incomplete deductive principles and evidence to arrive at the 'best explanation'. Here, folk theoretical principles are combined with information acquired through experimentation using analogical reasoning to infer causal relationships.

10.1.4.1 Hot–Cold Distinction

In contemporary Mayan society the hot–cold distinction is a recurrent feature of causal theories of health and illness.[13] As a concept likely adopted from European colonizers (Foster, 1994), indigenous healer diagnoses refer to the hot–cold distinction to varying degrees (Waldram, 2020). In addition to interindividual variability, environmental variables also appear to play a role in terms of the adoption of the hot–cold distinction as a basis for diagnosis. Supporting the socioecological approach, García-Hernández et al. (2021) found that in Mexican traditional medicine, temperate areas tend to have more cold-associated illnesses with a focus on hot medicinal plants. Similarly, there is also suggestive evidence that warm areas tend to have more hot illnesses with a focus on cold medicinal plants.[14]

10.1.4.2 Animism and Agency

Another fundamental distinction is that between living and non-living entities. Animistic reasoning and agentic reasoning focus on the behaviors attributable to life forces and autonomous agency.[15] Rather than a single force (e.g., *a* soul/spirit), some Mayan traditions have assumed multiple animating forces, with upwards of 13 (Zonacantán) to 39 being inferred (Chamula; Foster, 2005, p. 203; Grube & Nahm, 1994; Houston & Stuart, 1989). For instance, one model assumes that three souls perform separate function (*yolia*, *tonalli*, and *ihiyotl*; see Figure 10.3; Furst, 1995; L ópez Austin, 1980).[16] Summarizing contemporary healing practices, Waldram (2020) notes, 'The mind-body-spirit is not typically treated as an integrated whole, and although the connections between the parts are understood the *iloneleb'* [healers] often treat them separately,' (p. 213).

In that each of these animating forces performs a specialized function, they are analogous to organs.[17] According to this account, sickness is a result of losing parts of the soul or souls, with groups such as the Maya and Mazatec using terms related to illness and dying interchangeably (Giovanni & Heinrich, 2009; Maffi, 1994). *Susto* is often presented as a canonical case, wherein a health seeker is believed to have lost a soul (Armijos et al., 2014; Burman, 2010; Cepeda-Chamorro et al., 2018; Muñoz-Morán, 2011). *Susto* can be caused by immaterial forces such as interactions with souls of dead people, the Devil, failing to provide adequate offerings to deities, or intrusions into sacred spaces

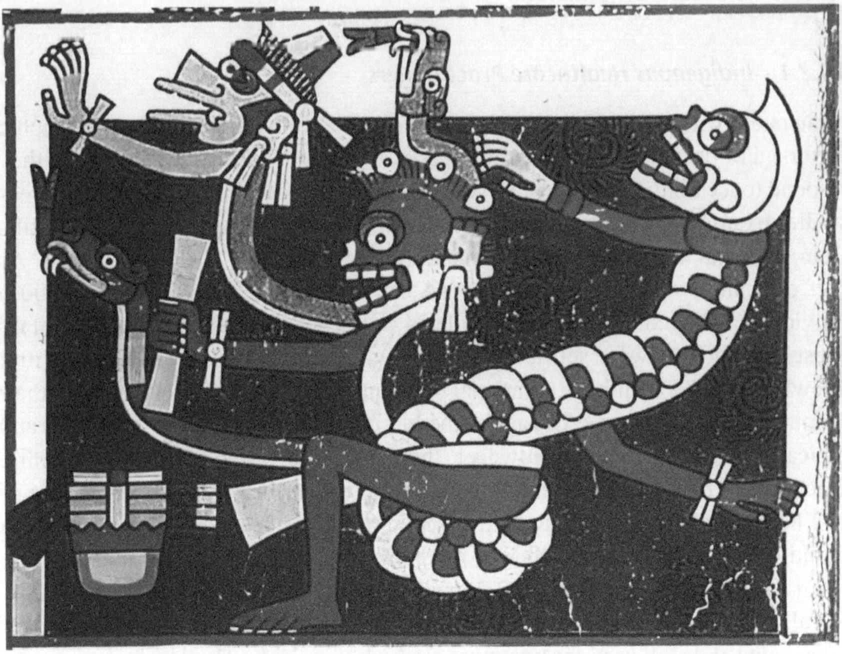

FIGURE 10.3 From left to right: *yolia* (serpent), *tonalli*, *ihiyotl* relative to the living spine (far right). Section of *Codex Laud* (López Austin, 1980).

Source: Image retrieved from www.famsi.org/research/pohl/jpcodices/laud/img_laud44.html.

(Bianchetti, 2014; Rösing, 1993; Rubel, 1964; Thomas et al., 2009; Vega, 2008). Material causes of *susto* have also been proposed including being attacked by a predator, experiencing violence, or being startled (Armijos et al., 2014; Remorini & Palermo, 2016).

10.2 Indigenous Mesoamerican Medicine

The absence of scientification of indigenous healthcare practices does not invalidate them. Mesoamerican healers' practices appear to stem from trial-and-error, with theoretical explanations being secondary to observed efficacy (Schoenherr & Beaudoin, 2027).[18] As different healers practice in diverse settings, the patients, pathologies, and availability of resources can lead to distinct kinds of skill sets and approaches to healing. Diverse groups of practitioners have been observed in Mesoamerican such as *empiricos* who focus on health outcomes *curanderos* who place greater emphasis on formal training and theoretical causal explanations, e.g., hot–cold distinctions. For instance, Mazatec and other communities differentiate between bonesetters (*chjota chjine b'ekjaoninda*), herbalists (*chjota chjine xka*), midwives (*chjine kjindi*), and shamans (*chjota chjine*; Abse, 2007; Mellado Campos, 1994). Here, I provide an overview of practitioners and their practices.

10.2.1 Indigenous Healthcare Practitioners

Healers are often defined by varying experiences, motivations, and demographic factors. For instance, early studies report that some healers believe that they respond to a calling (Fabrega & Silver, 1973; Metzger & Williams, 1963), whereas studies examining the practices of healers suggest that many acquire their skills from personal need and local demand (Hinojosa, 2020; Waldram, 2020). As part of a multi-year, multi-site study (Adams & Hawkins, 2007), Yukes (2007) provides a more comprehensive profile of indigenous healers (see Table 10.1).[19] Most practitioners were self-taught (70%) with clinical classes (30%), ancestral knowledge (30%), and observational learning with peers (26%) defining their training and experiences.[20] The age of the sample is relatively old (57 years old) and typically quite experienced. However, the experience varied considerably within practitioners of the same type. For instance, *curadero* (healers) saw an average of 232 health seekers, with a standard deviation of 425 health seekers.[21] Yukes also found differences in the number of medicinal plants that healers could identify. *Curadero* were able to identify 22.2 medical plants on average (compared to 20.1 for all practitioners). Thus, in the absence of formal training, the acquisition of knowledge and skill used for treatment are highly variable. This stochastic process conforms to a socioecological approach: practitioners acquire their knowledge from interaction with their physical, biological, and social environment.[22]

TABLE 10.1 Traditional Practitioners' Profiles

ID	*Practitioner Expertise*			*Exp. (Yrs.)*	*Age*	*Source of Training*						*# Plants*	*Min. walking to municipal center*
	Comadrona	*Curandera*	*Huesera*			*Self*	*Clinic*	*Obs.*	*Par.*	*Anc.*	*Div.*		
N03	32.5	27.5		40	65	1	0	0	0	0	0	24	25
N05	10	1.5		40	70	1	1	0	0	0	0	3	5
N06		15	4.5	**	38	1	0	1	0	0	0	26	2
N07	9	**		9	63	1	0	0	0	0	0	6	15
N08	3	30	40	40	70	1	0	0	0	0	0	8	15
N09	17.5	50	15	26	56	1	0	0	0	0	0	12	12
N10	10	1	0	5	35	1	1	0	0	0	0	2	15
N11	45	1,408	0	12	46	1	0	1+	0	1	0	44	15
N12	10		0	45	70	1	0	0	0	0	0	11	7
N13	10	9	1.5	30	60	0	0	1	0	0	0	19	15
N15	48			15	50	1	1	1	1	0	0	11	8
N16	50	480	2.5	5	38	0	1	0	1	0	1	30	7
N19	42	42	1.5	24	55	0	0	0	1	1	0	38	5
N20	102	6		50	92	1	0	1	0	0	0	34	35
N22	36	30		20	55	1	0	0	0	0	0	19	6
N23	42	1,095	1.5	45	60	0	1	0	1	1	0	31	5
N24	**			55	75	0	0	0	0	1	0	12	40
N25	102			3	60	1	0	1	0	0	0	3	30
N26	36	42	2.5	20	45	0	1	0	0	1	0	73	35
N28	24	626	1	29	48	1	1	0	0	0	0	8	5
N29	36	36	1	7	52	1	0	0	0	0	0	8	5
N30	84	48		8	43	1	0	0	0	1	0	14	30
N31	**			30	70	0	0	0	0	1	0	27	**
M	37.5	232.2	5.46	25.4	57.2	.70	.30	.26	.17	.30	.04	20.1	15.3
SD	29.5	425.7	11.1	16.2	13.8	.47	.47	.45	.39	.47	.21	16.6	11.8

Source: Adapted from Tables 1 and 2 (pp. 47–48), Yukes (1997). N represents informant number. Tables reorganized and standardized, mean (M) and standard deviation (SD) computed by the author.

Note:
***Additional is classified as a* cura los ojos (5.5).

Similar results have been observed in other communities. In his study of bonesetters, Hinojosa (2020) found that healers in one area (San Juan Comalapa) acquired their skills through their own experiences of pain and experimentation on others within their own communities.[23] This idiosyncratic experience can be supplemented by learning from experienced bonesetters (Paul & McMahon, 2001). Thus, in unstructured learning environments, indigenous healers engage in a form of self-directed learning that can be supplemented with an apprenticeship.

10.2.2 Diagnostic and Treatment Practices

Medical expertise reflects the core competency of any healer. In addition to knowledge, four practices define medical expertise in Mayan healthcare: pulsing, *jilok*, prayer, and pharmacology (Balick et al., 2008; Hatala & Waldram, 2016; Hinojosa, 2020; Waldram, 2013, 2020). As with any form of abductive reasoning, these practices are not necessarily discrete. Instead, diagnostic and therapeutic practices can overlap in a process of healer sensemaking. This section treats them discretely for ease of comprehension.

10.2.2.1 Physical Diagnosis

Physical diagnosis stands as the fundamental activity of Mayan healers (Holland, 1962; Huber & Anderson, 1996; Orellana, 1987). Pulsing is a traditional practice that is used to gather broad, diagnostic information about the patient. As one practitioner notes, '*el pulso me dice todo*' (the pulse tells me all; p. 133; Balick et al., 2008; see also Berger-González et al., 2016). Pulsing focuses on the wrist/thumb/hand, forehead, and feet as well as over the heart/chest with variability in terms of healers' preference (Waldram, 2020). In general, informants note that pulsing starts at the radial artery on the wrist above the thumb, with healthy individuals having steady, moderate pulse (Balick et al., 2008). Ill patients are described as having a 'thin and weak or fat and rapid' pulse, requiring that the healer move higher up the arm. Using this method, one experienced practitioner used it to diagnose 42 conditions, divided into 5 different kinds: physiological conditions and states, insanity, spiritual/cultural, and winds.[24]

A mild form of massage that uses downward motions, or *jilok*, is also used to gather diagnostic evidence, often coupled with breathing on the hands (Waldram, 2013, 2015, 2020). Together, pulsing and *jilok* provide healers with critical knowledge about the physiology and anatomy of the health seeker. Despite these consistent themes, the use of empirical methods can vary based on regional traditions. In his study, Hinojosa (2020) found that practitioners in one region (San Juan Comalapa) adopted an empirical approach that assumes a physiological etiology based on folkbiological theories of the human body. Replicating Waldram's findings, physical diagnosis using palpitation and massaging was coupled with physical treatments. However, Hinojosa (2020) also found that some bonesetters used both manual methods and supernatural practices in two lakeside communities (San Pedro La Laguna, San Juan La Laguna). These methods typically relied on artifacts used by family members and distant ancestors or those that were revealed to them in dreams.

Evidencing satisficing syncretism defined by trial-and-error, observational learning, and apprenticeships, contemporary healers additionally incorporate elements of the BWM medical paradigm including supplementary x-rays obtained by health seekers (often at the encouragement of the bonesetter; Hinjosa, 2004), herbal mixtures, commercial pharmaceuticals, and sweat bath (*tuj*). Other studies have found that midwives who have received formal training are also more likely to refer women to BWM practitioners than those without training – though most pregnant women did not see these providers (Goldman & Glei, 2003). Such practices embodied a pluralistic healthcare ecosystem that is heavily reliant on the agency of the health seeker within a therapeutic network.

10.2.2.2 Prayer Diagnostics and Therapeutics

Prayer provides another diagnostic resource for indigenous healers. As people are linked to the material and immaterial world, prayer provides a clear demonstration of an explicit attempt to bridge the two. The nonhuman entities that are believed to be part of the Mayan world act as critical informational and therapeutic resources.

Research demonstrates the utility of prayer for Mayan healers (Berger-González et al., 2016; Kunow, 2003). The efficacy of participant prayer is supported by empirical research (cf. remote prayer, Masters & Speilmans, 2007). Outside of the Maya and indigenous communities, prayer and meditation have been found to have a variety of analgesic and anxiolytic effects (Breslin & Lewis, 2008; Gossman et al., 2004; Wachholtz & Paragament, 2005). One long-term study demonstrated the benefits of continued use of these practices three years later (Miller et al., 1995).

Rather than these results being based on the act of praying, insight into participants' prayer efficacy can be gained by examining parallel practices such as meditation. Meditation has a variety of beneficial effects including improved decision-making. For instance, if stress (e.g., threats) narrows the focus of attention, leading to the reliance on biased responses, forms of meditation such as prayer can reduce (this bias) by reducing stress and anxiety (Hoge et al., 2013; Sun et al., 2015; Zeidan et al., 2014). Meditation has been found to have similar effects for problem-solving (Ding et al., 2015; Ostafin & Kassman, 2012; Raingruber & Robinson, 2007; Ren et al., 2011). Meditative practices such as prayers might increase the likelihood that healers will identify a solution.

Other typical cognitive and behavioral processes can also provide plausible explanations for certain health beliefs and practices. Periods of inactivity such as sleep can improve recall and insight problem-solving (Lewis et al., 2018; Müller & Pilzecker, 1900; Stickgold & Walker, 2013; Wamsley, 2014).[25] These results might also provide a plausible interpretation for the knowledge and insight attributed to immaterial sources such as ancestral and spirit guidance.

10.2.2.3 Medicinal Plants and Pharmacology

Despite the modest knowledge of medicinal plants observed in some regions (e.g., Yukes, 2007), interregional ethnobotanical surveys suggest an expansive indigenous pharmacopeia (e.g., Comerford, 1996). In one ethnobotanical survey, researchers identified indigenous knowledge of 169 medicinal plant species in Belize. The researchers found that the majority of plants were used to treat infections (145), the digestive system (88), the nervous system (57), and the muscular system (40), with moderate numbers for treating the skin (24) or poisons (23; Arnason et al., 2022). While the therapeutic function for each plant varied, healer consensus was greater than 50%. This study also supports similar results obtained from traditional Mexican healers (Heinrich et al., 1998). Thus, even in the absence of formal training, experimentation and communication through informal social networks can lead to the acquisition of extensive knowledge of therapeutics.

10.3 Integrating Healthcare within National and Global Systems

Healers serve communities. They are also part of a larger healthcare ecosystem. The introduction and integration of BWM within most modern states has led to heterarchical healthcare systems defined by integration and interference between indigenous practices and those of BWM (Arnold, 1993; Crozier, 2007; Hill, 2009; Lavellee & Poole, 2010; Lowes & Montero, 2021; Sutphen & Andrews, 2003). Here, I provide a brief review of the healthcare ecosystems in Mesoamerica, primarily focusing on Guatemala with some reference to Belize and Mexico.

10.3.1 Formalization, Accreditation, and State-Power

In addition to improving the well-being of people, healthcare – especially, public health – has been used as an instrument of colonialism through demonstrations of competency, superiority, and integration into larger world systems (Baer et al., 2013; Carey, 2023; Few, 2015 for discussion in this volume, see Chan et al., 2027; Schoenherr & Beaudoin, 2027).

Historically, governmental and nongovernmental organizations have attempted to regulate practitioners and healthcare delivery (Adams, 2020; Saltman, 2002; for recent reviews in Latin America, see Carter, 2023; Dalton & Weatherford, 2022), with professionalization reinforcing the dominance of select groups of healers (Coburn, 1993, 2006; Haber, 1991; Starr, 1982). In Latin America, Guatemala stands as a clear example of this process (Carey & Crafts, 2023; Cerón, 2019; Hoyler et al., 2018). As the modern Guatemalan state emerged, *curanderos* were often targeted by the state. Nevertheless, records suggest that police forces distinguished between legitimate and illegitimate practitioners. Moreover, despite arrests, many healers escaped (Carey, 2023, p. 68). This tacit acknowledgment of a form of legitimacy parallels those observed during early colonial period, suggesting that either the methods, intent, or community recognition provide some criteria. Despite their presence, no regulation currently exists for *empiricos* and *curanderos* in Guatemala.

The Guatemalan Ministry of Health (GOH) has adopted a three-tier BWM-based public health system. In rural villages, health posts provide basic primary care and vaccinations. In small cities and towns, health centers provide a wider array of primary care and some emergency care services. Finally, in large cities and department capitals, hospitals provide specialized care and emergency services. In theory, the three-tiered system should provide coverage for approximately 70% of the country's population (Ipplolito et al., 2017). In practice, limited material, financial, and human resources result in shortfall of coverage, especially for those in the lowest income groups and those in rural areas (e.g., Annis, 1981; Kragel et al., 2018; Kroger, 1983; Lindblade et al., 2011; Owen et al., 2010; PAHO, 2007).

Like Guatemala, the Ministry of Health of Belize has established a multi-tier system including a national referral hospital (Belize City), three regional hospitals, and three community hospitals. In Belize, clinics, health centers, and health posts provide additional primary care (Mac Arthur et al., 2014). In parallel with the national system, the Mayan Healers Association of Belize (MHAB) has also been established to validate traditional healers' competencies. Starting in 1999, the MHAB was created by healers to address the loss of indigenous knowledge (and language) by encouraging these practices and work as an advocate for governmental agencies. MHAB partnerships with Canadian academics also enabled the healers to purchase land (50 acres) and transplant medicinal plants to this site.

To be designated as an MHAB member, healers are required to pass tests of both knowledge and reputation within the community to practice (Waldram, 2009; Waldram et al., 2009). The requirement of reputation underscores the participatory nature of healthcare delivery in Mayan communities. Reputation is defined by multiple features. For instance, Vrettas (2020) notes that MHAB practitioners must

> Not ask a patient or their family for money and instead accepting whatever is offered;
>
> not disclosing when a sickness is caused by *obeah* (witchcraft) to reduce the likelihood of revenge feuds;
>
> not performing *obeah*-related practices;
>
> not criticizing other members; and keeping to the traditional apprenticeship model of training new healers (where the person interested in becoming a healer selects a master and pays them to share their knowledge in a one-on-one setting).
>
> *(p. 5)*

In the creation of these principles, we see the incorporation of local beliefs and values, ones that would be unlikely to be contained – or accepted – within the BWM tradition yet are consistent with basic ethical principles such as beneficence, nonmaleficence, and confidentiality. We additionally see the process of professionalization recapitulated, echoing the precedents of ancient traditions, paralleling the processes observed in BWM, and facilitated by other professionals (e.g., Waldram).

These efforts can be contrasted against those found in Guatemala. Rather than a practitioner-driven approach, the MoH has attempted to regulate traditional birth attendants (midwives), through training and validation (Berry, 2006, 2010; Maupin, 2008, 2009, 2011; Westreich, 1990). As Edvalson et al. (2013) state, the approach consists of formal curriculum that consists of developing basic skills, i.e., competencies. However, the curriculum contains messages emphasizing the legal risks associated with the provision of care including those associated with maternal death (Cosminsky, 1982; Greenberg, 1982; Hinojosa, 2004; Maupin, 2008). Similarly, by providing licenses to midwives, the state is attempting to regulate the delivery of healthcare. While midwives seek out this training to attain legitimacy, both their perception and empirical studies found no significant differences in the quality of care for those midwives who did and who did not complete formal training (Goldman & Glei, 2000, 2003). This is satisficing syncretism at the institutional level, such that formal certification is adopted because it is the most accessible means of securing practice legitimacy within a state-regulated ecosystem.

10.3.2 Language, Knowledge, and Education

The limited avenues for training and education in a Mayan dialectic create assimilative pressures that are typically defined in terms of attempted paternalistic re-education, persecution, and persuasive communication. Unsurprisingly, indigenous languages are often targeted due to their role in communication, both in terms of a continuity of the indigenous cultural traditions and as a repository of knowledge. They understandably have tightly coupled associations with identity, especially in Mayan society.

Studies have demonstrated that language is a significant barrier to innovation adoption. For instance, many indigenous practitioners such as midwives have only a limited ability to communicate in Spanish (Greenberg, 1982; Kruske & Barclay, 2004; Lang & Elkin, 1997; Maupin, 2008). By failing to offer education and training programs in a language that is intelligible to practitioners, program developers have effectively created unnecessary barriers to program delivery (Schoenherr & Hamstra, 2024). This is equally true to heal seekers (Berry, 2008; Chary et al., 2016; Chomat et al., 2018; Ippolito et al., 2017; Strader et al., 2024; Van Dijk et al., 2013).

The loss of language associated with cultural assimilation represents a shift in epistemological authority away from indigenous populations. For instance, Semotiuk et al. (2012) note both a decline in interest in learning traditional practices and knowledge related to Mayan medicine as well as a decrease in use of Mayan dialect (Q'eqchi' and Mopán). Their informants attributed such changes to formal education (44%), travel (24%), and interaction with people outside of the community (16%; for similar patterns in Belize, see Dickerson, 2008).

Language academies have emerged to preserve and restore these vital connections to the past and the environment (Figure 10.4). Beyond retaining traditional knowledge, the delivery of healthcare and healthcare education in indigenous languages facilitates health communication and can improve the therapeutic alliance between healers and health seekers (e.g., Flood et al., 2018; Shtanko et al., 2024).

In a pluralistic healthcare system, it might seem that healers and health seekers must choose between treatments and therapeutic traditions as their time and attention are limited. For instance, in a study of rural indigenous communities in Oaxaca, Giovanni et al. (2011) obtained a negative correlation between formal education and medicinal plant knowledge (cf. Aparicio Aparicio et al., 2021;

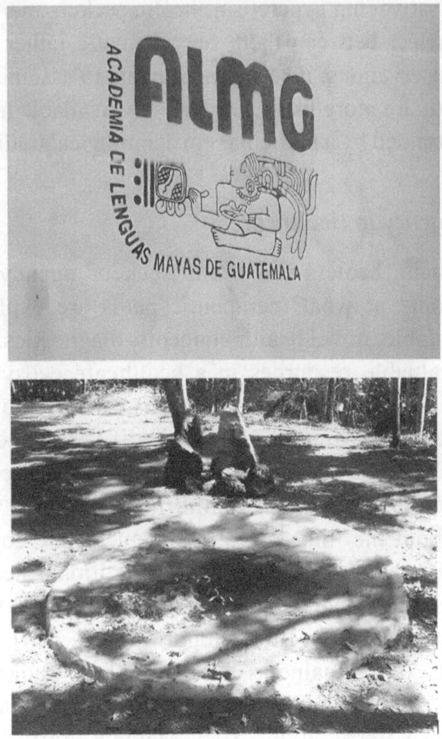

FIGURE 10.4 Mayan language school (*Academia de Lenguas Mayas de Guatemala*) logo (left). A nearby ceremonial area was used for learning traditional ceremonies (right). Peten, Guatemala, December 2012.

Source: Photo credit author.

Jiménez-Balam et al., 2019). This finding is consistent with general historical trend of a decrease in specific knowledge of nature (Kesebir & Kesebir, 2017; Wolff et al., 1999) as well as other studies linking reduction of local plant knowledge to the process of urbanization (Arjona-García et al., 2021). Outside of the Maya homeland, this process has been observed elsewhere in Central America such that changes in cultural norms account for shifts in medicinal knowledge beyond that of individual (e.g., Reyes-García et al., 2014).

The division between health-related and unrelated knowledge is necessarily complex. Healers and health seekers are likely to form these categories as a result of direct and indirect feedback from therapeutic products and practices and the folk wisdom of their community. For instance, in a survey of a Mazatec community, Giovanni et al. (2011) found that knowledge of pharmaceuticals and medicinal plants were *positively* correlated. They qualify this finding by noting that while the community differentiated between 'medicine from the shop' (*xki-tienda*) and medicinal plants (*xka-xki*), their choice in therapeutics stemmed from practical criteria (e.g., access, cost, efficacy) rather than epistemological categories. This is one of the clearest examples of satisficing syncretism: health seekers maintain parallel knowledge systems and select between them on pragmatic rather than ideological grounds. From these observations, it seems reasonable to assume that those individuals interested in health are more likely to retain any available health knowledge rather than remain constrained by a particular epistemological tradition.

10.3.3 Medical Pluralism and Agency in Healthcare

In a pluralistic healthcare ecosystem, healers and health seekers' agency and health literacy are key determinants of what therapeutic paths are explored and ultimately selected. Once available, novel health concepts, diagnostics, and therapeutic techniques become valuable resources in a healthcare ecosystem (Cosminsky & Scrimshaw, 1980; Hall-Clifford, 2015; Hawkins, 2007; Hinojosa, 2020; King et al., 2015). For instance, Leyn (2007) notes that if health seekers recognized an illness and had knowledge of a plant-based remedy, they chose the plant-based remedy. Pharmacies, clinics, and public health offices were sought if there was uncertainty about the illness, the treatment, or the cost of alternative treatment. Similarly, Hoyer et al. (2018) found traditional healers repeatedly referenced germ theory, a concept that had been adopted from BWM. They also found that indigenous illness diagnostic categories (e.g., *chij*) were interpreted using BWM concepts (e.g., malnourishment). When traditional healers recognized that they could not cure an illness, they often referred health seekers to BWM resources (see also Berry, 2006, 2010; Maupin, 2008, 2009, 2011; Hinojosa, 2020). That traditional healers simultaneously incorporate BWM concepts (e.g., germ theory) and refer out to BWM practitioners when their own resources are insufficient, while BWM practitioners prescribe local plants, demonstrated the bidirectional nature of satisficing syncretism across the healthcare ecosystem.

The exchanges between indigenous medicine and BWM are not asymmetric. BWM practitioners also utilized indigenous knowledge by recommending/prescribing local medicinal plants. Summarizing this, Hoyer et al. claim that:

> the health system within [the region] ties together the work of biomedical and traditional practitioners so that neither can function as effectively without the other… An intervention that works together with both types of practitioners, as opposed to a focus on one with a mere appreciation of the other, can positively impact its sustainability. Furthermore, in resource-poor areas [Concepción Huista], engaging with practitioners from both systems enables the strengths of each system to contribute and compensate for the limitations of the other

10.3.4 Telehealth and Mobile Health in Remote Locations

The adoption and adaptation of healthcare innovations by Mayan communities is also evident in the use of smartphones and telehealth services. Unlike Belize which is comparatively small, the varied geography of Guatemala and southern Mexico presents challenges for healthcare delivery, limiting health seekers' access of health outposts to rural populations (Gutiérrez-Peláez et al., 2022; Pelcastre-Villafuerte et al., 2017). Wireless communication provides a straightforward means to increase and facilitate healthcare delivery remotely.

Mobile phones, smartphone applications, and networks that support them represent critical innovations that can support healthcare. By using mobile phones, health seekers and practitioners can connect to a larger network of professionals, monitor illnesses remotely, and access knowledge where services are available in remote areas. Illustrating these benefits, Martinez et al. (2018) compared traditional birth attendants (midwives) with and without access to a mobile health (mHealth) application in Guatemala. To ensure intelligibility regardless of literacy, to help midwives the application uses an image-based list of common maternal and perinatal complications that have been grouped based on the type of consultation. When a specific birth complication is selected, the mobile application automatically communicates with an on-call clinical team by text message or voice call. In their study, they found that referrals increased for those who had access to the application (33.5/100 births) relative to those who did not (20/100 births). However, while they did observe differences in maternal deaths (2 vs. 1) and neonatal deaths (7 vs. 3) in the early access and late access conditions, neither reached statistical significance (for other studies of mHealth, see Stroux et al., 2016).[26] Despite such promising results, caution is warranted as research has demonstrated that users can come to overtrust software applications and might not understand the basis for the recommendations.

10.4 Patient Adoption and Compliance

The focus on practitioner competencies and health technologies can often obscure the fact that health seekers must be at the center of any healthcare system. Health seekers will determine what products, procedures, and practitioners are selected. Instead of thinking of illness as something affecting and perceived by an individual in isolation, HCPs must also acknowledge that health seekers are connected to a larger social network of peers, elders, and healers. As noted above, in societies defined by collectivistic norms, the embeddedness of an individual within a community requires that we consider a therapeutic network as a whole.

10.4.1 Health as a Network

As Mayan society is defined by high levels of social embeddedness with concurrent emphasis on independent self (Section 10.1.3.3), the effective delivery of care requires understanding how health agency is represented and understood by health seekers in a social network. Rather than an exclusive focus on individual autonomy, therapeutic groups must also be considered as a unit of analysis (Schoenherr et al., 2027).

In his study of healthcare practices in Guatemala, Harvey (2011) uses a music metaphor (*polyphony*) to capture the multidirectional influences that are present in the healthcare context. Rather than members of the healthcare team being the primary locus, Harvey emphasizes the role of health seekers' companions in developing an illness narrative and contributing to treatment selection. Together, health seekers and their companions engage in a process of sensemaking, attempting to identify the causes of an illness, the reliability of healers and institutions, and the efficacy of treatment alternatives (Battles et al., 2006; Jordan et al., 2009). Companions are believed to be important sources of health information in symptom identification as they can detect changes in a health seeker's well-being.

Berger-González et al. (2016) have similarly characterized healthcare interactions as a collective, interdependent therapeutic unit. Here, the goal is to preserve the health of a *system*:

> The therapeutic unit brings all participants into a single coherent system. This system rests in a symbolic platform of shared beliefs that sustain relationships and enhance the quality of social interactions. *The presence of each element is equally important*, strengthened by their interactions and *the constant feedback each element provides to the system.* The interactions between healer, wellness seeker, and family members are mediated through the treatment requirements and responsibilities, as well as the classification of the disease in terms of origin and prognosis… *The healer distributes the responsibilities and particular tasks among members of the network* following the directions [they get] directly from the spiritual realm.
>
> *(p. 363; italics added)*

While the equality of each element in the network is highly speculative,[27] the centrality of the family and community networks is a critical observation. This conforms to Hinojosa's (2020) account of bonesetters: while their competencies are unique and sought after by members of the community, they are also *members* of that community with their knowledge shaped by interaction within a social network. Such patterns are consistent with the concept of a therapy management group, wherein health seeker and healer are embedded within a larger, social network (e.g., Janzen, 1978). For instance, women's involvement in women's support groups (WSG) has been linked to their self-esteem and increased health-seeking behavior (Schooley et al., 2009).

Social networks can also be disrupted. Many individuals sustained themselves with cyclical agricultural work. Seasonal migration of agricultural workers introduces additional complications into healthcare delivery and usage. Without stability, healthcare resources can be strained in communities and create uncertainty for health seekers (Gragnolati & Marini, 2003). Although mobile healthcare projects have the potential to increase stability (Martinez et al., 2018), infrastructure and the inherent limitations of services create constraints on the quality and reliability of care received by these individuals.

By claiming that health seekers are agents, this does not mean that their role is equal to that of healers and HCPs. Despite the emphasis on equality and interdependence provided by the above accounts, Waldram (2015) highlights relational *asymmetries*, noting that the 'patient is somewhat dialogically passive… [they play] a role that is rarely if ever a dominant one … During the actual treatment, there is virtually no dialogue between the patient and *ilonel* [healer]' (pp. 197–198). These observations conform to the notion of the sick role and underscore the importance of specific relational models that are available for the delivery of care (for a review, see Schoenherr et al., 2027).

10.4.2 Selection, Integration, and Contestation in a Pluralistic System

The concept of medical pluralism is frequently used to denote the existence of distinct, relatively homogenous healthcare traditions. When viewed as an instance of the process of cultural evolution, health beliefs and practices can be selected, integrated, and disintegrated in a single healthcare ecosystem, i.e., syncretic processes. Evidence from studies in contemporary Mesoamerica supports this proposal.

In their study of rural healthcare, Ippolito et al. (2017) found that health seekers' decisions to use health services were based on both the cost and proximity.[28] Health seekers who attended the health post believed that private care was superior, with health seekers raising concerns that the uncertainty in the clinics' hours of operation and waiting times created significant barriers. Health seekers also believed that consultations with physicians who spoke their dialect were preferable to nurse-clinicians and Spanish speakers. They were also more likely to use private clinic services if medications were not prescribed at the health post or diagnostic tests were required. These patterns of behavior reinforce the importance of health seekers, beliefs, agency, and health literacy.

Similar results have been obtained in studies of women's reproductive health. Using archival data, Ishida et al. (2012) found that indigenous women were less likely to have their contraceptive needs met (49%) than ladino women (72%), and less likely to make use of institutional prenatal care (36%) compared to ladino women (73%; see also Seiber & Bertrand, 2002). Previous studies have also demonstrated that increases in availability of contraceptives and education lead to higher rates of contraception adoption (Bertrand et al., 2001; De Broe & Hinde, 2006). In parallel, other factors such as religious beliefs (e.g., Catholicism) might also lead to reduced contraception use (Terborgh et al., 1995; Santiso-Galvez & Bertrand, 2004). Supporting these results, Richardson et al. (2016) found that contraception use was also affected by lack of knowledge of available methods, infertility concerns, spousal and community attitudes toward family planning, and belief that the use of contraception is a sin (Grace, 2010). Other studies have suggested that information concerning contraception is also acquired through social networks, with direct or indirect agents in one's social network associated with contraception adoption (Lindstrom & Hernández, 2006; Lindstrom & Muñoz-Franco, 2005). Thus, even when health services are available, prevalence of use within a community, peer, and familial attitudes will affect the perceived suitability of healthcare practices.

10.4.2.1 Contesting Epistemologies of Health and Illness

The coexistence of health beliefs, diagnostic methods, and therapies in no way implies that they are judged to be equally legitimate. For instance, European folk theories introduced by Spanish colonizer have been attributed to the rejection of BWM (Logan, 1973). In Guatemala, Harvey (2011) illustrates this with what he refers to as 'mobile medicine', described as an alternative form of public healthcare (see also Hersch-Martinez, 1997; Little, 2002). Mobile medicine includes indigenous health practices and BWM, favoring the former. He notes that multiple language groups (K'iche', Kaqchikel, or Tz'utujil) defined medicine (*kunab'al*) as natural, obtained from local plants in the forest (*pa le k'ajchela*) or hills (*pa le juyub'*). He also notes that these practices were limited to indigenous areas where language and health beliefs were shared. However, the term 'natural' also needs qualification based on conversational pragmatics, as some natural products were not indigenous to Guatemala, although they were cultivated within neighboring regions with nonpharmaceutical medicines. Moreover, vitamins and other supplements and over-the-counter medicines such as Vicks were used alongside them.

According to Harvey, mobile medicine practices use specific forms of health communication. He identified three general context-dependent persuasive communication paradigms, referred to as frames.[29] Frame 1 consisted of rote public announcements using loudspeakers. These presentations promoted medicines and therapeutics for common illnesses without complex dosage instructions and were typically presented in busy areas (e.g., bus terminals, town squares), lasting between 2 and 5 minutes. Frame 2 consisted of public health talks that occurred on buses. Due to the physical constraints of the space, demonstrations were not possible. These talks lasted between 15 and 20 minutes, consisting of generally accepted therapeutics that had less complex dosage instructions. Frame 3 consisted of both a public health talk and a demonstration of healthcare products. These presentations typically occurred on street corners, in open-air markets, and in town squares, lasting between 30 and 45 minutes. The length of the demonstration can be attributed to the need for greater persuasion, as they concerned the least accepted therapeutics with the most complex dosage instructions.

Unlike many other health communication strategies (Schoenherr & Le-Bouar, 2024), Frame 3 presentations were dramatic, interactive modes for the transmission of information, often using physical demonstrations, i.e., metonymic devices such as clothes or plastic bags representing an organ and dye to represent blood or infection (Harvey, 2011). They often involved presentation of a local plant and solicited the knowledge of the audience. Destigmatization was also a theme, with demonstrations often containing comedic elements and apologies for discussing matters that might be viewed as socially inappropriate.

Attempts were also made to delegitimize BWM therapeutics, to show that they contaminate the body, with presenters reciting warning label side-effects to reinforce these concerns. These presentations also contained misinformation and disinformation about the 'non-natural' BWM therapeutics. Presumably, such information could directly or indirectly affect health seekers' beliefs and behaviors, e.g., *sleeper effects*. However, acceptance of anti-BWM messaging is also likely the result of sharing those beliefs initially or having doubts about the diagnostic and therapeutic practices. The lingering distrust of colonial/governmental institutions coupled with low health literacy in health seekers can result in a failure to utilize health resources when they are available (Kelm, 1998).

10.5 Conclusions

Focusing on abstract competencies and evidence-based medicine can obscure the inherent variability associated with healthcare delivery. Health seekers, healers, and healthcare institutions are embedded in dynamic formal and informal social networks. Evaluating the adoption of healthcare products and practices must account for the sociocultural dimension of the implementation context. In healthcare ecosystems defined by medical pluralism, additional challenges are present due to heterarchical structures and heterogenous norms and practices. HCPs, educators, and administrators must ensure that they understand the dynamic relationships that define these situations.

Mayan and neighboring communities have existed for millennia, developing complex frameworks for understanding their world and place in it. The adoption and adaptation of diagnostic and treatment methods based on external medical paradigms as well as ancestral and spiritual knowledge using locally available medicinal plants represent embedded socioecological processes. Despite reduction in knowledge of medicinal plants in recent generations, it remains clear that 'forest medicine', its practitioners, and other empirically derived approaches to healthcare make important contribution to the healthcare ecosystems of the Americas. Claims of the 'dominance' of BWM (Baer et al., 2013) must be viewed in this light. In this chapter, I have attempted to demonstrate that they are overstated.

Traditionally, BWM has often been defined as comparatively rigid relationships defined by asymmetries in power (e.g., doctor–patient, doctor–nurse), which would subordinate alternative medical paradigms. This both assumes the perceived legitimacy of BWM practitioners and ignores the agency of health seekers, who do not necessarily define themselves as 'patients'. In indigenous and rural communities, BWM is neither exclusively nor predominantly used by health seekers due to limited availability, geographic boundaries, and inconsistent beliefs. Acknowledging and learning from these adaptations must inform health professionals' education and healthcare delivery locally, as well as providing general lessons about the function and structure of healthcare ecosystems.

10.5.1 Socioecology of Health: Fluid Ontologies and Knowledge Creation

It is tempting to identify a deep historic connection between indigenous medicines, as some have made between Mayan and East Asian[30] health epistemologies (e.g., France & Rodrigeuz, 2019; Garcia et al., 1999). Such narratives suggest that the first people to populate the Americas brought illness models with them as they migrated from Northern East Asia and that they persist. However, innovations can also be the result of adoption and adaptation of cultural variants from other traditions (e.g., hot–cold distinction; Foster, 1987). Convergent evolution is also highly likely as certain practices (e.g., pulsing) are present in many medical traditions (Ayurveda, East Asian, Egyptian, Greek, and Unani; Amber et al., 1993; Hall, 2001; Kuriyama, 1997; Steiner, 1987). There is no reason to think that a group, such as the Maya who independently invented the concept of zero, would not independently create complex health beliefs and systems of care that are comparable to any other healthcare tradition.

Like most people, the health beliefs of indigenous groups of Mesoamerica are defined by fluid ontologies[31] where boundaries between the material and immaterial world are permeable rather than static. Similarly, pragmatism defines the adoption of therapeutic methods. Here, I have referred to this as *satisficing syncretism* in that healers and health seekers are more interested in satisfactory outcomes than coherent, internally consistent explanations of cause–effect relationships, allowing them to use varied heuristic to draw from available beliefs in a healthcare ecosystem. Health seekers search for and adopt those methods that are cognitively accessible to them. Healers are equally reliant on the available resources of their environments as well as the demands from heal seekers in terms of the kinds of illnesses they experience as well as how they wish to be treated. *Empiricos* and *curanderos* embody the process of learning and practice, with their knowledge representing an often-idiosyncratic process of abductive reasoning. Learning from trial-and-error, apprenticeships, and each other, there is far greater emphasis on pragmatism than adhering to orthodoxy.

Despite the focus on the Maya peoples, these observations are likely true of any population. The pragmatism of healers and health seekers is necessary to use the means available to them to preserve health and eliminate illness. The division often implied by medical pluralism between indigenous medicine, 'complimentary and alternative' medicines, and BWM traditions appears impractical in this light (Hollenberg & Muzzin, 2010). HCPs might segregate beliefs, creating epistemological hierarchies, but principles of cognitive science favor the idea that these beliefs represent heterarchical structures that are drawn based on perceived contextual relevance.

Regardless of the formality of the institutional structures that healers work within, they must always adapt to resource limitations and characteristics of the patient populations they serve. Even in Western societies, most health seekers who adopt BWM are unlikely to understand the biological, physiological, and pharmacological features, i.e., they have minimal health literacy. Concurrently, healers *within* a community of practice do not always agree on the diagnosis and treatment recommendations despite maintaining high confidence in their delivery of care (e.g., Millington et al., 2018; Schoenherr et al., 2018). Rather than viewing these issues in terms of health literacy and patient compliance, HCPs must consider broader concerns of the compatibility of the mental models of healers and healer seekers. While this might not always be possible in practice, ensuring that members of a healthcare team are representative of the community will promote more effective collaborative care.

10.5.2 Heterarchical Medical Pluralism and Colonialism

Colonists brought with them new pathologies, treatments, and ideas and practices related to health and illness. The resulting medical pluralism can be beneficial. If biomedical principles were followed, evidence-based practices should examine the efficacy of a treatment regardless of its historical, theoretical, or practical origins. Instead, colonialism is about dominance, exploiting resources, controlling populations and practitioners, supplanting 'traditional' beliefs, and institutionalized re-educating communities to create hierarchical relationship between traditional medicine and BWM (de Sahagun, 1938). However, the persistence of – and often preference for – traditional medicine suggests that it occupies an important niche within the healthcare ecosystem. Healthcare is therefore defined by a heterarchical structure from the perspective of healers.

Heterarchies have specific sets of features including resources, mental models, authorities, and institutions. In the Mayan heartland, *curanderos* and midwives clearly represent the core of these practices. The repeated observations of reluctance of members of indigenous communities to obtain care from state-based public health services reinforce division of social organizations and paradigms. However, the fact that some BWM-based therapeutics (e.g., aspirin) are associated with 'natural' treatments demonstrates this as they have been medicalized within indigenous communities. Concurrently, the aims of bioprospecting also demonstrate that BWM is receptive to indigenous innovations, if they can be legitimated using its own instruments and criteria (Reeser, 2014). Thus, the boundaries of heterarchies represent mental models that are psychologically distinct to health seekers and healers.

Perhaps the best contemporary illustration of heterarchical structures in the Mayan healthcare ecosystem is that of midwifery. Midwives are represented across cultures, yet their autonomy has been consistently challenged (Ehrenreich & English, 2010; Fahy, 2007; Kananoja, 2021; Lay, 2000; Starr, 1982). Superficially, this appears to support claims of dominance of BWM and a hierarchical structure in healthcare (Baer et al., 2013). By attempting to introduce state legitimation through 'formal recognition… a registration system, [and] … licenses' (de Bocaletti et al., 1999; p. 11–12), midwifery is anchored further within a healthcare ecosystem of the state. Nevertheless, the WHO's recognition of the centrality of midwives to healthcare (World Health Organization (WHO), 2000) and the preferences of local women for traditional maternal attendants provide evidence suggesting a pluralistic healthcare ecosystem defined by heterarchical structure.

By drawing parallels with research in cognitive science, this chapter links practices that are often seen as irrational/transrational with practices that are beneficial to medical judgment and decision-making. Practices such as prayer used by indigenous healers likely represent an important adaption to decision-making. Rather than viewing them as intrinsically linked to Mayan medicine, HCPs practicing within the BWM tradition can take lessons from these approaches. Regardless of whether insights obtained by healers are attributed to immaterial forces (spirits), meditative practices have been demonstrated to facilitate problem-solving and could facilitate the recall of relevant patterns and information during healthcare delivery. The practice can also be likened with the metacognitive monitoring practices such as 'stop-and-think' used in surgical practices to promote reflection at critical decision points in healthcare delivery (Schoenherr et al., 2024).

10.5.3 Shifting from Informal Practice to Formalization

Regardless of the origins of indigenous traditions, both Mayan and BWM practitioners seek to develop core competencies. Rather than a stochastic search process, or semi-formalized apprenticeships, contemporary medicine is grounded in formal training. Whether in terms of an apprenticeship model that assumes that learners can acquire knowledge through exposure to models or a curriculum guided by competency-based design principles (Schoenherr & McConnell, 2024), learners are formally assessed and granted a status as practitioners.

As the review in this chapter demonstrates, formal education structures have existed historically in Mesoamerica and have emerged in contemporary society. Educational practices formalizing healer competencies are evidenced in Mayan society (Miles, 1957; Orellana, 1987) and later in Aztec society (Guerra, 1966) providing a clear demonstration of processes that were likely analogous to medicalization, professionalization, and institutionalization. While such social organization and structures do not appear to be on the order of those in East Asia (e.g., China's Imperial Examination System; Schoenherr & Beaudoin, 2027), they nevertheless provide evidence for converging cultural evolution that is not dependent on BWM (cf. Baer et al., 2013). What form they might have taken is of course not clear due to the influence of colonization.

The categorization and systematization of indigenous knowledge is also evidenced in contemporary Mayan communities. The creation of organizations like the MHAB in Belize demonstrates that there is interest in developing a formalized credentialing process for healers. The inclusion of community members in the legitimation of healers presents a distinctive process that underscores the interdependence between healers and health seekers. Such an approach provides a novel model for legitimating practitioners and assuring health seekers of the consistency of the healthcare services they receive by focusing on the efficacy of individual practitioners.

Notes

1 Research in psychology tends to different kinds of folk knowledge, e.g., folkbiology, theory of mind, folk sociology, naïve physics. Each contributes to human survival through understanding the world and predicting outcomes.
2 2000 BCE marks the end of the archaic period.
3 Referred to as *yalba winik* or *pach kah winikob*.
4 Social or public representations are the materialized beliefs and concepts within an epistemic community. The process of objectification facilitates the creation of a shared understanding of the world (Moscovici).
5 For comparable examples of the reliance on indigenous practitioners, see Schoenherr and Beaudoin (2026) for a discussion of colonial Taiwan under Imperial Japan's rule.
6 In its original formulation, heterarchy was used to describe the dynamic neuroanatomy of the human brain, such that no one region dominated memory or decision-making, with

cognition reflecting distributed systems (McCulloch, 1945; Hawkins, 2021; Rumelhart et al., 1986).

7 In Guatemala, the dual-naming system (i.e., Spanish and Mayan, e.g., Ixil) also reflects a clear demonstration of heterarchies in the region.

8 This general term is adopted here for ease of comprehension. As I noted below, there are numerous specific terms that vary across regions that describe a variety of practitioners.

9 Alternatively referred to as *Chol Q'ij* in K'iche' Maya.

10 It is perhaps unsurprising given that the 260-day cycle approximates the period of human development in the womb. Although alternative accounts for the systems adopted have been proposed (cf. Nuttail, 1928; Merill, 1945; Lamstrom, 1973; Aveni, 1980).

11 It is also unsurprising that Mayan kings (exemplar individuals) would have pseudo-calendars based on their life events.

12 Traditional Korean Medicine has a similar concept, constitutional medicine (Schoenherr & Beaudoin, 2027).

13 The hot–cold distinction is evidenced in both traditional Mayan and East Asian medicine (García-Hernández et al., 2023; see Schoenherr & Beaudoin, 2027).

14 The presence of the hot–cold distinction can be accounted for by psychological processes. For instance, so-called double-function words referring to both psychological and physiological traits are quite common across cultures (e.g., someone can be physically *cold* or have a *cold* personality; Asch, 1955; see also Asch & Nerlove, 1960; Lesser & Drouin, 1975). In this case, the hot–cold distinction stems from our ability to discriminate temperature, allowing it to act as a primary metaphor. Indeed, evidence suggests that the exact features of this distinction differ across cultures (e.g., Africa, see Lubben et al., 1999; Messer, 1981). Consequently, generative analogies and metaphors likely provide the basis for models of illness and disease (see Schoenherr & LeBouar, 2024).

15 These are often understood as metaphors or 'stances' that are not necessarily perceived to be literally true; rather, they function like heuristics (Schoenherr & Thomson, 2021).

16 Parallels can be observed in Western thought with natural philosophers assuming that 'animal spirits' controlled the body of human and nonhuman animals while only humans have a soul, i.e., human spirit.

17 For similar accounts in East Asian medicine, see Schoenherr and Beaudoin (2026).

18 For similar observations in East Asia, see Schoenherr and Beaudoin (2026).

19 I have calculated the overall distribution of learning experiences and practices engaged in by these healers to facilitate comprehension.

20 Only one of these was classified as an apprenticeship.

21 If we account for the two outlying practitioners (>1,000 patients), the mean is greatly reduced ($M = 96.3$) but the standard deviation remains quite high ($SD = 188$).

22 An interesting feature of this data is that experience ($r = .05$) and practitioner age ($r = -.15$) are not significantly related to knowledge of plants. However, age and experience were correlated ($r = .77$). The number of patients was associated with the number of plants a midwife is aware of ($r = .21$); however, this was not the case for healers ($r = -.06$).

23 Hinojosa's (2020) observations of bonesetters mirror early commentaries (and contemporary jokes) about surgeons in the BWM tradition.

24 Crucially for my purpose, the categorization methods used were *not* natural categories of indigenous practices. Rather, Arvigo and colleagues (Arvigo & Balick, 1998; Avrigo et al., 1994) used categories derived from TEAM (Hsu & Peacher, 1982).

25 Referred to as *offline memory reprocessing* (Lewis et al., 2018; Stickgold & Walker, 2013; Warmsley, 2014).

26 Given the small sample size and associated variability in the cases represented in the sample, it is difficult to determine whether such promising results would generalize outside of this use case.

27 There are many kinds of relational models that can inform the interactions of individuals including equivalence, equality, hierarchical, and proportionality (e.g., Fiske, 1991). Within the excerpt the distribution of responsibility by the healer minimally implies a proportionality rule, the primacy of the information obtained from the spiritual realm implies an epistemic authority, if not for the spirits, then for the medium that transmits the message.

28 For issues associated with accessibility, see Nieblas-Bedolla et al., (2019) and Owen et al., (2010).

29 Here, I have renumbered Harvey's frames in ascending order from simplest to most complex, i.e., the terms for Frame 1 and Frame 3 have been substituted.

30 As Schoenherr and Beaudoin (this volume) note, rather than 'Traditional Chinese Medicine' (TCM), the collection of traditions should be referred to as Traditional East Asian Medicine (TEAM) due to the multiple regional and epistemological influences on TEAM.

31 Goldman and Ballard (1998) use this term to describe societies within Papua New Guinea.

Bibliography

Abascal Miguel, L., Lopez, E., Sanders, K., Skinner, N. A., Johnston, J., Vosburg, K. B., ... & Diamond-Smith, N. (2022). Evaluating the impact of a linguistically and culturally tailored social media ad campaign on COVID-19 vaccine uptake among indigenous populations in Guatemala: A pre/post design intervention study. *BMJ Open*, *12*(12), e066365.

Abse, E. (2007). *Toward Where the Sun Hides: The Rise of Sorcery and Transformations of Mazatec Religious Life*. Doctoral dissertation. Department of Anthropology, University of Virginia.

Adams, T. L. (2020). Health professional regulation in historical context: Canada, the USA and the UK (19th century to present). *Human Resources for Health*, *18*(1), 72.

Adams, W. R., & Hawkins, J. P. (Eds.). (2007). *Health Care in Maya Guatemala: Confronting Medical Pluralism in a Developing Country*. University of Oklahoma Press.

Aissen, J., England, N. C., & Maldonado, R. Z. (Eds.). (2017). *The Mayan Languages*. Taylor & Francis.

Allen, L., Hatala, A., Ijaz, S., Courchene, E. D., & Bushie, E. B. (2020). Indigenous-led health care partnerships in Canada. *CMAJ*, *192*(9), E208–E216.

Amber, R., & Babey-Brooke, A. M. (1993). *Pulse Diagnosis: Detailed Interpretations for Eastern and Western Holistic Treatments*. Aurora Press.

Amzat, J., Razum, O., Amzat, J., & Razum, O. (2014). Medical pluralism: Traditional and modern health care. In Amzat, J. & Razum, O. (Eds.), *Medical Sociology in Africa*, 207–240.

Anderson, E. N. (2002). On Maya medicine and the biomedical gaze. *Current Anthropology*, *43*, 789–793.

Annis, S. (1981). Physical access and utilization of health services in rural Guatemala. *Social Science & Medicine. Part D: Medical Geography*, *15*(4), 515–523.

Aparicio Aparicio, J. C., Voeks, R. A., & Silveira Funch, L. (2021). Are mixtec forgetting their plants? Intracultural variation of ethnobotanical knowledge in Oaxaca, Mexico. *Economic Botany*, 75, 215–233.

Argens, L., Brophy, C., Weisser, W. W., & Meyer, S. (2023). Functional group richness increases multifunctionality in intensively managed grasslands. *Grassland Research*, *2*(3), 225–240.

Arjona-García, C., Blancas, J., Beltrán-Rodríguez, L., López Binnqüist, C., Colín Bahena, H., Moreno-Calles, A. I., ... & López-Medellín, X. (2021). How does urbanization affect perceptions and traditional knowledge of medicinal plants? *Journal of Ethnobiology and Ethnomedicine*, *17*(1), 48.

Armijos, C., Cota, I., & González, S. (2014). Traditional medicine applied by the Saraguro yachakkuna: A preliminary approach to the use of sacred and psychoactive plant species in the southern region of ecuador. *Journal of Ethnobiology and Ethnomedicine*, *10*(1), 10–26.

Arnason, J., Cal, V., Pesek, T., Awad, R., Bourbonnais-Spear, N., Collins, S., ... & Ferrier, J. (2022). A review of ethnobotany and ethnopharmacology of traditional medicines used by Q'eqchi'Maya Healers of Xna'ajeb'aj Ralch'o'och', Belize. *Botany*, *100*(2), 219–230.

Arnold, D. (1993). *Colonizing the Body: State Medicine and Epidemic Disease in Nineteenth-Century India*. University of California Press.

Atran, S. (1999). Itzaj Maya folkbiological taxonomy: Cognitive universals and cultural particulars. *Folkbiology*, *119*, 203.

Arvigo, R., & Balick, M. (1998). *Rainforest Remedies: One Hundred Healing Herbs of Belize*. 2nd ed. Lotus Press.

Arvigo, R., Epstein, N., & Yaquinto, M. (1994). *My Apprenticeship with a Maya Healer*. HarperSanFrancisco.

Asamoah, G. D., Khakpour, M., Carr, T., & Groot, G. (2023). Exploring indigenous traditional healing programs in Canada, Australia, and New Zealand: A scoping review. *Explore*, *19*(1), 14–25.

Asch, S. E. (1955). On the use of metaphor in the description of persons. In Werner, H. (Ed.), *On Expressive Language; Papers Presented at the Clark University Conference on Expressive Language Behavior*. (Clark University Monographs in Psychology and Related Disciplines.) (pp. 29–38). Clark University Press.

Asch, S. E., & Nerlove, H. (1960). The development of double function terms in children: An exploratory investigation. In B. Kaplan & S. Wapner (Eds.), *Perspectives in Psychological Theory*. International Universities Press.

Ashdown, B. K., & Gibbons, J. L. (2012). Faith development and collectivism among emerging adults in Guatemala and the United States. *Advances in Psychology Study*, *1*, 22–28.

Aveni, A. F. (1980/2001). *Skywatchers: A Revised and Updated Version of Skywatchers of Ancient Mexico*. University of Texas Press.

Baer, H. A. (2011). Medical pluralism: An evolving and contested concept in medical anthropology. In Singer et al. (Eds)., *A Companion to Medical Anthropology* (pp. 405–423). Wiley-Blackwell.

Baer, H. A., Singer, M., & Susser, I. (2013). *Medical Anthropology and the World System: Critical Perspectives*. Bloomsbury Publishing.

Balick, M. J., De Gezelle, J. M., & Arvigo, R. (2008). Feeling the pulse in Maya medicine: An endangered traditional tool for diagnosis, therapy, and tracking patients' progress. *Explore*, *4*(2), 113–119.

Bassie-Sweet, K. (2014). *Maya Sacred Geography and the Creator Deities*. University of Oklahoma Press.

Battles, J. B., Dixon, N. M., Borotkanics, R. J., Rabin-Fastmen, B., & Kaplan, H. S. (2006). Sensemaking of patient safety risks and hazards. *Health Services Research*, *41*(4p2), 1555–1575.

Béhar, M. (1968). Food and nutrition of the Mayas before the conquest and at the present time. In *Biomedical Challenges Presented to the American Indians*, Scientific Publication No. 165 (pp. 114–119). Washington, DC: Pan American Health Organization.

Benson, P., Colom, A., Dasgupta-Tsikinas, S. N., Flood, D., Hall-Clifford, R., King, N., ... & Wise, P. (2015). *Privatization and the New Medical Pluralism: Shifting Healthcare Landscapes in Maya Guatemala*. Lexington Books.

Berdanier, C. D. (2019). Corn, niacin, and the history of pellagra. *Nutrition Today*, *54*(6), 283–288.

Berger-González, M., Gharzouzi, E., & Renner, C. (2016). Maya healers' conception of cancer as revealed by comparison with Western medicine. *Journal of Global Oncology*, *2*(2), 56–67.

Berger-Gonzalez, M., Scotti, F., Garcia, A. I., Hesketh, A., Hitziger, M., Thompson, I., & Heinrich, M. (2022). Green Health in Guatemala: How can we build mutual trust and partnerships to develop an evidence-base for local medicines and realize their potential? *Botany*, *100*(2), 109–126.

Berlin, B., & Berlin, E. A. (2004a). Community autonomy and the Maya ICBG project in Chiapas, Mexico: How a bioprospecting project that should have succeeded failed. *Human Organization*, *63*(4), 472–486.

Berlin, B., Berlin, E. A., Fernandez Ugalde, J. C., Garcia Barrios, L., Puett, D., Nash, R., ... & Gonzalez-Espinoza, M. (1999). The Maya ICBG: Drug discovery, medical ethnobiology, and alternative forms of economic development in the Highland Maya region of Chiapas, Mexico. *Pharmaceutical Biology*, *37*(1), 127.

Berlin, E. A., & Berlin, B. (2004b). Prior informed consent and bioprospecting in Chiapas. In Riley, M. (Ed.), *Indigenous Intellectual Property Rights: Legal Obstacles and Innovative Solutions* (pp. 341–372). AltaMira Press.

Berry, N. S. (2006). Kaqchikel midwives, home births, and emergency obstetric referrals in Guatemala: Contextualizing the choice to stay at home. *Social Science and Medicinei*, *62*, 1958–1969.

Berry, N. S. (2008). Who's judging the quality of care? Indigenous Maya and the problem of "not being attended". *Medical Anthropology*, *27*(2), 164–189.

Berry, N. S. (2010). *Unsafe Motherhood: Mayan Maternal Mortality and Subjectivity in Post-War Guatemala*. Berghahn Books.

Bertrand, J. T., Seiber, E., & Escudero, G. (2001). Contraceptive dynamics in Guatemala: 1978–1998. *International Family Planning Perspectives*, 27, 112–136.

Bhatt, S. (2012). Health care issues facing the Maya people of the Guatemalan Highlands: The current state of care and recommendations for improvement. *Journal of Global Health Perspectives*, *1*, 1–7.

Bianchetti, M. C. (2014). Curanderos, especializaciones y afecciones que rigen aún hoy en el área andina centro oeste suramericano. *Scripta Ethnologica*, *36*, 129–164.

Bogin, B., Wall, M., & MacVean, R. B. (1992). Longitudinal analysis of adolescent growth of ladino and Mayan school children in Guatemala: Effects of environment and sex. *American Journal of Physical Anthropology, 89*(4), 447–457.

Bramley, D., Hebert, P., Tuzzio, L., & Chassin, M. (2005). Disparities in indigenous health: A cross-country comparison between New Zealand and the United States. *American Journal of Public Health, 95*(5), 844–850.

Braswell, G. E. (2004). *The Maya and Teotihuacan: Reinterpreting Early Classic Interaction.* University of Texas Press.

Breslin, M. J., & Lewis, C. A. (2008). Theoretical models of the nature of prayer and health: A review. *Mental Health, Religion and Culture, 11*(1), 9–21.

Bressani, R. (1990). Chemistry, technology, and nutritive value of maize tortillas. *Food Reviews International, 6*(2), 225–264.

Broom, A., Doron, A., & Tovey, P. (2009). The inequalities of medical pluralism: Hierarchies of health, the politics of tradition and the economies of care in Indian oncology. *Social Science and Medicine, 69*(5), 698–706.

Brown, C. T., & Witschey, W. R. (2001). The geographic analysis of ancient Maya settlement and polity. In *Electronic Cultural Atlas Initiative Conference*, January 2001 (pp. 1–18).

Bunniss, S., & Kelly, D. R. (2010). Research paradigms in medical education research. *Medical Education, 44*(4), 358–366.

Bunzel, R. (1952). *Chichicastenango: A Guatemalan Village*. Publications of the American Ethnological Society XXII. J.J. Augustin Publisher.

Burman, A. (2010). The strange and the native: Ritual and activism in the aymara quest for decolonization. *The Journal of Latin American and Caribbean Anthropology, 15*(2), 457–475.

Bybee, E. R., Hawkins, J. P., MacDonald, J. H., & Adams, W. R. (2013). Saved from being lynched: Reinvention of customary law in Nahualá. In Hawksin, J. P. & Adams, W. R. (Eds.), *Crisis of Governance in Maya Guatemala: Indigenous Responses to a Failing State*, 86–114.

Cancian, F. (1965). *Economics and Prestige in a Maya Community: The Religious Cargo System in Zinacantan.* Stanford University Press.

Canuto, M. A., Estrada-Belli, F., Garrison, T. G., Houston, S. D., Acuña, M. J., Kováč, M., ... & Shrestha, R. (2018). Ancient lowland Maya complexity as revealed by airborne laser scanning of northern Guatemala. *Science, 361*(6409), eaau0137.

Carey, D., Jr. (2023). *Health in the Highlands: Indigenous Healing and Scientific Medicine in Guatemala and Ecuador*. University of California Press.

Carey, D., Jr., & Crafts, L. (2023). Indígenas and international influences of modern medicine in twentieth century Guatemala. In Amstrong-Fumero & Fallaw (eds.), *The Transnational Construction of Mayanness: Reading Modern Mesoamerica Through US Archives*, 145.

Carmack, R. M. (Ed.). (1988). *Harvest of Violence: The Maya Indians and the Guatemalan Crisis*. University of Oklahoma Press.

Carter, E. D. (2023). *In Pursuit of Health Equity: A History of Latin American Social Medicine*. UNC Press Books.

Cepeda-Chamorro, C., Flórez-Meza, V., & Vásquez-Truisi, M. L. (2018). Saberes y prácticas del cuidado de la salud en niños indígenas: Una perspectiva desde la etnia guambiana. *Investigaciones Andina, 20*(37), 177–196.

Cerón, A. (2019). Neocolonial epidemiology: Public health practice and the right to health in Guatemala. *Medicine Anthropology Theory, 6*(1).

Chan, C. B., Gramlich, L., Littlechild, L. M., Lightning, R., Ganske, J., & Thorlakson, J. (2026). Innovations in health professions education in Canada to address the Truth and Reconciliation Commission of Canada's calls to action and the health inequities experienced by Indigenous peoples. In Schoenherr, J. R. (Ed.), *Fundamentals and Frontiers of Medical Education and Decision-Making: Implementation and Innovation.*

Chary, A., Flood, D., Austad, K., Moore, J., King, N., Martinez, B., ... & Rohloff, P. (2016). Navigating bureaucracy: Accompanying indigenous Maya patients with complex health care needs in Guatemala. *Human Organization*, *75*(4), 305–314.

Chary, A., Hawkins, J., Flood, D., Martinez, B., Colom, M., & Austad, K. (2022). Medical students' experiences of compulsory rural services in Guatemala: A qualitative study. *Rural and Remote Health*, *22*(2), 1–11.

Chase, A. F., Chase, D. Z., Zorn, E., & Teeter, W. (2008). Textiles and the Maya archaeological record: Gender, power, and status in classic period Caracol, Belize. *Ancient Mesoamerica*, *19*(1), 127–142.

Chomat, A. M., Kring, B., & Bekker, L. P. (2018). Approaching maternal health from a decolonized, systemic, and culturally safe approach: Case study of the Mayan-Indigenous populations of Guatemala. In Schwartz, A. (Ed.), *Maternal Death and Pregnancy-Related Morbidity among Indigenous Women of Mexico and Central America: An Anthropological, Epidemiological, and Biomedical Approach* (pp. 483–511). Springer.

Clarke, M. E. (2022). Myth, ritual, and the classic-period Maya sweat bath. *Res: Anthropology and Aesthetics*, *77*(1), 48–68.

Cleary, M. R. (2000). Democracy and indigenous rebellion in Latin America. *Comparative Political Studies*, *33*(9), 1123–1153.

Coburn, D. (1993). State authority, medical dominance, and trends in the regulation of the health professions: The Ontario case. *Social Science & Medicine*, *37*(7), 841–850.

Coburn, D. (2006). Medical dominance then and now: Critical reflections. *Health Sociology Review*, *15*(5), 432–443.

Colmant, S. A., Eason, E. A., Winterowd, C. L., Jacobs, S. C., & Cashel, C. (2005). Investigating the effects of sweat therapy on group dynamics and affect. *The Journal for Specialists in Group Work*, *30*(4), 329–341.

Comerford, S. C. (1996). Plantas medicinales de dos curanderos Mayas de San Andrés, Petén, Guatemala. *Economic Botany*, *50*, 327–336.

Commission for Historical Clarification. (1999). Guatemala: Memory of Silence. *Report of the Commission for Historical Clarification Conclusions and Recommendations*. United Nations.

Cook, G. (2007). Heterarchy and homoarchy in Maya village politics. In Bondarenko, D. M. & Nemirovskiy, A. A. (Eds.), *The History of Civilizations*, 67.

Cooper, F., & Stoler, A. L. (1989). Tensions of empire: Colonial control and visions of rule. *American Ethnologist*, *16*(4), 609–621.

Copeland, N. (2014). Mayan imaginaries of democracy: Interactive sovereignties and political affect in postrevolutionary Guatemala. *American Ethnologist*, *41*(2), 305–319.

Coreil, J., Augustin, A., Holt, E., & Halsey, N. A. (1994). Use of ethnographic research for instrument development in a case-control study of immunization use in Haiti. *International Journal of Epidemiology*, *23*(Suppl. 1), S33–S37.

Cosminsky, S. (1977). Part four: Childbirth and midwifery on a Guatemalan finca. *Medical Anthropology*, *1*(3), 69–104.

Cosminsky, S. (1982). Childbirth and change: A Guatemalan study. In: MacCormack, C. (Ed.), *Ethnography of Fertility and Birth* (pp. 205–230). Academic Press.

Cosminsky, S. (2001). Maya midwives of Southern Mexico and Guatemala. In Huber, B. R. & Sandstrom, A. R. (Eds.), *Mesoamerican Healers* (pp. 179–210). University of Texas Press.

Cosminsky, S., & Scrimshaw, M. (1980). Medical pluralism on a Guatemalan plantation. *Social Science and Medicine. Part B Medical Anthropology*, *14*(4), 267–278.

Crozier, A. (2007). *Practising Colonial Medicine: The Colonial Medical Service in British East Africa*. Bloomsbury Publishing.

Crumley, C. L. (1995). Heterarchy and the analysis of complex societies. In Ehrenreich R. M., Crumley C. L., & Levy J. E. (Eds.), *Heterarchy and the Analysis of Complex Societies: Archeological Papers no. 6* (pp. 1–6). American Anthropological Association.

Crumley C. L. (2015). Heterarchy. In Scott R. A., & Buchmann M. C. (Eds.), *Emerging Trends in the Social and Behavioral Sciences: An Interdisciplinary, Searchable, and Linkable Resource* (pp. 1–14). Wiley Online Library.

Dalton, D. S., & Weatherford, D. J. (Eds.). (2022). *Healthcare in Latin America: History, Society, Culture*. University Press of Florida.

De Broe, S., & Hinde, A. (2006). Diversity in fertility patterns in Guatemala. *Population, Space and Place*, *12*(6): 435–459.

de Bocaletti, E., Schumacher, R., Hurtado, E., Bailey, P., Matute, J., McDermott, J., … & Salgado, R. (1999). Perinatal mortality in Guatemala: Community study. *MotherCare*.

de Sahagun, B. (1938). *Historia General de las Cosas de Nueva España. 5* vols, Robredo, P. (Ed.), M6xico.

de Sahagun, B. (1950–1963). *Florentine Codex. General History of the Things of New Spain. 13* vols, trans. by Dibble, C. E. & Anderson, A. J. O. University of Utah.

DeMarrais, E. (2013). Understanding heterarchy: Crafting and social projects in pre-Hispanic Northwest Argentina. *Cambridge Archaeological Journal*, *23*(3), 345–362.

Dickerson, C. M. (2008). *A Look at Bush Medicine in a Pharmaceutical World: Three Traditional Healers in Belize Face Globalization*. Texas State University.

Diemont, S. A., & Martin, J. F. (2009). Lacandon Maya ecosystem management: Sustainable design for subsistence and environmental restoration. *Ecological Applications*, *19*(1), 254–266.

Diemont, S. A. W., Martin, J. F., Levy Tacher, S. I., Nigh, R. B., Ramirez-Lopez, P., & Golicher, J. D. (2006). Lacandon Maya forest management: Restoration of soil fertility using native tree species. *Ecological Engineering*, *28*, 205–212.

Ding, X., Tang, Y. Y., Cao, C., Deng, Y., Wang, Y., Xin, X., … & Posner, M. I. (2015). Short-term meditation modulates brain activity of insight evoked with solution cue. *Social Cognitive and Affective Neuroscience*, *10*(1), 43–49.

Dirlik, A. (2002). Rethinking colonialism: Globalization, postcolonialism, and the nation. *Interventions*, *4*(3), 428–448.

Douglas, P. M., Demarest, A. A., Brenner, M., & Canuto, M. A. (2016). Impacts of climate change on the collapse of lowland Maya civilization. *Annual Review of Earth and Planetary Sciences*, *44*, 613–645.

Dunning, N., Beach, T., Farrell, P., & Luzzadder-Beach, S. (1998). Prehispanic agrosystems and adaptive regions in the Maya lowlands. *Culture & Agriculture*, *20*(2–3), 87–101.

Dussault, G., & Franceschini, M. C. (2006). Not enough there, too many here: Understanding geographical imbalances in the distribution of the health workforce. *Human Resources for Health*, *4*, 1–16.

Earle, D. (2008). Maya caves across time and space: Reading-related landscapes in K'iche' Maya text, ritual and history. In Staller, J. E. (Ed.), *Pre-Columbian Landscapes of Creation and Origin* (pp. 67–94). Springer.

Edmonson, M. S. (1988). *The Book of the Year: Middle American Calendrical Systems*. University of Utah Press.

Edvalson, R. A., Edvalson, J. J., Hawkins, J. P., McDonald, J. H., & Adams, W. R. (2013). Barriers to political empowerment of Nahualese midwives. In Hawkins, J. P., McDonald, J. H., & Adams, W. R. (Eds.), *Crisis of Governance in Maya Guatemala: Indigenous Responses to a Failing State* (pp. 175–194). University of Oklahoma Press.

Ehrenreich, B., & English, D. (2010). *Witches, Midwives, & Nurses: A History of Women Healers*. The Feminist Press at CUNY.

Fabrega, H., & Silver, D. B. (1973). *Illness and Shamanistic Curing in Zinacantan*. Stanford University Press.

Fahy, K. (2007). An Australian history of the subordination of midwifery. *Women and Birth*, *20*(1), 25–29.

Farahani, A., Chiou, K. L., Harkey, A., Hastorf, C. A., Lentz, D. L., & Sheets, P. (2017). Identifying 'plantscapes' at the classic Maya village of Joya de Cerén, El Salvador. *Antiquity*, *91*(358), 980–997.

Ferrier, J., Pesek, T., Zinck, N., Curtis, S., Wanyerka, P., Cal, V., ... & Arnason, J. T. (2020). A classic Maya mystery of a medicinal plant and Maya hieroglyphs. *Heritage*, *3*(2), 275–282.

Few, M. (2015). *For All of Humanity: Mesoamerican and Colonial Medicine in Enlightenment Guatemala*. University of Arizona Press.

Feyisetan, B. J., Asa, S., & Ebigbola, J. A. (1997). Mothers' management of childhood diseases in Yorubaland. The influence of cultural beliefs. *Health Transition Review*, *7*(2), 221–234.

Figueroa, J. C., Paniagua-Avila, A., Sub Cuc, I., Cardona, S., Ramirez-Zea, M., Irazola, V., ... & Fort, M. P. (2022). Explanatory models of hypertension in Guatemala: Recognizing the perspectives of patients, family members, health care providers and administrators, and national-level health system stakeholders. *BMC Public Health*, *22*(1), 2320.

Fischer, E. F. (1999). Cultural logic and Maya identity: Rethinking constructivism and essentialism. *Current Anthropology*, *40*(4), 473–499.

Fiske, A. P. (1991). *Structures of Social Life: The Four Elementary Forms of Human Relations*. Free Press.

Fiske, A. P. (1993). Social errors in four cultures: Evidence about universal forms of social relations. *Journal of Cross-Cultural Psychology*, *24*(4), 463–494.

Fiske, A. P. (2012). Metarelational models: Configurations of social relationships. *European Journal of Social Psychology*, *42*(1), 2–18.

Flood, D., Chary, A., Rohloff, P., & Henderson, B. (2018). Language as health: Healing in indigenous communities in Guatemala through the revitalization of Mayan languages. In Avineri, N., Graham, L. R., Johnson, E. J., Riner, R. C., & Rosa, J. (Eds.), *Language and Social Justice in Practice* (pp. 136–144). Routledge.

Foley, J. M. (2017). *When Worlds Collide: Understanding the Effects of Maya-Teotihuacán Interaction on Ancient Maya Identity and Community*. Vanderbilt University.

Foster, G. M. (1987). On the origin of humoral medicine in Latin America. *Medical Anthropology Quarterly*, *1*(4), 355–393.

Foster, G. M. (1994). *Hippocrates' Latin American Legacy: Humoral Medicine in the New World.* Gordon and Breach.

Foster, L. V. (2005). *Handbook to Life in the Ancient Maya World.* Oxford University Press.

France, H., & Rodriguez, C. (2019). Traditional Chinese medicine in Canada: An indigenous perspective. *Chinese Medicine and Culture*, *2*(1), 1–5.

Fryberg, S. A., Covarrubias, R., & Burack, J. A. (2018). The ongoing psychological colonization of North American indigenous people: Using social psychological theories to promote social justice. In Hammack, P. L. (Ed.), *The Oxford Handbook of Social Psychology and Social Justice* (pp. 113–128). Oxford University Press.

Furst, J. L. M. (1995). *The Natural History of the Soul in Ancient Mexico.* Yale University Press.

Gall, A., Anderson, K., Adams, J., Matthews, V., & Garvey, G. (2019). An exploration of healthcare providers' experiences and perspectives of Traditional and complementary medicine usage and disclosure by Indigenous cancer patients. *BMC Complementary and Alternative Medicine*, *19*, 1–9.

Gallego-Pérez, D. F., Declercq, E., Saper, R. B., Barnes, L. L., & Wardle, J. (2023). Characterizing therapeutic pluralism policies in Latin America: A qualitative content analysis. *Journal of Integrative and Complementary Medicine*, *29*(6–7), 439–450.

García, H., Sierra, A., & Balam, G. (1999). *Wind in the Blood: Mayan Healing and Chinese Medicine*. North Atlantic Books.

García Ortega, M. (2021). Multi-ethnic borders: Mexico-Guatemala-Belize migrations of agricultural sugar workers. *Estudios Fronterizos*, *22*.

García-Hernández, K. Y., Vargas-Guadarrama, L. A., & Vibrans, H. (2023). Academic history, domains and distribution of the hot-cold system in Mexico. *Journal of Ethnobiology and Ethnomedicine*, *19*(1), 50.

García-Hernández, K. Y ., Vibrans, H ., Colunga-GarcíaMarín, P., Vargas-Guadarrama, L. A., Soto-Hernández, M., Katz, E., & Luna-Cavazos, M. (2021). Climate and categories: Two key elements for understanding the Mesoamerican hot-cold classification of illnesses and medicinal plants. *Journal of Ethnopharmacology*, *266*, 113419.

Garza, M., & Abascal Miguel, L. (2025). Health disparities among indigenous populations in Latin America: A scoping review. *International Journal for Equity in Health*, *24*(1), 119.

Gilliland, J. A., Shah, T. I., Clark, A., Sibbald, S., & Seabrook, J. A. (2019). A geospatial approach to understanding inequalities in accessibility to primary care among vulnerable populations. *PloS One*, *14*(1), e0210113.

Giovannini, P., & Heinrich, M. (2009). Xki yoma' (our medicine) and xki tienda (patent medicine)—interface between traditional and modern medicine among the Mazatecs of Oaxaca, Mexico. *Journal of Ethnopharmacology*, *121*(3), 383–399.

Giovannini, P., Reyes-Garcia, V., Waldstein, A., Heinrich, M., (2011). Do pharmaceuticals displace local knowledge and use of medicinal plants? Estimates from a cross-sectional study in a rural indigenous community, Mexico. *Social Science & Medicine*, *72*, 928–936.

Giralt, A. (2012). A decade after Guatemala's agreement on identity and rights of Indigenous peoples: Mayan-Tz'utujil women's views on health, healing, and disease. *Health Care for Women International*, *33*(5), 440–456.

Girón, A. B. S. (2007). Taking matters into one's hands: Lynching and violence in post-civil war Guatemala. *Urban Anthropology and Studies of Cultural Systems and World Economic Development*, 36, 357–379.

Glei, D. A., & Goldman, N. (2000). Understanding ethnic variation in pregnancy-related care in rural Guatemala. *Ethnicity & Health*, *5*(1), 5–22.

Glei, D. A., Goldman, N., & Rodríguez, G. (2003). Utilization of care during pregnancy in rural Guatemala: Does obstetrical need matter? *Social Science & Medicine*, *57*(12), 2447–2463.

Goldman, L., & Ballard, C. (1998). *Fluid Ontologies: Myth, Ritual, and Philosophy in the Highlands of Papua New Guinea*. Bergin & Garvey.

Goldman, N., & Glei, D. A. (2000). *Evaluation of Midwifery Care: A Case Study of Rural Guatemala*. MEASURE Evaluation, Carolina Population Center, University of North Carolina.

Goldman, N., & Glei, D. A. (2003). Evaluation of midwifery care: Results from a survey in rural Guatemala. *Social Science & Medicine*, *56*(4), 685–700.

Goldstein, M. S. (2004). The persistence and resurgence of medical pluralism. *Journal of Health Politics, Policy and Law*, *29*(4), 925–945.

Goodnight, C. J., & Stevens, L. (1997). Experimental studies of group selection: What do they tell us about group selection in nature? *The American Naturalist*, *150*(S1), s59–s79.

Grace, K. (2010). Contraceptive use and intent in Guatemala. *Demographic Research*, *23*, 335–364.

Gragnolati, M., & Marini, A. (2003). *Health and Poverty in Guatemala*. The World Bank.

Graham, E., & Isendahl, C. (2018). *Neotropical Cities as Agro-Urban Landscapes: Revisiting 'Low-Density, Agrarian-Based Urbanism'*. Uppsala University Press.

Grandin, G., & Oglesby, E. (2011). *The Guatemala Reader: History, Culture, Politics*. Duke University Press.

Grauer, K. C. (2021). Heterarchical political ecology: Commoner and elite (meta) physical access to water at the ancient Maya city of Aventura, Belize. *Journal of Anthropological Archaeology*, *62*, 101301.

Green, B., & Colucci, E. (2020). Traditional healers' and biomedical practitioners' perceptions of collaborative mental healthcare in low-and middle-income countries: A systematic review. *Transcultural Psychiatry*, *57*(1), 94–107.

Green, L. (1999). *Fear as a Way of Life: Mayan Widows in Rural Guatemala*. Columbia University Press.

Greenberg, L., (1982). Midwife training programs in Highland Guatemala. *Social Science and Medicine*, *16*, 1599–1609.

Greene, S. (2004). Indigenous people incorporated? Culture as politics, culture as property in pharmaceutical bioprospecting 1. *Current Anthropology*, 45, 211–237.

Griffiths, K., Coleman, C., Lee, V., & Madden, R. (2016). How colonisation determines social justice and Indigenous health—a review of the literature. *Journal of Population Research*, *33*, 9–30.

Grossman, P., Niemann, L., Schmidt, S., & Walach, H. (2004). Mindfulness-based stress reduction and health benefits: A meta-analysis. *Journal of Psychosomatic Research*, *57*(1), 35–43.

Grube, N., & Nahm, W. (1994). A census of Xibalba: A complete inventory of way characters on Maya ceramics. In B. Kerr & J. Kerr (Eds.), *The Maya Vase Book*, Vol. 4 (pp. 686–715). Kerr Associates.

Guerra, F. (1966). Aztec medicine. *Medical History*, *10*(4), 315–338.

Gutiérrez-Peláez, K., Aranda, Z., Jiménez-Peña, A., & Mata-González, H. (2022). How inequity threatens the lives of pregnant women: Barriers to accessing health services during an incomplete miscarriage in rural southern Mexico. *BMJ Case Reports CP*, *15*(5), e248819.

Haber, S. (1991). *The Quest for Authority and Honor in the American Professions, 1750–1900*. University of Chicago Press.

Hall, T. (2001). Pulse diagnosis and tonification in Japanese acupuncture. *Acupuncture Today*, *2*, 1–10.

Hall-Clifford, R. (2015). Capitalizing on care: Marketplace quasi-pharmaceuticals in the Guatemalan health-seeking landscape. In Chary, A., & Rohloff, P. (Eds.), *Privatization and the New Medical Pluralism: Shifting Healthcare Landscapes in Maya Guatemala* (pp. 36–47). Lexington Books.

Hamilton, N., & Chinchilla, N. S. (1991). Central American migration: A framework for analysis. *Latin American Research Review*, *26*(1), 75–110.

Han, G. S. (2002). The myth of medical pluralism: A critical realist perspective. *Sociological Research Online*, *6*(4), 65–80.

Harvey, T. S. (2011). Maya mobile medicine in Guatemala: The "other" public health. *Medical Anthropology Quarterly*, *25*(1), 47–69.

Hatala, A. R., & Waldram, J. B. (2016). The role of sensorial processes in Q'eqchi'Maya healing: A case study of depression and bereavement. *Transcultural Psychiatry*, *53*(1), 60–80.

Haug, G. H., Gunther, D., Peterson, L. C., Sigman, D. M., Hughen, K. A., & Aeschlimann, B. (2003). Climate and the collapse of Maya civilization. *Science*, *299*, 1731–1735.

Hawkins, J. (2021). *A Thousand Brains: A New Theory of Intelligence*. Basic Books.

Hawkins, J. P. (2007). *Health Care in Maya Guatemala: Confronting Medical Pluralism in a Developing Country*. University of Oklahoma Press.

Heinrich, M., Ankli, A., Frei, B., Weimann, C., & Sticher, O. (1998). Medicinal plants in Mexico: Healer's consensus and cultural importance. *Social Science & Medicine*, *47*, 1859–1871.

Hendon, J. A. (1999). Multiple sources of prestige and the social evaluation of women in pre-His-panic Mesoamerica. In Robb, J. E. (Ed.), *Material Symbols: Culture and Economy in Prehistory* (pp. 257–276). Center for Archaeological Investigations, Southern Illinois University.

Hersch-Martínez, P. (1997). Medicinal plants and regional traders in Mexico: Physiographic differences and conservational challenge. *Economic Botany*, *51*(2), 107–120.

Hill, D. M. (2009). Traditional medicine and restoration of wellness strategies. *International Journal of Indigenous Health*, *5*(1), 26–42.

Hill, M. D., Fernández Salvador, C., Pelfini, A., Salas, M., & Rosés, M. A. (2022). Medical pluralism and ambivalent trust: Pandemic technologies, inequalities, and public health in Ecuador and Argentina. *Critical Public Health*, *32*(1), 19–30.

Hinojosa, S. Z. (2020). *Maya Bonesetters: Manual Healers in a Changing Guatemala*. University of Texas Press.

Hinojoas, S. Z. (2004). Bonesetting and radiography in the Southern Maya Highlands. *Medical Anthropology*, *23*(4): 263–293.

Hinojosa, S. Z. (2002). "The hands know": Bodily engagement and medical impasse in Highland Maya bonesetting. *Medical Anthropology Quarterly*, *16*(1), 22–40.

Hinojosa, S. Z., (2004). Authorizing tradition: Vectors of contention in Highland Maya midwifery. *Social Science and Medicine*, *59*, 637–651.

Hitziger, M., Berger Gonzalez, M., Gharzouzi, E., Ochaíta Santizo, D., Solis Miranda, R., Aguilar Ferro, A. I., ... & Krütli, P. (2017). Patient-centered boundary mechanisms to foster intercultural partnerships in health care: A case study in Guatemala. *Journal of Ethnobiology and Ethnomedicine*, *13*, 1–13.

Hodell, D. A., Curtis, J. H., & Brenner, M. (1995). Possible role of climate in the collapse of classic Maya civilization. *Nature, 375*(6530), 391–394.

Hofstede, G. (1980). *Culture's Consequences: International Differences in Work-Related Values*. Sage Publications.

Hoge, E. A., Bui, E., Marques, L., Metcalf, C. A., Morris, L. K., Robinaugh, D. J., ... & Simon, N. M. (2013). Randomized controlled trial of mindfulness meditation for generalized anxiety disorder: Effects on anxiety and stress reactivity. *The Journal of Clinical Psychiatry, 74*(8), 16662.

Holland, W. R. (1962). *Highland Maya Folk Medicine: A Study of Culture Change*. PhD dissertation. Department of Anthropology, University of Arizona.

Hollenberg, D., & Muzzin, L. (2010). Epistemological challenges to integrative medicine: An anti-colonial perspective on the combination of complementary/alternative medicine with biomedicine. *Health Sociology Review, 19*(1), 34–56.

Houston, S. D., & Stuart, D. (1989). *The Way Glyph: Evidence for "Co-Essences" Among the Classic Maya* (Vol. *30*). Center for Maya Research.

Hoyler, E., Martinez, R., Mehta, K., Nisonoff, H., & Boyd, D. (2018). Beyond medical pluralism: Characterising health-care delivery of biomedicine and traditional medicine in rural Guatemala. *Global Public Health, 13*(4), 503–517.

Hsu, H-Y, & Peacher, W. G. (1982). *Chinese Herb Medicine and Therapy*. Oriental Healing Arts Institute of the USA.

Huber, B. R., & Anderson, R. (1996). Bonesetters and curers in a Mexican community: Conceptual models, status, and gender. *Medical Anthropology, 17*(1), 23–38.

Hutson, S. R., Hanks, B. K., & Anne Pyburn, K. (2012). Gender, complexity, and power in prehistory. In Bolger, D. (Ed.), *A Companion to Gender Prehistory*, 45–67.

Immerman, R. (1982). *The CIA in Guatemala*. University of Texas Press.

Ippolito, M. M., Chary, A., Daniel, M., Barnoya, J., Monroe, A., & Eakin, M. (2017). Expectations of health care quality among rural Maya villagers in Sololá Department, Guatemala: a qualitative analysis. *International Journal for Equity in Health, 16*(1), 47.

Ishida, K., Stupp, P., Turcios-Ruiz, R., William, D. B., & Espinoza, E. (2012). Ethnic inequality in Guatemalan women's use of modern reproductive health care. *International Perspectives on Sexual and Reproductive Health*, 38, 99–108.

Janzen, J. M. (1978). *The Quest for Therapy in Lower Zaire*. University of California Press.

Jiménez-Balam, D., Alcalá, L., & Salgado, D. (2019). Maya children's medicinal plant knowledge: Initiative and agency in their learning process. *Learning, Culture and Social Interaction, 22*, 100333.

Jordan, M. E., Lanham, H. J., Crabtree, B. F., Nutting, P. A., Miller, W. L., Stange, K. C., ... & McDaniel, R. R. (2009). The role of conversation in health care interventions: Enabling sensemaking and learning. *Implementation Science, 4*, 1–13.

Joyce, R. A., & Hendon, J. A. (2012). Heterarchy, history, and material reality: "Communities" in late classic Honduras. In Canuto, M. A. & Yaeger, J. (Eds.), *Archaeology of Communities: A New World Perspective* (pp. 143–160). Routledge.

Kananoja, K. (2021). *Healing Knowledge in Atlantic Africa: Medical Encounters, 1500–1850*. Cambridge University Press.

Katz, S. H., Hediger, M. L., & Valleroy, L. A. (1974). Traditional maize processing techniques in the New World: Traditional alkali processing enhances the nutritional quality of maize. *Science, 184*(4138), 765–773.

Kellogg, S. (2005). *Weaving the Past: A History of Latin America's Indigenous Women from the Prehispanic Period to the Present*. Oxford University Press.

Kelm, M. E. (1998). *Colonizing Bodies: Aboriginal Health and Healing in British Columbia, 1900–1950*. UBC press.

Kennett, D. J., Breitenbach, S. F., Aquino, V. V., Asmerom, Y., Awe, J., Baldini, J. U., ... & Haug, G. H. (2012). Development and disintegration of Maya political systems in response to climate change. *Science, 338*(6108), 788–791.

Kesebir, S., & Kesebir, P. (2017). A growing disconnection from nature is evident in cultural products. *Perspectives on Psychological Science, 12*(2), 258–269.

King, N., Chary, A., & Rohloff, P. (2015). Leveraging resources in contemporary Maya midwifery. In Chary, A., & Rohloff, P. (Eds.), *Privatization and the New Medical Pluralism: Shifting Healthcare Landscapes in Maya Guatemala* (pp. 88–94). Lexington Books.

Kirmayer, L. J., Lemelson, R., & Barad, M. (Eds.). (2010). *Understanding Trauma: Integrating Biological, Clinical, and Cultural Perspectives*. Cambridge University Press.

Kleinman, A. (1980). *Patients and Healers in the Context of Culture: An Exploration of the Borderland Between Anthropology, Medicine, and Psychiatry*. University of California Press.

Klein, C. F. (1995). Wild woman in colonial Mexico: An encounter of European and Aztec concepts of the other. In Farago, C. (Ed.), *Reframing the Renaissance: Visual Culture in Europe and Latin America*. (pp. 245–63). Yale University Press.

Knight, N. (2008). Yukatek Maya children's attributions of belief to natural and non-natural entities. *Journal of Cognition and Culture, 8*(3–4), 235–243.

Knight, N., Sousa, P., Barrett, J. L., & Atran, S. (2004). Children's attributions of beliefs to humans and God: Cross-cultural evidence. *Cognitive Science, 28*(1), 117–126.

Kodicek, E., Braude, R., Kon, S. K., & Mitchell, K. G. (1959). The availability to pigs of nicotinic acid in tortilla baked from maize treated with lime-water. *British Journal of Nutrition, 13*, 363–384.

Koss-Chioino, J., Leatherman, T. L., & Greenway, C. (Eds.). (2003). *Medical Pluralism in the Andes* (p. 16). London: Routledge.

Kragel, E. A., Beyer, L. N., & Boyd, D. L. (2018). Barrier to healthcare access faced by Indigenous women in the Guatemalan Highland. *International Journal of Indigenous Health, 13*, 104–121.

Krause, S., Beach, T. P., Luzzadder-Beach, S., Cook, D., Bozarth, S. R., Valdez, F., Jr., & Guderjan, T. H. (2021). Tropical wetland persistence through the Anthropocene: Multiproxy reconstruction of environmental change in a Maya agroecosystem. *Anthropocene, 34*, 100284.

Kroeger, A. (1983). Anthropological and socio-medical health care research in developing countries. *Social Science of Medicine, 17*, 147–161.

Kruske, S., & Barclay, L. (2004). Effect of shifting policies on traditional birth attendant training. *Journal of Midwifery and Women's Health, 49*, 306–310.

Krys, K., Vignoles, V. L., De Almeida, I., & Uchida, Y. (2022). Outside the "cultural binary": Understanding why Latin American collectivist societies foster independent selves. *Perspectives on Psychological Science, 17*(4), 1166–1187.

Krys, K., Zelenski, J. M., Capaldi, C. A., Park, J., van Tilburg, W., & Uchida, Y. (2019). Putting the "we" into well-being: Using collectivism-themed measures of well-being attenuates well-being's association with individualism. *Asian Journal of Social Psychology, 22*, 256–267.

Kunow, M. A. (2003). *Maya Medicine: Traditional Healing in Yucatan*. UNM Press.

Kuriyama, S. (1997). Pulse diagnosis in the Greek and Chinese traditions. In Kawakita, Y. (Ed.), *History of Diagnostics* (pp. 43–67). The Taniguchi Foundation.

Lang, J. B., & Elkin, E. D. (1997). A study of the beliefs and birthing practices of traditional midwives in rural Guatemala. *Journal of Nurse Midwifery, 42*, 25–31.

Lavallee, L. F., & Poole, J. M. (2010). Beyond recovery: Colonization, health and healing for Indigenous people in Canada. *International Journal of Mental Health and Addiction, 8*, 271–281.

Law, D. (2020). Contact and Mayan languages. In Hickey, R. (Ed.), *The Handbook of Language Contact* (2nd ed., pp. 613–623). Wiley-Blackwell.

Lay, M. M. (2000). *The Rhetoric of Midwifery: Gender, Knowledge, and Power*. Rutgers University Press.

Lee, J., Houser, R. F., Must, A., de Fulladolsa, P. P., & Bermudez, O. I. (2012). Socioeconomic disparities and the familial coexistence of child stunting and maternal overweight in Guatemala. *Economics & Human Biology, 10*(3), 232–241.

Lehman, B. J., David, D. M., & Gruber, J. A. (2017). Rethinking the biopsychosocial model of health: Understanding health as a dynamic system. *Social and Personality Psychology Compass, 11*(8), e12328.

Leonti, M., Cabras, S., Castellanos, M. E., Challenger, A., Gertsch, J., & Casu, L. (2013). Bioprospecting: Evolutionary implications from a post-olmec pharmacopoeia and the relevance of widespread taxa. *Journal of Ethnopharmacology, 147*(1), 92–107.

Leslie, C. (1980). Medical pluralism in world perspective. *Social Science & Medicine. Part B: Medical Anthropology, 14*(4), 191–195.

Lesser, H., & Drouin, C. (1975). Training in the use of double-function terms. *Journal of Psycholinguistic Research, 4*(4), 285–302.

Lewis, M. E., & Myhra, L. L. (2018). Integrated care with indigenous populations: Considering the role of health care systems in health disparities. *Journal of Health Care for the Poor and Undererved, 29*(3), 1083–1107.

Lewis, P. A., Knoblich, G., & Poe, G. (2018). How memory replay in sleep boosts creative problem-solving. *Trends in Cognitive Sciences, 22*(6), 491–503.

Leyn, J. (2007). The Sickness Was Too Strong. In Adams, W. R. & Hawkins, J. P. (Eds.), *Health Care in Maya Guatemala: Confronting Medical Pluralism in a Developing Country*, 100–122.

Lincoln, J. (1942). *The Maya Calendar of the Ixil of Guatemala*. Carnegie Institution Pub. No. 528, 97–128.

Lindblade, K. A., Johnson, A. J., Arvelo, W., Zhang, X., Jordan, H. T., Reyes, L., … & Padilla, N. (2011). Low usage of government healthcare facilities for acute respiratory infections in Guatemala: Implications for influenza surveillance. *BMC Public Health, 11*, 885.

Lindstrom, D. P., & Hernández, C. H. (2006). Internal migration and contraceptive knowledge and use in Guatemala. *International Family Planning Perspectives*, 146–153.

Lindstrom, D. P., & Muñoz-Franco, E. (2005). Migration and the diffusion of modern contraceptive knowledge and use in rural Guatemala. *Studies in Family Planning, 36*, 277–288.

Little, W. E. (2002). *Mayas in the Marketplace: Tourism, Globalization, and Cultural Identity*. University of Texas Press.

Little, E. E., Polanco, M. A., Baldizon, S. R., Wagner, P., & Shakya, H. (2019). Breastfeeding knowledge and health behavior among Mayan women in rural Guatemala. *Social Science & Medicine, 242*, 112565.

Logan, M. H. (1973). Humoral medicine in Guatemala and peasant acceptance of modern medicine. *Human Organization, 32*(4), 385–396.

Lohse, J. C., & Valdez Jr, F. (Eds.). (2010). *Ancient Maya Commoners*. University of Texas Press.

López Austin, A. (1980). *Cuerpo Humano e Ideología: Las Concepiones de los Antiguos Nahuas*. 2 tomos. IIA-UNAM.

Lowes, S., & Montero, E. (2021). The legacy of colonial medicine in Central Africa. *American Economic Review, 111*(4), 1284–1314.

Lubben, F., Netshisaulu, T., & Campbell, B. (1999). Students' use of cultural metaphors and their scientific understandings related to heating. *Science Education, 83*(6), 761–774.

Lutz, C. H. (1994). *Santiago de Guatemala, 1541–1773: City, Caste, and the Colonial Experience*. University of Oklahoma Press.

Mac Arthur, I., Nelson, J., & Woodye, M. (2014). *Quality Improvement of Health Care in Belize: Focusing on Results*. Inter-American Development Bank..

Maffi, L. (1994). *A Linguistic Analysis of Tzeltal Maya Ethnosymptomatology*. Doctoral dissertation, University of California, Berkeley.

Malmstrom, V. H. (1973). Origin of the Mesoamerican 260-day calendar. *Science, 181*(4103), 939–941.

Magnani, L. (1992). Abductive reasoning: Philosophical and educational perspectives in medicine. In *Advanced Models of Cognition for Medical Training and Practice* (pp. 21–41). Springer Berlin Heidelberg.

Magnani, L. (1997). Basic science reasoning and clinical reasoning intertwined: Epistemological analysis and consequences for medical education. *Advances in Health Sciences Education, 2*, 115–130.

Mann, C. C. (2005). *1491: New Revelations of the Americas before Columbus*. Knopf.

Marcus, J. (2004). Maya commoners: The stereotype and the reality. In Lohse, J. C. & Valdez, F. (Eds.), *Ancient Maya Commoners* (pp. 255–284). University of Texas Press.

Marrone, S. (2007). Understanding barriers to health care: A review of disparities in health care services among indigenous populations. *International Journal of Circumpolar Health, 66*(3), 188–198.

Martinez, B., Ixen, E. C., Hall-Clifford, R., Juarez, M., Miller, A. C., Francis, A., ... & Rohloff, P. (2018). mHealth intervention to improve the continuum of maternal and perinatal care in rural Guatemala: A pragmatic, randomized controlled feasibility trial. *Reproductive Health, 15*, 1–12.

Martinez-Fernandez, A., Lobos-Medina, I., Diaz-Molina, C. A., Chen-Cruz, M. F., & Prieto-Egido, I. (2015). TulaSalud: An m-health system for maternal and infant mortality reduction in Guatemala. *Journal of Telemedicine and Telecare, 21*, 283–291.

Martínez Hernández, J. (Ed.). (1929). *Diccionario de Motul: Maya-Español*. Compañía Tipográfica Yucateca, Mérida.

Martini, C. (2023). Abductive reasoning in clinical diagnostics. In *Handbook of Abductive Cognition* (pp. 467–479). Springer International Publishing.

Masters, K. S., & Spielmans, G. I. (2007). Prayer and health: Review, meta-analysis, and research agenda. *Journal of Behavioral Medicine, 30*, 329–338.

Maupin, J. N., (2008). Remaking the Guatemalan midwife: Health care reform and midwifery training programs in Highland Guatemala. *Medical Anthropology, 27*, 353–382.

Maupin, J. N. (2009). 'Fruit of the accords': Healthcare reform and civil participation in Highland Guatemala. *Social Science and Medicine, 68*, 1456–1463.

Maupin, J. N. (2009). Remaking the Guatemalan midwife: Health care reform and midwifery training programs in Highland Guatemala. *Medical Anthropology*, *28*(4), 353–382.
Maupin, J. N. (2011). Divergent models of community health workers in Highland Guatemala. *Human Organization*, *70*, 44–53.
McCulloch, W. S. (1945). A heterarchy of values determined by the topology of nervous nets. *Bulletin of Mathematical Biophysics*, *7*, 89–93.
McKivett, A., & Paul, D. (2024). Recreating the future—Indigenous research paradigms in health professional education research. *Medical Education*, *58*(1), 149–156.
Médecins Sans Frontières. (1999). *Guatemala: After the War, a Health System in Ruins*. MSF Activity Report 1999. Médecins Sans Frontières.
Medina-Elizalde, M., & Rohling, E. J. (2012). Collapse of classic Maya civilization related to modest reduction in precipitation. *Science*, *335*(6071), 956–959.
Mellado Campos, V. (1994). *La medicina tradicional de los pueblos indígenas de México*. Instituto Nacional Indigenista.
Melville, M. B., & Lykes, M. B. (1992). Guatemalan Indian children and the sociocultural effects of government-sponsored terrorism. *Social Science & Medicine*, *34*(5), 533–548.
Merrill, R. H. (1945). Maya sun calendar dictum disproved. *American Antiquity*, *10*(3), 307–311.
Messer, E. (1981). Hot-cold classification: Theoretical and practical implications of a Mexican study. *Social Science & Medicine*, *15B*, 133–145.
Metz, B. E. (1998/1999). *Without Nation, Without Community: The Transformation of Q'eqchi' Maya Political Life Under Guatemalan State and Religious Penetration* (doctoral dissertation/related publication).
Metzger, D., & Williams, G. (1963). Tenejapa medicine I: The curer. *Southwestern Journal of Anthropology*, *19*(2), 216–234.
Miles, S. W. (1957). The sixteenth-century Pokom Maya. A documentary analysis of structure and archaeological setting. *Transactions of American Philosophical Society 47*, 731–781.
Miller, C. A. (2013). *Earth. Water. Sky. The Liminal Landscape of the Maya Sweatbath.*
Miller, J. J., Fletcher, K., & Kabat-Zinn, J. (1995). Three-year follow-up and clinical implications of a mindfulness meditation-based stress reduction intervention in the treatment of anxiety disorders. *General Hospital Psychiatry*, *17*(3), 192–200.
Millington, S. J., Arntfield, R. T., Guo, R. J., Koenig, S., Kory, P., Noble, V., ... & Schoenherr, J. R. (2018). Expert agreement in the interpretation of lung ultrasound studies performed on mechanically ventilated patients. *Journal of Ultrasound in Medicine*, *37*(11), 2659–2665.
Minkov, M., Dutt, P., Schachner, M., Morales, O., Sanchez, C., Jandosova, J., & Mudd, B. (2017). A revision of Hofstede's individualism–collectivism dimension: A new national index from a 56-country study. *Cross Cultural & Strategic Management*, *24*, 386–404.
Minocha, A. A. (1980). Medical pluralism and health services in India. *Social Science & Medicine. Part B: Medical Anthropology*, *14*(4), 217–223.
Mirza, N. A., Akhtar-Danesh, N., Noesgaard, C., Martin, L., & Staples, E. (2014). A concept analysis of abductive reasoning. *Journal of Advanced Nursing*, *70*(9), 1980–1994.
Moriarty, R. J. (1970). A general syllogy of Maya medicine. *Katunob*, *7*, 43–58.
Müller, G. E., & Pilzecker, A. (1900). Experimentelle Beiträge zur Lehre vom Gedächtnis. *Zeitschrift für Psychologie*, Ergänzungsband *1*, 1–300.

Muñoz-Morán, O. (2011). *El diablo y la enfermedad: precisiones en cuanto al concepto de susto/espanto entre los indígenas de Michoacán, Mexico.* Nuevo Mundo-Mundos Nuevos.

Nash, J. C. (1970). *In the Eyes of the Ancestors: Belief and Behavior in a Mayan Community.* Yale University Press.

Nieblas-Bedolla, E., Bream, K. D., Rollins, A., & Barg, F. K. (2019). Ongoing challenges in access to diabetes care among the indigenous population: Perspectives of individuals living in rural Guatemala. *International Journal for Equity in Health, 18*, 1–10.

Nigenda, G. (2013). Servicio social en medicina en México: una reforma urgente y posible. *Salud Pública de México, 55*(5), 519–527.

Nigh, R. (2002). Maya medicine in the biological gaze: Bioprospecting research as herbal fetishism. *Current Anthropology, 43*(3), 451–477.

Nolan-Ferrell, C. A. (2012). *Constructing Citizenship: Transnational Workers and Revolution on the Mexico-Guatemala Border, 1880--1950.* University of Arizona Press.

Nuttall, Z. (1928). Nouvelles lumières sur les civilisations américaines et le système du calendrier. *Proceedings of the 22nd ICA*, 119–148.

Nyembezi, A., Ngcobo, S., & Lehmann, U. (2024). Collaboration between traditional health practitioners and biomedical health practitioners: Scoping review. *African Journal of Primary Health Care & Family Medicine, 16*(1), 1–11.

O'Gorman, R., Sheldon, K. M., & Wilson, D. S. (2008). For the good of the group? Exploring group-level evolutionary adaptations using multilevel selection theory. *Group Dynamics: Theory, Research, and Practice, 12*(1), 17.

Oishi, S. (2014). Socioecological psychology. *Annual Review of Psychology, 65*, 581–609.

Oishi, S., & Graham, J. (2010). Social ecology: Lost and found in psychological science. *Perspectives on Psychological Science, 5*(4), 356–377.

Orellana, S. L. (1987). *Indian Medicine in Highland Guatemala.* University of New Mexico Press.

Ortiz de Montellano, B., (1975). Empirical Aztec medicine. *Science, 188*, 215–220.

Ortiz de Montellano, B. (1976). Curanderos: Spanish shamans or Aztec scientists? *Grito del Sol, 1*(2), 21–28.

Ortner, S., & Whitehead, H. (1981). *Sexual Meanings. The Cultural Construction of Gender and Sexuality.* New York.

Ostafin, B. D., & Kassman, K. T. (2012). Stepping out of history: Mindfulness improves insight problem solving. *Consciousness and Cognition, 21*(2), 1031–1036.

Owen, K. K., Obregón, E. J., & Jacobsen, K. H. (2010). A geographic analysis of access to health services in rural Guatemala. *International Health, 2*, 143–149.

PAHO. (2007). *Pan American Health Organization Health Systems Profile of Guatemala.* PAHO/WHO.

Paul, B. D., & McMahon, C. E. (2001). Mesoamerican bonesetters. In *Mesoamerican Healers* Huber, B. E., & Sandstrom, A. (Eds.), (pp. 243–269). University of Texas Press.

Pelcastre-Villafuerte, B. E., Meneses-Navarro, S., Ruelas-González, M. G., Reyes-Morales, H., Amaya-Castellanos, A., & Taboada, A. (2017). Aging in rural, indigenous communities: An intercultural and participatory healthcare approach in Mexico. *Ethnicity & Health, 22*(6), 610–630.

Potter, D. R., & King, E. M. (1995). A heterarchical approach to lowland Maya socioeconomies. *Archeological Papers of the American Anthropological Association, 6*(1), 17–32.

Pushpangadan, P., George, V., Ijinu, T. P., & Chithra, M. A. (2018). Biodiversity, bioprospecting, traditional knowledge. Sustainable development and value added products: A review. *Journal of Traditional Medicine & Clinical Naturopathy*, *7*(01), 1–7.

Raingruber, B., & Robinson, C. (2007). The effectiveness of Tai Chi, yoga, meditation, and Reiki healing sessions in promoting health and enhancing problem solving abilities of registered nurses. *Issues in Mental Health Nursing*, *28*(10), 1141–1155.

Redvers, N., & Blondin, B. S. (2020). Traditional Indigenous medicine in North America: A scoping review. *PloS One*, *15*(8), e0237531.

Reed, N. A. (2001). *The Caste War of Yucatan: Revised Edition*. Stanford University Press.

Reeser, D. C. (2014). *Medical Pluralism in a Neoliberal State: Health and Deservingness in Southern Belize*. University of South Florida.

Reilly, F. K. (1986). Olmec iconographic influences on the symbols of Maya rulership: An examination of possible sources. In Fields, V. M. (Ed.), *Sixth Palenque Round Table* (pp. 151–166). University of Oklahoma Press.

Remorini, C., & Palermo, M. L. (2016). "Los míos...¡ todos asustados!": Vulnerabilidad infantil y trayectorias de desarrollo en los Valles Calchaquíes salteños. *Mitológicas*, *31*.

Ren, J., Huang, Z., Luo, J., Wei, G., Ying, X., Ding, Z., ... & Luo, F. (2011). Meditation promotes insightful problem-solving by keeping people in a mindful and alert conscious state. *Science China Life Sciences*, *54*, 961–965.

Reyes-Foster, B. M. (2014). Maya geography and culture: Ancient and contemporary. In Smith, C. (Ed.), *Encyclopedia of Global Archaeology* (pp. 4710–4715). Springer.

Reyes-García, V., Paneque-Gálvez, J., Luz, A., Gueze, M., Macía, M., Orta-Martínez, M., ... & Pino, J. (2014). Cultural change and traditional ecological knowledge: An empirical analysis from the Tsimane'in the Bolivian Amazon. *Human Organization*, *73*, 162–173.

Richardson, E., Allison, K. R., Gesink, D., & Berry, A. (2016). Barriers to accessing and using contraception in highland Guatemala: the development of a family planning self-efficacy scale. *Open Access Journal of Contraception*, *7*, 77–87.

Rösing, I. (1993). *Mundo Ankari. 5. Rituale zur Rufung des Regens: Zweiter Ankari-Zyklus: Kollektivrituale der Kallawaya-Region in den Anden Boliviens*. Zweitausendeins.

Ross, N. J., & Rangel, T. F. (2011). Ancient Maya agroforestry echoing through spatial relationships in the extant forest of NW Belize. *Biotropica*, *43*, 141–148.

Roys, R. L. (1933). *The Book of Chilam Balam of Chumayel*. Carnegie Institution of Washington.

Rubel, A. J. (1964). The epidemiology of a folk illness: Susto in Hispanic America. *Ethnology*, *3*(3), 268–283.

Rumelhart, D. E., Hinton, G. E., & McClelland, J. L. (1986). A general framework for parallel distributed processing. *Parallel Distributed Processing: Explorations in the Microstructure of Cognition*, *1*(45–76), 26.

Saltman, R. B. (2002). Regulating incentives: The past and present role of the state in health care systems. *Social Science & Medicine*, *54*(11), 1677–1684.

Sanford, V. (2003). *Buried Secrets: Truth and Human Rights in Guatemala*. Palgrave Macmillan.

Santiso-Galvez, R. and Bertrand, J. T. (2004). The delayed contraceptive revolution in Guatemala. *Human Organization*, *63*, 57–67.

Scarborough, V. L. (1998). Ecology and ritual: Water management and the Maya. *Latin American Antiquity*, *9*(2), 135–159.

Schaller, M. (2020). Evolutionary psychology meets socio-ecological psychology: The motivational psychologies of disease-avoidance and parental care. *Current Opinion in Psychology, 32*, 6–11.

Schirmer, J. G. (1998). *The Guatemalan Military Project: A Violence Called Democracy*. University of Pennsylvania Press.

Schlesinger, S., & Kinzer, S. (2005). *Bitter Fruit: The Story of the American Coup in Guatemala*. Harvard University, David Rockefeller Center for Latin American Studies.

Schoenherr, J. R. (2022a). Vaccination, values, and health information search behaviour in the New Folk medicine. In *2022 IEEE International Symposium on Technology and Society (ISTAS)* (Vol. *1*, pp. 1–10). IEEE.

Schoenherr, J. R. (2022b). Folkmedical technologies and the sociotechnical systems of healthcare. *IEEE Technology and Society Magazine*, *41*(3), 38–49.

Schoenherr, J. R. & Beaudoin, J. (2027). Medical heterarchies in East Asian medical education: The evolving landscape of health professions education in East Asia. In Schoenherr, J. R. (Ed.), *Fundamentals and Frontiers of Medical Education and Decision-Making: Innovation, Implementation, and Translational Research*. Routledge.

Schoenherr, J. R., & Dopko, R. L. (2019). Heterarchical social organizations and relational models: Understanding gender biases in psychological science. *Theory and Psychology, 29*(2), 258–281.

Schoenherr, J. R. & Grubesic, R. (in preparation). *Physical and technological Barriers to healthcare utilization in the South Texas colonías*.

Schoenherr, J. R., & Hamstra, S. J. (2024). Validity in health professions education: From assessment instruments to program innovation and evaluation. In J. R. Schoenherr & McConnell, M. M. (Eds.), *Fundamentals and Frontiers of Medical Education and Decision-Making: Educational Theory and Psychological Practice* (pp. 80–107). Routledge.

Schoenherr, J. R., Mahias-Ito, I., & Li, X. (2026). Collective competence in the health professions: Learning, thinking, and deciding in groups. In Schoenherr, J. R. (Eds), *Fundamentals and Frontiers of Medical Education and Decision-Making: Innovation, Implementation, and Translational Research*. Routledge.

Schoenherr, J. R., & McConnell, M. M. (2024). Human-Centered Design in Health Professions Education. In *Fundamentals and Frontiers of Medical Education and Decision-Making: Educational Theory and Psychological Practice*, *3*(1).

Schoenherr, J. R., & Le-Bouar, C. (2024). Representing and communicating health information: Fundamentals of persuasive health communication. In J. R. Schoenherr & M. M. McConnell (Eds.), *Fundamentals and Frontiers of Medical Education and Decision-Making* (pp. 270–312). Routledge.

Schoenherr, J. R., & Thomson, R. (2021). Persuasive features of scientific explanations: Explanatory schemata of physical and psychosocial phenomena. *Frontiers in Psychology, 12*, 644809.

Schoenherr, J. R., Waechter, J., & Lee, C. H. (2024). Quantifying expertise in the healthcare professions: Cognitive efficiency and metacognitive calibration. In *Fundamentals and Frontiers of Medical Education and Decision-Making* (pp. 213–244). Routledge.

Schoenherr, J. R., Waechter, J., & Millington, S. J. (2018). Subjective awareness of ultrasound expertise development: Individual experience as a determinant of overconfidence. *Advances in Health Sciences Education, 23*, 749–765.

Schooley, J., Mundt, C., Wagner, P., Fullerton, J., & O'Donnell, M. (2009). Factors influencing health care-seeking behaviours among Mayan women in Guatemala. *Midwifery, 25*, 411–421.

Seiber, E. E., & Bertrand, J. T. (2002). Access as a factor in differential contraceptive use between Mayans and ladinos in Guatemala. *Health Policy and Planning, 17*, 167–177.

Semotiuk, A. J., Cus, M., & Semotiuk, N. L. (2012). Modern education and culture impact on both language and botanical healing traditions of the Maya in Belize. In *International Symposium on Medicinal and Aromatic Plants IMAPS2010 and History of Mayan Ethnopharmacology IMAPS2011 964* (pp. 205–210).

Senteio, C., Fields, S. D., Pritam Singh, R. K., Namata Kamoga, R. M., Andrews, E., Gandsman, D., ... & Snow, S. (2025). Overcoming health misinformation in marginalized groups: a systematic review. *International Journal for Equity in Health, 24*(1), 323.

Serna-Saldivar, S. O., Rosell, C. M., Bajerska, J., & El Sheikha, A. F. (2015). Nutritional and nutraceutical features of regular and protein fortified corn tortillas. In Rosell, C. M., Bajerska, J., & El Sheikha, A. F. (Eds.), *Bread and Its Fortification: Nutrition and Health Benefits*. CRC Press.

Sheets, P., Dixon, C., Lentz, D., Egan, R., Halmbacher, A., Slotten, V., ... & Lamb, C. (2015). The sociopolitical economy of an ancient Maya village: Ceren and its sacbe. *Latin American Antiquity, 26*, 341–361.

Shih, C. C., Su, Y. C., Liao, C. C., & Lin, J. G. (2010). Patterns of medical pluralism among adults: Results from the 2001 national health interview survey in Taiwan. *BMC Health Services Research, 10*, 1–9.

Shiva, V. (2007). Bioprospecting as sophisticated biopiracy. *Signs: Journal of Women in Culture and Society, 32*, 307–313.

Shtanko, Y., Litenski, M. N., Clarke, R., Hernandez, S., & Oliveira, J. B. (2024). Examining the cultural appropriateness and acceptability of a traditional birth attendants' training program in rural Guatemala. *Cureus, 16*(9), e69940.

Simon, B., Fletcher, J. A., & Doebeli, M. (2013). Towards a general theory of group selection. *Evolution, 67*, 1561–1572.

Smallwood, R., Woods, C., Power, T., & Usher, K. (2021). Understanding the impact of historical trauma due to colonization on the health and well-being of indigenous young peoples: A systematic scoping review. *Journal of Transcultural Nursing, 32*, 59–68.

Soejarto, D. D., Fong, H. H. S., Tan, G. T., Zhang, H. J., Ma, C. Y., Franzblau, S. G., ... & Dietzman, G. R. (2005). Ethnobotany/ethnopharmacology and mass bioprospecting: Issues on intellectual property and benefit-sharing. *Journal of Ethnopharmacology, 100*(1–2), 15–22.

Spence, M. W. (1996). Commodity or gift: Teotihuacan obsidian in the Maya region. *Latin American Antiquity, 7*, 21–39.

Stanton, T. W. (2000). *Heterarchy, Hierarchy, and the Emergence of the Northern Lowland Maya: A Study of Complexity at Yaxuna, Yucatan, Mexico (400 BC–AD 600)*. Southern Methodist University.

Starr, P. (1982/2017). *The Social Transformation of American Medicine: The Rise of a Sovereign Profession and the Making of a Vast Industry*. Hachette.

Steiner, R. P. (1987). Tibetan medicine: Part II: Pulse diagnosis in Tibetan medicine: Translated from the first chapter for the Fourth Tantra (rGyud-bzi). *American Journal of Chinese Medicine, 15*, 165–170.

Stickgold, R., & Walker, M. P. (2013). Sleep-dependent memory triage: Evolving generalization through selective processing. *Nature Neuroscience, 16*(2), 139–145.

Strader, A. V., Sotz, M., Gilbert, H. N., Miller, A. C., Lee, A. C., & Rohloff, P. (2024). A biosocial analysis of perinatal and late neonatal mortality among Indigenous Maya Kaqchikel communities in Tecpán, Guatemala: A mixed-methods study. *BMJ Global Health, 9*(4), e013940.

Stroux, L., Martinez, B., Coyote Ixen, E., King, N., Hall-Clifford, R., Rohloff, P., ... & Clifford, G. D. (2016). An mHealth monitoring system for traditional birth attendant-led antenatal risk assessment in rural Guatemala. *Journal of Medical Engineering & Technology, 40*(7–8), 356–371.

Struthers, R., Eschiti, V. S., & Patchell, B. (2004). Traditional indigenous healing: Part I. *Complementary Therapies in Nursing and Midwifery, 10*, 141–149.

Sugiyama, S., & Sugiyama, N. (2020). Interactions between ancient Teotihuacan and the Maya world. In Hutson, S. R., & Ardren, T. (Eds.), *The Maya World* (pp. 689–711). Routledge.

Summer, A., Guendelman, S., Kestler, E., & Walker, D. (2017). Professional midwifery in Guatemala: A qualitative exploration of perceptions, attitudes and expectations among stakeholders. *Social Science & Medicine, 184*, 99–107.

Sun, S., Yao, Z., Wei, J., & Yu, R. (2015). Calm and smart? A selective review of meditation effects on decision making. *Frontiers in Psychology, 6*, 120409.

Sutphen, M. P., & Andrews, B. (Eds.). (2003). *Medicine and Colonial Identity*. Routledge.

Tataryn, D. J. (2002). Paradigms of health and disease: A framework for classifying and understanding complementary and alternative medicine. *The Journal of Alternative & Complementary Medicine, 8*(6), 877–892.

Tedlock, B. (1982). Sound texture and metaphor in Quiche Maya ritual language. *Current Anthropology, 23*(3), 269–272.

Tedlock, B. (1982). *Time and the Highland Maya*. University of New Mexico Press.

Terborgh, A., Rosen, J. E., Galvez, R. S., Terceros, W., Bertrand, J. T., & Bull, S. E. (1995). Family planning among indigenous populations in Latin America. *International Family Planning Perspectives, 21*, 143–149 + 166.

Thomas, T. L., DiClemente, R., & Snell, S. (2014). Overcoming the triad of rural health disparities: How local culture, lack of economic opportunity, and geographic location instigate health disparities. *Health Education Journal, 73*(3), 285–294.

Thomas, E., Vandebroek, I., Van Damme, P., Semo, L., & Noza, Z. (2009). Susto etiology and treatment according to Bolivian Trinitario people: a "masters of the animal species" phenomenon. *Medical Anthropology Quarterly, 23*(3), 298–319.

Treviño, C. V. (1984). El médico mexica. In Lo´pez Austin, A., & Viesca Treviño, C. (coord), *México antiguo. 1* vols. (pp. 217–230). Universidad Nacional Autónoma de México; Academia Nacional de Medicina.

Treviño, C. V. (2001). Curanderismo in Mexico and Guatemala its historical evolution from the sixteenth to the nineteenth century. In Huber, B. R., & Sandstrom, A. R. (Eds.), *Mesoamerican Healers* (pp. 47–65). University of Texas Press.

Uskul, A. K., & Oishi, S. (2020). What is socio-ecological psychology? *Current Opinion in Psychology, 32*, 181–184.

Valeggia, C. R., & Snodgrass, J. J. (2015). Health of indigenous peoples. *Annual Review of Anthropology, 44*(1), 117–135.

Van Dijk, M., Ruiz, M. J., Letona, D., & García, S. G. (2013). Ensuring intercultural maternal health care for Mayan women in Guatemala: A qualitative assessment. *Culture, Health & Sexuality, 15*(sup3), S365–S382.

Vega, A. (2008). La pérdida del alma y la etiología de un taxón tradicional: el" susto" entre los migrantes Aymara de Buenos Aires. In *V Jornadas de Sociología de la UNLP (La Plata, 10 al 12 de diciembre de 2008)*.

Venosa, A. R., Baroneza, J. E., & Fernandes, R. A. F. (2027). Medical Education in Brazil: A History of An Evolving Pluralistic Health Care System. In J. R. Schoenherr (Ed.), *Fundamentals and Frontiers of Medical Education and Decision-Making: Innovation, Implementation, and Translational Research* (pp. 310–335). Routledge.

Vignoles, V., Owe, E., Becker, M., Smith, P., Easterbrook, M. J., Brown, R., … & Bond, M. H. (2016). Beyond the 'east– west' dichotomy: Global variation in cultural models of selfhood. *Journal of Experimental Psychology: General*, *145*, 966–1000.

Vogt, E. Z. (1976). *Tortillas for the Gods: A Symbolic Analysis of Zinacantan Rituals*. Harvard University Press.

Vrettas, D. (2020). *Searching for a Cure: Health Care Behaviour Among the Q'eqchi'Maya in Southern Belize* (Doctoral dissertation, University of Saskatchewan).

Wachholtz, A. B., & Pargament, K. I. (2005). Is spirituality a critical ingredient of meditation? Comparing the effects of spiritual meditation, secular meditation, and relaxation on spiritual, psychological, cardiac, and pain outcomes. *Journal of Behavioral Medicine*, *28*, 369–384.

Waldram, J. B. (2013). Transformative and restorative processes: Revisiting the question of efficacy of indigenous healing. *Medical Anthropology*, *32*(3), 191–207.

Waldram, J. B. (2015). "I don't know the words he uses": Therapeutic communication among Q'eqchi Maya Healers and their patients. *Medical Anthropology Quarterly*, *29*(3), 279–297.

Waldram, J. B. (2020). *An Imperative to Cure: Principles and Practice of Q'eqchi'Maya Medicine in Belize*. University of New Mexico Press.

Waldram, J. B., Cal, V., & Maquin, P. (2009). The Q'eqchi' Healer's Association of Belize: An endogenous movement in heritage preservation and management. *Heritage Management*, *2*(1), 35–54.

Waldram, J. B., & Hatala, A. R. (2015). Latent and manifest empiricism in Q'eqchi'Maya healing: A case study of HIV/AIDS. *Social Science & Medicine*, *126*, 9–16.

Wamsley, E. J. (2014). Dreaming and offline memory consolidation. *Current Neurology and Neuroscience Reports*, *14*, 1–7.

Watson, S. E., Schnell, J. T., Morell-Hart, S., Scherer, A. K., & Dussol, L. (2023). Health care in the marketplace: Exploring maya medicinal plants and practices at piedras negras, Guatemala. *Ancient Mesoamerica*, *34*(2), 383–406.

Weiner, A. B. (1976). *Women of Value, Men of Renown: New Perspectives in Trobriand Exchange*. University of Texas Press.

Westreich, L. (1990). Modern, medical training confronts Guatemalan poverty. *Minnesota Medicine*, *73*, 19–22.

Wichmann, S. (2006). Mayan historical linguistics and epigraphy: A new synthesis. *Annual Review of Anthropology*, *35*(1), 279–294.

Williams, G. C. (1966). *Adaptation and Natural Selection*. Princeton University Press.

Wilson, N. W., Couper, I. D., De Vries, E., Reid, S., Fish, T., & Marais, B. J. (2009). A critical review of interventions to redress the inequitable distribution of healthcare professionals to rural and remote areas. *Rural and Remote Health*, *9*(2), 1–21.

Wolff, P., Medin, D. L., & Pankratz, C. (1999). Evolution and devolution of folkbiological knowledge. *Cognition*, *73*(2), 177–204.

World Health Organization (WHO). (2000). *Nurses and midwives for health: A WHO European Strategy for Nursing and Midwifery Education*. WHO.

Young, J. C., & Garro, L. Y. (1982). Variation in the choice of treatment in two Mexican communities. *Social Science & Medicine*, *16*(16), 1453–1465.

Yukes, J. (2007). "No one wants to become a healer": Herbal medicine and ethnobotanical knowledge in Nahualá. In W. R. Adams & J. P. Hawkins (Eds.), *Health Care in Maya Guatemala: Confronting Medical Pluralism in a Developing Country* (pp. 44–59). University of Oklahoma Press.

Zeidan, F., Martucci, K. T., Kraft, R. A., McHaffie, J. G., & Coghill, R. C. (2014). Neural correlates of mindfulness meditation-related anxiety relief. *Social Cognitive and Affective Neuroscience*, *9*(6), 751–759.

11

MEDICAL EDUCATION IN SUB-SAHARAN AFRICA

Emiola Oluwabunmi Olapade-Olaopa, Akinyele O. Adisa, Funmilayo E. Olopade, Taiwo A. Lawal, Nazik Hammad, Jehu Erapu Iputo, and Ajovi B. Scott-Emuakpor

Acknowledgement: The authors thank Mr. Jesusogo Akinyemi for his technical assistance in the preparation of this manuscript.

11.1 Introduction

> Whatever device is created for dealing with the sheer volume of health work (in Africa), it must not be one which compromises the standards of university medical school education.
>
> *(Brown, 1961)*

The roots of the challenges faced by SSA health systems today were established in the colonial times when health facilities were primarily for the purpose of providing health care for the Europeans (Church Missionary Society Archive). Two parallel health systems were thus inevitably created. One system was run by qualified European doctors, who provided health services to the colonizing Europeans, while the other system was operated by herbalists, dispensers, and a few missionary health centres and private clinics, and they provided care to the indigenous populations. Some of these facilities in the second system were run by African doctors who returned after training overseas (Iliffe, 1998; Monekosso, 2014).

The education of health professionals, especially doctors, plays a major role in determining the quality of healthcare systems globally. The philosophy of educating health professionals must therefore continuously evolve to respond effectively to the changing and ever increasingly complex health needs of communities. Medical education in SSA was initially based on colonial training models. Later, efforts were made to base medical education on indigenous knowledge and experience. It was recognized much later that a modern approach that meets the current demands

DOI: 10.4324/9781003498155-11

of SSA, and which meets globally accepted standards was required. However, despite the growing numbers of medical schools in sub-Saharan Africa, there is evidence that the medical education system still faces many challenges.

According to a World Health Organization (WHO) report in 2006 (WHO, World Health Report, 2006), SSA has about 11% of the world's population, bears over 24% of the global disease burden, but is home to only 3% of the global health workforce, and spends less than 1% of the world's financial resources on health. It is therefore not surprising that the health systems of most of the countries in SSA are not able to adequately cope with the needs of their population. To address this challenge, many countries are scaling up training programmes and refining the education strategies of health professionals, and this is in addition to the overhaul of the healthcare systems. These efforts are said to have resulted in a 129% increase in the numbers of doctors, nurses, midwives, etc. in SSA by 2018. However, when this increase is adjusted for the growth of the population, it translates only to a 4.9% increase in real growth in Human Resource for Health (HRH) density across the continent (Okoroafor et al., 2022). In addition to this relative shortage of healthcare workers, there are many other challenges which negatively influence the effectiveness of SSA healthcare systems. Most of these challenges are common to countries across the subcontinent. Prominent amongst these challenges are insufficient funding, infrastructural deficiencies, rapidly increasing population, political instability, and internal conflicts, all of which negatively influence both medical education and healthcare delivery (Mullan & Frehywot, 2007). The continuous (internal and external) migration of all cadres of health professionals is a special problem as it continues to drain the limited resources of poor countries, thus making their development even more difficult (Mullan, 2005). Innovative ways have been developed to address these challenges, especially in the areas of medical instruction, retention of trained HRH, funding, and capacity building with a view to strengthening national health systems. This chapter provides an abridged view of the current state of medical education on the subcontinent.

11.1.1 Essential History of Medical Education in Sub-Saharan Africa from Pre-Independence to Date

Biomedical education was introduced in sub-Saharan Africa early in the 20th century. Since then, medical education has developed in overlapping phases on the subcontinent, primarily because of ill-defined and incoherent healthcare policies, influenced by political and economic changes on the subcontinent (Monekosso, 2014).

- **Pre-Independence Period (1890–1960)**

In the early stages of this phase, medical education was introduced into SSA by colonizing Europeans. At the same time, missionaries have recognized that healthcare services had become a major part of evangelism, for winning converts. Also, World War I made the colonizing Europeans realize the urgent need for the training of indigenous healthcare personnel. In the most populous SSA nation, Nigeria, this consideration led to the establishment of the Yaba Medical College in 1939 which, at first, trained medical assistants but was later upgraded to train assistant medical officers (Scott-Emuakpor, 2010). As alluded to above, initially the emphasis was on training Africans as medical assistants, nursing aides, and field assistants, who would work under European doctors, to provide health care for European and African civil servants, military personnel, and their families. As the colonies sought independence, the agitation by nationalists for the establishment of tertiary institutions that would produce the skilled graduates considered essential for the economic development of these countries post-independence (Mellanby, 1958). Medical schools that would produce African doctors to address the health problems of the local population were considered essential components of these new institutions. By 1960, the number of schools established in SSA for this purpose had grown to 13 in 8 countries. These schools were well-planned, well-staffed, and well-equipped medical schools, but with markedly limited training spaces and they were usually started as colleges of universities in the colonizing countries, and then later upgraded to full-fledged independent tertiary institutions. Postgraduate/speciality programmes were not available on the continent during this period and, African doctors could only pursue such training abroad after practising for a minimum of five years.

- **Post-Independence Period (1961–1980)**

The post-independence governments of African nations gave priority to education and healthcare systems to boost their growth and economic development. Indeed, in some countries, medical schools and teaching hospitals were created at the same time as the new regions/states. These schools were well-planned, funded, and staffed as part of the national development plans of these countries and had high student application and thus stiff competition from the outset (Monekosso, 2014). This drive for rapid increase in the number of home-grown graduates (including HRH) produced 51 medical schools in sub-Saharan Africa by 1980 (Table 11.1).

- **The Locust Years (1975–1990)**

The political and economic upheavals that afflicted SSA for almost two decades, from 1975 to 1990 disproportionately affected the health and education systems. This resulted in massive emigration of high-quality medical specialists and nurses alongside other highly trained intellectuals and scientists. Across the continent, very few new medical schools were founded during this period and there was a general deterioration of the infrastructure of the existing institutions, especially

TABLE 11.1 Medical Schools Established in Sub-Saharan Africa from Pre-Independence to 1980

S/N	*Country*	*School Name*	*Founding Date*
Medical Schools Founded Prior to 1960			
1	Madagascar	Universite d'Antanarivo	1896
2	Senegal	Faculté de Médecine, Pharmacie et d'Odontologie	1918
3	South Africa	Faculty of Health Sciences, University of Cape Town	1919
4	South Africa	Wits Medical School, University of the Witwatersrand	1919
5	Uganda	School of Medicine, Makerere University College of Health Sciences	1923
6	Sudan	Faculty of Medicine, University of Khartoum	1924
7	Nigeria	Yaba Medical School	1930–1948
8	South Africa	University of Pretoria	1943
9	Nigeria	College of Medicine, University of Ibadan	1948
10	Democratic Republic of Congo	Université de Kinshasa	1954
11	Democratic Republic of Congo	Université de Lubumbashi	1956
12	Rhodesia (Salisbury)	College of Health Sciences, University of Zimbabwe	1963
13	South Africa	Faculty of Health Sciences, Stellenbosch University	1956
Medical Schools Founded 1961–1980			
14	Cote d'Ivoire	UFR Sciences Médicales d'Abidjan	1962
15	Nigeria	University of Lagos	1962
16	Angola	Faculdade de Medicina, Agostinho Neto	1963
17	Ethiopia	Faculty of Medicine, Addis Ababa University	1963
18	Mozambique	Faculty of Medicine, Eduardo Mondlane University	1963
19	Rwanda	Faculty of Medicine, National University of Rwanda	1963
20	Congo	Université de Kisangani	1963
21	Tanzania	School of Medicine, Muhimbili University of Health and Allied Sciences	1968

22	Madagascar	Tananrive	1963(Preclinical only)
23	Ghana	University of Ghana Medical School	1964
24	Burundi	Bujumbura	1964(Preclinical only)
25	Zambia	School of Medicine, University of Zambia	1966
26	Guinea	Faculté de Médecine Pharmacie et Odontostomatologie, Université de Conakry	1967
27	Nigeria	Ahmadu Bello University	1967
28	Nigeria	College of Medicine, University of Nigeria, Enugu Campus	1967
29	Kenya	University of Nairobi	1967
30	Benin	Faculté des Sciences de la Santé de Cotonou	1968
31	Burundi	Faculty of Medicine, University of Burundi	1968
32	Liberia	A.M. Dogliotti College of Medicine	1968
33	Cameroon	Faculté de Médecine et des Sciences Biomédicales, Université de Yaoundé	1969
34	Mali	Faculty of Medicine, Pharmacy and Odontostomatologie	1969
35	Nigeria	College of Medicine, University of Nigeria, Enugu Campus	1970
36	Togo	Faculté Mixte de Médecine et de Pharmacie (FMMP), Université de Lome	1970
37	South Africa	School of Medicine, Faculty of Health Sciences, University of the Free State	1971
38	Gabon	Faculté de Médecine et des Sciences de la Santé	1972
39	Nigeria	College of Health Sciences, Obafemi Awolowo University	1972
40	Nigeria	University of Benin	1973
41	Niger	Faculte des Sciences de la Sante, Universite Abdou Moumouni	1974
42	Republic of Congo	Université Marien Ngouabi de Brazzaville	1975
43	Ghana	School of Medical Sciences, Kwame Nkrumah Univ of Science and Tech	1975

(*Continued*)

TABLE 11.1 (Continued)

S/N	*Country*	*School Name*	*Founding Date*
44	Central African Republic	Faculté de Sciences de la Santé de l'Université de Bangui	1976
45	Nigeria	College of Health Sciences, University of Ilorin	1977
46	Nigeria	College of Medical Sciences, University of Maiduguri	1978
47	Nigeria	University of Jos	1978
48	Nigeria	University of Maiduguri College of Medical Sciences	1978
49	South Africa	University of Limpopo, Medunsa Campus	1978
50	Sudan	Faculty of Medicine, University of Gezira	1978
51	Nigeria	College of Health Sciences, University of Port Harcourt	1979

the science laboratories, which had grave implications for biomedical research and learning in SSA (Monekosso, 2014).

- **Period of Rejuvenation (1990–2020)**

The return of relative political stability and economics in this period saw another phase of rapid growth in the number of medical schools in sub-Saharan Africa. A survey conducted by the sub-Saharan African Medical School Study (SAMSS) in 2009 found 168 medical schools, the majority of which were established after 1990. The expansion also saw the creation of many faith-based and private schools, in addition to the traditional public-owned medical schools, such that many countries now have more than one medical school (Mullan & Frehywo, 2007). In addition to this increase in the number of schools, several governments have also increased the number of students admitted into their medical schools to meet the rising demand for access to medical training, often without providing the additional resources needed.

11.1.2 Development of Postgraduate Medical Education (PGME) Programmes

Graduates of medical schools across Africa usually undergo compulsory internship, national service, or other programmes before independent practice or entry into a postgraduate training programme in their countries or overseas (Chen et al., 2012). However, postgraduate training in medical and surgical specialities has taken a longer period to gain ground than undergraduate training in sub-Saharan Africa. The seed for local postgraduate medical training in SSA was first sown in West Africa in the 1960s by the Association of West African Surgeons. Many countries, especially those in the East and Southern sub-regions, initially adopted the Master of Medicine (MMed) as the university designation. Like undergraduate medical training and postgraduate academic programmes most PGME programmes were structured and affiliated to the colonial heritage of individual countries (Table 11.2).

The establishment of the West African Postgraduate Medical College (WAPMC) as the local professional certification body for both medical and surgical PGME in the sub-region in 1973 initiated the harmonization of the francophone and anglophone PGME training programmes in the sub-region in both of its constituent colleges (the West African College of Physicians and the West African College of Surgeons). This model of certification of professional PGME has since been adopted in other regions in the subcontinent and the postgraduate medical colleges are often formed to incorporate similar specialities such as the College of Surgeons of East, Central, and Southern Africa, and the East, Central, and Southern Africa College of Physicians. Some countries have also established national postgraduate colleges or boards that regulate the training of specialists in the country. These countries include Nigeria, Sudan, Ghana, and South Africa. The period of residency

TABLE 11.2 Percentage Ownership and Geographic Distribution of Medical Schools in Sub-Saharan Africa

		Ownership		*Geographic Region*			
		Public	*Private*	*W. Africa*	*C. Africa*	*E. Africa*	*S. Africa*
PGME programmes	General surgery	53	27	58	38	33	89
	Ob. Gy.	52	27	58	38	31	89
	Pediatrics	53	23	58	38	31	89
	Internal medicine	51	27	55	25	33	89
	Surgical sub-specialities	41	23	50	0	23	89
	Medical sub-specialities	33	23	45	13	13	78
	Anesthesiology	36	5	38	13	15	89
	Radiology	34	14	40	13	13	89
	Psychiatry	31	9	38	0	S	89
	General/family practice	30	14	33	13	10	100
	Pathology	29	5	40	13	4	67
	Other	28	14	18	13	27	56
	Mean	**39.25**	**17.58**	**44.25**	**18.08**	**20.25**	**84.41**
Other health professions education programmes	Nursing	65	73	58	50	73	89
	Public health	59	36	53	50	52	78
	Pharmacy	45	45	53	38	44	22
	Dentistry	34	41	38	25	35	33
	Clinical/health officers	34	23	28	13	35	44
	Medical laboratory	23	23	18	0	35	0
	Healthcare management	17	23	15	0	19	44
	Physiotherapy	14	14	10	0	15	44
	Other	30	27	15	13	35	78
	Mean	**35.67**	**33.89**	**32**	**21**	**38.11**	**48**

Source: Adapted from Chen et al. (2012).

training differs across countries and specialities and typically ranges from four to seven years (Chen et al., 2012; Talib et al., 2019), with surgical specialities usually requiring comparatively longer training. PGME programmes are coupled to colleges or schools of medicine in some countries while they are undertaken in general/tertiary hospitals in other countries (Chen et al., 2012).

In recent times, the requirement that clinical teachers in medical schools must acquire a research doctorate has been controversial. This requirement was borne out of concerns about the academic research content of residency training programmes, which are often not as structured as those anchored by universities. On the other hand, academic degrees or paper-based qualifications that do not incorporate skills acquisition are deemed inadequate for postgraduate medical education (PGME) and the certification of technical competence (Ajao & Alao, 2016). An alternative that has been proposed is incorporation of a research-based academic program, such as the higher doctorate degree of Doctor of Medicine (UK version) or a Ph.D, that is tied to skills acquisition in a formal residency training programme for interested residents. A major advantage is that the products of such residency training, combined with an MD of Ph.D degree from an affiliated university, can function better as teachers for undergraduate and postgraduate medical programmes and as clinician-scientists in their day-to-day activities in teaching hospitals.

11.1.3 National Medical Educators' Associations

The need to harmonize capacity-building efforts through medical education within countries has resulted in the formation of national associations of educators in South Africa and in Nigeria. These associations were formed to focus attention on the peculiar needs of individual nations rather than the generic international and regional needs.

- **Southern African Association of Health Educationalists**

The Southern African Association of Health Educationalists (SAAHE) was founded in 2004 as an umbrella body for health-science educators in all public and private institutions in South Africa. Like similar bodies, SAAHE aims to improve the teaching and learning, and the research capacity of health-science educators in South Africa, but its membership now cuts across the countries of Southern Africa. The Association has six regional chapters and nearly 400 members who are mostly medical educators, but an increasing number of other health professions educators are joining its fold.

- **National Association of Medical Educators (Nigeria)**

In Nigeria, the National Association of Medical Educators was established in 2009 as an umbrella body for all teachers in medical schools in the country. Most of the founding members were graduates of the medical education training programmes run by the Foundation for Advancement of International Medical Education and Research (FAIMER, now Intealth) and the National Open University of Nigeria (NOUN). The Association held a medical education workshop and conference in 2012 which was attended by national and international stakeholders in health professions education in Nigeria. Its members have since contributed to the development of the 2012 National Medical and Dental Curriculum Template (12) and the 2022 National Universities Commission (NUC) Core Curriculum Minimum Academic Standards (Disciplines – NUC CCMAS).

11.1.4 Contributions of Alumni and the Diaspora to the Development of Medical Education in SSA

The role of Alumni of SSA's HTPIs to the improvement of medical education on the subcontinent is less well-known when compared to their financial contributions to their families and communities (Glytsos, 2002). They also make significant contributions to the sub-region's health system through the establishment of training centres (Karekezi & Khamlichi, 2019; Taslakian et al., 2022), policymaking and advocacy (Scott-Emuakpor, 2010), participating in joint research projects (Tegally et al., 2022), and organizing medical outreaches and missions (Wojczewski et al., 2015).

The efforts in medical education are through their involvement in institutional capacity-building projects such as at the Medical Education Partnership Initiative (MEPI), organization of training workshops on curricula development/reform (Hammad et al., 2023), research in medical education projects (Manirakiza et al., 2020). Equally important are the efforts of numerous individual alumni/Diasporan medical education experts who support the development of medical education in SSA Health Professionals Training Institutions (HPTIs). In this regard, the funding support provided by international funding programmes for educational projects at African higher education institutions such as the Carnegie African Diaspora Fellowship Program (Carnegie African Diaspora Fellowship Program | IIE – The Power of International Education) is crucial to sustain these individual initiatives.

But perhaps the most under-stated (and unrewarded) contribution of SSA alumni to medical education in the region are those directed at mentoring undergraduate and postgraduate students, researchers and faculty and guiding their quest to acquire the much-needed competences for career progression in all specialities. Without a doubt, the value and impact of this guidance have become even more significant with the resurgence of the brain drain that has depleted the pool of mentors locally.

11.2 International Collaborative Medical Education Projects

Political independence notwithstanding international partnerships have continued to play a major role in the growth and development of medical education in sub-Saharan

Africa. Global initiatives such as the WHO's *Global Competency and Outcomes Framework* for universal health coverage (World Health Organization (WHO), 2022) that are initiated by international contributors also provide a common point of reference for healthcare professionals. However, the most significant changes are likely to be the results of continuing relationships between medical schools and their parent colonial institutions, as well as the development of new networks with other medical schools both in Europe, the United States, and in the subcontinent (Olapade-Olaopa et al., 2014). The contributions of these relationships to medical education in SSA have mainly been through the establishment of medical school associations/networks, institutional strengthening grants, and collaborative medical education research and capacity-building projects, of which the major ones are highlighted below.

11.2.1 Medical School Associations

Medical school associations have been major contributors to the development of medical education in sub-Saharan Africa. These associations have the mission of fostering a high standard of medical education in the subcontinent that will produce highly trained personnel to overcome health challenges that are unique to the region. The mission and activities of these associations have resulted in the improvement of the quality of graduates from SSA medical schools. These associations have facilitated networking and the exchange of ideas and experiences between their member schools through scientific meetings and bilateral/regional faculty and student interactions (Khogali, 2014; Monekosso, 1975). Other shared activities include cooperation in areas such as social responsibility, quality assurance and accreditation, curricula reform and development of pedagogical skills, funding opportunities, scientific activities, and research, staff training and assessment, and the governance of the institutions. These associations also represent SSA medical schools in global medical education and international organizations such as the World Federation for Medical Education (WFME), WHO, the World Health Assembly, the Conference of Universities on Global Health (CUGH), and the African Union. Medical school associations in SSA have contributed to several initiatives directed at upscaling production and retention of physicians and designing curricula for socially accountable health professionals' education (HPE; Olapade-Olaopa et al., 2014; Boelen, 2004) and inter-professional education. Thus, these medical school associations have a unique view of the current challenges facing HPE and health systems in Africa, especially as regards contemporary demand for training and retention of physicians.

The earliest medical school networks in SSA have, perhaps inevitably, continued their strong colonial leanings. This is clearly understandable, as colonizing countries always wished to retain their influence in SSA countries previously under their control, the independence of these nations notwithstanding. For instance, Chen et al. (2012) reported that the language of instruction in PGME institutions was either

English (45.75%), French (36.5%), or Arabic (9.33%). In this regard, and perhaps because of colonial heritage, anglophone medical schools are related more to the Association of Medical Schools in Africa (AMSA) whose founding was supported by the Association of American Medical Colleges (AAMC). On the other hand, medical schools in the francophone countries have a stronger association with the International Conference of Deans of French-Speaking Faculties of Medicine (CIDMEF) which has its roots in the Francophone University Agency (AUF). More recently, Finland facilitated the establishment of medical school networks in Southern Africa.

11.2.2 Association of Medical Schools in Africa (AMSA)

The need for a Forum for medical schools in Africa to network and exchange ideas was realized soon after the establishment of the first few institutions (Khogali, 1966). This Forum was initiated at a meeting of five medical schools at the University of Ibadan in 1961, which was facilitated by the Association of American Colleges with the aid of a grant provided by the Rockefeller Foundation (Table 11.3). These meetings were held yearly with an increasing number of medical schools participating. This resulted in the formation of the AMSA in 1965 (Khogali, 1966). Unfortunately, due to the economic downturn in the continent and the brain drain affecting its members in the 1980s, the association was inactive for many years. AMSA was revitalized in 2014 at the end of a process initiated in the mid-2000s by WHO-AFRO. This process took advantage of the partnerships and opportunities provided by the series of medical education projects on the subcontinent during the period, especially, the sub-Saharan African Medical Schools Survey (SMSS) and the African Medical Education Symposium (AMES), and the MEPI (Olapade-Olaopa et al., 2014; Mullan et al., 2011; Eyal et al., 2015). Since its revitalization, AMSA has resumed its activities at both the continental and global levels.

11.2.3 Federation of Associations of Medical Students in Africa (FAMSA)

FAMSA is an independent, non-political federation of medical students' associations in Africa. A by-product of AMSA, it was founded in 1968 as a Nigerian, Ghanaian, and Ugandan initiative to foster the spirit of friendship and cooperation among African medical students (FAMSA). Interestingly, FAMSA has fared better than its parent association and survived the political and socio-economic upheavals of the sub-region by remaining intact. As evidence of this, FAMSA held its 50th Congress in Ibadan, Nigeria, in September 2018, which was attended by over 200 delegates from medical schools across sub-Saharan Africa. This achievement is probably due, at least in part, to the early establishment of a permanent secretariat for the association which provided it with an anchor during the years of instability in the subcontinent.

TABLE 11.3 AMSA Founding Member Medical Schools – December 1963, Kampala, Uganda

	University/Medical School	*Country*
	Full Members	
1	University of Khartoum	Sudan
2	University of Leopoldville (Kinshasha)	Democratic Republic of Congo
3	Makarere University	Uganda
4	University of Ibadan	Nigeria
5	University of Lagos	Nigeria
6	University of Cheikh Anta Diop (Dakar)	Senegal
	Observers	
7	University of Dar-Es-Salam	Tanzania
8	University of Addis Ababa	Ethiopia

12.2.4 International Conference of Deans of French-Speaking Faculties of Medicine (CIDMEF)

The francophone counterpart of AMSA, the CIDMEF was founded in 1981 in Abidjan. Like its parent university association, the Francophone University Agency or Agence Universitaire de la Francophonie (AUF), it is a worldwide network of French-speaking medical schools with the objective of promoting 'health medicine in the French-speaking world in a spirit of solidarity, sharing and freedom'. CIDMEF hopes to achieve this by promoting medical and public health research and strengthening cooperation between medical schools in executing their primary function, i.e., education, research, and service provision. The organization also provides the schools with the opportunity to cooperate in their various functions. This engenders a uniformity of standards in the structure and function of medical schools across the French-speaking world that enables them to provide their faculties and students with the opportunity for mobility across these institutions.

11.2.5 Consortium of New Southern African Medical Schools (CONSAMS)

The founding of this consortium in 2011 was supported by Finland as the Consortium of New Southern African Medical Schools (CONSAMS), a network of three 'new' African medical schools and two international partnering schools with similar objectives to AMSA and CIDMEF. It was expanded in 2015 to include other SSA medical schools that were within 10–15 years of graduating their first cohort of medical students. To reflect this change, its name was changed from 'Southern Africa' to 'Sub-Saharan Africa' but its objectives remained unchanged.

11.3 Medical School Surveys

There have been two major surveys of medical schools in SSA in the post-colonial era. These were to determine the number, characteristics, the state of the teaching and learning infrastructure, and the staffing and student levels in these schools.

11.3.1 Survey of Sub-Saharan African Medical Schools

The first survey of sub-Saharan African Medical Schools was done by the Association of African Universities in 1974 and was financed by the Canadian Development Agency (Monekosso, 1975). This project involved the 25 existing medical schools, all of which were sent questionnaires. Twenty of the institutions were later visited for physical evaluation. The project reported that the medical schools were generally modelled after the four colonial traditions of SSA, viz. British, French, Belgian, and Portuguese. Of significance was the report that the schools were all university-oriented and were primarily directed at producing generalist healthcare professionals. They also varied considerably in size, numbers of staff and students (although they all generally had small class sizes), and adequate teaching and learning infrastructure (i.e., research laboratories, classrooms, and well-stocked libraries). Despite these variations, no school was self-sufficient, and each school had its strengths, which it had utilized in tackling its challenges. The report concluded that fora such as AMSA, where these schools meet to exchange ideas and resources (human and material), would be beneficial to them all as they would not only exchange resources but also share their innovative solutions to their common and idiosyncratic problems. This would enhance the quality of medical training in the subcontinent and thus the quality of graduates produced and the effectiveness of healthcare systems in SSA. This report may have contributed to the formation of CIDMEF a few years later.

11.3.2 Sub-Saharan African Medical Schools Study (SAMSS)

SAMSS was a multinational, multi-institutional collaborative project funded by the Bill and Melinda Gates Foundation (Mullan et al., 2011). It aimed at establishing a baseline understanding of medical schools in sub-Saharan Africa to inform future policies, plans, and investments (Figure 11.1). This study had four primary components: a comprehensive literature review, a series of key informant interviews, site visits to ten medical schools, and a survey of all identified sub-Saharan African medical schools. The project was executed by a team of funded medical educators, researchers, and policymakers (Mullan et al., 2011).

SAMSS identified 168 medical schools in SSA, and its findings showed that medical education was being prioritized in the regions as part of overall strengthening of the health system. In contrast to the earlier survey by Monekosso, this study found that the leading challenges to medical education scale-up were

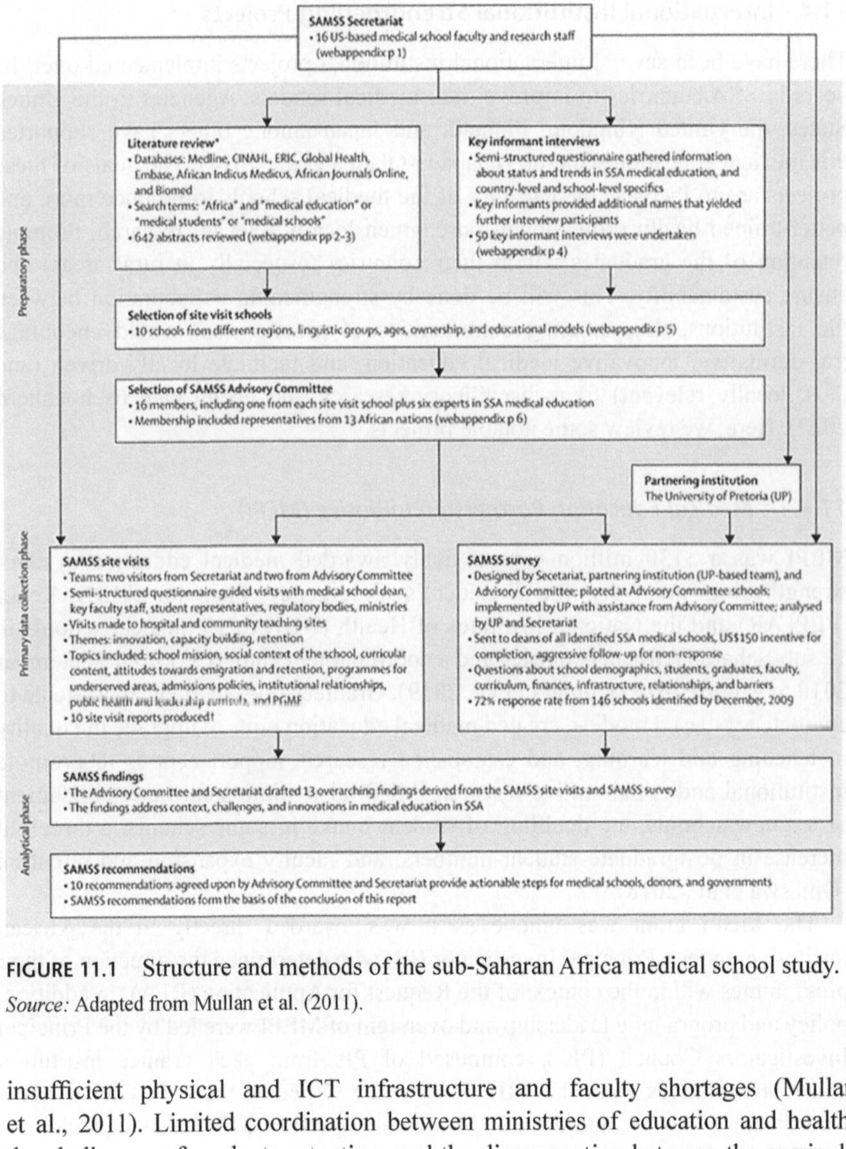

FIGURE 11.1 Structure and methods of the sub-Saharan Africa medical school study. *Source:* Adapted from Mullan et al. (2011).

insufficient physical and ICT infrastructure and faculty shortages (Mullan et al., 2011). Limited coordination between ministries of education and health, the challenges of graduate retention, and the disconnection between the curricula and needs of the community/nation were also observed. SAMSS equally identified several innovative models of medical education in the region (Mellanby, 1958). These included the adaptation of new curricular innovations such as problem-based and community-engaged learning, the growth of PGME in many schools, growing research experience and funding, and a robust set of international partnerships. As noted previously, a major outcome of SAMSS was the revitalization of AMSA in 2014.

11.4 International Institutional Strengthening Projects

There have been several international institutional projects implemented over the years in SSA countries to improve their medical schools. Agencies in the United States, the United Kingdom, Finland, and Japan among others have supported this medical education scale-up (Olapade-Olaopa et al., 2014). The goals of these projects are to increase the capacity of the medical schools to produce more and better-trained health professionals, strengthen locally relevant research, promote retention of the graduates within their countries (especially in rural areas) and ensure sustainability. This will be done by strengthening collaboration between the institutions, thus creating communities of practice that would encourage transformative, innovative medical education, and facilitate locally driven (and thus, locally relevant) trans-disciplinary research and health care (Schoenherr, 2027). Here, we review some notable projects.

11.4.1 Medical Education Partnership Initiative (MEPI)

MEPI was a $130 million competitively awarded medical education system-strengthening grant by the President's Emergency Plan for AIDS Relief (PEPFAR) and the National Institutes of Health (NIH) to 13 medical schools in 12 sub-Saharan African countries and a coordinating centre (CC) from September 2010 to August 2015 (Kilmarx et al., 2019). Grantees revised medical curricula to competency-based models, created medical education units to upgrade the quality of teaching and learning, and established research support centres to promote institutional and collaborative research. MEPI also stimulated the establishment of ten new schools, the doubling of student intake in some schools, a threefold increase in postgraduate student numbers, and faculty expansion and retention (Omaswa et al., 2018).

The MEPI grant was unique as it was awarded directly to the African institution under a Principal Investigator (PI) who determined the direction of their programmes within the context of the Request for Application (RFA). In addition, policy and programme leadership and oversight of MEPI were led by the Principal Investigators Council (PIC), composed of PIs from each grantee institution and representatives from the NIH, HRSA, the Office of the U.S. Global AIDS Coordinator (OGAC), and the CC (Mullan et al., 2012). MEPI also expanded the activities of the programme to institutions beyond the original 13 medical schools who received grants, as representatives from more than 50 medical institutions and other education leaders attended the yearly MEPI Symposium. By this, MEPI encompassed about 60 African schools, representing approximately 25% of the 240 schools of medicine in sub-Saharan Africa by the end of the project (Omaswa et al., 2018).

11.4.1.1 African Forum for Research and Education in Health (AFREhealth)

The African Forum for Research and Education in Health (AFREhealth) is an independent body that emerged from the MEPI and the Nursing Education Partnership Initiative (NEPI) which were funded by PEPFAR–NIH in 2010 and 2011 (Omaswa et al., 2018). The Forum was launched in August 2016 at the annual MEPI Symposium held in Nairobi, Kenya, as an Africa-initiated, owned, and led initiative intended to take charge of the continent's future in HPE following the completion of its two parent projects (Sewankambo et al., 2018). The Forum is open to all health professions education and research institutions and health professions educators and researchers both on the continent and in the Diaspora, regardless of whether they participate in MEPI or NEPI or not. Similar to other such networks/ associations in SSA, AFREhealth's stated objectives are the following: capacity building in teaching and learning HPE and research in Africa, sharing best practices, and improving health outcomes across the subcontinent. Unlike the other international professional networks on the continent, AFREhealth's mission is to be inter-professional, sustain the gains of MEPI/NEPI and expand them to more schools across Africa. To achieve this goal, the Forum has brought together health professionals including physicians, nurses, pharmacists, and dentists in the belief that the complex health problems facing the continent can only be solved by all health professions working together as a team.

In pursuance of its objectives, since its founding, AFREhealth holds an annual symposium which is attended by its members, partners, and other stakeholders. This is where participants share best practices and new innovations in HPE relevant to the African environment. During the COVID-19 pandemic, the Forum also used its networks to carry out multinational SSA collaborative research projects (Nachega et al., 2020) and to evaluate the opportunities and challenges of collaborative initiatives within the Global South and between the Global North and Global South (Eichbaum et al., 2021).

11.4.1.2 Medical Education for Equitable Services to All Ugandans Consortium (MESAU)

This countrywide consortium of five medical schools was formed in 2011 with the support of Johns Hopkins University (the United States), and its aim was to improve health outcomes in their communities and Uganda as a whole. The five medical schools were those of Busitema University, Gulu University, Kampala International University, Makerere University, and Mbarara University of Science and Technology. Despite the initial reservations about this project, it has gained acceptance due to the significant benefits to schools participating in the network.

11.4.2 MEDUNAM (2011–2013)

The MEDUNAM I and II projects were initiated to take advantage of the sustainable partnership between the University of Oulu (Finland), the University of Namibia (UNAM), and Lurio University (UniLurio) in Mozambique provided by CONSAMS to produce a lasting effect on the health systems in Southern Africa (Jacobson et al., 2015). MEDUNAM I focused on improving the medical training in the African institutions by revising their curricula (including the inclusion of community-based learning) and improving their teaching and assessment methods. Following the success of MEDUNAM I, II was directed at integrating inter-professional medical education at all levels of instruction as a critical step towards improving student training and administrative/management processes in the schools.

11.5 National and International Medical Education Capacity-Building Projects

The need for faculty in medical schools to acquire medical education skills was recognized in SSA much later than it was in the developed countries (Mullan et al., 2011). The situation was worsened by the fact that, until recently, the few physicians interested in acquiring specific skills in medical education had to undertake their training overseas (Olapade-Olaopa et al., 2014). In the beginning, these were short courses in curriculum development and teaching and assessment methods, but later degree courses became more accessible. However, the beginning of the 21st century brought a multitude of locally sited collaborative medical education capacity-building efforts by various stakeholders which have included the universities, postgraduate medical colleges, medical education associations, and medical education research projects. These efforts have mostly been limited to a few weeks of certificated training workshops in medical education skills. However, a few degree-awarding programmes have now been established in the region.

11.5.1 Ibadan's Master's Degree Programme in Biomedical Education

The first postgraduate biomedical education (BME) programme in West Africa was established in Ibadan in 2009 as an online professional Master's degree programme in BME. The programme was a collaboration between six universities in SSA and the Universities of Liverpool and Swansea in the United Kingdom. Three of the institutions were from Nigeria, i.e., Ibadan (which was the host university), Jos and Ahmadu Bello (Zaria), whilst the others were the universities of Sierra Leone, The Gambia, and the Kwame Nkrumah University of Science and Technology, Ghana. The first 24 students from these Universities were admitted in 2009 and graduated in 2011. This programme changed into the distance learning academic Master's degree course in BME which is based in the Faculty of Clinical Sciences, College of Medicine, University of Ibadan (COMUI). The course is open to graduates from all health professional/science courses and its duration is a minimum of four semesters. This change to an academic course is to ensure that students with good grades at the end of the course will be eligible to proceed to M.Phil., M.Phil./ Ph.D. and Ph.D. programmes in BME.

11.5.2 FAIMER Regional Institutes in Africa

The FAIMER was established in 2000 by the Educational Commission for Medical Graduates (ECFMG) to improve global health by improving health professions education mainly in developing countries. As part of this strategy, the International FAIMER Institute (IFI) was established in 2011. The programme consists of a two-year sandwich programme for health professions educators that focuses on the development of educational, leadership, and management skills and knowledge, as well as the development of a professional community of practice. Building on this programme, FAIMER has collaborated with key individuals and institutions (medical schools and universities) at the local level to develop FAIMER Regional Institutes (FRIs). These are centres of medical education activity where the interactions among educators are intended to improve local health professions education systems. To date, there are 11 regional institutes in developing regions in Asia, Africa, and Latin America (Table 11.4). The core curriculum of the IFI is offered through the FRIs, but it is adapted to the local context. In addition to the core curriculum, FAIMER is developing new curricula in response to emerging regional and global health professions education needs. Certificates of both the international and regional FAIMER institutes are considered equivalent in distinction and prestige.

Two of these regional institutes are in Africa; the sub-Saharan African-FAIMER Regional Institute (SAFRI) which was established in 2008 (and which is currently suspended) and the Eastern African FAIMER Regional Institute (EAFRI) which was established in 2023. These regional institutes are to serve health professions educators in Southern, East, and Central African Community member states primarily but will also consider applicants from other regions of Africa.

11.6 Innovations in Medical Education Curriculum Reform from Sub-Saharan Africa

The current challenges faced in health care are severe and varied worldwide, and demand that medical/dental schools produce graduates that can respond to the peculiar needs of their communities. The philosophy of medical education is therefore being constantly modified to address the changing needs of societies being served by healthcare professionals. Concurrently, the health professions must also adapt to utilize modern methods of teaching, assessment, and patient management to achieve this goal.

TABLE 11.4 FAIMER Regional Institutes (www.faimer.org/faimer-regional-institutes/)

S/N	*Faimer Regional Institute (FRI)*	*Medical School/University/ Corporation*	*Country*	*Language of Instruction*	*Years of Operation*
1	GSMC-FRI	Seth G S Medical College (GSMC), Mumbai	India	English	2005 to present
2	CMCL-FRI	Christian Medical College Ludhiana (CMCL)	India	English	2006 to present
3	Brazil-FRI	Universidade Federal do Ceara, Fortaleza	Brazil	Portuguese	2007–2017
4	PSG-FRI	PSG Institute of Medical Sciences and Research, Coimbatore	India	English	2007 to present
5	SAFRI	SAFRI Corporation, Cape Town	South Africa	English	2008–2021
6	CMU-FRI	China Medical University, Shenyang	China	English	2013 to present
7	MAHE-FRI	Manipal Academy of Higher Education, Manipal	India	English	2015 to present
8	SMU-FRI	SMU-FRI Southern Medical University, Guangzhou	China	English	2016 to present
9	FRILA	Pontificia Universidad Catolica de Chile, Santiago	Chile	Spanish	2018 to present
10	ASU-MENA-FRI	Ain Shams University Faculty of Medicine, Cairo	Egypt	English	2019 to present
11	FRIENDSHIP	Universitas Gadjah Mada, Yogyakarta	Indonesia	English	2019 to present
12	EAFRI	Makerere University College of Health Sciences, Kampala, and Mbarara University of Science and Technology, Mbarara	Uganda	English	2023 to present

In consideration of this fact, the post-independence era in SSA has brought about a wave of curriculum revisions in the medical schools across the region. This has occurred primarily because of the desire of these schools to ensure that their graduates possess skill sets that fit the needs of their communities while maintaining international standards. It is therefore important for medical education on the subcontinent to reflect cultures and customs and thus ensure that the graduates imbibe the overriding African values that emphasize communal mutual dependence, relationships, solidarity, and caring (cited). As such SSA medical schools require re-orientation away from their colonial traditions, with recourse to the needs of their communities, to make the graduates more socially responsive, allowing them to be better fit for practice. This re-orientation does not diminish adherence to a minimum global standard.

In this regard, the two most common philosophies adopted by many African schools are the following: community-based education (CBE) and, more recently, competency-based medical education (CBME). Both have resulted in the development of innovative methods of medical instruction in SSA that have been globally accepted.

11.6.1 Innovations in Community-Based Education from Sub-Saharan Afr1ca

CBE involves the use of the community as the learning environment and encourages health professionals to work in underserved communities and rural areas to give them access to improvements in preventive and curative aspects of health care (Amalba et al., 2020). It also improves recruitment of students from these areas into universities/medical schools (Amalba et al., 2020; Iputo, 2008). The community-based model of medical education is now a major component of health professions training curricula globally as it enshrines the concept of medical schools producing graduates equipped with the skills required by their communities, thus making them fit for purpose, and encouraging retention. This is particularly important in SSA because a large percentage of the population live in rural or suburban communities and have no access to large teaching academic hospitals, which are usually located in big cities, and are unable to provide the wholesome training required to produce fit-for-purpose healthcare workers (HCW) HRH for community needs. If properly coordinated and implemented, community-based medical education strategies may solve the perennial problem of shortage of places for graduates to do their mandatory year of rotating house-jobs. The community can serve as the clinical laboratory, supervised by experienced doctors, where Surgical, Obstetrics and Gynecology, Internal Medicine, and Child Care can be learned confidently.

11.6.2 The Ibarapa Project and Ibarapa Community and Primary Healthcare Programme

Community-based medical education was pioneered by the Ibarapa Project of the University of Ibadan Medical School in 1963. The founders of this project recognized the need for a learning environment that would make health professionals and health-science training relevant to the needs of their host community. This realization might have been stimulated by the success of the programme of home-based psychiatric care of mentally ill patients established in its region in 1954 due to the scarcity of in-patient care facilities (Lambo, 1962; Boroffka & Olatatwura, 1977). This finding, and the later appointment of the psychiatrist, TA Lambo, onto the staff of the University, contributed to the acceptance of the importance of socio-cultural interactions in the care of patients and therefore the need to incorporate training in the community into the learning experience of health professions students.

The Ibarapa Project was the first model of vertical integration of primary, secondary, and tertiary health care with the specific objectives of improving learning and assessment in undergraduate and PGME. Funded by the Rockefeller Foundation, and with technical support from the Liverpool School of Tropical Medicine and London School of Tropical Medicine and Hygiene, the Ibarapa Project was the product of a unique collaboration for health development between the three different tiers of government in Nigeria, viz. Federal (represented by the University of Ibadan), State (Western Nigeria), and Local (Ibarapa community). Interestingly, this programme of community-based healthcare and health education system was birthed 25 years before the WHO Alma-Ata Declaration (September 1978) that identified primary health care as the key to attaining the goal of 'Health for All' around the world.

The success of the Ibarapa Project resulted in its later evolution into the Ibarapa Community and Primary Healthcare Programme, which has hosted postings of undergraduate/Master's/diploma students from health-related departments, strategic interactions with 'non-health'-related departments, and several academic visits from international students of several countries (Asojo et al., 2014). The programme has also stimulated the development of other CBE programmes in the University of Ibadan such as the Community Dentistry and Ophthalmology programmes (Aderinokun, 2000).

11.6.3 Walter Sisulu University Health Professions Training Programme

The Walter Sisulu University (WSU) Faculty of Health Sciences was founded in 1985 with the objective of equipping doctors with the knowledge, clinical skills, and professional attitudes that would enable them to provide quality health care in the rural and disadvantaged communities of South Africa. This Health Professions Training Programme advanced the philosophy of CBE further as it was the first to be developed based on the hypothesis that recruiting and training health professions students in their local environment would increase their retention in the rural areas (Iputo, 1996). Accordingly, most students are recruited from local communities, using admission processes that look beyond academic achievements and assess the candidates' personal psycho-social attributes (Larkins et al., 2018; van der Merwe et al., 2015). The main attributes assessed are thinking skills, communication skills, interpersonal skills, and motivation to work in the local rural communities. Uniquely, the local communities are active participants in the selection of students into the programmes.

A curriculum combining CBE with problem-based learning (PBL) in small groups was adopted (Iputo et al., 1996a; 1996b). Teaching and learning are organized around community and patient health needs. Education is embedded in the health system and takes place in the community and the primary healthcare clinics instead of predominantly in university and hospital settings. Community-based practitioners are recruited and trained as teachers and mentors.

The WSU curriculum is based on the bio-psycho-social model of training, i.e., the biomedical dimension and the population medicine dimension. The biomedical dimension emphasizes the knowledge of pathology, physiology, therapeutics, and the acquisition of motor skills. The population medicine dimension calls for emotional intelligence – how people involved in the clinical encounter are handled as important and interested parties in the management of the clinical encounter. This population aspect is developed further during the longitudinal community clerkship rotation, where students rotating through the academic health centres follow their patients from the clinics to their homes which enable the student to develop a complete picture of the clinical encounter. Together, the student, the patient, the family, and the community develop a management plan unique to clinical encounters.

The WSU model of medical education has been a major contributor to health professions training in South Africa and has significantly increased retention of fit-for-purpose physicians in rural areas (Iptuo, 2008). More than 2000 doctors have graduated from the training programme. Most of these graduates are from the rural areas of the Eastern Cape and Kwazulu Natal, and 80% of them are working within those two regions. In the Eastern Cape, more than 50% of the health workforce graduated from WSU (over 1000 graduates), with the vast majority working in the primary care disciplines and settings. These findings have confirmed that the WSU policy of recruiting locally and training locally has led to higher retention of primary care physicians in the rural areas. Furthermore, the programme has enabled WSU to partner with health-systems actors to produce locally relevant competencies bringing fulfilment to the WSU motto – 'globally competent and locally relevant' physicians.

11.6.4 Innovation in Competency-Based Medical Education from Sub-Saharan Africa

CBME is defined as the design, implementation, and evaluation of education programmes, and teaching and assessment methods across the medical continuum that use the competencies or observable abilities of learners (Eliasz et al., 2023; Ma, 2024; Schoenherr, 2027a; Schoenherr & McConnell, 2024). In contrast to time-based educational methods, CBME is a learner-centred, active, and lifelong learning experience that incorporates feedback between the teacher and the learner to enable the acquisition of the desired competency outcomes. It de-emphasizes time-based training and promises greater accountability, flexibility, and learner-centredness (Frank et al., 2010). 'The intended outcome of CBME is a health-professional who can practice medicine at a globally accepted level of proficiency, in accord with local conditions, to meet local needs' (McGaghie, 1978).

Sub-Saharan African (SSA) needs medical/dental graduates that can respond to the peculiar needs of their communities (Wilcox et al., 2015). In a quest to achieve this reality, the CBME model was initially adopted by two notable schools in SSA: the COMUI, Nigeria, and College of Health Sciences, Makerere University, Uganda (Kiguli-Malwadde et al., 2014). Since then, several other SSA medical schools have revised their medical curricula to incorporate new competencies and to align their teaching, learning, and assessment methods with outcome-based philosophy.

- **The 2010 MBBS/BDS-Revised Curricula of the COMUI, Nigeria**

From 2001 to 2010, the COMUI undertook a comprehensive review of its 60-year-old traditional MBBS/BDS curricula that it inherited from its parent university, the University of London, in 1948 (Olapade-Olaopa et al., 2010). The aim of the ten-year project was to produce an instrument for medical and dental instruction that meets current and future national health needs and global standards (Box 11.1). This was done through a series of overlapping processes divided broadly into preparatory, review, reform, and implementation phases.

The preparatory phases comprised capacity building of selected faculty in medical education (who were later to play key roles in the curriculum revision process; Afolabi & Olapade-Olaopa, 2006), and an extensive needs assessment of the host community, major employers, and other relevant stakeholders in the university's medical education system was undertaken to determine the kind of medical/dental graduates they desired.

BOX 11.1 THE 2010 COLLEGE OF MEDICINE UNIVERSITY OF IBADAN, NIGERIA, MBBS/BDS CURRICULUM

The modifications made to achieve stated aims of the curriculum revision are summarized below.

1. **Modifications to Teaching and Assessment:** Horizontal integration was done at either the preclinical or clinical school while vertical integration involves an interplay of disciplines in both schools. Competency-Based Assessment of the students was also integrated at the affected levels and were both formative and summative.

2. **Modification to Learning**
   A. **Competency-Based Learning:** Each department identified well-defined measurable, specific learning objectives to direct teaching, learning, and assessment of subjects.

B. Prioritization of Learning: Subject contents were allotted 50%, 30%, and 10% of the instruction time for 'must-know', should-know', and 'may-know' topics, respectively. Assessment is also to be based on this prioritization.

C. Self-Directed Learning: The new curriculum incorporated 12 term papers/projects in different disciplines and e-learning platforms at all levels of training. These learning methods will also expose the students early to the culture of research.

3. Other Novel Modifications

A. Community Orientation: Provisions were made for increased students' contact with the community from preclinical levels.

B. Allotment of Credits Units to Each Course all of Which were Compulsory:

C. Intercalation: Students can take a break from the MBBS/BDS course at 500 level to undertake MSc and Ph.D courses and return to complete the MBBS course.

D. Remediation: Students are allowed a maximum of three (3) attempts only at each part of the MBBS/BDS Final Examinations.

The curriculum review phases involved the review of the existing medical and dental curricula by academic and non-academic staff and student representatives (Olapade-Olaopa et al., 2022). This exercise identified the strengths and weaknesses of the old instrument as well as the mode of instruction best suited to ensure the acquisition of the necessary skills to serve the host community and stakeholders. Following these phases, an integrated, system-based, person-centred, community-oriented, and competency-driven curriculum was selected as the preferred method of instruction that would produce doctors that will meet present and future healthcare needs in Nigeria. During the revision phases, the necessary modifications were made to the traditional curricula to achieve this new philosophy of teaching and assessment (Table 11.5). After synchronization of submissions from departments, the revised curriculum was approved by the (COMUI) Academic Board and then ratified by the University Senate as the new (2010) MBBS/BDS curriculum of the University.

The final phases of the curriculum revision were the implementation phases. This was supervised by the newly formed College Medical Education Unit and recorded several challenges and successes. Academic and non-academic staff had the challenge of changing their orientation and participating in pedagogical sessions alongside running activities of the old curriculum. Many teachers also complained about increased time commitments in teacher–student contact time. In addition, the first sets of students admitted under the revised curriculum felt

TABLE 11.5 Comparison of the Old (Traditional) Curriculum with the 2010 College of Medicine, University of Ibadan MBBS/BDS Curriculum

<table>
<tr><th>School</th><th>Old Curriculum</th><th>2010 Curriculum</th><th>Comment</th></tr>
<tr><td>Preclinical School</td><td>Course/Posting</td><td>Course/Posting</td><td></td></tr>
<tr><td>200 level (1st and 2nd Semesters)</td><td>Anatomy | Physiology | Biochemistry | Epidemiology and Biostatistics | Demography</td><td>Integrated Core Basic Sciences (Anatomy, Physiology, Biochemistry)</td><td>Course to be taught in coordinated system-based modules to achieve integration</td></tr>
<tr><td></td><td></td><td>GIP</td><td>Orientation to the University/CMU</td></tr>
<tr><td></td><td></td><td>Medicine as a Profession: Introduction to Critical Care Medicine, Family Medicine, Psychology, Applied Medical Sciences</td><td>To give students a broad based knowledge in applied medical sciences and an early orientation to medicine as a profession</td></tr>
<tr><td></td><td></td><td>Multidisciplinary Healthcare Delivery: Introduction to the roles of various healthcare specialists in MHD, Complimentary and Alternate Medicine, Human Nutrition, Preventive and Social Medicine I (Public Health Science), Medicine in the Community, Critical Care Medicine, Family Medicine, Psychology</td><td>To give students a broad based knowledge in applied medical sciences and an early orientation to multidisciplinary healthcare delivery</td></tr>
<tr><td></td><td></td><td>Mid-Semester Vacations</td><td></td></tr>
<tr><td>300 level (1st Semester)</td><td>Anatomy | Physiology | Biochemistry | Psychology</td><td>Block posting I (Introductory Pathology and Pharmacology)</td><td>To give early introduction to the Applied Basic Sciences</td></tr>
<tr><td></td><td></td><td>Clinical Application of Core Basic Science Human Nutrition Family Medicine</td><td>Clinical applications of core basic subjects will be taught in system-based modules</td></tr>
<tr><td></td><td></td><td>Revision Core Basic Science</td><td></td></tr>
<tr><td></td><td>Self-Revision</td><td>Self-Revision</td><td></td></tr>
</table>

	Part I MBBS Examinations (Anatomy, Physiology, Psychology, Biochemistry)	Part I MBBS Examinations (Anatomy, Physiology, Biochemistry, CAB, Psychology, AMS, MAP, PHS, CAM)	Candidates that fail 3 attempts at this exam shall exit and may aim for a BSc. in one of the core basic sciences or in certain instances the BSc Medical Science
		Vacation	
Clinical School	*Course/Posting*	*Course/Posting*	
300 level (2nd Semester)	Introductory Posting in Pathology and Pharmacology	Clinical Introductory Posting	Orientation to Clinical School with sessions in A and E Dept. GOPD
	Medicine I	Integrated Clinical Posting 1: Medicine I and Surgery I	Integrated posting involves teaching in General Medicine and Surgery
	Surgery I	Block Posting II	
	Block Posting I	Block Posting II	Integrated posting that involve teaching of core basic and basic system pathology and Pharmacology
	Vacation	Vacation	
400 level (1st Semester)	Block Posting II	Integrated Clinical Posting II	Taken in 1st Semester of 300 level
	Medicine II	Radio-diagnosis and Therapy I	Integrated posting involves system-based teaching in Radiology, Speciality Medicine and Surgery, Paediatrics and OBGYN with vertical integration with the basic sciences (Pathology and Pharmacology). Also includes integrated Infectious disease posting
	Surgery II	Junior Paediatrics	
	Block Posting II	Medicine II	
	Vacation	Surgery II	
400 level (2nd Semester)	Gynaecology	OBGYN I	
	Junior Paediatrics	Special Surgical Posting I	
	Special Posting I	Infectious Diseases Posting	
	Vacation	Preventive and Social Medicine II (Community Medicine I)	

(*Continued*)

TABLE 11.5 (Continued)

School	*Old Curriculum*	*2010 Curriculum*	*Comment*
500 level (1st Semester)	Block Posting III	Vacation	
	Part II MBBS Exams (Pathology and Pharmacology)	Block Posting Revision	
	Junior OBGYN	Part II MBBS Examinations (Pathology and Pharmacology, CAB, CAM and MHD)	To include clinically oriented questions Candidates that fail 3 attempts at this exam shall exit and may transfer to a suitable BSc. course in CMUI/UI or the BSc. Medical Sciences
	Senior Paediatrics	OBGYN II	
	Radiology	Senior Paediatrics	
	Vacation	Family Medicine I	
500 level (2nd Semester)	Block Posting II	Revision OBGYN	
	Senior OBGYN	Preventive and Social Medicine III (Community Medicine II)	
	Outside Posting	Revision Paediatrics	
	Paediatrics/OBGYN Revision	Psychiatry I	
		Self-Revision	
	Part III MBBS Examination (Paediatrics and OBGYN)	Part III MBBS Examination (Paediatrics and OBGYN) – To include applied basic science questions	Candidates that fail 3 attempts at this exam shall exit and may transfer to a suitable BSc. course in CMUI/UI or the BSc. Medical Sciences

600 level (1st Semester)	Community Medicine	Vacation	
	Special Posting II	Family Medicine II Special Surgical Posting II	
	Elective Posting	Radio-diagnosis and Therapy II Elective Clinical/Research Posting	
	Vacation	Psychiatry II	
600 level (2nd Semester)		Vacation	
	Medicine III	Preventive and Social Medicine IV (Community Medicine III)	
	Surgery III	Medicine III and Surgery III	Include revision of other clinical and PHS subjects
	Psychiatry	Self-Revision	
	Revision		
	Part IV MBBS Examination – Medicine, Surgery and Preventive and Social Medicine	Part IV MBBS Examinations – Medicine (to include Psychiatry as a separate clinical examination), Surgery and Preventive and Social Medicine	Candidates that fail 4 attempts at this examination shall exit and may transfer to a suitable BSc. course in CMUI/UI or the BSc. Medical Sciences

Source: Adapted from Olapade-Olaopa et al. (2010).

TABLE 11.6 AMSA Essential Professional Duties for Sub-Saharan Medical/Dental Graduates

S/N	*Essential Professional Duties*
Basic Elective Care	
1	Ability to independently obtain clinical information from a patient in a logical and organized manner and utilize such information to formulate a clinical diagnosis and develop a prioritized list of differential diagnoses (problem-oriented medical record)
2	Ability to apply basic, clinical, and social science knowledge to identify key clinical and social problems to formulate and intimate treatment of common medical and surgical conditions and ensure follow-up (holistic bio-psycho-social assessment)
3	Ability to appropriately request and interpret common investigations/tests
Basic Emergency Care	
4	Ability to promptly identify and triage acutely ill patients and initiate resuscitative measures/treatment of common emergencies including providing basic life support and basic trauma care
5	Ability to identify patients requiring a higher level of medical care and safely transfer them to the appropriate facility
6	Ability to perform minor diagnostic and therapeutic surgical procedures
Administrative and Entrepreneurial Skills	
7	Ability to prescribe appropriate medications and give other instructions safely
8	Ability to complete/write common medico-legal documents (e.g., sick and death certificates, referral letters, etc.)
9	Ability to hand-over and take-over patient care safely
10	Ability to manage/coordinate services in a primary healthcare setting
Communication	
11	Ability to document and present clinical cases accurately including concise summaries (use of problem-oriented medical record)
12	Ability to explain tests and other procedures to patients and/or relations and obtain an informed consent
13	Ability to communicate effectively with colleagues, patients, and relations (e.g., breaking bad news/counselling a dying patient)
Inter-professional Activities	
14	Ability to recognize the role of other healthcare professionals and functions as an effective member of the multidisciplinary healthcare delivery system
Self-directed Learning Activities	
15	Ability to seek, retrieve, and utilize information from resource centres and to utilize this to improve patient care
16	Ability to identify, execute, and publish simple research and audit projects
Social Responsibilities	
17	Ability to practice with sound ethical behaviour, recognizing the patient as a person, and to treat him/her with respect and with understanding of local social and cultural considerations
18	Ability to understand health systems and medical jurisprudence in the locality

Source: Adapted from Olapade-Olaopa et al. (2016).

vulnerable in these 'uncharted waters' and were anxious about the outcome of the implementation, whilst the older students felt abandoned during the process and worried about the value of their certificates that were based on the older curriculum (Anyanwu et al., 2022).

The 2010 revised curriculum also recorded several successes. Most important has been the increase in depth of the students' understanding of the basic sciences and their interest in research (Olapade-Olaopa et al., 2022). These have been typified by the distinctions recorded in examinations of the basic science subjects (Anatomy, Physiology, and Biochemistry) for the first time in several years, and the number of students and graduates winning national and international prizes for their research projects (Olopade et al., 2016).

The 2010 CMUI-revised CBME curriculum has since served as the template for the Nigeria Medical Undergraduate Curriculum adopted by the ministries of education and health in 2012, and other national and international institutions involved in the training of health professionals. More importantly, its principles of teaching and assessment were the template for the recently published core Curriculum Minimal Academic Standards of the NUC, for all courses in Nigeria (Disciplines – NUC CCMAS).

11.6.5 Innovation in Essential Professional Duties

Although the CBME focuses on equipping the graduate with the competencies that are relevant to the host community (Lurie et al., 2009), medical practice depends on the physician's ability to independently integrate competencies from several competency domains in multiple combinations to meet the needs of individual communities (Ten Cate et al., 2010). It is now recognized that the effectiveness of graduates is measured by their ability to utilize competencies to effectively carry out specific professional activities that the public expects all physicians to be able to carry out independently upon graduating, i.e., entrustable professional activities (Ten Cate et al., 2010). However, the peculiarities of general medical and dental practice in individual communities make it necessary to define general clinical situations found in routine medical/dental practice in individual communities that are essential for safe medical and dental practices, and which graduates should be trusted to perform competently, i.e., essential professional duties (EPDs). This is particularly important in SSA as doctors often practice unsupervised after the mandatory period of internship in most countries in the subcontinent.

Determination of EPDs for each community is an important health-systems objective as this will give direction to health education and healthcare strategies. This is because EPDs are professional activities of international standard that are locally relevant, and which clarify the roles of the different cadres of HCWs in their local health system and are thus natural targets for health professionals training curricula (Olapade-Olaopa et al., 2016).

- **AMSA EPDs for an SSA Medical/Dental Graduate**

The AMSA recently developed the EPDs for SSA medical and dental graduates to address the health-systems challenges of the subcontinent (Olapade-Olaopa et al., 2016). This framework is expected to guide the training of physicians so they can perform their redefined professional duties and roles (Olapade-Olaopa et al., 2016).

The AMSA EPDs defines the basic duties that are required for contemporary safety and effective medical and dental practice in the region. They were developed by a committee of seasoned medical educators and have been grouped into those required for basic patient care, basic emergency care, basic administrative skills, communication, inter-professional relationships, self-directed learning, and social responsibilities on the continent (Table 11.6). Twenty-one EPDs were initially identified by these educators and then evaluated for their relevance and suitability by faculty, medical/dental students, and members of the public in several SSA countries. Nineteen of these EPDs were selected by this process as being most appropriate for newly graduated doctors and dentists in SSA and were proposed for adoption. These 19 EPDs were evaluated by medical educators from all over SSA at a Medical Education Workshop at the 2015 MEPI Symposium held in Harare, Zimbabwe, and scored on a scale of 0–5 (0 = not relevant and 5 = relevant; (Olapade-Olaopa et al., 2015). A cut-off score of 75% was used to select the EPDs to be accepted. This final selection process chose 18 EPDs as being most appropriate for newly graduated doctors and dentists in SSA and was proposed for adoption. These 18 EPDs were accepted by AMSA and published in 2016 (Olapade-Olaopa et al., 2016).

11.7 Current Challenges for Medical Education in Sub-Saharan Africa

Despite the gains made in medical education in SSA, challenges remain. The problems of political instability, civil unrest, corruption, and food insecurity across SSA have contributed to limiting the development of medical education and healthcare systems (Greysen et al., 2011). Notwithstanding the spirited efforts to improve medical education in SSA, gaps still exist in attaining global best practices. Prominent amongst these are the following: inadequate production of doctors due to the limited funding of, and access to, medical schools, inability of the average family to bear the cost of medical education, limited number of medical faculty especially in the basic sciences, brain drain, and constantly changing government policies. Whilst these challenges occur globally, they are particularly severe and unrelenting in SSA.

11.7.1 Inconsistent and Poorly Coordinated Governance Policies

The variable commitment of governments in SSA to their health and education system has limited the attainment of global health education standards and made the maintenance of those standards already attained difficult (Olapade-Olaopa, 2022; Mash et al., 2014). Furthermore, there is poor coordination between the government ministries and agencies that are involved in implementing multi-sectoral policies with the implementation strategies being determined mainly by the primary agency's culture and viewpoint rather than the overall goal (Olapade-Olaopa et al., 2014; Ssennyonjo et al., 2022). Inevitably, there is a continuing disconnect between the goals of health professionals training and those of the health and education systems and the host communities.

11.7.2 Poorly Funded Educational and Health Systems

Despite the best efforts of governments, the educational and health systems in SSA are severely underfunded, leading to significant challenges in both sectors (Financing Education in sub-Saharan Africa: Meeting the Challenges of Expansion, Equity, and Quality). This has resulted in a detrimental cycle of inadequate training of health professionals, lack of progress in local biomedical science research, compromised health care, which has limited development in both sectors and the SSA economy (Mullan et al., 2011). This situation was made worse by the global economic crisis caused by the COVID-19 pandemic, which resulted in the 2.1% contraction of Africa GDP in 2020 (African Economic Outlook, 2021).

In the realm of HPTIs, particularly government-owned medical schools, inadequate funding stands as a major hurdle. Insufficient financial support hampers the maintenance and modernization of training facilities and the fair compensation of highly skilled academic staff, which fuels brain drain (Toyin-Thomas et al., 2023). This deficiency has diverted tertiary institutions from their core roles of knowledge dissemination and liberal education, ultimately diminishing the quality of medical education and proficiency (EO Olapade-Olaopa, PG School). Scarce local research funding has resulted in overbearing foreign influence over research priorities, sidelining critical domestic health, science, and economic needs. Additionally, until recently, the lack of a national Intellectual Property Policy further jeopardized the financial gains from local research endeavours funded by foreign grants. The restriction on realistic tuition fees in most government-owned institutions, due to societal perceptions of tertiary education as a public service, adds to the funding constraints and limits educational enhancement.

The inadequacies of the healthcare system compound the issue by impeding the practical/clinical training of health professionals. SSA's healthcare system faces significant breakdowns due to inadequate funding, staffing shortages, inconsistent policies, and deficient infrastructure (Olapade-Olaopa, 2022). The dual role of teaching hospitals (as academic and service institutions dividing responsibilities between ministries of education and health) whilst being under the control of Ministries of Health, makes their administration disjointed and inefficient. Strained relationships between medical schools, teaching hospitals, and local authorities further undermine effective healthcare delivery. These cumulative shortcomings result in a dysfunctional healthcare system, ultimately impacting the training and retention of healthcare workers.

11.7.3 Poor Host Environment

The 'poor host environment' in SSA encompasses several critical challenges that hinder development in most countries across various sectors, particularly in education and health on which medical education relies. The subcontinent's unstable political climate has led to a shift from long-term development plans to short-term projects driven by political expediency or limited administrative tenures. This lack of sustained planning inhibits meaningful development of the education and health systems. Furthermore, security concerns, including civil wars, terrorism, banditry, and population shifts due to climate-induced migration, have led to shifting disease patterns and increased psychological distress among citizens and HCWs. These challenges have not only resulted in a partial or total breakdown of the education system in some countries, they have also triggered changes in carefully nurtured community dynamics around medical schools, affecting community-oriented learning approaches where these are still functioning.

SSA's inadequate basic infrastructure in areas of power, water, internet access, sanitation, and transportation networks further undermines sustainable development efforts. Insufficient technological and industrial foundations hinder progress across sectors, including education and health, which require robust infrastructure to thrive and contribute to the region's growth.

11.7.4 Quality of Human Capital

The non-standardized educational curricula in SSA, which is supposed to provide the foundation before learners enter higher educational institutions, are also challenging. The outcome is an overall variability of human educational capital being admitted for training in the health professions. Another challenge that has affected the quality of human capital is the disconnection between the socio-economic development of African nations and the internationally standardized curricula of the tertiary institutions. Hence, it appears that SSA graduates are sometimes better prepared for practice in Western countries than within the limitations of their local communities.

11.7.5 Infrastructural Difficulties

Physical infrastructure for medical training in SSA flourished from the 1960s until the 1980s. Since then, however, investment in infrastructure has dwindled, and this has affected training and retention of HRH (Greyson, 2011). Currently, there is limited funding to support or renovate facilities. This deficiency of infrastructure is coupled with rapidly expanding staff and student populations resulting in overcrowded classes and congested offices, which reduce productivity and impede adequate teaching and learning. Therefore, teachers and learners require additional efforts to ensure the students acquire the necessary attitudes, skills, and knowledge to be fit for purpose upon graduation (Olopade et al., 2016).

11.7.6 Limited Access to Health Professionals Training

The recent rapid expansion in medical schools in SSA notwithstanding, multifaceted admission processes and relatively small class sizes reduce access to medical education in most countries (Mullan, 2003). This is because the existing training institutions cannot satisfy the numbers currently required for African populations making access to these schools extremely competitive. In Nigeria for the year 2023, less than 80,000 medical school spaces were available for the nearly half-a-million applicants, i.e., 16% availability. Although most medical schools in SSA are public, an increasing number of private schools (for-profit and not-for-profit faith-based) are being established. These private schools are much more expensive than public schools and have much smaller classes; they are therefore unaffordable to most citizens. Furthermore, whilst faith-based institutions do not limit admissions to their adherents, the schools often comply with the religious, social, and dietary norms of the proprietor, which may discourage some students from applying to these schools. As such, there is a reduction in student numbers and patient load with implications for laboratory, clinical, and community-based health-professionals teaching and research, and the number and quality of the graduates (Cancedda et al., 2015).

11.7.7 Limited Accreditation and Quality Assurance Systems

A central feature of health professions education is accreditation (Ma, 2024; Schoenherr, 2027a; Schoenherr & Beaudoin, 2027; Schoenherr & McConnell, 2024). Although progress has been made towards implementation of curriculum and the strengthening of capacity and quality of HRH and matching competencies with population needs, standardized accreditation of medical programmes is not universal in SSA. A recent review of accreditation mechanisms in African countries showed that whilst 31 countries (79%) have an accreditation framework for health training institutions, 7 countries do not have any such mechanism (Okoroafor et al., 2022). Algeria, Benin, Burkina Faso, Congo, Mali, Mauritania, and Togo (18% of the countries) did not have an accreditation mechanism and Chad was in the process of establishing an accreditation mechanism. Another challenge for the accreditation system in SSA is the duality of academic and professional regulatory bodies which superintend health professional training. These often issue diverging guidelines which make it difficult to develop harmonized curricula for academic and professional training of students (Olapade-Olaopa, 2022).

11.7.8 Faculty Recruitment, Retention, and Development and Brain Drain

Multiple challenges define the recruitment and retention processes of HRH in SSA. These issues include preference for employment in tertiary hospitals or local international/non-governmental agencies rather than secondary or primary healthcare centres mainly due to remuneration differences; movement away from regions perceived to be hostile socially, economically, or politically; the lure of living in the urban rather than rural areas; and brain drain. This internal and external migration of HRH has caused significant economic losses to nations in SSA (Olapade-Olaopa, 2022). It has also reduced the efficiency of healthcare delivery and dampened the morale of the retained HRH who are overworked (Connell et al., 2007). The external brain drain has worsened over the years and is particularly concerning in Nigeria. A UK report showed that 13,609 Nigerian HRH were granted working visas in 2022. This has led to severe alteration in the already poor doctor–patient ratio of 1:5000 in Nigeria as against the WHO recommendation of 1:600.

11.7.9 The Threat of Non-Physician Clinicians

Most SSA countries have accepted the use of non-physician clinicians (NPCs) to treat common diseases as part of the strategy to resolve the mismatch of the burden of disease and the inadequate number of trained (HCW; Mullan et al., 2005). This is because they can be quickly trained and produced in large numbers, whilst the production and retention of doctors and nurses can only be scaled-up in the longer term (*Tasks shifting: rational redistribution of tasks among health workforce teams: Global recommendations and guidelines*. Geneva, Switzerland: World Health Organisation, 2008; Mullan et al., 2011; Cancedda et al., 2015). However, an often-unrecognized consequence of the un-coordinated expansion of NPCs is its effect in diluting the efforts to improve the training and quality of physicians. This is because these task-shifting efforts may reduce important direct physician-patient care in practice and the patient load available for training medical students (Olapade-Olaopa et al., 2016). Paradoxically, these effects also increase the workload of physicians who are now saddled, not only with the additional responsibilities of the supervision and training of NPCs but also have to manage the complications of inadequate and/or improper treatment of patients by the NPCs (Mullan et al., 2007; Munga et al., 2012).

11.8 Future Challenges and Prospects

Universal health coverage (one of the United Nations Sustainable Development Goals (UN, 2015) requires that populations have access to a well-functioning healthcare system that is well-staffed by well-trained HRH (Zurn et al., 2021;

Campbell et al., 2013). This can only be achieved by increasing the training and certification of healthcare workers and by integrating all the SDGs into higher education in order to equip future HPE graduates with necessary attitudes, skills, and knowledge (Amorós Molina et al., 2023). It has been projected that SSA needs additional 6.1 million healthcare workers by 2030 to attain universal health coverage (WHO Global Strategy, 2016; WHO, the State of the Health Workforce in the WHO African Region, 2021). However, the challenges of producing these additional quantities of quality HRH, along with ensuring their employment, equitable distribution, and retention, will require significant investments and political support from SSA governments (Olapade-Olaopa, 2022; Frenk et al., 2010). Some of the important challenges and prospects that should be focused on to achieve this goal are listed below.

11.8.1 Role of Governments in Health Professions Education in SSA

Governments must, in conjunction with representatives of HRH, develop and implement policies that promote capacity building and equitable distribution and retention of HRH. SSA governments should also engage researchers, health professional educators, and other stakeholders in the health and education systems to develop socially responsive and accountable programmes which are inclusive and impactful. In addition, SSA governments should support innovative approaches to medical education which must fit the socio-cultural norms and values of each country. The policies driving these programmes must be implemented in a stable enabling environment, unaffected by transitions in government leadership. It is important that these policies include those that will standardize the training of NPCs and regulate their practice in SSA (similar to what occurs in developed countries (American Academy of Physician Assistants (AAPA)). This will formalize their roles and career paths, as well as their relationship to the established cadres of health workers (Yaya et al., 2013). The policies will also reduce NPCs tendency to work unsupervised and/or offer services outside their scope or training (Munga et al., 2012).

11.8.2 Slowing the Brain Drain

The extensive investment in time and resources needed to train and to produce competent healthcare professionals demands that we mobilize effective means in ensuring their retention once they have been trained. Educating more doctors with greater competencies in SSA, only to have them depart at a continued high rate, is an enormous loss for the region. Averting this pattern should begin with admitting candidates to medical schools who are interested in serving the community. However, many students in schools whose curricula are designed with an eye towards the epidemiology and technology of industrial countries would have decided to migrate even before they graduate. Expanding locally based postgraduate training programmes and addressing medical practice issues might improve the retention of graduates, but graduates who see only limited opportunity, bad management, and poor terms of service in practice will still want to emigrate (Burch et al., 2011). To combat this, national authorities have the responsibility of providing support for medical doctors that will make local practice a reasonable option for the patients (Toyin-Thomas et al., 2023). This is especially true for rural areas. Discourses are ongoing in SSA and the recipient (High Income) countries on how to mitigate brain drain and its effects on the donor countries and this on global health security (Do Health, 2010; Blacklock et al., 2012). Despite these initiatives by donor countries and the WHO voluntary code that restricts the migration of individual HCW from countries with shortages (Eckenwiler, 2009), international labour, health, and education may need to support compulsory measures to compensate of donor countries that been proposed by some authors (Gostin et al., 2013; Mackey& Liang, 2012).

11.8.3 Granting Universities/Medical Schools Autonomy

Despite the proliferation of private medical schools in SSA, the majority of HRH in the region are produced by public health professional training institutions that are generally inadequately funded. SSA governments should consider ending the present culture of financial and administrative dependence on government by granting these institutions (administrative and financial) autonomy which would encourage adoption of corporate governance that would increase their access to both private and corporate private sector funds. Such autonomy would also reduce government influence on these institutions and preserve their academic freedom. This is because autonomy confers on each university the capacity to govern itself, thus the right to select or admit its own students, decide its curricula and areas of research focus, and most importantly, determine methods and terms of employment (especially remuneration). Each university/medical school would then develop its own character and culture which should be espoused by its vision and mission documents, and which will guide its academic activities, staff employment, and research outlook (Smego et al., 2010).

11.8.4 Increasing Access to Health Professions Education

The shortage of healthcare workers in SSA prescribes an urgent need to increase the quantity and quality of HRH being produced in SSA. This problem is not unique to SSA (for a discussion of India, see Khan, 2027). It will therefore be necessary to increase access to HPE by increasing class sizes in both public and private medical schools and modifying the admission criteria to expand the pool of eligible candidates. In this wise, the WSU bio-psycho-social admission criteria could be adopted (Ipto, 2008; Larkins et al., 2015). In addition, similar to what obtains in developed countries, SSA governments and private finance institutions should provide student loans with low interest rates, while institutions should be encouraged to establish substantial partnerships with major (private) individual and corporate endowments. Part of these latter funds should be used to provide scholarships and grants to deserving students. Innovative efforts should also be directed at removing the bottleneck that exists at the internship level in some SSA countries. This could include expanding the spaces available for training by adopting the CBE model as part of these programmes.

11.8.5 Curriculum Review

Health professions education curricula need to continually evolve to meet global standards while being locally relevant (Adisa et al., 2019). For example, outcomes from local research should be translated to evidence-based practice and policy changes. Curricula must change from 'science-based' to 'competency-based' so that graduates can be fit for purpose (Frank et al., 2010). This entails matching educational experience to clearly defined societal and patient needs. Training must include objectives related to PBL, CBE, and multidisciplinary team-based learning (Olapade-Olaopa et al., 2016). The curriculum should also adopt medicine and art as interlinked social constructs. In such an approach, health professions education will feature components of local literature, folklore, music, drama, and poetry which will make health education attractive to the local community (Lawal & Ogunbiyi, 2019). These address the priority health concerns of the community and are foundational to health communication (Daboval et al., 2025; Schoenherr & LeBour, 2024). As socially responsive curricula are implemented on a countrywide level, the corollary is that accreditation indices must be appropriate to the health-system needs used to develop the curriculum. Further development of CBE and CBME that suit the health and education needs of SSA and that are adaptable to the health and educational systems of individual countries is required.

11.8.6 Continuing Capacity Building of Faculty

For effective introduction of CBME curricula, especially with increasing student population, medical school executives and faculty must be committed to its implementation and to training in the relevant and valid assessment methods for the various competencies (McKenzie-White et al., 2022). After completion of formal medical specialist training, medical educators need to update their skills and knowledge. To solve peculiar medical education and health challenges in SSA, this interaction should include all related disciplines (medical and non-medical). Such inclusive groups would be charged with developing practical domestic approaches to resolving medical education and healthcare challenges (Adisa et al., 2019).

11.8.7 Technology Advancement in Medical Education

Information technology has transformed medical education elsewhere and has the potential to bring high-quality education to SSA through the installation of VSAT community training centres. Therefore, SSA medical colleges must develop interactive robust content which will enable real-time/offline teaching and learning. An example of a tech-based healthcare solution is simulation technology adapted for clinical procedures, mimicking diseases, and replacing humans with virtual cadavers (Adisa et al., 2019). SSA needs these programmes for improvement in medical education because actual interaction with patients for training is declining globally.

11.8.7 Maximising the Contributions of Alumni and the Diaspora

The Alumni and Diaspora remain a huge resource for SSA as they can contribute their expertise, funding, and networking with other stakeholders for the improvement of medical education across the subcontinent. Governments and HPTIs should therefore continue to develop and implement policies and programmes that would provide an enabling environment to maximize the benefit of this huge human resource. Towards this goal, national and international alumni networks, and their relations with their administrative and regulatory bodies of their countries and institutions, should be strengthened, whilst their individual and corporate efforts should be further encouraged to increase their participation in the development and implementation of medical education strategies in their home HPTIs and countries specifically, and in SSA generally. In this regard, the support given by the Nigerian government to organizing Nigerians in the Diaspora should be adopted by other SSA countries. Similarly, the agreements Egypt has reached with several countries that allows its Diaspora to return home for sabbaticals of up to three years is worthy of replication (Wojczewski et al., 2015). These efforts are likely to encourage the current trend of Diaspora health workers forming professional associations whose objective is to support their countries of origin. It is, however, imperative that every effort is made to forge a harmonious relationship between the local actors (medical educators, administrators, and regulators) and those in the Diaspora to avoid potential conflicts that may sabotage these mutually beneficial projects.

Alumni and Diaspora physicians also constitute an excellent reserve of teaching Faculty who can support local Faculty through online and in-person teaching (Kamarulzaman et al., 2022). African universities are urged to 'identify and prioritize the academic areas, skill sets, and expertise gap as part of their differentiated approach to diaspora involvement'. They should also collect data on Diaspora engagement and evaluate the contribution of the Diaspora. In addition to teaching, Diaspora faculty can assume important roles in mentoring learners and young faculty and brokering opportunities in medical education innovation and research. This engagement, if fully harnessed, has the potential to modify some of the push factors for brain drain such as lack of mentorship, opportunities for professional development and intellectual stimulation. The African Diaspora straddles a world of privilege in which they have unique knowledge of the local realities in SSA together with an insider view of the Global North. However, Diaspora medical educators are at risk of adopting a harmonization approach to medical education prioritizing Western pedagogical approaches that may not suit local needs. Creation of communities of practice, self-reflection, and humility on both sides can help avoid potential conflicts. While SSA institutions may not be able to afford the 'reverse brain programs' of incentivizing the actual return of Diaspora faculty, incentives such as offering adjunct faculty positions (paid or unpaid), academic recognition, and opportunities to collaborate on teaching and research can provide mutual benefits and facilitate bi-directional learning. African Diaspora faculty can also be a great ally in de-colonizing global health and ensuring that local solutions and local agenda dictate the trajectory of medical education and health care on the continent.

11.8.8 Artificial Intelligence

Learning analytics and artificial intelligence (AI) have been framed as 'disruptive technology' that can revolutionize both education and decision-making in the health professions (for a review in this volume, see Schoenherr, 2027). For instance, the benefits of AI are that it can provide more personalized training where resources (e.g., medical educator time) are limited. In SSA, this could be of immense benefit as HRH are not sufficient in the required numbers. Large Language Models (LLM) that are capable of sentiment analysis and reproduction can be utilized in life-sized mannequins to train students on medical procedures and the diverse range of patients emotions before they are introduced to actual patient care (Liu et al., 2020). Such mannequins can also be used to simulate patients with any medical condition for the purpose of teaching real-time history taking or assessment of knowledge by creating clinical scenarios via natural language processing (Manning, 2022).

There are, however, several challenges to the use of AI in SSA. The cost of this technology is high and deploying it for most medical schools in SSA could really be difficult (Biderman et al., 2023). Moreover, clinicians will undoubtedly need to commit time and some effort to learn how best to understand when, where, and how to incorporate the use of these technologies into their practice. For HRH who are already overstretched, this could initially be an over-reach for them and a potential source of stress. However, the benefits of SSA health care must be viewed against caution. Like all AI, there can be issues associated with implementation (Schoenherr, 2027a; Schoenherr & Hamstra, 2024). There is also the possibility of bias that can be introduced from the training data, since the most likely training data used would have been obtained from countries outside SSA. When unfamiliar datasets are introduced to AI-driven devices, it can even lead to AI hallucination

(Birhane et al., 2023; Dilmegani, 2023). As AI is being adopted, the HRH in SSA must be aware of these potential conflicts of datasets.

11.9 Challenges of Artificial Intelligence

The main use of AI in medical education is for learning support, however, there are several challenges associated with its use. Some of these are described below.

1. ***AI system performance:*** This is the challenge with the innovation itself and includes the technical difficulties in acquiring a large sample size needed for the development of the model, the prerequisite for a qualified and experienced content specialist to design the curriculum for machine learning and the communication difficulties relative to the knowledge gap between physicians and engineers (Chan & Zary, 2019).
2. ***Effectiveness and effectiveness verification:*** Useful feedback should essentially assist students in identifying conceptual misunderstandings, critique their performance, and be structured enough to help students achieve their learning objectives (Mason & Bruning, 2001). Could AI compromise the quality of this feedback, especially since the feedback generated is based on the knowledge and model of the AI system, which currently still needs improvement? A major case in point is the concept of 'clinical reasoning'. Clinical problems are ill-structured and multifaceted, as such, clinicians must obtain a detailed history and try to piece the information together to derive logical differentials. Since this is more complex than stringing symptoms and labelling a diagnosis, it would be a large sample comparison between traditional methods and AI to yield probable results (Chan & Zary, 2019). Also, a single coding error could yield completely incorrect responses from the machine, and what fail-safe methods are there in the system to detect possible errors quickly?
3. ***AI training data sample:*** Sufficient and globally representative training data will be required to avoid bias in machine learning and hence with feedback (Chan & Zary, 2019). Using this technology in SSA could be especially problematic as the training data would most likely have been obtained from outside SSA and lead to error in machine responses or even to AI hallucination.
4. ***AI and ethical issues:*** As healthcare delivery evolves in complexity, clinical decisions should not be made solely on technical and medical grounds (Lo, 2012). Some decisions will be made based on the patient's expectations and empathy from the clinician, something that AI is severely limited in or is incapable of achieving (Wartman & Combs, 2019).
5. ***Need for technical expertise:*** HRH in SSA, who are already overstretched will need to commit time to learn the uses and functionality of the system, and this would yet pose an initial source of significant stress on everyone involved.

6. ***Cost of AI tools and applications:*** The initial costs of purchase, installation, and driving the technology could be unaffordable for several SSA countries. Maintenance costs and training support staff for maintenance and repairs of the equipment could also be another major source of expenditure which could limit their use in SSA.
7. ***Data privacy and security:*** The use of AI in health care requires large amounts of patient data, which raises concerns about data privacy and security. Then there are also still concerns about using AI for students' assessments and examinations because of issues with secure communication and the possibility of examination cheating (Sarrayrih, 2013).

11.9.1 Sustainability of Innovations

Historically, SSA health professions education projects have been funded by external bodies as has been highlighted above. Different from colonial-era educational initiatives, most of the externally supported medical education investments of today emphasize African leadership and are aware of local/national needs. Nonetheless, sustainability is an issue in all these projects. SSA must therefore be careful to build sustainability into these programmes to ensure that they continue to run effectively in the future. In this regard, institutional commitment and, particularly, increased support from national governments and the private sector will be of utmost importance. Several local drug therapies have also been developed over the decades and reached a peak during the COVID-19 pandemic. However, the national government needs to show interest in these innovations to ensure their further development as commercially viable products.

11.10 Conclusion

The development of HPE in SSA has been undeniably eventful. From the philosophy of establishment, through the several decades of challenges, to the changing and ever progressively complex health needs of communities, significant advances have been achieved. In the evolution of medical education in SSA, innovative and competency-based programmes have been developed, regional and international collaborations have been formed, and associations to drive best practices and build institutional strengths are in existence and are expanding in capacity. However, there are still systemic problems of poor funding, infrastructural difficulties, limited access to health professionals training, and Faculty training, recruitment, and retention. To overcome these challenges and move closer to acceptable standards, governments in SSA and HRH must engage in defining roles in HPE, must find ways of creating a conducive work environment that encourages retention and discourages the brain drain, must increase access to HPE and continuing capacity building, and must embrace fit-for-purpose technology advancements in medical education and healthcare delivery.

References

Aderinokun, G. A. (2000). Review of a community oral health programme in Nigeria after ten years. *African Journal of Biomedical Research*, *3*(3), 123–128.

Adisa, A. O., Orunmuyi, A. T., Lawal, T. A., Afolami, J. I., Sigbeku, O. F., Odukogbe, A. A., ... & Olapade-Olaopa, E. O. (2019). Strategies for health professionals education in Nigeria for 2050. *African Journal of Medicine and Medical Sciences*, *48*(Supplement 1), 211–215.

Afolabi, B. B., & Olapade-Olaopa, E. O. (2006). International training in medical education--the FAIMER institute 2002 fellowship experience.

Ajao, O. G., & Alao, A. (2016). Surgical residency training in developing countries: West African college of surgeons as a case study. *Journal of the National Medical Association*, *108*(3), 173–179.

Amalba, A., Abantanga, F. A., Scherpbier, A. J., & van Mook, W. N. (2020). The Role of community-based education and service (COBES) in undergraduate medical education in reducing the mal-distribution of medical doctors in rural areas in Africa: a systematic review. *Health Professions Education*, *6*(1), 9–18.

Amoros Molina, A., Helldén, D., Alfvén, T., Niemi, M., Leander, K., Nordenstedt, H., ... & Biermann, O. (2023). Integrating the United Nations sustainable development goals into higher education globally: a scoping review. *Global Health Action*, *16*(1), 2190649

Anyanwu, J. C., Olopade, F. E., Kolars, J. C., & Olapade-Olaopa, E. O. (2022). Perception of students on the learning environment during early stages of curriculum reform at the college of medicine, university of Ibadan. *African Journal of Medicine and Medical Sciences, 52*(4), 229–237.

Asojo, O. A., Asuzu, M. C., & Adebiyi, A. O. (2014). Ibarapa programme: half a century of rural health service, training, and international cooperation in Nigeria. *PLoS Neglected Tropical Diseases*, *8*(10), e3201.

Biderman, S., Schoelkopf, H., Anthony, Q. G., Bradley, H., O'Brien, K., Hallahan, E., ... & Van Der Wal, O. (2023, July). Pythia: a suite for analyzing large language models across training and scaling. In *International Conference on Machine Learning* (pp. 2397–2430). PMLR.

Birhane, A., Kasirzadeh, A., Leslie, D., & Wachter, S. (2023). Science in the age of large language models. *Nature Reviews Physics*, *5*(5), 277–280.

Blacklock, C., Heneghan, C., Mant, D., & Ward, A. M. (2012). Effect of UK policy on medical migration: a time series analysis of physician registration data. *Human Resources for Health*, *10*, 1–9.

Boelen, C. (2004). Building a socially accountable health professions school: towards unity for health. *Education for Health*, *17*(2), 223–231.

Boroffka, A., & Olatawura, M. O. (1977). Communty psyciatry in Nigeria—the current status. *International Journal of Social Psychiatry*, *23*(4), 275–280.

Brown, A. (1961). Medical education in Nigeria. *Academic Medicine*, *36*(9), 1036–1041.

Burch, V. C., McKinley, D., Van Wyk, J., Kiguli-Walube, S., Cameron, D., Cilliers, F. J., ... & Morahan, P. S. (2011). Career intentions of medical students trained in six sub-Saharan African countries. *Education for Health*, *24*(3), 614.

Campbell, J., Buchan, J., Cometto, G., David, B., Dussault, G., Fogstad, H., ... & Tangcharoensathien, V. (2013). Human resources for health and universal health coverage: fostering equity and effective coverage. *Bulletin of the World Health Organization*, *91*, 853–863.

Cancedda, C., Farmer, P. E., Kerry, V., Nuthulaganti, T., Scott, K. W., Goosby, E., & Binagwaho, A. (2015). Maximizing the impact of training initiatives for health professionals in low-income countries: frameworks, challenges, and best practices. *PLoS Medicine*, *12*(6), e1001840.

Chan, K. S., & Zary, N. (2019). Applications and challenges of implementing artificial intelligence in medical education: integrative review. *JMIR Medical Education*, *5*(1), e13930.

Chen, C., Buch, E., Wassermann, T., Frehywot, S., Mullan, F., Omaswa, F., ... & Olapade-Olaopa, E. O. (2012). A survey of sub-saharan African medical schools. *Human Resources for Health, 10*, 1–23.

Connell, J., Zurn, P., Stilwell, B., Awases, M., & Braichet, J. M. (2007). Sub-saharan Africa: beyond the health worker migration crisis?. *Social Science & Medicine*, *64*(9), 1876–1891.

Daboval, T., Ferreti, E., & Barkova, A. (2027). Validity in health professions education: from assessment instruments to program innovation and evaluation. In Schoenherr, J. R. (ed.) *Fundamentals and Frontiers of Medical Education and Decision-Making: Innovation, Implementation, and Translational Research.* Routledge.

Department of Health, Republic of South Africa. (2010). Employment of foreign health professionals in the south African health sector. Retrieved September 18, 2023 from: www.hrhresourcecenter.org/node/3361.html

Dilmegani, C. (2023). Large language models: complete guide in 2023. AIMultiple research, [Online]. https://research. aimultiple. com/large-language-models

Eckenwiler, L. A. (2009). Care worker migration and transnational justice. *Public Health Ethics*, *2*(2), 171–183.

Eichbaum, Q., Sam-Agudu, N. A., Kazembe, A., Kiguli-Malwadde, E., Khanyola, J., Wasserheit, J. N., ... & Nachega, J. B. (2021). Opportunities and challenges in North-South and South-South global health collaborations during the COVID-19 pandemic: the AFREhealth-CUGH experience (as reported at the CUGH 2021 satellite meeting). *Annals of Global Health*, *87*(1), 90.

Eliasz, K. L., Nick, M. W., Zabar, S., Buckvar-Keltz, L., Ng, G. M., Riles, T. S., & Kalet, A. L. (2023). Viewing readiness-for-residency through binoculars: mapping competency-based assessments to the AAMC's 13 core entrustable professional activities (EPAs). *Teaching and Learning in Medicine*, *35*(4), 436–441.

Eyal, N., Cancedda, C., Kyamanywa, P., & Hurst, S. A. (2015). Non-physician clinicians in sub-Saharan Africa and the evolving role of physicians. *International Journal of Health Policy and Management*, *5*(3), 149.

Frank, J. R., Snell, L. S., Cate, O. T., Holmboe, E. S., Carraccio, C., Swing, S. R., ... & Harris, K. A. (2010). Competency-based medical education: theory to practice. *Medical Teacher*, *32*(8), 638–645.

Frenk, J., Chen, L., Bhutta, Z. A., Cohen, J., Crisp, N., Evans, T., ... & Zurayk, H. (2010). Health professionals for a new century: transforming education to strengthen health systems in an interdependent world. *The Lancet*, *376*(9756), 1923–1958.

Glytsos, N. P. (2002). The role of migrant remittances in development: evidence from mediterranean countries. *International Migration*, *40*(1), 5–26.

Gostin, L. O., Friedman, E. A., Buse, K., Waris, A., Mulumba, M., Joel, M., ... & Sridhar, D. (2013). Towards a framework convention on global health. *Bulletin of the World Health Organization, 91*, 790–793.

Greysen, S. R., Dovlo, D., Olapade-Olaopa, E. O., Jacobs, M., Sewankambo, N., & Mullan, F. (2011). Medical education in sub-Saharan Africa: a literature review. *Medical Education*, *45*(10), 973–986.

Hammad, N., Ndlovu, N., Carson, L. M., Ramogola-Masire, D., Mallick, I., Berry, S., & Olapade-Olaopa, E. O. (2023). Competency-based workforce development and education in global oncology. *Current Oncology, 30*(2), 1760–1775.

Iliffe, J. (1998). *East African Doctors: A History of the Modern Profession* (Vol. *95*). Cambridge University Press.

Iputo, J. E. (2008). Faculty of health sciences, walter sisulu university: training doctors from and for rural South African communities. *Medicc Review, 10*(4), 25–29.

Iputo, J. E., & Nganwa-Bagumah, A. B. (1996a). The innovative medical curriculum of the university of Transkei medical school. Part I. Problem-based learning. *South African Medical Journal= Suid-Afrikaanse tydskrif vir geneeskunde, 86*(6), 649–651.

Iputo, J. E., & Nganwa-Bagumah, A. B. (1996b). The innovative medical curriculum of the university of Transkei medical school. Part II. Community-based learning. *South African Medical Journal= Suid-Afrikaanse tydskrif vir geneeskunde, 86*(6), 651–652.

Jacobson, C., Wessels, Q., Pires P, Vainio O. (2015). Together towards seven-star doctors the MEDUNAM project at the university of Oulu. In *Higher Education Institutions Partnering for Development and Change – Reflections of the First Round of the Finnish HEI ICI Programme* (pp. 113–123).

Kamarulzaman, A., Ramnarayan, K., & Mocumbi, A. O. (2022). Plugging the medical brain drain. *The Lancet, 400*(10362), 1492–1494.

Karekezi, C., & El Khamlichi, A. (2019). Takeoff of African neurosurgery and the world federation of neurosurgical societies rabat training center alumni. *World Neurosurgery, 126*, 576–580.

Khogali, A. (1966). The association of medical schools in Africa. *Academic Medicine, 41*(10), 999–1000.

Kiguli-Malwadde, E., Olapade-Olaopa, E. O., Kiguli, S., Chen, C., Sewankambo, N. K., Ogunniyi, A. O., ... & Omaswa, F. (2014). *Competency-Based Medical Education in Two Sub-Saharan African Medical Schools*. Advances in Medical Education and Practice, pp. 483–489.

Kilmarx, P. H., Katz, F., Razak, M. H., Palen, J., Cheever, L. W., & Glass, R. I. (2019). The medical education partnership initiative: strengthening human resources to end AIDS and improve health in Africa. *Academic Medicine, 94*(11), 1704–1713.

Lambo, T. A. (1962). The importance of cultural factors in treatment (with special reference to the utilization of the social environment). *Acta Psychiatrica Scandinavica, 38*, 176–182.

Larkins, S., Johnston, K., Hogenbirk, J. C., Willems, S., Elsanousi, S., Mammen, M., ... & Neusy, A. J. (2018). Practice intentions at entry to and exit from medical schools aspiring to social accountability: findings from the training for health equity network graduate outcome study. *BMC Medical Education, 18*, 1–12.

Larkins, S., Michielsen, K., Iputo, J., Elsanousi, S., Mammen, M., Graves, L., ... & Neusy, A. J. (2015). Impact of selection strategies on representation of underserved populations and intention to practise: international findings. *Medical Education, 49*(1), 60–72.

Lawal, T. A., Ogunbiyi, A. O., & Olapade-Olaopa, E. O. (2019). Total health for all in Nigeria 2050 and beyond: strategies for reforming health professionals' education. *African Journal of Medicine and Medical Sciences, 48*(Supplement 1), 143–148.

Liu, F., Cui, J., Liu, X., Chen, K. W., Chen, X., & Li, R. (2020). The effect of tai chi and Qigong exercise on depression and anxiety of individuals with substance use disorders: a systematic review and meta-analysis. *BMC Complementary Medicine and Therapies, 20*, 1–11.

Lo, B. (2012). *Resolving Ethical Dilemmas: A Guide for Clinicians*. Lippincott Williams & Wilkins.

Lurie, S. J., Mooney, C. J., & Lyness, J. M. (2009). Measurement of the general competencies of the accreditation council for graduate medical education: a systematic review. *Academic Medicine*, *84*(3), 301–309.

Ma, T. (2024). 2 considerations for implementation of a competency-based education program for preclerkship courses. In Schoenherr, J. R., & McConnell, M. (eds.), *Fundamentals and Frontiers of Medical Education and Decision-Making: Educational Theory and Psychological Practice*. Routledge.

Mackey, T. K., & Liang, B. A. (2012). Rebalancing brain drain: exploring resource reallocation to address health worker migration and promote global health. *Health Policy*, *107*(1), 66–73.

Manirakiza, A., Rubagumya, F., Fehr, A. E., Triedman, A. S., Greenberg, L., Mbabazi, G., ... & Hammad, N. (2020). Oncology training in rwanda: challenges and opportunities for undergraduate medical students (The EDUCAN Project). *Journal of Cancer Education*, *35*, 359–365.

Manning, C. D. (2022). Human language understanding & reasoning. *Daedalus*, *151*(2), 127–138.

Mash, R. J., De Villiers, M. R., Moodley, K., & Nachega, J. B. (2014). Guiding the development of family medicine training in Africa through collaboration with the medical education partnership initiative. *Academic Medicine, 89*(8), S73–S77.

Mason, B. J., Bruning, R. (2001). *Providing Feedback in Computer-Based Instruction: What the Research Tells Us*. Center for Instructional Innovation, University of Nebraska–Lincoln.

McGaghie, W. C. (1978). Competency-based curriculum development in medical education. An Introduction. Public Health Papers No. 68.

McKenzie-White, J., Mubuuke, A. G., Westergaard, S., Munabi, I. G., Bollinger, R. C., Opoka, R., ... & Kiguli, S. (2022). Evaluation of a competency based medical curriculum in a Sub-Saharan African medical school. *BMC Medical Education*, *22*(1), 724.

Mellanby, K. (1958). *The Birth of Nigeria's Uuniversity*. Methuen.

Monekosso, G. L. (1975). *Report of a Survey on African Medical Schools (July-December, 1974)*. Association of African Universities.

Monekosso, G. L. (2014). A brief history of medical education in Sub-Saharan Africa. *Academic Medicine*, *89*(8), S11–S15.

Mullan, F. (2003). The future of medical education: a call for action. *Health Affairs*, *22*(4), 88–90.

Mullan, F. (2005). The metrics of the physician brain drain. *New England Journal of Medicine*, *353*(17), 1810–1818.

Mullan, F., & Frehywot, S. (2007). Non-physician clinicians in 47 sub-Saharan African countries. *The Lancet*, *370*(9605), 2158–2163.

Mullan, F., Frehywot, S., Omaswa, F., Buch, E., Chen, C., Greysen, S. R., ... & Neusy, A. J. (2011). Medical schools in sub-Saharan Africa. *The Lancet*, *377*(9771), 1113–1121.

Mullan, F., Frehywot, S., Omaswa, F., Sewankambo, N., Talib, Z., Chen, C., ... & Kiguli-Malwadde, E. (2012). The medical education partnership initiative: PEPFAR's effort to boost health worker education to strengthen health systems. *Health Affairs*, *31*(7), 1561–1572.

Munga, M. A., Kilima, S. P., Mutalemwa, P. P., Kisoka, W. J., & Malecela, M. N. (2012). Experiences, opportunities and challenges of implementing task shifting in underserved remote settings: the case of Kongwa district, central Tanzania. *BMC International Health and Human Rights*, *12*, 1–12.

Nachega, J. B., Sam-Agudu, N. A., Budhram, S., Taha, T. E., Vannevel, V., Somapillay, P., ... & AFREhealth COVID-19 Research Collaboration Working Group. (2020). Effect of SARS-CoV-2 infection in pregnancy on maternal and neonatal outcomes in Africa: an AFREhealth call for evidence through multicountry research collaboration. *The American Journal of Tropical Medicine and Hygiene*, *104*(2), 461.

Okoroafor, S. C., Ahmat, A., Asamani, J. A., Millogo, J. J. S., & Nyoni, J. (2022). An overview of health workforce education and accreditation in Africa: implications for scaling-up capacity and quality. *Human Resources for Health*, *20*(1), 37.

Olapade-Olaopa, E. O. (2006). College of medicine, university of Ibadan 2004 college lecture "curriculum change and the college of medicine, university of Ibadan".

Olapade-Olaopa, E. O. (ed.) (2010). *MBBS CMUI Curriculum*. Office of the Provost. College of Medicine, University of Ibadan.

Olapade-Olaopa, E. O. (2022). *Imperatives of Transforming Health Professions Education in Nigeria: 2nd Emeritus Professor Oladipo Akinkugbe Distinguished Lecture*. University of Medical Sciences.

Olapade-Olaopa, E. O., Baird, S., Kiguli-Malwadde, E., & Kolars, J. C. (2014). Growing partnerships: leveraging the power of collaboration through the medical education partnership initiative. *Academic Medicine*, *89*(8), S19–S23.

Olapade-Olaopa, E. O., Sewankambo, N. K., & Iputo, J. (2015, July). Consensus on African physician competencies. In Presentation at: the 2015 MEPI Symposium.

Olapade-Olaopa, E. O., Sewankambo, N. K., & Iputo, J. E. (2016). Defining Sub-Saharan Africa's health workforce needs: going forwards quickly into the past: comment on "non-physician clinicians in Sub-Saharan Africa and the evolving role of physicians". *International Journal of Health Policy and Management*, *6*(2), 111.

Olapade-Olaopa, E. O., Sewankambo, N., Iputo, J. E., Rugarabamu, P., Amlak, A. H., Mipando, M., Monekosso, G. L.. (2016). Essential professional duties for the sub-Saharan medical/dental graduate: an association of medical schools of Africa initiative. *African Journal of Medicine and Medical Sciences*, *45*(3), 221–227.

Olopade, F. E., Adaramoye, O. A., Raji, Y., Fasola, A. O., & Olapade-Olaopa, E. O. (2016). Developing a competency-based medical education curriculum for the core basic medical sciences in an African medical school. *Advances in Medical Education and Practice*, 389–398.

Omaswa, F., Kiguli-Malwadde, E., Donkor, P., Hakim, J., Derbew, M., Baird, S., ... & de Villiers, M. (2017). Medical education partnership initiative gives birth to AFREhealth. *The Lancet Global Health*, *5*(10), e965–e966.

Omaswa, F., Kiguli-Malwadde, E., Donkor, P., Hakim, J., Derbew, M., Baird, S., ... & De Villiers, M. (2018). The medical education partnership initiative (MEPI): innovations and lessons for health professions training and research in Africa. *Annals of Global Health*, *84*(1), 160.

Sarrayrih, M. A., & Ilyas, M. (2013). Challenges of online exam, performances and problems for online university exam. *International Journal of Computer Science Issues (IJCSI)*, *10*(1), 439–443.

Schoenherr, J. R. (2027a). Innovation and implementation in the health professions: Translating research in education and healthcare delivery. In Schoenherr, J. R. (Ed.), *Fundamentals and Frontiers of Medical Education and Decision-Making: Innovation, Implementation, and Translational Research* (pp.1–76). Routledge.

Schoenherr, J. R. (2027b). Human-centered artificial intelligence in health professions education and decision-making: A sociotechnical systems perspective. In Schoenherr, J. R. (eds.), *Fundamentals and Frontiers of Medical Education and Decision-Making: Innovation, Implementation, and Translational Research* (pp. 132–188). Routledge.

Schoenherr, J. R., & Beaudoin, J. (2027). Medical heterarchies in East Asian medical education: the evolving landscape of health professions education in East Asia. In Schoenherr, J. R. (ed.), *Fundamentals and Frontiers of Medical Education and Decision-Making: Innovation, Implementation, and Translational Research* (pp. 462–509). Routledge.

Schoenherr, J. R., & Hamstra, S. J. (2024). Validity in health professions education: from assessment instruments to program innovation and evaluation. In Schoenherr, J. R., & McConnell, M. (eds.), *Fundamentals and Frontiers of Medical Education and Decision-Making: Educational Theory and Psychological Practice*. (pp. 80–107) Routledge.

Schoenherr, J. R., & McConnell, M. M. (2024). Human-Centered Design in Health Professions Education. *Fundamentals and Frontiers of Medical Education and Decision-Making: Educational Theory and Psychological Practice*, 3(1).

Schoenherr, J. R., Chiou, E., & Goldshtein, M. (2023). Building trust with the ethical affordances of education technologies: a sociotechnical systems perspective. In Llinas, *et al.* (eds.), *Putting AI in the Critical Loop* (pp. 127–165). Elsevier.

Schoenherr, J. R., & Le Bouar, C. (2024). Communication in healthcare settings: from normal interpersonal processes to social networks during health crises. In Schoenherr, J. R., & McConnell, M. (eds.), *Fundamentals and Frontiers of Medical Education and Decision-Making: Educational Theory and Psychological Practice* (pp. 270–312). Routledge.

Scott-Emuakpor, A. (2010). The evolution of health care systems in Nigeria: which way forward in the twenty-first century. *Nigerian Medical Journal*, *51*(2).

Sewankambo, N. K., & Donkor, P. (2018). Linkage of the medical education partnership initiative (MEPI) and the nursing education partnership initiative (NEPI) to the African forum for research and education in health (AFREhealth). *Annals of Global Health*, *84*(1), 1.

Smego Jr, R. A., D'Alessandri, R. M., Linger, B., Hunt, V. A., Ryan, J., Monnier, J., ... & Thompson, W. (2010). Anatomy of a new US medical school: the commonwealth medical college. *Academic Medicine*, *85*(5), 881–888.

Ssennyonjo, A., Van Belle, S., Ssengooba, F., Titeca, K., Bakubi, R., & Criel, B. (2022). Not for us, without us: examining horizontal coordination between the ministry of health and other sectors to advance health goals in Uganda. *Health Policy and Planning*, *37*(10), 1221–1235.

Talib, Z., Narayan, L., & Harrod, T. (2019). Postgraduate medical education in sub-Saharan Africa: a scoping review spanning 26 years and lessons learned. *Journal of Graduate Medical Education*, *11*(4s), 34–46.

Taslakian, E. N., Garber, K., & Shekherdimian, S. (2022). Diaspora engagement: a scoping review of diaspora involvement with strengthening health systems of their origin country. *Global Health Action*, *15*(1), 2009165.

Tegally, H., San, J. E., Cotten, M., Moir, M., Tegomoh, B., Mboowa, G., ... & Schubert, G. (2022). The evolving SARS-CoV-2 epidemic in Africa: insights from rapidly expanding genomic surveillance. *Science*, *378*(6615), eabq5358.

ten Cate, T. J. O., Snell, L., & Carraccio, C. (2010). Medical competence: the interplay between individual ability and the health care environment. *Medical Teacher*, *32*(8), 669–675.

Toyin-Thomas, P., Ikhurionan, P., Omoyibo, E. E., Iwegim, C., Ukueku, A. O., Okpere, J., ... & Wariri, O. (2023). Drivers of health workers' migration, intention to migrate and non-migration from low/middle-income countries, 1970–2022: a systematic review. *BMJ Global Health*, *8*(5), e012338.

Van der Merwe, L. J., Van Zyl, G. J., Gibson, A. S. C., Viljoen, A., Iputo, J. E., Mammen, M., ... & Volmink, J. (2016). South African medical schools: current state of selection criteria and medical students' demographic profile. *South African Medical Journal*, *106*(1), 76–81.

Wartman, S. A., & Combs, C. D. (2019). Reimagining medical education in the age of AI. *AMA Journal of Ethics*, *21*, E146–E152.

Willcox, M. L., Peersman, W., Daou, P., Diakité, C., Bajunirwe, F., Mubangizi, V., ... & Mant, D. (2015). Human resources for primary health care in sub-Saharan Africa: progress or stagnation? *Human Resources for Health, 13*, 1–11.

Wojczewski, S., Poppe, A., Hoffmann, K., Peersman, W., Nkomazana, O., Pentz, S., & Kutalek, R. (2015). Diaspora engagement of African migrant health workers–examples from five destination countries. *Global Health Action, 8*(1), 29210.

World Health Organization (WHO). (2014). Experts discuss improvement of medical education and training in Africa. Retrieved August 23, 2023 from www.afro.who.int/news/experts-discuss-improvement-medical-education-and-training-africa

World Health Organization (WHO). (2022). Global competency and outcomes framework for universal health world health organization. Retrieved August 23, 2023 from www.who.int/publications/i/item/9789240034662

Yaya Bocoum, F., Kouanda, S., Kouyaté, B., Hounton, S., & Adam, T. (2013). Exploring the effects of task shifting for HIV through a systems thinking lens: the case of Burkina Faso. *BMC Public Health, 13*, 1–10.

Zurn, P., Zapata, T., & Okoroafor, S. C. (2021). The importance of strengthening the health workforce in Nigeria to improve health outcomes. *Journal of Public Health, 43*(Supplement 1), i1–i3.

Appendix: List of Websites

1. www.ampltd.co.uk/digital_guides/church_missionary_society_archive_general/editorial%20introduction%20by%20rosemary%20keen.aspx
2. https://saahe.org.za/
3. https://nuc-ccmas.ng/disciplines/
4. www.iie.org/programs/carnegie-african-diaspora-fellowship-program/
5. https://famsanet.org/
6. www.cidmef.u-bordeaux2.fr/
7. https://consams.org/
8. www.fic.nih.gov/programs/Pages/medical-education-africa.aspx
9. https://afrehealth.org/
10. https://chs.mak.ac.ug/page/mesau
11. www.open.ac.uk/africa/heat/resources/case-studies/ibadan-university-msc-biomedical-education-nigeria
12. www.faimer.org/faimer-regional-institutes/
13. https://uis.unesco.org/sites/default/files/documents/financing-education-in-sub-saharan-africameeting-the-challenges-of-expansion-equity-and-quality-en_0.pdf
14. https://sdgs.un.org/goals
15. www.assapa.org/
16. https://unesdoc.unesco.org/query?q=Conference:%20%22International%20Conference%20on%20Academic%20Freedom%20and%20University%20Autonomy,%20Sinaia,%20Romania,%201992%22&sf=sf:*
17. https://unesdoc.unesco.org/query?q=Corporate:%20%22UNESCO%20European%20Centre%20for%20Higher%20Education%22&sf=sf:*

12

THE EVOLVING LANDSCAPE OF HEALTH PROFESSIONS EDUCATION IN EAST ASIA

Heterarchies in East Asian Medicine and Medical Education

Jordan Richard Schoenherr and Jenna Beaudoin

12.1 Introduction

A key assumption of accreditation of health professions education is that standardization is necessary to ensure the practitioners can provide effective and consistent care to patients. Competency-based medical education (CBME) provides a seemingly straightforward means to achieve this: competencies are identified, milestones are created, and education interventions and assessment instruments are developed to monitor learner performance (Frank et al., 2010; Hakins et al., 2015; Lockyer et al., 2017; Ma, 2024; Schoenherr et al., 2023; Schoenherr & McConnell, 2026; Schoenherr et al., 2026; Touchie & ten Cate, 2016).

The recent World Health Organization (WHO) (World Health Organization (WHO), 2022) competency-based framework is an ambitious attempt to achieve this on a global scale. By isolating competencies that *all* healthcare professionals (HCPs) should develop and maintain, a common standard could be used across borders to ensure that all practitioners can be assessed using the same standards. However laudable, this perspective risks overlooking regional differences in how local educational traditions and traditional knowledge might compliment, conflict, or compete with biomedical Western medicine (BWM; Schoenherr, 2027a, 2027b). It also disregards critical differences in the availability of resources used to promote health and prevent and treat illnesses.

Without exception, all human populations have developed indigenous healthcare practices (e.g., Abdullahi, 2011; Adhikari & Paul, 2018; Chan et al., 2026; Kananoja, 2021; Murdock, 1980; Murdock et al., 1978; Moore, 1988; Oyebode et al., 2016; Ozioma & Chinwe, 2019; Redvers & Blondin, 2020; Saad et al., 2005; Venosa et al., 2027), many of which continued to be used – or reclaimed – in contemporary societies due to their alignment with folk beliefs, availability of

DOI: 10.4324/9781003498155-12

resources, and comparatively limited cost (Chan et al., 2027). Crucially, rather than being displaced by BWM, these healthcare systems often exist in parallel, creating healthcare ecosystems defined medical pluralism (e.g., Baer et al., 1997/2013; Broom et al., 2009; Kaptchuk & Eisenber, 2001; Stevenson et al., 2003; Schoenherr, 2027b). Regardless of whether HCPs share these beliefs, ensuring effective health communication and adoption of treatment recommendations must account for how attitudes and beliefs affect the adoption of healthcare practices (Schoenherr & Le-Bouar, 2024).

East Asia has one of the longest-lived and well documented healthcare traditions in recorded history. Evolving from informal, unsystematic knowledge and practices shared by non-specialist healers similar to those of other indigenous traditions into formal, systematized knowledge and set of healthcare practices that require training, assessment, and licensure by HCPs. Beyond its potential efficacy, Traditional East Asian Medicine (TEAM) presents a topic of interest to HCPs as it constitutes a distinct, formal system of healthcare delivery and medical education with its own set of practitioners and selection criteria. Due to globalization and migration of the East Asian diaspora, TEAM concepts, therapeutics, and practices have been adopted outside their societies of origin. By acknowledging the features of TEAM, it challenges the notion that traditional approaches to healing necessarily represent heterodoxic ethnomedicines (e.g., Baer et al., 1997/2013). Concurrently, TEAM has responded to sociopolitical factors which have shaped how knowledge and social institutions are formally organized (e.g., DiMoia, 2008, 2013; Lo, 2002; Lei, 2014; Soon, 2024; Suh, 2015, 2020; Taylor, 2004).

12.1.1 Overview

In this chapter, we provide a selective review of medical education landscape in East Asia, its historical development, and consider associated modern practices. Collectively, these countries reflect unique, interrelated pluralistic systems that include both heterogeneous folk medicines and formal TEAM systems that precede and parallel BWM[1] systems. How the comparatively recent introduction of BWM knowledge and practices have been assimilated and accommodated by the diverse populations within East Asia provides insight into the social networks and practices of healthcare.

In Section 12.2, the general process of cultural evolution is described with a review of studies that have identified how procedural and declarative knowledge have been transmitted in East Asian healing traditions. In Section 12.3, a historical review of informal and formal medical knowledge is provided for China, Japan, Korea (North and South), Taiwan, and Vietnam to illustrate how individual approaches to TEAM have emerged – and merged – within this region. This overview highlights different approaches to the integration of TEAM and BWM that range from relatively distinct, parallel systems to a fully integrated system. This review is supplemented with a quantitative analysis to demonstrate the relative use of TEAM and BWM. The chapter concludes by briefly noting that the view that BWM has dominated in East Asian ignores historical precedence and oversimplifies how TEAM and BWM relate to one another in each country.

12.2 East Asia Therapeutic Traditions: Transmission and Socialization

Cultural evolution is a ubiquitous process, wherein behaviors, beliefs, conventions, and technological and social innovations are adopted within a population (Boyd & Richerson, 1996; Henrich & McElreath, 2003; Henrich et al., 2008; Jablonka & Lamb, 2014; Mesoudi et al., 2006; Morgan et al., 2015). Adoption of innovations can occur for numerous reasons, including an understanding of the functional affordance[2] of the innovation, blind imitation of group members, or due to the symbolic value of possessing and displaying technology, i.e., prestige technologies (Hayden, 1998; Liu, 2017; Schoenherr, 2017) and the healthcare professions education (Schoenherr, 2027a; Schoenherr et al., 2024).

Like all innovations, education innovations must be adapted to sociocultural niches through implementation processes (Schoenherr & Hamstra, 2024). While BWM is often framed as a coherent, evidence-based approach to healthcare, this greatly oversimplifies the reality of how education, research, and practice have emerged within healthcare systems historically (Coburn, 2006; Friedson, 1970/2007; Schoenherr, 2019; Schoenherr & Hamstra, 2017; Starr, 1982). Practitioners and institutions vary in the extent to which they adopt and adapt "standard practices" (Sinclair, 1997) and differ in their diagnoses of diseases (Allison et al., 2014; Drinnan et al., 1998; Millington et al., 2018).[3] Moreover, by reducing patients to their biology and physiology, BWM ignores relevant psychological and cultural dimensions, e.g., affective responses, mental models of illness, and social networks (Borrell-Carrió et al., 2004; Wade et al., 2017; see McConnell, 2024; Schoenherr & Le-Bouar, 2024). If critical dimensions of health and illness are ignored, health seekers might become more dependent on alternative approaches to diagnosis and treatment whether in terms of novel technologies (e.g., websites and mobile phone applications; Schoenherr, 2021, 2022) or alternative healthcare traditions outside of their cultural traditions, i.e., complimentary/alternative medicines or CAM (Ernest, 2000; Frass et al., 2012; Kessler et al., 2001; Tangkiatkumjai et al., 2020; World Health Organization (WHO), 2019).

Rather than focusing on a specific innovation in a particular institution, an understanding of cultural evolution of health professions education requires an examination of the beliefs and practices that are evidenced in different sociocultural contexts. By examining the evolution of indigenous medical education traditions and the specific adoption and adaption of Western indigenous medicine (i.e., BWM) in East Asia countries, greater insight can be obtained concerning the factors affecting health professions education and healthcare delivery.

12.2.1 Traditional Medical Practice and Education: Transmission and Cultural Evolution

Cultural evolution is a defining feature of TEAM and health professions education. For instance, in her work on the social history of Traditional Vietnamese Medicine (TVM), Thompson (2017) identifies division of medicinal categories (*thuốc*) into *thuốc Bắc* and *thuốc Nam,* where *Bắc* means North (and China/Chinese) and *Nam* refers to South (and Vietnam/Vietnamese). Each of these frameworks represents a distinct approach to healthcare, with cultural exchanges flowing between Vietnam to China in terms of knowledge and materia medica (see also Monnais et al., 2011). For instance, remedies used in *thuốc Bắc* tend to require more animal-based ingredients than *thuốc Nam*, with contemporary Vietnamese practitioners attributing the use of animals to the Chinese tradition (Nguyen, 1993). Indeed, changes in TVM and traditional *Chinese* medicine (TCM) can also be attributed to sociopolitical factors (Chee, 2021; Lei, 2014). Moreover, even within China, many different medical traditions exist, suggesting that even TCM is not homogenous tradition (Farquhar & Lai, 2021)[4]. As we will discuss below, a similar pattern of exchange is also evidenced between ancient Korea, Japan, and Taiwan.

As TEAM encountered BWM, it faced many challenges to its legitimacy. Paradigms assume an association between theory, methods, and data (Laudan, 1978). Here, "theory" describes causal relationships in physiological and anatomical systems, energies (e.g., *qi*, chemical/electrical), symptoms, and treatment (Figure 12.1b). As the BWM approach began to provide a more coherent theoretical account of the causal mechanisms of illness and disease, there were increased calls for the rejection of traditional medicine which became *seen as* TCM (e.g., China; Lei, 2014). Rather than eliminating the TCM paradigm, TCM practitioners suggest that while the causal relationships described by the paradigm might be erroneous, the correlation between symptoms and treatment efficacy remained valid.[5] "Symptom differentiation" emerged as an approach to identify the co-occurrence of symptoms which allowed for the selection of an appropriate therapeutics (Figure 12.1a). In this way, medical pluralism can arise by minimizing the inconsistencies created by focusing on divergent causal explanations.

12.3 Comparison of Medical Education Landscape

Health professions education might appear to be a well-demarcated domain. However, it has been influenced by the epistemologies, ontologies, and educational practices and philosophies of the societies it has emerged within. Supporting this, differences have been noted in Eastern and Western modes of knowledge acquisition and perception (for a review, see Henrich, 2020).[6] For instance, Eastern epistemologies approaches are often defined by wholistic/relational perception of the environment and a focus on social and physical context, whereas Western

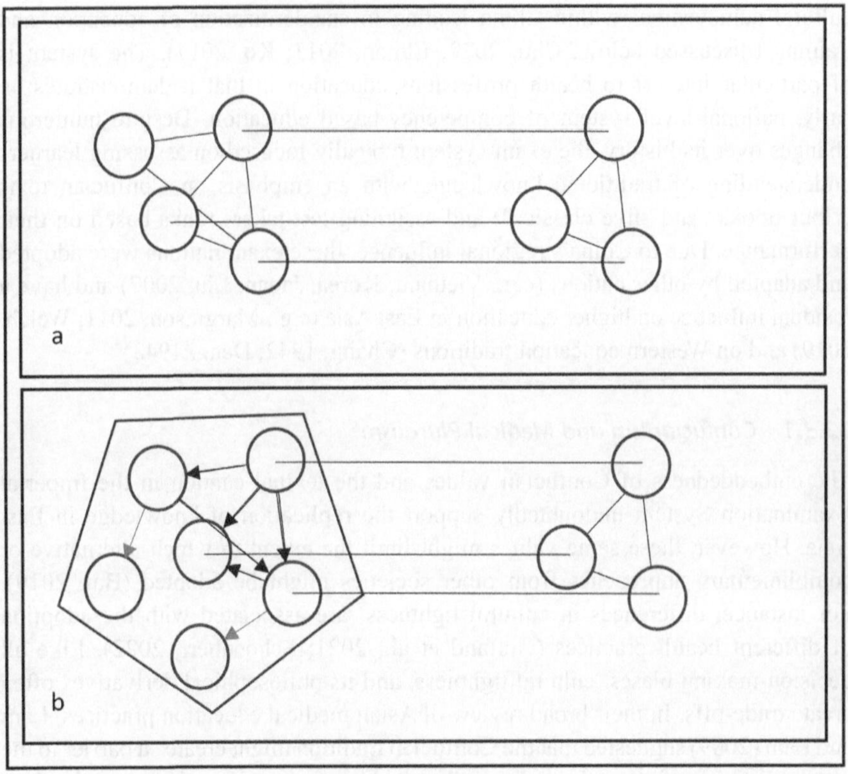

FIGURE 12.1 Models of 'symptom differentiation' and disease. *Symptom differentiation* (a) assume that there are co-occurrences of symptoms (lines). A therapeutic model is selected on experience such as previous trial-and-error from TEAM practitioners. As a correlational model, it does not state the causal relationships between therapeutic efficacy, symptoms, and underlying basis of illness. *Disease models* (b) assumes that there are causal relationships between features of an illness (arrows). Therapeutic model is selected based on causal relationships. As a causal model, it potentially makes predictions of other features that have not been observed. TEAM and Western biomedical models are both described in these terms.

Abstract representation of East Asia medical approach that shows one-to-one mappings of symptoms and features (denoted with circles) and associations (denoted by lines). An abstract representation of BWM approach that prioritizes the integration of features with causal connections (denoted with arrows of solid of shaded lines) and overall theory (denoted by a hexagon boundary).

epistemologies tend to focus on analytic perception, decontextualize information, and the individual (Nisbett, 2004).

Cognitive biases have co-evolved with education philosophies. In East Asia, the Confucian tradition has co-evolved with state-based educational institutions. The Chinese Imperial Civil Service Examination System represents an important cultural achievement within China leading to standardization of education and training (discussed below; Chu, 2022; Elman, 2013; Ko, 2017). The system is of particular interest to health professions education in that it demonstrates an early, national-level system of competency-based education. Despite numerous changes over its history, the exam system typically focused on assessing learners understanding of traditional knowledge, with an emphasis on Confucian texts ("four books" and "five classics") and assigning test-takers ranks based on their performance. Due to China's regional influence, these examinations were adopted and adapted by other nations (e.g., Vietnam, Korea, Japan; Liu, 2007) and have a residual influence on higher education in East Asia (e.g., Marginson, 2011; Welch, 2019) and on Western education traditions (Chang, 1942; Deng, 1943).

12.3.1 Confucianism and Medical Pluralism

The embeddedness of Confucian values and the textual cannon in the Imperial Examination System undoubtedly support the replication of knowledge in East Asia. However, these same values might limit the extent to which alternative or complimentary approaches from other societies might be adopted (Bai, 2019). For instance, differences in cultural tightness[7] are associated with the adoption of different health practices (Gelfand et al., 2021; Schoenherr, 2022). Like all decision-making biases, cultural tightness, and its philosophical derivatives often create trade-offs. In their broad review of Asian medical education practices, Lam and Lam (2009) suggested that the Confucian tradition might create "a barrier to the implementation of education reforms," as its basis is "rote learning, examination-oriented mindset, and the superior status of the teacher" (p. 1313; see also Bai, 2010; Lam et al., 2006). As teacher-centered learning is the dominant educational paradigm, learner-centered educational innovations might not be as well received, i.e., cultural scaffolding (LeBel et al., 2018; O'Regan et al., 2016; Schoenherr et al., 2027).

The introduction of collaborative learning activities such as problem-based learning (PBL) into the medical education curriculum in East Asia provides an illustration. Commentators have suggested that the low rate of adoption of PBL is attributable to educators having issues effectively integrating it into the curriculum (Chen et al., 2017), resulting in PBL being used as a supplementary instructional method (Liu et al., 2005). Nevertheless, even if PBL as a method has been implemented in a modified form, it does suggest that educational practices are adapted and, as we note below, pluralistic medical traditions can combine methods from both TEAM and BWM.

12.3.2 Pluralistic Health Professions Education Systems of East Asia

A healthcare *system* is defined by organizations, institutions, resources, and people who activities are dedicated to improving health. For instance, Chi et al. (1996)

notes in a discussion of TEAM in Taiwan, a healthcare system is defined by (1) systematic health knowledge and technology, (2) HCPs who possess and use health knowledge and technology, and (3) dedicated resources for healthcare use and delivery such as drugs and equipment. Thus, pluralistic medicine is evidenced when distinct collections of these practices (paradigms) are present in a single healthcare ecosystem (Wagstaff, 2007).

When BWM arrived in East Asia, it was one of many possible therapeutic approaches in a diverse healthcare ecosystem (e.g., Ayurveda; Jaiswal & Williams, 2017). In contrast to the rootless BWM system, TEAM had well-established methods, educational institutions, and accreditation system.[8] With the existence of two distinct paradigms, a heterarchical structure has emerged.[9] While not explicitly framed as heterarchies, pluralistic medical systems have been described with similar attributes (e.g., Baer & Coulter, 2008; Bourhealut & Mulvale, 2006; Coburn, 2006; Ernst, 2002; Khan, 2006; Kleinman, 1980; Schoenherr, 2027b; Stevenson et al., 2003; Whalberg, 2007).

With the recognition of the WHO that indigenous medical traditions play an important role in healthcare delivery by increasing access to health services, utilizing local resources, and promoting self-sufficiency in less developed countries (World Health Organization (WHO), 2019), there is an increased drive to integrate BWM and traditional medicines. However, traditional approaches to healthcare are often placed in subordinate relationships to BWM. For instance, Baer et al. (1997/2013) claim that

> biomedicine enjoys *a dominant status* over heterodox and ethnomedical systems. The dominant status is legitimatized by laws that give biomedicine *a monopoly* over certain medical practices and limit or prohibit the practice of other types of healing. Various heterodox medical systems… may have their own professional associations, schools, hospitals, and clinics and thus *replicate* the organizational structure of biomedicine.
>
> *(p. 48–49; italics added)*

This account suggests that even when medical pluralism is observable, that indigenous approaches to healthcare are subordinate to BWM. Moreover, the replication of BWM structures implies that the BWM approach is the principal influence for the organization of indigenous approaches to healthcare. A comparison of the number of BWM practitioners relative to TEAM could be interpreted to support such an assertion (for reviews, see Fan et al., 2012; He et al., 2022; Park et al., 2016). However, this misrepresents how these healthcare education and delivery systems have evolved, interacted, and blended over time. For instance, China's centralized examination systems including TCM, and its influences elsewhere in East Asia, demonstrate that BWM is not the sole or primary influence for the development of healthcare traditions. In parallel, the persistence of other indigenous medical traditions in China (Farquhar & Lai, 2021) and heterogeneity of TEAM suggest that the BWM dominance does not accurately represent the realities of healthcare ecosystems in East Asia.

As we will demonstrate below, medical pluralism in contemporary East Asia takes on a variety of forms. However, there are several consistent features. In their survey of TEAM practices in China, Japan, Korea, and Taiwan, Park et al. (2016) note that they all require a national licensing exam. The need for licensure clearly demonstrates legitimated national systems in these countries, reflecting a heterarchical structure. For instance, a review of South Korean health information seeking behavior also demonstrates that folk psychological, faith healing, and shamanistic rituals are used in conjunction or can be used to replace BWM (Han et al., 2018; Kim, 1999; Ock et al., 2009; Park et al., 2019), although there can be tension concerning the ambiguous legitimacy of some of these practices (e.g., Yun, 2019; for a broad survey in Asia, see Rhi et al., 1995). Moreover, at the level of formal institutions, the healthcare systems of China, South Korea, and Taiwan as "dual" healthcare systems where TEAM and BWM occur in parallel whereas Japan represents a unified system where traditional medicine (*kanpo*) is integrated with BWM (Na, 2012; for discussion of attempted integrate of TEAM and BWM, see Dobos & Tao, 2011; Eisenberg, 2011; Lei, 2014; Xu & Yang, 2009; Yoon & Kim, 2013).

Contemporary accounts have also suggested that while the causal model provided by TEAM is incorrect, the pragmatic value of the relationship between symptoms and therapy retains considerable value (Figure 12.1). Thus, we suggest that Baer et al.'s (1997/2013) account notably ignores (or misinterprets) the East Asia models of healthcare education and delivery that existed before the colonial era and have adapted to – rather than replicated – the BWM approach (Figure 12.2).

To simplify the analysis, we define healthcare systems reviewed in this chapter along three dimensions: structural permeability, regulatory centralization, and institutional stability. *Structural permeability* defines the degree to which formal mechanisms allow practitioners to access resources, credentials, or diagnostic tools across paradigms. *Regulatory centralization* defines the degree to which a single accreditation authority governs both TEAM and BWM. Finally, *institutional stability* defines the degree to which the relationship between TEAM and BWM reflects settled equilibrium versus active institutional competition. Stability is evidenced by the absence of documented inter-professional legitimacy disputes, state-managed practitioner categories, and consistent policy direction, while instability by practitioner grievances, contested licensing equivalence, and sustained reform pressure (for a comparable history in the US, see Starr, 1982). Combining these dimensions produces six observable dimensional clusters that describe the East Asian countries considered here.

In an analogous manner to population migration (Figure 12.3), we assume that the ideas that define TEAM have diffused across a large geographic region as humans have adapted their behavior and social organization to the environment.

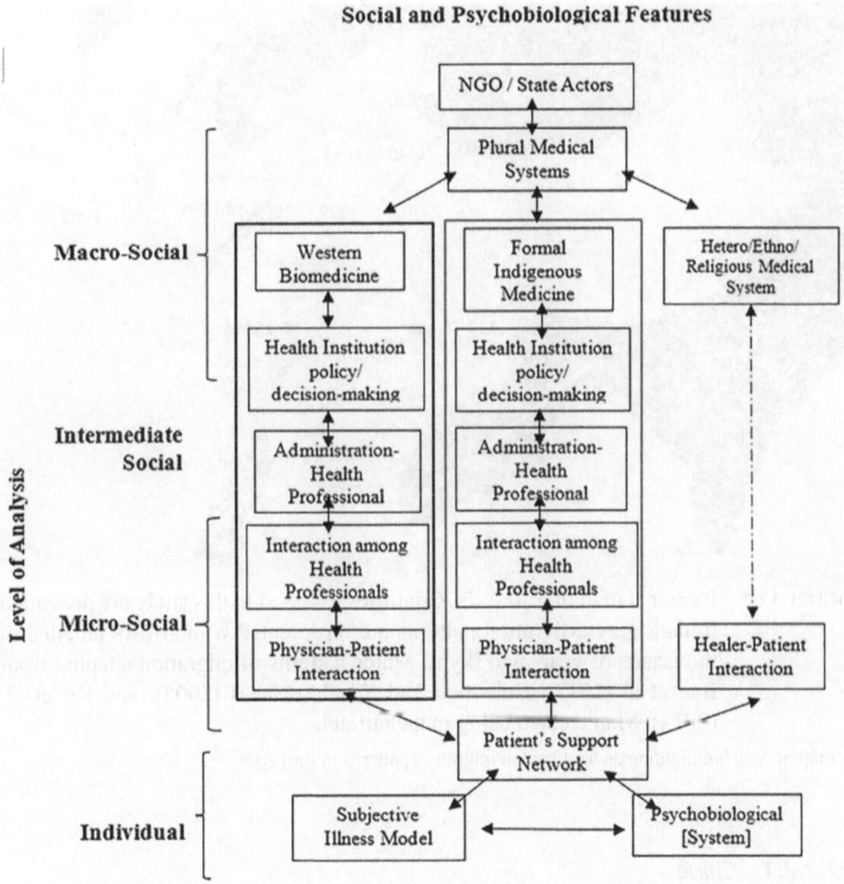

FIGURE 12.2 Levels of health systems. Adapted and modified from Baer et al. (2013) to include formalized healthcare systems beyond that of Western biomedicine (left). The black border demarcating the BWM represents low-permeability approach whereas grey border demarcating the formal indigenous medicine (here, TEAM) represents a semi-permeable approach (middle).

A diagram demonstrating the levels of health systems. Three systems are shown, represented in three vertical structures: Western biomedicine (left), formal indigenous system (e.g., TEAM), and folk medical approach (right).

In the next section, we review evidence from the evolution of TEAM education and practices in five regions to illustrate the process of assimilation and accommodation of the BWM approach. As a comprehensive review would constitute another volume, we selectively emphasize similarities and differences between each regional TEAM approach.

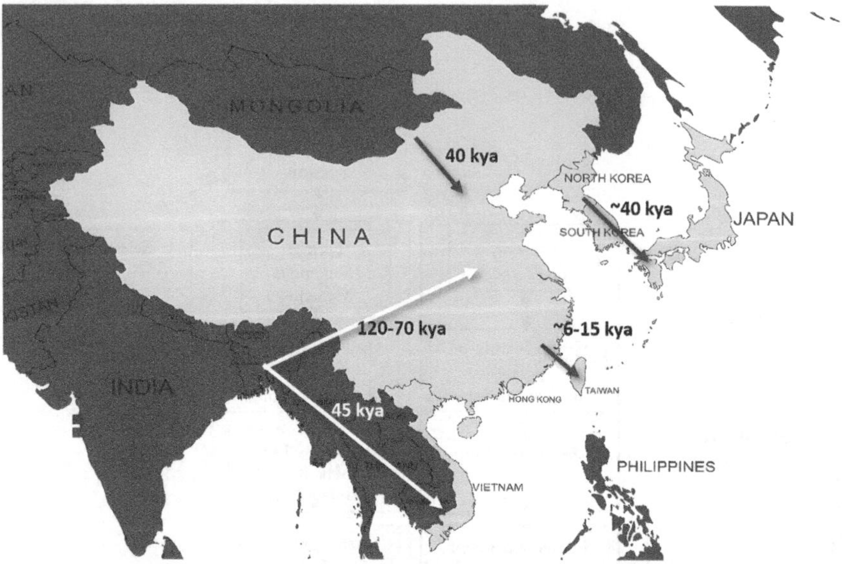

FIGURE 12.3 Regional map of East Asia. Countries assessed in this study are presented in dark grey. Migration patterns are represented with arrows labelled in thousands of years ago (kya). Major patterns of migration adapted from Bae et al (2017), Bellwood and SanchezMazas (2005), and Ko et al. (2014). Map created using mapchart.net.

A map of Asia highlighting ancient human migration patterns in East Asia.

12.3.2.1 China

Despite attempts at progressive centralization of power, considerable regional diversity has been – and continues to be – evidenced within China's geopolitical boundaries (e.g., Blum & Jensen, 2002). Consequently, "Traditional Chinese Medicine" (TCM) is best understood as an aggregate of numerous regional cultural innovations that have been adopted and adapted inside and outside of China (Hinrichs, & Barnes, 2022; Farquhar & Lai, 2021; Liming et al., 2015; Park et al., 2012),[10] with the "*Chinese*" framing of TEAM representing a comparatively recent nationalistic trend in response to the expansion of BWM into China and the complimentary benefit of reinforcing a national identity (Chee, 2021; Lei, 2014; 4).[11] Thus, we use the term TCM in this section to refer to the practices that occurred within ancient and contemporary China while acknowledge that many subcultures and neighboring societies have influenced TCM. We discuss these influences in subsequent sections.

BOX 12.1 BASIC FORCES WITHIN TEAM

The central assumption of the Ying-Yang doctrine is that two complimentary forces must remain in *balance* in the universe. *Yin* is described as a passive force (rest) associated with cold, whereas *Yang* is described as active force (movement) associated with heat, both aspects of *qi*. They exist within a dynamic state rather than being separable forces. The influence of ying and yang is seen as cyclical, within the universe, seasonally, in the shift from day to night, and in the body. A healthy state is defined as someone who has yin and yang in balance, with illness attributed to an imbalance. Yet, despite the prioritization of balance, considerable weight is given to cures that are gradual and long-lasting (aligning with *yin*) rather than those that are rapid and destabilize the system (aligning with *yang*; e.g., Kwan, 2002; Lam, 2001). This basic approach is also observed in other distal cultures (e.g., for a discussion in its relation to Mesoamerica, see Schoenherr, 2027b).[12]

The *Wuxing* doctrine assumes that all substances can be classified into five elements, representing phases of matter ordered from wood, fire, earth, metal, to water. Each organ of the body is associated with these elements/states: liver, heart, spleen, lung, and kidney, respectively. Therapeutic techniques often take the form of promotion of the function of one organ by facilitating the one preceding it in the cycle (e.g., liver-wood promotes heart-fire) or address restraint of subsequent functions (e.g., liver-wood restrains spleen-earth). This approach is prescriptive for the world outside the body: an emphasis on plants and herbs. The interconnectedness of the natural world and the human body consequently places greater emphasis on the preservation of environment.

12.3.3 TEAM and TCM Epistemological Framework

TEAM and TCM can be considered a family resemblance structure,[13] with practitioners subscribing to many – but not necessarily all – knowledge and practices. The core medical practices of TEAM and TCM include herbal medicine, acupuncture, moxibustion, and (less frequently) religious and spiritual healing. Paralleling these practices, an explanatory model emerged that accounted for, and informed, the success of TCM methods. Two major frameworks inform the illness models of TCM and other approaches to TEAM: the *ying-yang* (阴阳学说) and *Wuxing* Xueshuo (Five Elements/Phases Doctrine; 五行学说; see Box 12.1). This information was formalized in a series of texts, starting with the Yellow Emperor's Inner Cannon (黄帝内經).

While an explanatory framework might suggest an emphasis on internal coherence and consistency, these recommendations are viewed in more pragmatic terms, leading to inconsistencies in application and recommendations for reformulation of the relationships based on empirical research (Deng, 1988). Like many theoretical frameworks, the *ying-yang* and *wuxing* doctrines are best viewed "not as immutable laws, but as *heuristic* models found from clinical experience to be useful guides for diagnosis and therapy" (Hong, 2014; p. 121; italics in original). The pragmatism of this approach has undoubtedly been influenced by the awareness of, and challenges from, the introduction of other therapeutic traditions (e.g., Ayurveda, BWM), with evidence suggesting that less emphasis is placed on some of these distinctions in other forms of TEAM (e.g., Zhuang Medicine; Farquhar & Lai, 2021).

12.3.4 Professionalization and Education

Like all traditional medicines, healers initially acquired knowledge and practiced through informal channels (Schoenherr, 2027b). However, professionalization emerged with the creation of Imperial China's medical bureau which not only served the imperial palace but also provided healthcare services for the state (Leung, 1987; Needham & Lu, 1962; cf. Aricanli, 2013). Starting in the Northern Wei (386–534 CE) and continuing into the Song Dynasty (960–1279 CE), medical education grew into a formalized, state-wide system including a medical examination system, referred to as the Imperial Medical Service (Taiyiju 太醫局). Later, the Imperial Academy of Medicine established three levels of examination including monthly quizzes, quarterly exams, and a joint exam held at six-year interval (Chang, 2015). Like the Imperial Civil Service Examination, it provided a pathway to acquire and maintain status within Chinese society.

In addition to the exchanges with other societies in East Asia (discussed below), BWM and associated educational institutions were introduced into China in the early 1900s including the creation of the Shanghai German Medical Hall in 1907, Peking Union Medical College in 1912, and Private West China Union Medical College in 1914 (Jin et al., 2020).

The adoption of BWM in 1929 by the Chinese state created a significant risk to traditional practitioners when the government threatened to abolish TEAM. This external threat galvanized TCM practitioners, who advocated for their practices and profession they referred to as *guoyi* (國醫; National Medicine; Lei, 2014). In addition to formal channels, individual agents also continued to influence the introduction and status of BWM. During the war between communist and nationalist forces, Canadian doctor Norman Bethune worked as a battlefield surgeon for communist forces while they fought against the invasion of Imperial Japan during the Pacific War (Ross & Del Maestro, 2023). His contribution to battlefield medicine in China continues to be respected and commemorated by the Chinese government (Figure 12.4).

Following the conclusion of the civil war in 1949 (Kucherenko & Schoenherr, 2027), the People's Republic of China adopted the Soviet model of medical education which included both independent medical schools as well as the

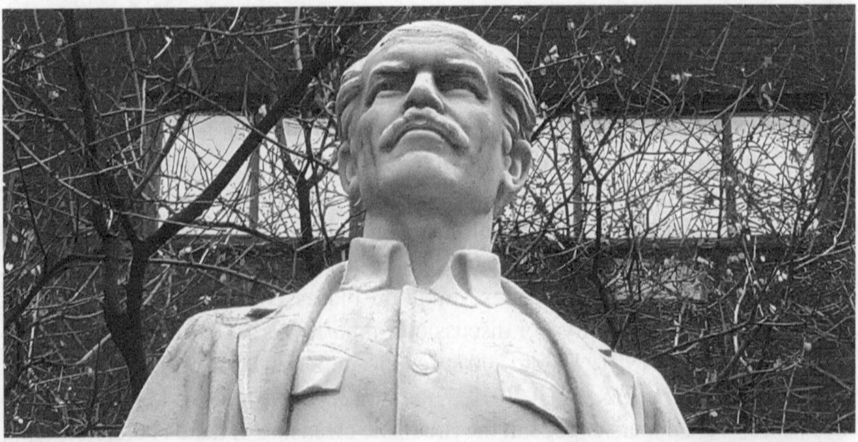

FIGURE 12.4 Statue of Norman Bethune in his communist uniform. Downtown Montréal, Québec, Canada. Photo Credit to Jordan Richard Schoenherr.

A statue of Norman Bethune, underneath trees.

Feldsher system, an alternative, shorter, and lower-level education for medical practitioners (Hsieh et al., 2019). This progress was interrupted by the Cultural Revolution (1966–1976). Practitioners referred to as "barefoot doctors" who were often farmers with basic medical knowledge became the primary healers during this time. By 1998, education reform resumed, and stand-alone medical institutions were merged into comprehensive universities to increase the number of qualified physicians (Wang, 2021; Wu et al., 2014; Zhu et al., 2016).

In the decades that followed, China has achieved several key medical education milestones. In 2008, a clinical medical education accreditation process was established, and in 2013 the government launched a plan to standardize the quality of medical education (Wang, 2021). The new education model includes five years of undergraduate education followed by three years of residency (Hsieh et al., 2019). China has also become more integrated within the global community of medical educators.[14] In 2020, China joined the international medical accreditation circle when the World Federation for Medical Education (WFME) recognized China's Committee for the Accreditation of Medical Education (Wang, 2021).

After millennia of evolution, pluralism is explicitly represented in the Chinese medical landscape. Chinese physicians can be divided into four categories: Western clinical medicine, dental, TCM, and public health. Rather than formal syncretism, the boundaries between these approaches to healthcare are maintained, defining a heterarchical structure: a medical practitioner in one category can not practice outside the bounds of their domain (Young & Garro, 1982; Zhang et al., 2020). Thus, while health seekers might have the ability to choose from among different healthcare traditions, distinct accreditation and regulatory systems maintain different groups of healers.

12.3.4.1 Japan

The islands of Japan were populated by multiple waves of colonist from the Korean peninsula and modern-day China via the Eastern Sea/Sea of Japan. Continued exchanges through the peninsula over millennia led to the transfer of TEAM knowledge, referred to as *kanpo* (*kan* = Chinese; *po* = medicine), as well as Confucianism and Buddhism.

Japan's indigenous religion, Shintoism, is an animistic belief system based on the worship of ancestors (*kami*). Torii gates and shrines denote areas of specific spiritual importance (Figure 12.5). Japanese tradition places considerable importance of physical and spiritual purity (for discussions of purity across cultures, see Douglas, 1966/2003; Fiske, 1991; Haidt, 2007; for the importance of purity in Japan and East Asia, see Burgess & Horii, 2012; Kitamura & Matsuo, 2021; Lee et al., 2015). In shrines, worshippers engage in the ritualistic cleansing of hands before entering. Worshippers can also purchase items (e.g., talismans and masks) to ward off evil spirits around them or in their homes (Figure 12.5).

Unlike Western epistemologies which tend to be comparatively analytic, reductive, and homogenous, Japanese and other East Asian epistemologies tend to be wholistic, integrative and pluralistic, or syncretic. Like other forms of TEAM, the emphasis in *kanpo* is on the health seeker outcomes, with individuals adopting practices liberally from secular and sacred sources, e.g., BWM, Shinto birth ritual, and Buddhist death ritual. Indeed, *kanpo* is influenced by other TEAM traditions, especially TCM (Lock, 1980a, 1980b; Ohnuki-Tierney, 1981, 1984). Conjointly, these traditions influenced healthcare practices in *kanpo* (Goble, 2011; Trambaiolo, 2013).

12.3.5 Professionalization and Education

BWM was introduced as a result of trade with the Portuguese and Spanish through Nagasaki, with German medicine and education being introduced later (Bowers, 1970, 1979, 1980; Hashimoto, 2013; Kim, 2014). By 1870, BWM was available in Japan following the establishment of the first government-run Western-style medical school, Daigaku To-ko (Eastern College; Onishi, 2018). Prior to the creation of BWM institutions, students who wished to become a doctor could do so by either becoming an apprentice to a practitioner of *kanpo*, or by studying medical texts under a doctor- or Confucian-scholar (Chen et al., 2017). In 1884, *The Regulation of Physician Licensing* (医師免許規則) was promulgated in Japan, requiring that all medical professionals graduate from a medical school or pass a licensing exam (Fujimoto, 1884). As the Japanese empire spread, Western healthcare norms and conventions were brought with it (see Taiwan; Section 12.3.5.3).

Japan's defeat and subsequent occupation by the U.S. at the end of Pacific War accelerated the adoption of Western medical paradigms and practices. In the postwar era, Japan's focus was on reforming and standardizing medical education, establishing a post-graduate system, accrediting medical institutions,

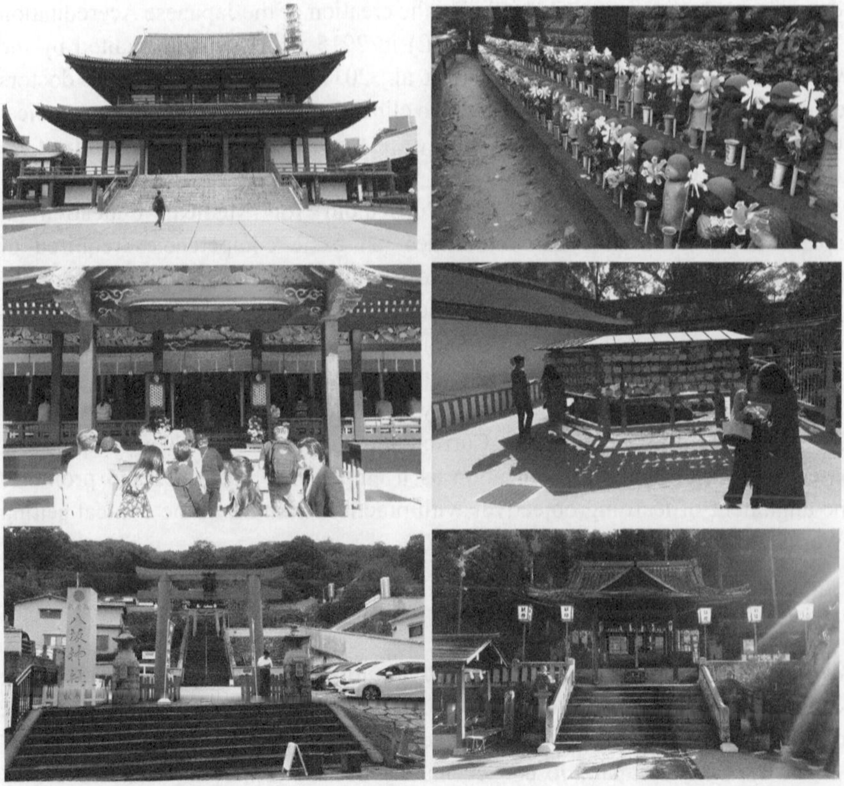

FIGURE 12.5 First row: Portions of the imperial Shinto Temple complex, Tokyo Japan. Second row: Shinto ceremony (left) and prayer cards (right), Dazaifu Tenmangu Shrine, Fukuoka, Japan. Third row: Shinto shrines. Entrances ways are typically marked with a tori. Nagasaki, Japan. Fourth row: Talisman and incense from Imperial Temple (Tokyo; left) and miniature mask (Daizafu; right). Photo credit author: Jordan Richard Schoenherr.

Portions of the imperial Shinto Temple complex, Tokyo Japan. Second row: Shinto ceremony and prayer cards, Dazaifu Tenmangu Shrine, Fukuoka, Japan. Third row: Shinto shrines. Entrances ways are typically marked with a tori. Nagasaki, Japan. Fourth row: Talisman and incense from Imperial Temple (Tokyo) and miniature mask (Daizafu).

and improving specialty training quality (Onishi, 2018). Starting in 1967, health insurance coverage also included *kampo*, initially only including four medicines. Today, coverage has expanded to over 148 prescriptions (Motoo et al., 2011).

Kanpo education was integrated into the curriculum of all 80 medical schools in Japan by 2005 (Moschik et al., 2012; Motoo et al., 2011; Muramatsu et al., 2012). As a major world economic power, Japan's health system is also tightly coupled with global trends in healthcare and education. For instance, in 2010 when the U.S. announced new requirements for foreign doctors, Japan reviewed its medical education evaluation system. This led to the creation of the Japanese Accreditation Council for Medical Education (JACME) in 2015 which was accredited by the WFME in 2017 (Onishi, 2018; Saiki et al., 2017). Currently, Japanese doctors require six years (four pre-clinical and two clinical years) of undergraduate medical education (UGME) as well as two years of post-graduate residency (Honda et al., 2022; Kozu, 2006).

The most recent Model Core Curriculum for Medical Education in Japan was released in 2022. It outlines ten basic competencies required of physicians: professionalism (respect diversity and humanity), generalism (multi-systemic view), lifelong learning, research (scientific innovation), problem-solving (using evidence-based medicine), making use of information technology, communication (building good relationships with patients), interprofessional collaboration, and medicine in society (striving to provide equitable care). Unsurprisingly, this Model Core Curriculum is consistent with a competency-based approach to medical education as it emphasizes outcomes and promotes the alignment of learning objectives with practical training in the clinical setting (World Health Organization (WHO), 2022).

12.3.5.1 Korea

Korea's early history is largely defined by multiple co-existing states, e.g., Three Kingdom's Period, North-South States Period. Following the overthrow of the long-lived Goryeo Dynasty (918 CE), the Joseon Dynasty was established (1392–1897 CE). Like Vietnam, Joseon eventually became a tributary state to China, while being effectively autonomous. The frequent and early exchanges between Korea and China often make it difficult to disentangle the unique contributions of Traditional Korean Medicine (TKM)[15] to TEAM due to limited early records (Kim, 1981). However, like other forms of TEAM, TKM developed distinctive features over time (Cha et al., 2007). For instance, some archaeological evidence has been interpreted as suggesting that acupuncture therapeutic models and techniques first emerged in ancient Korea (Kang & Cha, 2017; Yim et al., 2009)[16] although these instruments and medical knowledge (e.g., herbal medicine) might have only been recorded, adapted, and systematized later in China (Kang, 2011; see Figure 12.6).

As TCM texts reached the Korean peninsula, practitioners began to systematically document and adapt TEAM to local conditions, culminating in the publication of two medical treatises (Figure 12.7).[17] By the 17th century, TKM had developed a *constitutional medicine* approach that recognized individual differences, such that the same disease can require different treatments in different individuals, i.e., personalized medicine (Cha et al., 2007).

12.3.6 Professionalization and Education

During increasingly formalized exchanges between China and Korean societies, TEAM diffused into Korea through medical texts and practitioners, with

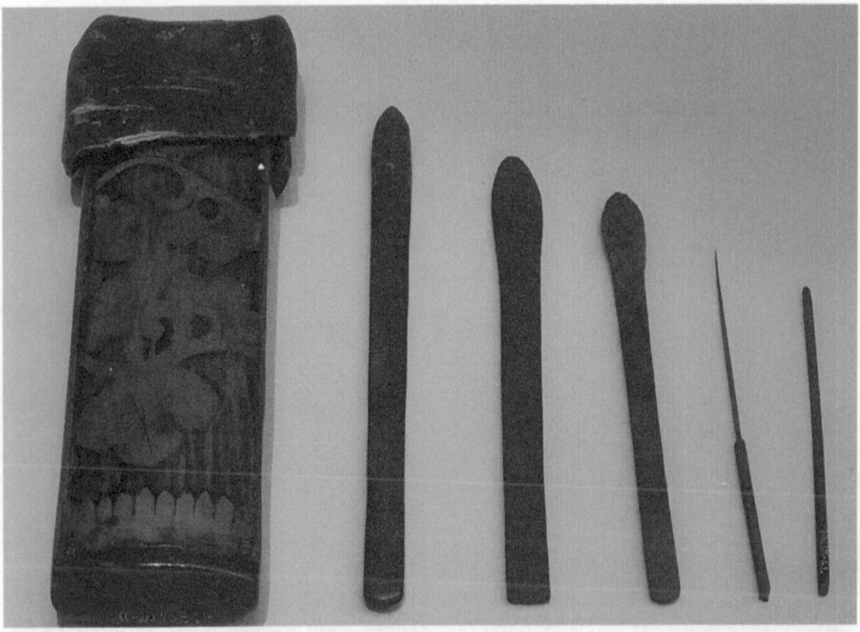

FIGURE 12.6 Acupuncture needle case (left) and acupuncture needles (right). Needles are inserted into key locations in the body as a form of therapy, typically used for pain relief and to stimulate natural responses of the body to illness. Photo credit Jeung Soyoung.

Acupuncture needle case with embossed features on the left and acupuncture needles of varied sizes and structures on the right.

practitioners in the Silla kingdom adapting the medical education knowledge and system of the Chinese Tang dynasty (Kim, 1981). As early as 692 CE in the Silla kingdom, medical education became formalized ("Uihak / 醫學"; Oh & Shin, 2023). Early texts (*History of Goryeo*; 高麗史) suggest that medical education and stated-based examination were occurring as early as the 11th century (Maeng, 2006).

Following the model established by the Goryeo kingdom, the Korean state founded the Bureau of Royal Medicine (*Jeon Eui Gam*; 전의감) in 1392 CE, investing it with the responsibility of administrating education and practice of medicine for the Royal Family. During the Joseon Dynasty, healthcare practitioners could receive training in state or private clinics. From the outset, a medical licensing examination (*uigwa*; 우이와) was established and continued until 1894, requiring completion of two stages to formally practice. However, outside of services to the royal court, healers were not required to pass formal examinations (Han et al., 2016; Kim, 2013; Lee, 2015). While a comparatively modern TKM medical school (*Donje*) was created in 1904, it was discontinued in 1907 (Pyo, 1987).

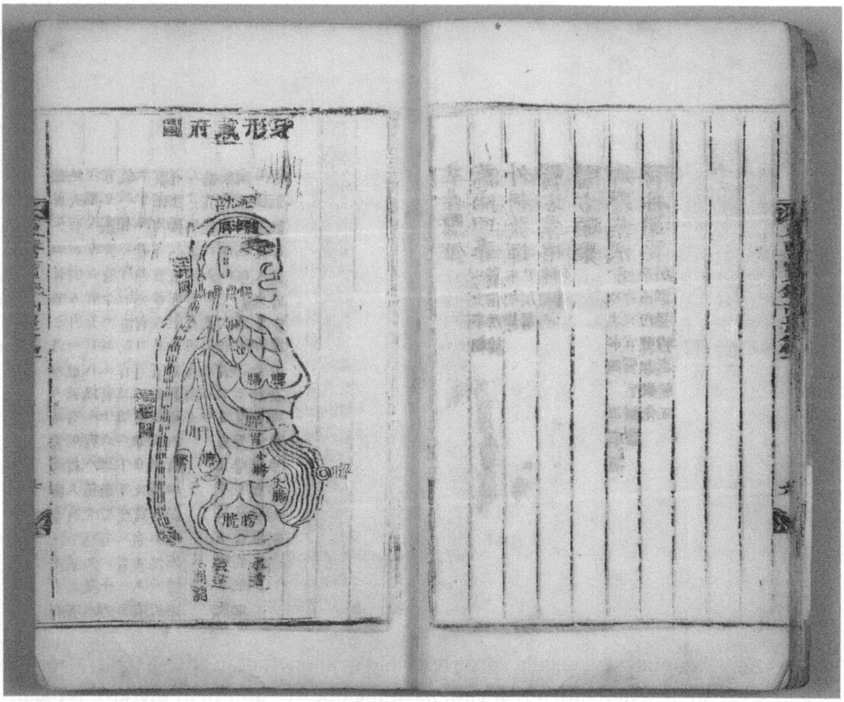

FIGURE 12.7 Dongeuibogam, National Museum of Korea, Seoul, South Korea.

Source: Photo from the Korean National Archive.

Interior to of the Dongeuibogam showing an abstract illustration of the internal structure of the human body.

Starting in 1905 following their victory over Russia, Japan began to exert increasing influence over the Korean peninsula, culminating in the annexation of the short-lived Korean Empire. By 1910, TKM was prohibited during the Imperial Japanese occupation, with BWM promoted by Japan. Following the defeat of Imperial Japan in 1945, the United States and Soviet Union partitioned Korea into North and South, and Korea's indigenous medical tradition resumed albeit in different forms. After North Korea's unsuccessful invasion of South Korea in 1950, a deep divide was created in the education and practice of TKM with the demilitarized zone as its physical instantiation.

12.3.6.1 South Korea

Contemporary medical education in S. Korea is defined by two separate, parallel healthcare services based on TKM[18] and BWM, respectively. Following the end of the Pacific War, TKM was renewed with the establishment of Dongyang Daehakwan (later, Dongyang College) in 1947 (Han et al., 2016). Despite being based on the traditional apprenticeship model, contemporary TKM's curriculum is defined by lectures, specialized courses, and hospital practicums that resemble BWM practices. TKM practitioners are additionally required to learn BWM clinical skills.

BWM was introduced to Korea through China and Japan, with the first BWM medical schools and hospitals open at the turn of the millennium (Lee & Kee, 1996). A period a rapid economic reform and grow between the 1970s and 1990s in S. Korea was paralleled with a growth in the number of medical schools, with over 40 medical schools currently in operation (World Health Organization (WHO), 2015). In 1994, the Korea Institute of Oriental Medicine was created for the conduct of TKM research, followed by the Bureau of TKM and Ministry of Health and Welfare (MOHW) in 1997 (Han et al., 2016). However, while TKM programs exist, Pusan National University School of Korean Medicine is the only department specifically dedicated to TKM. Consequently, healthcare education in S. Korea is defined by a pluralistic system, one that is largely dominated by BWM.

The rapid increase in the number of educational institutions led to a need for quality assurance, with the government recommending a restructuring of medical education into a four-year undergraduate program and a four-year graduate program (Ministry of Education and Human Resources, 2002). Not all institutions adopted this recommendation, resulting in three institutional approaches: a *six-year undergraduate system* defined by two years of basic medical education, two years of pre-clinical sciences, and two years of clerkship, the recommended *four-year graduate system* with one year of basic science, one year of pre-clinical service and two years of clerkship, and *hybrid model* (Kim & Kee, 2010).

Starting in 1998, the accreditation process in Korea was vested in the Korean Institute of Medical Education and Evaluation (KIMEE; Meng, 2020; Yoo et al., 2020).[19] However, not all medical institutions have adopted these practices equally. An early study found that medical schools could be classified based on the extent to which they meet the accreditation standards and that these rankings accounted for variation in student satisfaction (84.4%) and passing (54.2%; Yang, 2002).

Despite many parallels in BWM and TKM education, training in TKM is not considered equivalent to BWM due to the absence of international standards (Cho et al., 2008). Unsurprisingly, this gap is a concern for TKM practitioners (Kyeong et al., 2020) and learners, who perceived the learning environment to be worse than BWM institutions (Park et al., 2015; Kim et al., 2021). Thus, despite the pluralistic nature of the healthcare ecosystem in S. Korea, it represents a heterarchical structure, wherein BWM dominants (Baer et al., 1997/2013).

12.3.6.2 North Korea[20]

The division of North and South introduced a considerable ideological difference in the resulting states, in terms of communism-capitalist divide and between the emphasis placed on TKM and BWM. For instance, aspects of the nationalistic ideologies of Imperial Japan (i.e., purity in Shintoism) were Koreanized into a belief in Korean racial purity, with N. Koreans perceiving themselves as vulnerable to external social and physical influences including those from the West (Myers, 2011). The differences in healthcare training are also apparent in the difficulty defecting N. Korean doctors have had obtaining licensure in the S. Korea (Ha et al., 2019).

Despite the common use of TKM in both North and South Korea, the division of the two countries also led to different perceptions of health and illness as well as different prevalence and incidents of disease due to socioeconomic differences. The repeated famines reported in N. Korea (Goodkind & West, 2001; Noland et al., 2001) as well as further restrictions resulting from the COVID-19 pandemic of the early 2020s provide clear illustrations of the influence of socioecology on healthcare systems. Similarly, as there is no discernible journal dedicated to psychiatry (Kim & Jeon, 2020) along with the greater prevalence of somatization disorders in N. Korean defectors, researchers have suggested that the socialistic-materialistic philosophy of the North might affect how patients' symptoms are perceived by health seekers and diagnosed by HCPs (Park et al., 2014).

Immediately after liberation, responsibility for medical education was shared between the Ministry of Health and Bureau of Education, with the latter eventually assuming sole responsibility (Park & Park, 1998). Only two medical education institutions were operational during this time: Pyongyang Medical Center and Hamheung Medical College (Park, 2012). Provincial committees soon assumed control with small-scale organizations performing this role in other provinces. Autonomous organizations were formed in each region to allow for direct administration of medical education. Starting in 1946, a process of "centralization" and "systematization" defined N. Korean medical education with the central government restricting local self-governing bodies (Heo & Cho, 2014). This led to a shift from local governments being the primary financial contributors to medical education (62%) in 1945 to the central government (67%) in 1946.

The training of HCPs was also affected by the communist ideology of N. Korea that prioritized labor. Beyond communist tenets, the formal *Juche* state ideology (주체사상) emphasizes the need for national independence and loyalty to the leader undoubtedly influenced medical training. During the initial period of the formation of the N. Korea state, although some HCPs studied medicine exclusively, students could complete degrees at night or through correspondence, allowing them to work during the day. Revisions to the curriculum eventually led to the formal requirement of learning state ideology directed including loyalty to the Kim dynasty (Park & Park, 1998).

In N. Korea, medical pluralism is clearly evidenced in the organization of medical schools, which are divided into departments of clinical medicine (BWM), TKM, basic medicine (research), and hygiene (public health and education). However, this pluralism has the appearance of integration between the subdisciplines of medicine. Supporting this, studies suggest that the N. Korean government seeks to integrate BWM and TKM, especially in the domain of therapeutics (Lim et al., 2009). For instance, practitioners receiving instruction in BWM must complete courses in TKM. For a country which has separated itself from many avenues of trade, a clear benefit of TKM is its emphasis on locally available ingredients, thereby reducing dependency on other countries.

12.3.7 Taiwan

Taiwan's proximity to China has led to considerable cultural influence between the two societies (Chen, 2017; Jiao, 2007; Olsen & Miller-Antonio, 1992). Yet, the cultural norms and conventions of the indigenous Taiwanese have traditionally been far closer to Austronesia than mainland China throughout most of its history (Bellwood & SanchezMazas, 2005; Dawley, 2009; Trejaut et al., 2014). Like other societies in East Asia, the early inhabitants discovered and used the local plants and animals to promote health and treat illness, with much of this knowledge being retained in oral traditions and left unwritten (Chang & Goodenough, 1996; Li, 2013; Lo & Hu, 2023; Tsang, 2005). While BWM educational and medical practices dominate (Ho et al., 2017), contemporary Taiwanese society continues to provide and use traditional diagnostic and treatment methods, albeit biased toward a TCM approach (Chin et al., 2020; Chang et al., 2014; Lu et al., 2021; Tsai et al., 2006, 2008; Yeh et al., 2016).

12.3.7.1 Professionalization and Education

Following colonization by the Dutch, Spanish, and Qing empires, Taiwan was transferred to Imperial Japan in 1895[21] and remained in its possession until the end of the Pacific War (Ching, 2001; Ka, 2018; Tsurumi, 1977). In addition to introducing laws to regulate healthcare practices that excluded traditional medical practices (e.g., *The Regulation of Medical Practice in Taiwan*, in 1896), the colonial Japanese government also attempted to implement changes to the education system, eventually attempting to "Japanize" the Taiwanese in 1937. In healthcare, this resulted in the creation of two Western medical schools and 36 public hospitals (Chiang, 2007; Chiu et al., 2009; Hsiao et al., 1990; Lu & Chiang, 2011).

In parallel with these efforts to change Taiwanese society, Japanese researchers also documented Han (TCM) and indigenous medicinal plants for treating over 30 diseases (Liu, 2009). And while initially ignoring or suppressing Taiwanese Traditional Medicine (TTM), public health issues and an absence of other resources led the Japanese colonial government to reluctantly work with local practitioners, eventually allowing for licensure of their practices in 1901 with *a single* cohort on one occasion. While the examination legitimated those currently practicing TTM, the absence of further licensing created a finite supply of TTM practitioners that would continue to diminish throughout the remaining years of the Japanese occupation, i.e., from a high of approximately 1903 in 1901 to less than 12 by 1945 (Lin, 2004; cited in Liu & Chiang, 2018).

After the defeat of Imperial Japan, Taiwan reverted to Chinese rule. Soon after, the Chinese Civil War led to the retreat of Nationalist Forces to Taiwan in what was believed to be a temporary measure.[22] Seeking to maintain its independence, Taiwan largely allied itself with the West, leading to continued exposure to BWM marked by a change from the German-Japanese paradigm to an Anglo-American paradigm. However, Taiwanese healers have nevertheless continued to practice TEAM and work within a pluralistic medical system (Kleinman, 1980; Shih et al., 2010; Wu & Hu, 1980). For instance, recent estimates suggesting between 26 and 62.5%[23] of the population use TEAM (Chen et al., 2007; cf. Huang et al., 2018) with some studies finding an upward trend in its use (Yeh et al., 2016).

The influence of BWM is not only evidenced in the delivery of healthcare but is also apparent in curriculum development and accreditation practices. Starting in 1975, accreditation was the responsibility of the Ministry of Education. Following a critical review of medical education in Taiwan by the U.S. National Committee on Foreign Medical Education and Accreditation (NCFMEA 1998) that described the systems as "non-comparable" to the U.S., the Taiwan Medical Accreditation Council (TMAC) was created in 2000 to enact reforms. However, TCM practices remain important, with a greater contemporary focus on research.

Despite the existence of two healthcare traditions, the barrier between TEAM and BWM is more permeable than countries such as China and S. Korea. Taiwanese HCPs can obtain a dual major and complete both TEAM and BWM licensure exams (Kim et al., 2021). Current UGME education requirements require 2 years of premedical courses, 2.5–3 years of clinical courses, and 2.5–3 years of clerkship and internships. The Ministry of Examination administers licensing exams in two steps, assessing medical knowledge followed by a licensure exam (Chou et al., 2012; Lai, 2009).

Despite the dual-licensing system, HCPs can only practice either TCM or BWM, with two exceptions: BWM practitioners can use acupuncture, whereas TEAM practitioners can order BWM diagnostic tests (Kim et al., 2021). Thus, while not defined by the kind of syncretism evidenced in Japan, there is some overlap that distinguishes the Taiwanese system from China and S. Korea.

12.3.8 Vietnam

Despite the existence of few indigenous records, historical Chinese records suggest that TVM was defined by distinct methods. As we noted above, TVM (*thuốc Nam;* southern medicine) places a greater emphasis on herbal remedies relative to TCM (*thuốc Bắc*; northern medicine; Nguyen, 1993). TVM also included methods for the distillation of alcohol for medical purposes and identified over 100 medical plants (Chu, 2001). Despite their knowledge, healers were not assigned high status in Vietnamese society. This is partially attributable to a belief that their abilities were limited, captured in the popular saying "doctors can deal with illness, but cannot alter fate"[24] (Marr, 1987, p. 176). Healers were also prohibited from adopting any customs that would have identified them as a distinct profession including clothes, institutionalization, or developing any form of accreditation.

12.3.8.1 Professionalization and Education

The consolidation of Nguyen dynasty rule (1802 CE) led to significant changes in the status of healers in Vietnam. Soon after the Royal Medical Service was established (1805 CE), four grades of palace physicians were created and established in temples of medicine, with provincial medical organization and a medical school created later (Marr, 1987). Despite the presence of European clinicians and early interest in their methods, continued political unease between the Nguyen dynasty and the French limited the adoption of BWM (Thompson, 2001). For instance, researchers have attributed low vaccination rates to an absence of traditional practitioners, the ambivalence of colonial healthcare workers, and the haphazard efficacy of the available vaccination methods (Guenel, 1996; Thompson, 2001, 2016).

A century after the Royal Medical Service was created, the l'université de médecine de Hanoï[25] was established in 1902 by French colonials, allowing Vietnamese clinicians to receive a formal education in BWM. However, BWM practitioners remained in the minority, with census data from 1942 indicating that there were only .006 BWM doctors for every 1,000 persons (Long, 1973). Consequently, TVM remained the dominant healthcare tradition in Vietnam well into the 20th century. During the Pacific War, scarcity of pharmaceutical imports from Western and Chinese sources resulted in a resurgence of TVM which was supported by government initiatives that sought to formalize training (Wahlberg, 2006). By 2000, three groups of TVM practitioners existed: those with traditional training, those with formal training from academic institutions, and those who had acquired knowledge through informal apprenticeships (Bùi, 1999).

Despite the rise of BWM in Vietnam, medical education was – and is – defined by institutional variability, and an absence of accreditation standards (Ha & Siddiqui, 2022). In recent decades, this has led to calls for the establishment of a national medical licensing exam (Fan et al., 2012; Ha, 2023). Similarly, quotas were established by the Ministry of Education and Training and the Ministry of Health, with the number of medical students left to the discretion of the respective institutions after 2008 (MOH, 2008). However, student admissions are determined by multiple factors including examination results, direct recruitment that is not dependent on examination results, or by students entering into a contract with a municipality where they agree to practice after graduation (Fan et al., 2012).

Starting in 2015, the Ministry of Health developed a competency-based model. However, there is only limited evidence that this model has been implemented successfully (Dunong et al., 2019; World Bank, 2014).[26] While implementation of the curriculum is at the discretion of individual medical schools, their curriculum is based on a model curriculum developed by the Ministry of Education and approved by the Ministry of Health. In UGME, students can either enter a four- or six-year program, having passed an in-house university examination or the National Entrance Examination, respectively. Both programs are defined by two stages. Students must first complete a general education program including basic science and general courses, with 25% of the general science courses consisting of "political education," e.g., Marxist and Leninist Philosophy, History of the Vietnamese communist party, and Ho Chi Ming Ideology (MOET, 2001a, 2001b). In the second stage, professional education consists of basic and professional medicine courses, consisting of afternoon lectures. Students also attend clinical rotations in the morning and perform an average of one overnight on-call shift per week.

Graduate medical education (GME) consists of one of three tracks: academic, clinical, or residency training (Duong et al., 2021; Fan et al., 2012). In academic training, learners focus on conducting research and do not practice medicine. In clinical training, learners (approximately 90% of healthcare practitioners) must find and complete an 18-month internship in hospitals, reflecting an apprenticeship model. Once completed, they can then register for a medical license. Finally, in residency training, learners (approximately 10% of healthcare practitioners) complete specialized studies at one of Vietnam's major academic medical centers. Many educational institutions have also shifted the focus of their UGME programs toward competency-based designs based on Vietnam's MOH (Doung et al., 2021). The methods of teaching are consistent with BWM, consisting of Objective Structured Clinical Examinations, evidence-based, and collaborative learning (PBL and team-based learning (TBL)) approaches.

An early review of the medical education landscape by Fan et al. (2012) noted that "...it is very difficult to evaluate the overall quality of teaching and training," given that curriculum development is at the discretion of each university. Over a decade later, these observations largely remained true. Namely, while accreditation processes exist for health professions education, no central organization is dedicated to regulating the specific requirements of medical education (Ha & Siddiqui, 2022).

12.3.9 Summary of East Asian Medical Education Landscape

Rather than assuming that BWM has challenged, dominated, and displaced other indigenous healthcare systems (Baer et al., 1997/2013), traditional health professions education and healthcare delivery in East Asia has persisted, adapted, and reasserted in a changing world. Rather than displacing TEAM, BWM has influenced, is used in parallel, or has been integrated within TEAM practices and institutions. To further establish the relationship between TEAM and BWM, we reviewed available archival data on the TEAM and BWM workforce and other supporting statistics.

As Table 12.1 demonstrates, there is considerable variability in the healthcare and health professions landscape in East Asian countries. Multiple features remain apparent. First, the number of BWM practitioners is typically greater than TEAM practitioners. These statistics might be taken as evidence supporting a BWM-dominance account; however, the frequent integration of TEAM and BWM reviewed above suggests that this is an oversimplification. For instance, many practitioners use combinations of methods available in the healthcare ecosystem. Second, the number of both TEAM and BWM practitioners per 1,000 has increased over time. This observation is critical as it suggests that *both* methods of healthcare delivery continue to be viewed as legitimate paths for maintaining health and treating illnesses. While small in absolute terms, the increase in TEAM use might be motivated by a rebound in interest, dissatisfaction with BWM reductive therapeutic models, or due to financial and physical accessibility (for similar observations in the Americas, see Schoenherr, 2027b; Venosa et al., 2027). Supporting this, surveys have demonstrated that there is continued interest in traditional medicine use (Harmsworth & Lewith, 2011). However, some studies suggest that desire for interprofessional (TEAM–BWM) collaborative practice has been mixed (Leem et al., 2021; Min et al., 2012) in addition to reduced support for TEAM in specific populations (Chan et al., 2003). Thus, it might be the case that TEAM and BWM represent *distinct* paradigms in a healthcare ecosystem, each used for its perceived efficacy in promoting health and preventing and treating specific illnesses.

Another notable feature of this review concerns the adequacy of healthcare coverage in East Asia. The number of BWM practitioners exceeds the WHO recommendations of one physician per thousand, suggesting that the workforce is adequate in addressing the healthcare needs of the populations examined here (Abt Associates, 1991; cf. Hicks & Glenn, 1989, 1991; Miller et al., 1989). The smaller proportion of TEAM practitioners is not concerning in this light. Again, the observation that BWM practitioners often make use of, or refer health seekers to, practices and practitioners of TEAM qualifies the smaller number.

12.3.10 Heterarchical Typology in East Asia

As Table 12.1 illustrates, structural permeability and regulatory centralization together distinguish the broad system type, while institutional stability differentiates systems that share the same structural configuration. China and South Korea both exhibit low permeability and high centralization, yet differ fundamentally in stability: China's four-category practitioner system reflects a state-managed equilibrium with no sustained inter-paradigm competition, whereas South Korea's parallel licensing system is marked by documented practitioner grievances, contested equivalence between TKM and BWM credentials, and ongoing reform pressure (Kyeong et al., 2020; Park et al., 2015; Ha & Siddiqui, 2022). North Korea shares some of China's structural features but its stability is coerced centrally

TABLE 12.1 *Heterarchical Dimensions of TEAM–BWM Integration Across East Asian Healthcare Systems.*

Country	*TEAM Tradition*	*Structural Permeability*	*Regulatory Centralization*	*Institutional Stability*	*Primary System Formative Conditions*	*System Type*
China	TCM (中醫)	Low[1]	High	High	Nationalist consolidation of TCM against abolition threat, post-1949 Soviet-modelled restructuring, and ongoing state political mandate	Compartmentalized hierarchical (stable)
Japan	Kampo (漢方)	High	High	High	Meiji-era German-paradigm adoption, U.S. occupation-driven restructuring, and Anglo-American post-war realignment	Integrated hierarchical
South Korea	TKM (한의학)	Low	High	Low	Japanese colonial suppression of TKM, post-liberation North-South partition, and sustained BWM–TKM inter-professional contest	Compartmentalized heterarchical
Taiwan	TCM (中醫)	High	Low	High	Japanese colonial suppression and practitioner attrition, Nationalist retreat and Western geopolitical realignment, and NHI-stabilized dual system	Selectively permeable heterarchical
North Korea	Koryŏ Medicine (고려의학)	Low	High	High	Juche self-sufficiency doctrine, ideological mandate for BWM–Koryŏ integration, and resource constraints	Compartmentalized hierarchical (coerced)
Vietnam	TVM (Thuốc Nam)	Low	Low	Low	French colonial disruption of TVM institutions, wartime pharmaceutical scarcity driving TVM resurgence, and post-colonial governance deficit	Decentralized heterarchical

[1] Rating reflects formal architecture: China's Medical Practitioners Law (2021, Art. 14) enforces four-category scope restriction, supporting Low. Note that Shim (2018) classifies China as "interpenetrative pluralism" such that TEAM and biomedicine "cross over unconditionally in practice," describing de facto behaviour rather than the formal licensing structure.

rather than arrived through comparative consensus, i.e., integration is ideologically mandated rather than institutionally established. Consequently, it is distinguished as a Compartmentalized Hierarchical Coerced system. Vietnam, scoring low on all three dimensions, represents comparative deficit in governance, consistent with calls for national licensing and accreditation reform (Fan et al., 2012; Ha & Siddiqui, 2022). When viewed in these terms, this three-dimensional framework extends Crumley's (1995) observation that heterarchical systems differ in the reversibility of rank relations by adding regulatory centralization and institutional stability as independent axes. Where Shim's (2016) framework describes patterns of health-seeker utilization, the present framework describes the institutional conditions that constrain and enable those patterns, representing a distinct and complementary level of analysis. Specifically, Shim's interpenetrative system corresponds to high-permeability configurations, his subjugatory system to low-permeability, high-stability configurations, and his exclusionary system to low-permeability, low-stability configurations. Vietnam's structure is not addressed adequately by Shim's framework, nor the coerced stability of North Korea.

12.4 Conclusions

Health and illness present ubiquitous concerns for all human populations. Indigenous medicines are a ubiquitous feature of all societies, with specialist roles (healers) emerging through a process of convergent cultural evolution (Schoenherr, 2027b). While informal socialization and regulations exist, formal education and monitoring systems (e.g., accreditation and licensure) have been developed in multiple societies (for a review of medicine regulation, see Coderey & Pordié, 2019). Despite the apparent dominance of BWM of healthcare delivery and CBME (World Health Organization (WHO), 2019), traditional approaches to promoting health and treating illness remain relevant and responsive to health seekers' concerns. As our review has demonstrated, rather than representing a direct, unmediated relationship between practitioner and patient, East Asia societies formed social institutions dedicated to medical education that provided earlier, and distinct models of healthcare delivery that can be contrasted with BWM (cf. Baer et al., 2013).

12.4.1 A Healthcare Pluralism Defined by Heterarchical Structures

Previous frameworks have often glossed TEAM as "folk medicine." Folk medicine implies a relatively informal pre-paradigmatic approach to health and illness that is driven by *ad hoc* social cognitive processes rather than systematic social institutions (Baer et al., 2013). As our review has demonstrated, medical education as well as accreditation and licensing bodies have been a repeated feature of East Asian societies, such that TEAM has been systematized, monitored, and regulated in a manner that shares many features with the BWM for centuries. The replication of Chinese examination systems in multiple countries prior to the introduction of

BWM suggests that they satisfied a need, even if they were restricted to healers that exclusively served the elites of kingdoms and empires. The rise of BWM in East Asia cannot solely be attributed to its comparative efficacy. Rather, BWM's influence was accelerated by regional and international geopolitical force. Beyond the passive diffusion of knowledge brought through trade, Japanese colonialism accelerated the influence of BWM by supressing TEAM and restructuring healthcare in the region in the late 1800s and mid-1900s using "modern" Western methods. Japan's defeat at the end of the Pacific War reinforced this trend, especially in those countries who allied themselves with Western powers. Thus, in a comparable manner to scientific paradigms (Laudan, 1978; Kuhn, 1962/1996), externalities (e.g., conflict and colonialism) are determinants of the implementation of healthcare paradigms (Schoenherr, 2027a; Panova, 2019).

12.4.2 Structures of Healthcare Delivery and Education

To claim that BWM dominates healthcare in East Asia provides an oversimplistic account of how TEAM and BWM knowledge and practices have co-evolved. Healthcare in contemporary East Asia is undeniably defined by a heterarchical structure where multiple healthcare paradigms can exist in parallel (Schoenherr, 2027b). As this review suggests, not only is medical pluralism apparent in healthcare education systems including informal (folk medicine) and formal TEAM and the BWM approaches but is also evidenced in terms of how the relationship between TEAM and BWM is understood in each country.

In Japan, *kanpo* and BWM are well integrated, representing a *Centralized Hierarchical System*. Here, healthcare and health professions education represent a single system, with BWM representing the dominant theoretical paradigm and *kanpo* incorporated as a subspeciality of medicine. This is reinforced by a single, centralized accreditation system. This system could be interpreted as hierarchical, with TEAM subordinated to BWM.

Outside of Japan, other systems reflect clear heterarchical structures. The most obvious case is Vietnam. In Vietnam, no centralized accreditation system exists for BWM or TVM. The current system can be described as a *Decentralized Heterarchical System*, wherein there is comparatively little formal, centralized regulation and monitoring. Instead, groups (e.g., professionals and governmental representatives) introduce pressure for standardization and compliance.

In contrast to these two poles, other heterarchical models are evidenced. In Taiwan, despite the existence of parallel TEAM and BWM systems, there appears to be little conflict between approaches and greater flexibility for practitioners. The fact that two systems co-exist, and that some resources of each tradition can formally be used by practitioners of the other means that this system reflects as a *Selectively Permeable Heterarchical System*. China's recognition of four pathways for HCPs (e.g., (ethnic doctors), BWM, (TCM), and BWM–TEAM) additionally reflects a compartmentalized system.

In South Korea, there is greater separation and tension between TKM and BWM systems, reflecting a formal "dual system" (Kim et al., 2021). Based on these characteristics, this appears to reflect a *Compartmentalized Heterarchical System*. However, it is important to qualify this by noting that compartmentalization occurs at the level of institutionalized system and not health seekers. Health seekers remain free to select amongst the alternative therapeutic traditions of BWM and TKM.

Our approach is consistent with and complement's Shim's (2018) approach. Rather than the six systems we have defined based on the three heterarchical structural dimensions (permeability, centralization, and stability), Shim (2018) classified the Chinese system as *interpenetrative*, the (South) Korean system as *exclusionary*, and the Japanese system as *subjugatory* in terms of how TEAM and BWM are integrated. These categories can be mapped onto the diagonal of the our three-dimensional framework: Shim's interpenetrative system corresponds to high-permeability configurations, his subjugatory system to low-permeability, high-stability, high-centralization configurations, and his exclusionary system to low-permeability, low-stability configurations.

However, where Shim's typology describes patterns of health-seeker utilization, the present framework describes the *institutional* structures that constrain and enable those patterns, thereby operating at a distinct and complementary level of analysis. In the present study, three cases cannot be accommodated in Shim's framework. First, Vietnam's low scores on all three dimensions reflects a governance deficit rather than a stable pluralism. Second, North Korea's apparent stability is coerced rather than negotiated. Third, Taiwan's combination of high permeability and low centralization produces a configuration that Shim's single-axis typology cannot accommodate. By grounding the present typology in concept of heterarchy (Crumley, 1995, 2015) and extending it to regulatory and stability dimensions, we align this review with broader research on the social organization of complex systems while placing the evolution of these systems in their historical and political context.

The adoption of the concept of heterarchical structures has the additional benefit of increasingly alignment with the cognitive science (McCulloch, 1945): the brain organizes information heterarchical, leading to the possibility that health seekers hold multiple therapeutic and disease models that are not necessarily coherent or integrated. Thus, the external social structure is reflected, and influenced by, the cognitive structure of memory. Health seekers are unlikely to consider the "structure" of a system but rather seek care from practitioners using methods that are associated with the promotion of health or prevention of a specific illness. However, a heterarchy would influence health seeking behavior to the extent that each system – or individual treatment – is viewed as associated with others. If an illness experience is associated with only one illness model, health seekers are unlikely to consider alternatives therapeutic techniques.

The features of TEAM reviewed in this chapter represent a challenge to existing models of the social structure of healthcare. For instance, Baer et al. (1997/2013) provide an influential model of medical pluralism that places the formal BWM in contrast to informal folkmedicine. As the current review demonstrates, there is sufficient evidence that TEAM was formalized through processes analogous to accreditation prior to the introduction of BWM in East Asia, providing a parallel model of healthcare education and delivery. While there are fewer contemporary practitioners and educators within TEAM currently (Table 12.1), it would be a mistake to consider them "folk" practitioners in the traditional sense because they are educated and practice in formal healthcare systems[27] that (1) offers a distinct alternative (e.g., *generally* less expensive and invasive) relative to BWM, (2) might be selected due to its alignment with indigenous beliefs (e.g., Confucian norms, cultural tightness, and wholistic), and (3) that antedate and are more widespread than BWM. As we noted above, even when CBME approaches have been adopted, their implementation is significantly influenced by existing approaches to education (e.g., PBL; Kwan, 2019).

12.4.3 Lost in Translation: Successes and Failures of Implementing Western Medical Education

Our review demonstrates that the history of healthcare delivery and health professions education in East Asia is defined by four broad stages: (1) the emergence of indigenous practices in response to environmental conditions early humans encountered, (2) formalization of TEAM, heavily influenced by China and the 16th and 17th centuries and the gradual penetration of Western medical practices, (3) the amplification of BWM (specifically, the German–Japan paradigm) due to the influence of colonization by Imperial Japan, and (4) the dominance of the Anglo-American system after the defeat of Japan. Despite epistemological challenges and sociopolitical suppression, TEAM persists in East Asia.

The development of educational activities and assessment in the West are often simply referred to as "innovations." However, an innovation requires demonstrable widespread adoption, as well as consideration of how products and practices are modified during the implementation process (Schoenherr, 2027b; Schoenherr & Le-Bouar, 2024; Schoenherr & Hamstra, 2024). Innovations in contemporary medical education historically originate in the West and are adopted and adapted by practitioners in other countries. Many of these methods have proven effective. For instance, Hu et al. (2018) demonstrate that flipped classrooms have been successful in promoting improved learning outcomes in Chinese nursing education. However, as we have demonstrated, greater efforts must be directed toward understanding and communicating innovations in medical education in non-Western countries as they are likely to provide greater insight into the implementation process and resources that might be relevant to educational traditions in other cultures.

One such case is the adoption of PBL in Asian countries (PBL; Kwan, 2002, 2019). Originally developed at McMaster University (Canada), PBL has been widely adopted. However, its implementation and perceived success has varied considerably. Kwan (2016, 2019) presents a critical review of PBL adoption in modern Asia. First, Kwan differentiates four broad types of PBL that range from its use as a minor supplement (e.g., a case; Type I) to a traditional PBL approach that focuses on learners resolving realistic problems rather than focus on didactic lectures centered on the educators (Type IV). PBL was typically not adopted in its original form (Type IV) in East Asia. Kwan attributes this to issues with translation from English into Chinese, wherein most references to PBL *learning* referred to as PBL *teaching*. With "problem" also translated as question or difficult situation. Similarly, promotion (through conferences) also resulted in failures in knowledge translation which Kwan partially attributes to "conflicting sentiments: i.e., admiring and striving for innovation on one hand, but clinging and clenching to traditional comfort on the other hand" (p. 897). Indeed, multiple schools stopped providing PBL-based courses, although the focus was on hybridized versions of PBL.

For an education innovation to have implementation validity, it must ultimately be delivered in a consistent manner by competent personnel (Schoenherr & Hamstra, 2024). Kwan also suggests that these resources might not always be available in institutions that have large populations of students, such as in China. Others have suggested that hierarchical social structures and achievement motivations adversely affect adoption of these methods (Frambach et al., 2012). Nevertheless, these issues can be overcome. To address these concerns, Kwan suggests using senior students (*senpai* in Japanese) as a possible resources or complimentary methods of TBL, wherein larger classes are restructures into smaller teams or groups of learners (Schoenherr et al., 2027).

Despite the typical focus on BWM innovations adoption in East Asia, we must also acknowledge that cultural evolution is rarely unidirectional. We can also identify instance of where features of TEAM have influenced thinking outside of East Asia (Chang, 1942; Deng, 1943), if only through analogical reasoning. For instance, comparisons have been made between the Yin-Yang doctrine's notion of balance and the BWM concept of homeostasis, the function of sympathetic and parasympathetic nervous systems, and the relationship between anabolic and catabolic processes in the body (Koob, 1996; Sica et al., 2014; cf. Rodrigeuz et al., 2019). It is crucial to note that these high-level (dis)analogies do not correspond to the diagnoses derived from the Ying-Yang doctrine (Hong, 2014). Outside of institutional healthcare, many TEAM beliefs and practices have been brought by members of the East Asian diaspora to a global community and influenced the folk medical practices of health seekers in other countries (Shelton, 2020). Successful innovation in health professions education must make more effort in understanding the features of education innovation, the social, political, economic, and education systems in which assessment instruments, interventions, and instruction methods are embedded, and how implementation can result in adaptations that are significantly different as to represent wholly new innovations.

Acknowledgements

The authors would like to thank Dr. John P. DiMoia for reviewing a draft of this chapter, suggesting additional resources, and providing helpful feedback.

Notes

1 The cultural evolution approach here acknowledges that, while these systems that they have been influenced by healthcare practices and education methods adopted within the BWM approach.
2 Affordances reflect what a technology can do regardless of whether users are aware of this function.
3 For instance, Millington et al. (2018) observed high degrees of variability in experienced clinicians' ratings of the presentation of lung pathophysiologies using ultrasound.
4 As I discuss later, TCM is a relatively recent term that has sociopolitical implications. The heterogeneity is consequently a function of how categorical boundaries are defined, with many traditions better understood as part of the larger TEAM tradition rather than necessarily being part of TCM.
5 Correlation v. causation.
6 This dichotomy is used pragmatically, as the multidimensional nature of cross-cultural psychology is outside the scope of this chapter (for a review, see Henrich, 2020).
7 Cultural tightness refers to the value of conformity bias within a culture.
8 State-based examination systems.
9 Based on models of neurological organization (McCulloch, 1945), heterarchies are observed when multiple systems defined by their own exchange norms operate in parallel (Crumley, 1995, 2005, 2015; for a discussion of heterarchies in healthcare, see Schoenherr, 2025b).
10 While these traditions are also influenced by traditions outside East Asia (e.g., India), we restrict ourselves to those of East Asia.
11 Lei (2014) argues that comparatively recent political and nationalistic movements resulted in its being framed as "Chinese." As the title of his book frames it, TCM is neither donkey (cross-bred) or horse (pure bred). Lei also notes that these practitioners referred to their practice as "National Medicine" such that there was a co-evolution of the social institutions of TCM and the state.
12 Despite the current geographic distance, ancient humans who migrated to N. America could have conceivably brough this distinction with them from East Asia.
13 Wittgenstein assumes that members of a category share some features from a set. Here, typicality is determined by the number of shared features. These findings are supported by experimental studies (Rosch, 1973).
14 For instance, universities have established relationships with international partners, such as the Shanghai Jiao Tong University's and the University of Ottawa's Joint School of Medicine. The first author of this chapter contributed a peer reviewed paper to a journal that was re-launched in 2014.
15 Despite scholars referring to Korean medicine as either hanuihak (or hanbang), the TKM conventions is adopted for consistency.
16 While the Yanji District, Xiaoyingzi, and Tuman River where these artifacts were collected during the Japanese colonial period currently lies within (or demarcates) the borders of China, these borders would not have been relevant to the period of the artifacts use.

17 (Hyangyakjipseongbang (향약집성방) in 1443 and Dongeuibogam (동의보감) in 1663; e.g., Lee, 2011).
18 The Ministry of Health and Welfare refers to this simply as Korean medicine.
19 Formerly, Accreditation Board for Medical Education in Korea (ABMEK).
20 The tensions between North Korea and many other nations and a concomitant lack of transparency, limited information is available on North Korea's healthcare education and delivery system. The limited accessible publications and reports from defectors can provide some insight into this system.
21 Taiwan would be its first colony.
22 "Prepare for one year, counterattack in two years, sweep out the enemy in three years and succeed within five years."
23 Differences in percentage are likely attributable to the use interval use in the study.
24 Thầy chữa bệnh không chữa mệnh.
25 Đại Học Y Hà Nội; formerly, l'École de Médecine de l'Indochine).
26 As Schoenherr and McConnell (2024) note, competency-based approaches are generally largely underdeveloped despite formal requirements to the contrary.
27 Indeed, preferences for terms such as hanuihak suggest that "traditional" medicine has specific negative connotations.

Bibliography

Abdullahi, A. A. (2011). Trends and challenges of traditional medicine in Africa. *African Journal of Traditional, Complementary and Alternative Medicines*, *8*(5S), 115–123.

Abt Associates (1991). *Reexamination of the Adequacy of Physician Supply Made in 1980 by the Graduate Medical Education National Advisory Committee (GMENAC) for Selected Specialties*. National Technical information Service. Health Resources and Services Administration publication 240-89-0041 PB.

Adhikari, P. P., & Paul, S. B. (2018). History of Indian traditional medicine: A medical inheritance. *History*, *11*(1), 421.

Allison, K. H., Reisch, L. M., Carney, P. A., Weaver, D. L., Schnitt, S. J., O'Malley, F. P., ... & Elmore, J. G. (2014). Understanding diagnostic variability in breast pathology: Lessons learned from an expert consensus review panel. *Histopathology*, *65*(2), 240–251.

Aricanli, S. (2013). Plurality in Qing Imperial Medicine: Examining institutional formations beyond the Imperial Medical Bureau. *Asia Pacific: Perspectives*, *12*(1), 61–83.

Baer, H. A., & Coulter, I. (2008). Taking stock of integrative medicine: Broadening biomedicine or co-option of complementary and alternative medicine? *Health Sociology Review*, *17*(4), 331–341.

Baer, H. A., Singer, M., & Susser, I. (1997/2013). *Medical Anthropology and the World System: Critical Perspectives*. Bloomsbury Publishing USA.

Bai, L. (2010). Human capital or humane talent? Rethinking the nature of education in China from a comparative historical perspective. *Frontiers of Education in China*, *5*(1), 104–129.

Bai, Y. (2019). Farewell to Confucianism: The modernizing effect of dismantling China's imperial examination system. *Journal of Development Economics*, *141*, 102382.

Bellwood, P., & SanchezMazas, A. (2005). Human migrations in continental East Asia and Taiwan: Genetic, linguistic, and archaeological evidence. *Current Anthropology*, *46*(3), 480–484.

Blum, S. D., & Jensen, L. M. (Eds.). (2002). *China Off Center: Mapping the Margins of the Middle Kingdom*. University of Hawaii Press.

Borrell-Carrió, F., Suchman, A. L., & Epstein, R. M. (2004). The biopsychosocial model 25 years later: Principles, practice, and scientific inquiry. *The Annals of Family Medicine*, *2*(6), 576–582.

Bourgeault, I. L., & Mulvale, G. (2006). Collaborative health care teams in Canada and the USA: Confronting the structural embeddedness of medical dominance. *Health Sociology Review*, *15*(5), 481–495.

Bowers, J. Z. (1970). *Western Medical Pioneers in Feudal Japan*. Johns Hopkins University Press.

Bowers, J. Z. (1979). The adoption of German medicine in Japan: The decision and the beginning. *Bulletin of the History of Medicine*, *53*, 57–80.

Bowers, J. Z. (1980). *When the Twain Meet: The Rise of Western Medicine in Japan*. Johns Hopkins University Press.

Boyd, R., & Richerson, P. J. (1996, January). Why culture is common, but cultural evolution is rare. In *Proceedings-British Academy* (Vol. *88*, pp. 77–94). Oxford University Press Inc.

Broom, A., Doron, A., & Tovey, P. (2009). The inequalities of medical pluralism: Hierarchies of health, the politics of tradition and the economies of care in Indian oncology. *Social Science & Medicine*, *69*(5), 698–706.

Bùi, C. H. (1999). Integration of traditional medicine into the health care system. In B. C. Hoàng, T. Phó, & N. Huu (Eds.), *Vietnamese Traditional Medicine*, pp. 29–36. Hanoi: The Gioi Publishers.

Burgess, A., & Horii, M. (2012). Risk, ritual and health responsibilisation: Japan's 'safety blanket'of surgical face mask-wearing. *Sociology of Health & Illness*, *34*(8), 1184–1198.

Cha, W. S., Oh, J. H., Park, H. J., Ahn, S. W., Hong, S. Y., & Kim, N. I. (2007). Historical difference between traditional Korean medicine and traditional Chinese medicine. *Neurological Research*, 29(sup1), 5–9.

Chan, C.B., Gramlich, L., Littlechild, L., M., Lightning, R., Ganske, J., & Thorlakson, J. (2027). Innovations in health professions education in Canada to address the Truth and Reconciliation Commission of Canada's Calls to Action and the Health Inequities experienced by indigenous peoples. In Schoenherr, J. R. (Ed.), *Fundamentals and Frontiers of Medical Education and Decision-Making: Innovation, Implementation, and Translational Research*. Routledge.

Chan, M. F., Mok, E., Wong, Y. S., Tong, T. F., Day, M. C., Tang, C. K. Y., & Wong, D. H. C. (2003). Attitudes of Hong Kong Chinese to traditional Chinese medicine and Western medicine: Survey and cluster analysis. *Complementary Therapies in Medicine*, *11*(2), 103–109.

Chang, C. (2015). The Qing imperial academy of medicine: Its institutions and the physicians shaped by them. *East Asian Science, Technology, and Medicine*, *41*, 63–92.

Chang, K. C., & Goodenough, W. H. (1996). Archaeology of southeastern China and its bearing on the Austronesian homeland. In W. H. Goodenough (Ed.), *Prehistoric Settlement of the Pacific* (pp. 28–35). American Philosophical Society.

Chang, M. Y., Liu, C. Y., & Chen, H. Y. (2014). Changes in the use of complementary and alternative medicine in Taiwan: A comparison study of 2007 and 2011. *Complementary Therapies in Medicine*, *22*(3), 489–499.

Chang, Y. Z. (1942). China and English civil service reform. *The American Historical Review*, *47*(3), 539–544.

Chee, L. P. (2021). *Mao's Bestiary: Medicinal Animals and Modern China*. Duke University Press.
Chen, F. P., Chen, T. J., Kung, Y. Y., Chen, Y. C., Chou, L. F., Chen, F. J., & Hwang, S. J. (2007). Use frequency of traditional Chinese medicine in Taiwan. *BMC Health Services Research*, *7*(1), 1–11.
Chen, L. C., Reich, M., & Ryan, J. (2017). *Medical Education in East Asia: Past and Future*. Indiana University Press.
Chen, W. C. (2017). The early occupation of Taiwan. In J. Habu, P. V. Lape, & J. W. Olsen (Eds.), *Handbook of East and Southeast Asian Archaeology* (pp. 277–291). Springer.
Chen, X., Xiong, G., & Jiang, A. (1995). Integration of traditional teaching method and PBL in clinical teaching [in Chinese]. *Medical Education* (China), *11*, 26–28.
Chi, C. (1994). Integrating traditional medicine into modern health care systems: examining the role of Chinese medicine in Taiwan. *Social Science & Medicine*, 39(3), 307–321.
Chi, C., Lee, J. L., Lai, J. S., Chen, C. Y., Chang, S. K., & Chen, S. C. (1996). The practice of Chinese medicine in Taiwan. *Social sScience & Medicine*, 43(9), 1329–1348.
Chiang, T. L. (2007). *Health Care Policy in Taiwan*, 3rd ed. Yuan-Liu Publisher.
Chin, C. Y., Chen, Y. H., Wu, S. C., Liu, C. T., Lee, Y. F., & Tsai, M. Y. (2020). Complementary and alternative medicine use in breast cancer patients at a medical center in Taiwan: A cross-sectional study. *Integrative Cancer Ttherapies*, *19*, 1534735420983910.
Ching, L. T. (2001). *Becoming Japanese: Colonial Taiwan and the Politics of Identity Formation*. University of California Press.
Chiu, C.-H., Arrigo, L. G., & Tsai, D.-J. (2009). Historical context for the growth of medical professionalism and curriculum reform in Taiwan. *Kaohsiung Journal of Medical Sciences*, *25*, 510–514.
Cho, H. J., Choi, H. Y., Choi, H., & Ahn, S. Y. (2008). USMLE application and overseas expansion of TKM doctors. *Korean Journal of Oriental Medicine*, *14*(3), 149–154.
Chou, J. Y., Chiu, C. H., Lai, E., Tsai, D., & Tzeng, C. R. (2012). Medical education in Taiwan. *Medical Teacher*, *34*(3), 187–191.
Chu, L. T. (2001). An introduction to the history of traditional medicine and pharmaceutics in Vietnam. In *Historical Perspectives on East Asian Science, Technology, and Medicine* (p. 264).
Chu, S. (2022). The longer abolition of the Chinese imperial examination system (1900s–1910s). *International Journal of Asian Studies*, 20, 1–17.
Coburn, D. (2006). Medical dominance then and now: Critical reflections. *Health Sociology Review*, *15*, 432–443.
Coderey, C., & Pordié, L. (Eds.). (2019). *Circulation and Governance of Asian Medicine*. Routledge.
Crumley, C. L. (1995). Heterarchy and the analysis of complex societies. In R. M. Ehrenreich, C. L. Crumley, & J. E. Levy (Eds.), *Heterarchy and the Analysis of Complex Societies: Archeological Papers No. 6* (pp. 1–6). American Anthropological Association.
Crumley, C. L. (2005). Remember how to organize: Heterarchy across disciplines. In *Nonlinear Models for Archaeology and Anthropology* (pp. 35–50).
Crumley, C. L. (2015). Heterarchy. In R. A. Scott & M. C. Buchmann (Eds.), *Emerging Trends in the Social and Behavioral Sciences: An Interdisciplinary, Searchable, and Linkable Resource* (pp. 1–14). Wiley Online Library.
Dawley, E. N. (2009). The question of identity in recent scholarship on the history of Taiwan. *The China Quarterly*, *198*, 442–452.
Deng, S.-Y. (1943). Chinese influence on the western examination system. *Harvard Journal of Asiatic Studies*, *7*, 267–312.

Deng, T. (1988/2000). Practical diagnosis in traditional Chinese Medicine. *Clinical Acupuncture and Oriental Medicine, 1*, 174–177.

DiMoia, J. P. (2008). "알맞게 낳아서 훌륭하게 기르자!" (Let's Have the Proper Number of Children and Raise Them Well!): Family planning and nation-building in South Korea, 1961–1968. *East Asian Science, Technology and Society: An International Journal, 2*, 361–379.

DiMoia, J. P. (2013). *Reconstructing Bodies: Biomedicine, Health, and Nation-Building in South Korea since 1945*. Stanford University Press.

Dobos, G., & Tao, I. (2011). The model of western integrative medicine: The role of Chinese medicine. *Chinese Journal of Integrative Medicine, 17*, 11–20.

Douglas, M. (1966/2003). *Purity and Danger: An Analysis of Concepts of Pollution and Taboo*. Routledge.

Drinnan, M. J., Murray, A., Griffiths, C. J., & John Gibson, G. (1998). Interobserver variability in recognizing arousal in respiratory sleep disorders. *American Journal of Respiratory and Critical Care Medicine, 158*(2), 358–362.

Eisenberg, D. (2011). Reflections on the past and future of integrative medicine from a lifelong student of the integration of Chinese and Western Medicine. *Chinese Journal of Integrative Medicine, 17*, 3–5.

Elman, B. A. (2013). The civil examination system in late Imperial China, 1400–1900. *Frontiers of History in China, 8*(1), 32–50.

Ernst, E. (2000). Prevalence of use of complementary/alternative medicine: A systematic review. *Bulletin of the World Health Organization, 78*(2), 258–266.

Ernst, W. (Ed.). (2002). *Plural Medicine, Tradition and Modernity, 1800–2000*. Routledge.

Fan, A. P., Tran, D. T., Kosik, R. O., Mandell, G. A., Hsu, H. S., & Chen, Y. S. (2012). Medical education in Vietnam. *Medical Teacher, 34*(2), 103–107.

Farquhar, J., & Lai, L. (2021). *Gathering Medicines: Nation and Knowledge in China's Mountain South*. University of Chicago Press.

Fiske, A. P. (1991). *Structures of Social Life: The Four Elementary Forms of Human Relations*. Free Press.

Frambach, J. M., Driessen, E. W., Chan, L. C., & van der Vleuten, C. P. (2012). Rethinking the globalisation of problem-based learning: How culture challenges self-directed learning. *Medical Education, 46*(8), 738–747.

Frank, J. R., Snell, L. S., Cate, O. T., Holmboe, E. S., Carraccio, C., Swing, S. R., ... & Harris, K. A. (2010). Competency-based medical education: Theory to practice. *Medical Teacher, 32*, 638–645.

Frass, M., Strassl, R. P., Friehs, H., Müllner, M., Kundi, M., & Kaye, A. D. (2012). Use and acceptance of complementary and alternative medicine among the general population and medical personnel: A systematic review. *Ochsner Journal, 12*(1), 45–56.

Friedson, E. (1970). *Profession of Medicine*. Harper and Row.

Friedson, E. (1970/2007). *Professional Dominance: The Social Structure of Medical Care*. Harper a Transaction Publishers.

Fujimoto, Y. (1884). *A Comprehensive Collection of Great Japan's Laws with Corrections and Supplements*. Ryūeido.

Gelfand, M. J., Jackson, J. C., Pan, X., Nau, D., Pieper, D., Denison, E., ... & Wang, M. (2021). The relationship between cultural tightness–looseness and COVID-19 cases and deaths: A global analysis. *The Lancet: Planetary Health, 5*(3), e135–e144.

Goble, A. E. (2011). *Confluences of Medicine in Medieval Japan: Buddhist Healing, Chinese Knowledge, Islamic Formulas, and Wounds of War*. University of Hawai'i Press.

Goodkind, D., & West, L. (2001). The North Korean famine and its demographic impact. *Population and Development Review*, *27*(2), 219–238.

Guénel, A. (1996). La lutte antivariolique en Extrême-Orient: Ruptures et continuité. In A.-M. Moulin (Eds.), *L'Aventure de la vaccination: Fayard* (pp. 83–94). Anne Marie Moulin

Ha, S., Choi, H. R., Lee, J. K., & Lee, Y. H. (2019). Challenges experienced by north Korean refugee doctors in acquiring a medical license in South Korea: A qualitative analysis. *Journal of Continuing Education in the Health Professions*, *39*(2), 112–118.

Ha, T. M. (2023). A commentary on the National Medical Licensing Examination in Vietnam: Why, what, who and how. *MedEdPublish*, *13*(30), 30.

Ha, T. M., & Siddiqui, Z. S. (2022). Accreditation of medical education in Vietnam: From local to global excellence. *Pakistan Journal of Medical Sciences, 38*(4Part-II), 1077.

Haidt, J. (2007). The new synthesis in moral psychology. *Science*, *316*(5827), 998–1002.

Han, K. I., Shin, S. H., Lim, G. M., Lee, J. H., & Ko, Y. S. (2018). Reviewing research of Eastern-Western integrative medicine studies in Korea. *Journal of Korean Medicine Rehabilitation*, *28*(1), 53–60.

Han, S. Y., Kim, H. Y., Lim, J. H., Cheon, J., Kwon, Y. K., Kim, H., ... & Chae, H. (2016). The past, present, and future of traditional medicine education in Korea. *Integrative Medicine Research*, *5*(2), 73–82.

Harmsworth, K., & Lewith, G. T. (2001). Attitudes to traditional Chinese medicine amongst Western trained doctors in the People's Republic of China. *Social Science & Medicine*, *52*(1), 149–153.

Hashimoto, A. (2013). A 'German world'shared among doctors: A history of the relationship between Japanese and German psychiatry before World War II. *History of Psychiatry*, *24*, 180–195.

Hawkins, R. E., Welcher, C. M, Holmboe, E. S., Kirk, L. M., Norcini, J. J., Simons, K. B., & Skochelak, S. E. (2015). Implementation of competency-based medical education: Are we addressing the concerns and challenges? *Medical Education*, *49*, 1086–1102.

Hayden, B. (1998). Practical and prestige technologies: The evolution of material systems. *Journal of Archaeological Method and Theory*, *5*, 1–55.

He, P., Zhu, D., Man, X., Bai, Q., Huang, L., Shi, X., & Meng, Q. (2022). Strengthening of traditional Chinese medicine in the health system reform: effect on health outcomes and financial protection. *Evidence-Based Complementary and Alternative Medicine*, 2022(1), 7226674.

Henrich, J. (2020). *The WEIRDest People in the World: How the West became Psychologically Peculiar and Particularly Prosperous*. Penguin UK.

Henrich, J., Boyd, R., & Richerson, P. J. (2008). Five misunderstandings about cultural evolution. *Human Nature*, *19*, 119–137.

Henrich, J., & McElreath, R. (2003). The evolution of cultural evolution. *Evolutionary Anthropology: Issues, News, and Reviews: Issues, News, and Reviews*, *12*(3), 123–135.

Heo, Y. J., & Cho, Y. S. (2014). Formation of medical education in North Korea: 1945–1948. *Korean Journal of Medical History*, *23*(2), 239–268.

Hicks, L. L., & Glenn, J. K. (1989). Too many physicians in the wrong places and specialties? Populations and physicians from a market perspective. *Journal of Health Care Marketing*, *9*(4), 18–26.

Hicks, L. L., & Glenn, J. K. (1991). Rural populations and rural physicians: Estimates of critical mass ratios, by specialty. *The Journal of Rural Health*, *7*, 357–371.

Hinrichs, T. J. & Barnes, L. L. (2022). *Chinese Medicine and Healing: An Illustrated History*. Harvard University Press.

Ho, M. J., Shaw, K., Shih, J., & Chiu, Y. T. (2017). Mission and modernity: The history and development of medical education in Taiwan. In L. C. Chen, M. R. Reich, & J. Ryan (Eds.), *Medical Education in East Asia: Past and Future* (pp. 84–111). Indiana University Press.

Honda, M., Inoue, N., Liverani, M., & Nagai, M. (2022). Lessons learned from the history of postgraduate medical training in Japan: from disease-centred care to patient-centred care in an aging society. *Human Resources for Health*, 20(1), 54.

Hong, H. (2014). *The Theory of Chinese Medicine: A Modern Interpretation*. World Scientific.

Hsiao, W. C., Yaung, C. L., & Lu, J. R. (1990). Health care financing and delivery in the ROC: Current conditions and future challenges. *Indian Free China, 73*(2), 13–38.

Hsieh, C.-R., & Tang, C. (2019). The multi-tiered medical education system and its influence on the health care market-China's Flexner report. *Human Resources for Health, 17*(1), 50–50.

Hsu, E. (1999). *The Transmission of Chinese Medicine*. Cambridge University Press.

Hu, R., Gao, H., Ye, Y., Ni, Z., Jiang, N., & Jiang, X. (2018). Effectiveness of flipped classrooms in Chinese baccalaureate nursing education: A meta-analysis of randomized controlled trials. *International Journal of Nursing Studies, 79*, 94–103.

Huang, C. W., Hwang, I. H., Lee, Y. S., Hwang, S. J., Ko, S. G., Chen, F. P., & Jang, B. H. (2018). Utilization patterns of traditional medicine in Taiwan and South Korea by using national health insurance data in 2011. *PLoS One, 13*(12), e0208569.

Kucherenko, I. I., & Schoenherr, J R (2027). Medical education despite war: Innovation in the Health Professions during Armed Conflict. In Schoenherr, J. R. (Ed.), *Fundamentals and Frontiers of Medical Education and Decision-Making: Innovation, Implementation, and Translational Research*. Routledge.

Jablonka, E., & Lamb, M. J. (2014). *Evolution in Four Dimensions: Genetic, Epigenetic, Behavioral, and Symbolic Variation in the History of Life*. MIT Press.

Jaiswal, Y. S., & Williams, L. L. (2017). A glimpse of Ayurveda–The forgotten history and principles of Indian traditional medicine. *Journal of Traditional and Complementary Medicine, 7*(1), 50–53.

Jiao, T. (2007). *The Neolithic of Southeast China: Cultural Transformation and Regional Interaction on the Coast*. Cambria Press.

Jin, H., Dong, G., Zou, L., Shen, X., & Li, D. (2020). History and status quo of higher public health education in China. *Public Health Reviews, 41*, 12.

Ka, C. M. (2018). *Japanese Colonialism in Taiwan: Land Tenure, Development, and Dependency, 1895–1945*. Routledge.

Kananoja, K. (2021). *Healing Knowledge in Atlantic Africa: Medical Encounters, 1500–1850*. Cambridge University Press.

Kang, Y. (2011). The characteristics of Korean medicine based on time classification. *China Perspectives, 3*, 33–42.

Kang, I. U., & Cha, W. S. (2017). New perspectives on the origin of Korean acupuncture: Based on materials from Xiaoyingzi Tomb, Yanji and neighbouring region. *Korean Journal of Medical History, 26*(3), 339–378.

Kaptchuk, T. J., & Eisenberg, D. M. (2001). Varieties of healing. 1: Medical pluralism in the United States. *Annals of Internal Medicine, 135*(3), 189–195.

Kessler, R. C., Davis, R. B., Foster, D. F., Van Rompay, M. I., Walters, E. E., Wilkey, S. A., ... & Eisenberg, D. M. (2001). Long-term trends in the use of complementary and alternative medical therapies in the United States. *Annals of Internal Medicine, 135*(4), 262–268.

Khan, S. (2006). Systems of medicine and nationalist discourse in India: Towards "new horizons" in medical anthropology and history. *Social Science & Medicine, 62*(11), 2786–2797.

Kim, D.-J. (1981). *History of Korean Medicine*. Cheolsaudang.

Kim, H. E. (2014). *Doctors of Empire: Medical and Cultural Encounters between Imperial Germany and Meiji Japan* (Vol. *17*). University of Toronto Press.

Kim, H. K. (2013). *A Study on the Identity Formation of Korean Medicine in the Japanese Colonial Era*. Kyung Hee University.

Kim, H. W., & Jeon, W. T. (2020). Research output on mental health problems in North Korea between 2006 and 2017: A bibliographic analysis of North Korean medical journal articles. *Asian Journal of Psychiatry, 53*, 102228.

Kim, H., Jeon, P., Kim, S., Hong, J., & Kang, Y. (2021). Cross-cultural adaptation and validation of the Korean version of the Dundee ready education environment measure (DREEM). *Evidence-Based Complementary and Alternative Medicine*, 2021, 1–10.

Kim, H., Jeong, H., Jeon, P., Kim, S., Park, Y. B., & Kang, Y. (2016). Perception study of traditional Korean medical students on the medical education using the Dundee ready educational environment measure. *Evidence-Based Complementary and Alternative Medicine*, 2016, 1–7.

Kim, K. I. (1999). Culture and illness behavior in South Korea. *Transcultural Psychiatry, 36*(1), 65–77.

Kim, K. J., & Kee, C. (2010). Reform of medical education in Korea. *Medical Teacher, 32*(2), 113–117.

Kitamura, H., & Matsuo, A. (2021). Development and validation of the purity orientation–pollution avoidance scale: A study with Japanese sample. *Frontiers in Psychology, 12*, 590595.

Kleinman, A. (1980). *Patients and Healers in the Context of Culture: An Exploration of the Borderland between Anthropology, Medicine, and Psychiatry*. University of California Press.

Ko, A. M. S., Chen, C. Y., Fu, Q., Delfin, F., Li, M., Chiu, H. L., ... & Ko, Y. C. (2014). Early Austronesians: Into and out of Taiwan. *The American Journal of Human Genetics, 94*(3), 426–436.

Ko, K. H. (2017). A brief history of imperial examination and its influences. *Society, 54*, 272–278.

Koob, G. F. (1996). Drug addiction: The yin and yang of hedonic homeostasis. *Neuron, 16*, 893–896.

Kozu, T. (2006). Medical education in Japan. *Academic Medicine, 81*(12), 1069–1075.

Kuhn, T. S. (1962/1997). *The Structure of Scientific Revolutions*. University of Chicago press.

Kwan, C. Y. (2002). Teaching of human physiology as it relates to changes in medical education an Asian perspective based on the Yin-Yang principle. *Journal of Medical Education, 6*, 449–460.

Kwan, C. Y. (2016). Commentary: 5 decades of Skepticism about PBL in medical education: Reflection and outlook in the Asia Pacific Context. *Journal of Medical Education, 20*, 1–10.

Kwan, C. Y. (2019). A thorny path: The developmental course of problem-based learning for health sciences education in Asia. *Advances in Health Sciences Education, 24*, 893–901.

Kyeong, H. K., Ju, A. L., Ho-Yeon, G., Sunju, P., & Sangwoo, S. (2020). Traditional Korean Medicine education in the World. *Integrative Medicine Research, 9*(2).

Lai, C.-W. (2009). Experiences of accreditation of medical education in Taiwan. *Journal of Education and Evaluation in the Health Professions*, *6*(2), 1–3.

Lam, T. (2001). Strengths and weaknesses of traditional Chinese medicine and Western medicine in the eyes of some Hong Kong Chinese. *Journal of Epidemiology & Community Health*, *55*(10), 762–765.

Lam, T. P., & Lam, Y. Y. B. (2009). Medical education reform: The Asian experience. *Academic Medicine*, *84*, 1313–1317.

Lam, T. P., Wan, X. H., & Ip, M. S. M. (2006). Current perspectives on medical education in China. *Medical Education*, *40*, 940–949.

Laudan, L. (1978). *Progress and its Problems: Towards a Theory of Scientific Growth.* University of California Press.

LeBel, M. E., Haverstock, J., Cristancho, S., van Eimeren, L., & Buckingham, G. (2018). Observational learning during simulation-based training in arthroscopy: Is it useful to novices? *Journal of Surgical Education*, *75*(1), 222–230.

Lee, R. P. L. (1982). Comparative studies of health care systems. *Social Science and Medicine*, *16*, 629–642.

Lee, H. J. (2008). Study on the attitudes toward Korean oriental medicine and traditional Chinese medicine-based on the responses of the university students in Korea and China. *Journal of Physiology & Pathology in Korean Medicine*, *22*(6), 1383–1389.

Lee, J., Kim, K. I., Seo, J. H., Cheong, M. J., & Youn, I. (2021). Perception, attitude, and demand for Korean medicine and Western medicine collaborative treatment of medical occupational groups in Korea: A scoping review. *Integrative Medicine Research*, *10*(1), 100430.

Lee, J. C., & Kee, C. D. (1996). The rise of western medicine and the decline of traditional medicine in Korea, 1876–1910. *Korean Journal of Medical History*, *5*(1), 1–10.

Lee, K. L. (2011). The publication of Hyangyakjipseongbang and the Chosnization of the Chinese medicine. *Korean Journal of Medical History*, *20*, 225–262.

Leem, J., Kim, K. I., Seo, J. H., Cheong, M. J., & Youn, I. (2021). Perception, attitude, and demand for Korean medicine and Western medicine collaborative treatment of medical occupational groups in Korea: a scoping review. *Integrative Medicine Research*, *10*(1), 100430.

Lei, S. H. L. (2014). *Neither Donkey nor Horse: Medicine in the Struggle over China's Modernity*. University of Chicago Press.

Lee, S. W., Tang, H., Wan, J., Mai, X., & Liu, C. (2015). A cultural look at moral purity: Wiping the face clean. *Frontiers in Psychology*, *6*, 129142.

Leung, A. K. C. (1987). Organized medicine in Ming-Qing China: State and private medical institutions in the lower Yangzi region. *Late Imperial China*, *8*(1), 134–166.

Li, K. T. 2013. First farmers and their coastal adaptation in prehistoric Taiwan. In A. P. Underhill (Ed.), *A Companion to Chinese Archaeology* (pp. 612–633). Wiley.

Lim, B., Park, J., & Han, C. (2009). Attempts to utilize and integrate traditional medicine in North Korea. *The Journal of Alternative and Complementary Medicine*, *15*(3), 217–223.

Liming, C., Yanling, F., Lin, Z., Sijia, Z., Qing, F., Yihua, C., Tosha, Y., Daji, X., Mingyu, L., Sang, W. A., Woong, S. L., Seong, H. C., & Byung, W. L. (2015). Clinical application of traditional herbal medicine in five countries and regions: Japan; South Korea; mainland China; Hong Kong, China; Taiwan, China. *Journal of Traditional Chinese Medical Sciences*, *2*(3), 140–149.

Lin, J. G. (2004). *History of Chinese Medicine in Taiwan*. The National Union of Chinese Medical Associations.

Liu, H. (2007). Influence of China's imperial examinations on Japan, Korea and Vietnam. *Frontiers of History in China, 2*, 493–512.

Liu, M. S. (2009). *Prescribing colonization: The role of medical practices and policies in Japan-ruled Taiwan, 1895–1945*. Association for Asian Studies.

Liu, Y. (2017). Exotica as prestige technology: The production of luxury gold in Western Han society. *Antiquity, 91*(360), 1588–1602.

Liu, Y., Wang, Y., & Pei, J. (2005). Practical application of PBL teaching method [Chinese]. *Shanxi Yi Ke Da Xue Xue Bao (Ji Chu Yi Xue Jiao Yu Ban), 7*, 149–151.

Lo, M. C. (2002). *Doctors within Borders: Profession, Ethnicity, and Modernity in Colonial Taiwan* (Vol. *1*). Univ of California Press.

Lo, S. M., & Hu, J. M. (2023). Knowledge and practices of growing wild edible plants in 'Amis home gardens: Content and social distribution of a traditional ecological knowledge system of 'Etolan, southeastern Taiwan. In P. D'Arcy & D. D. Da-Wei Kuan (Eds.), *Islands of Hope: Indigenous Resource Management in a Changing Pacific*. ANU Press.

Lock, M. (1980a). The organization and practice of East Asian medicine in Japan: Continuity and change. *Social Science and Medicine, 14B*, 245–53.

Lock, M. M. (1980b). *East Asian Medicine in Urban Japan: Varieties of Medical Experience*. University of California Press.

Lockyer, J., Carraccio, C., Chan, M. K., Hart, D., Smee, S., Touchie, C., ... & ICBME Collaborators. (2017). Core principles of assessment in competency-based medical education. *Medical Teacher, 39*(6), 609–616.

Long, N. T. (1973). *Before the Revolution: The Vietnamese Peasants under the French*. Columbia University Press.

Lu, J. R., & Chiang, T. L. (2011). Evolution of Taiwan's health care system. *Health Economics, Policy and Law, 6*, 85–107.

Lu, M. C., Lo, H. C., Chang, H. H., Hsu, C. W., & Koo, M. (2021). Factors associated with the use of complementary therapies in Taiwanese patients with systemic lupus erythematosus: A cross-sectional study. *BMC Complementary Medicine and Therapies, 21*, 1–15.

Ma, T. P. (2024). Considerations for implementation of a competency-based education program for preclerkship courses. In J. R. Schoenherr, & M. M. McConnell (eds.), *Fundamentals and Frontiers of Medical Education and Decision-Making* (pp. 37–79). Routledge.

Maeng, W. et al. (2006). *General History of Korean Medicine*. Daesung Publish Company.

Marginson, S. (2011). Higher education in East Asia and Singapore: Rise of the Confucian model. *Higher Education, 61*, 587–611.

Marr, D. G. (1987). Vietnamese attitudes regarding illness and healing. In N. G. Owen (Ed.), *Death and Disease in Southeast Asia: Explorations in Social, Medical and Demographic History*. Asian Studies Association of Australia Southeast Asia Publications Series, no. 14. Oxford University Press.

McConnell, M. M. (2024). Emotions and clinical decision-making. In J. R. Schoenherr & M. M. McConnell (Eds.), *Fundamentals and Frontiers of Medical Education and Decision-Making* (pp. 139–168). Routledge.

McCulloch, W. S. (1945). A heterarchy of values determined by the topology of nervous nets. *Bulletin of Mathematical Biophysics, 7*, 89–93.

Meng, K. H. (2020). History of the medical education accreditation system in Korea: Implementation and activities in the early stages. *Journal of Educational Evaluation for Health Professions, 17, 1–18.*

Mesoudi, A., Whiten, A., & Laland, K. N. (2006). Towards a unified science of cultural evolution. *Behavioral and Brain Sciences, 29*(4), 329–347.

Miller, K. A., Miller, D. A., & Doeksen, G. A. (1989). A model to determine the feasibility of a pediatric practice. *American Journal of Diseases of Children, 143*(8), 919–923.

Millington, S. J., Arntfield, R. T., Guo, R. J., Koenig, S., Kory, P., Noble, V., ... & Schoenherr, J. R. (2018). Expert agreement in the interpretation of lung ultrasound studies performed on mechanically ventilated patients. *Journal of Ultrasound in Medicine, 37*(11), 2659–2665.

Min, H. J., Ryu, J. S., & Yun, Y. J. (2012). Changes in the attitudes of doctors toward cooperative practices between western medicine and traditional Korean medicine-a systematic review in Korean literature. *Journal of Society of Preventive Korean Medicine, 16*(1), 15–29.

Ministry of Education and Human Resources (2002). *Plans for the Introduction of Graduate Systems to Medical and Dental Programs*. Ministry of Education and Human Resources.

Ministry of Education and Training of Vietnam (MOET). (2001a). *Curriculum of General Practitioner Training Program – 4 Years*. Hanoi: MOET.

Ministry of Education and Training of Vietnam (MOET). (2001b). *Curriculum of General Practitioner Training Program – 6 years*. Hanoi: MOET.

Ministry of Health (MOH). (2008). *Decision on Quota for Training of Medical Students*. Hanoi: Ministry of Health of Vietnam.

Monnais, L., Thompson, C. M., & Wahlberg, A. (Eds.). (2011). *Southern Medicine for Southern People: Vietnamese Medicine in the Making*. Cambridge Scholars Publishing.

Moore, C. C. (1988). An optimal scaling of Murdock's theories of illness data—An approach to the problem of interdependence. *Behavior Science Research, 22*(1–4), 161–179.

Morgan, T. J., Uomini, N. T., Rendell, L. E., Chouinard-Thuly, L., Street, S. E., Lewis, H. M., ... & Laland, K. N. (2015). Experimental evidence for the co-evolution of hominin tool-making teaching and language. *Nature Communications, 6*(1), 6029.

Moschik, E. C., Mercado, C., Yoshino, T., Matsuura, K., & Watanabe, K. (2012). Usage and attitudes of physicians in Japan concerning traditional Japanese medicine (kampo medicine): A descriptive evaluation of a representative questionnaire-based survey. *Evidence-Based Complementary and Alternative Medicine, 2012*(1), 139818.

Motoo, Y., Arai, I., Hyodo, I., & Tsutani, K. (2009). Current status of Kampo (Japanese Herbal) medicines in Japanese clinical practice guidelines. *Complementary Therapies in Medicine, 17*, 147–154.

Motoo, Y., Seki, T., & Tsutani, K. (2011). Traditional Japanese medicine, Kampo: Its history and current status. *Chinese Journal of Integrative Medicine, 17*, 85–87.

Muramatsu, S-I, Aihara, M., Shimizu, I., Arai, M., & Kajii, E. (2012). Current status of Kampo medicine in community health care. *General Medicine, 13*, 37–45.

Murdock, G. P. (1980). *Theories of Illness: A World Survey*. University of Pittsburgh Pre.

Murdock, G. P., Wilson, S. F., & Frederick, V. (1978). World distribution of theories of illness. *Ethnology, 17*, 449–470.

Myers, B. R. (2011). *The Cleanest Race: How North Koreans see Themselves and Why It Matters*. Melville House.

Na, S. (2012). East Asian medicine in South Korea. *Harvard Asia Quarterly, 14*(4), 44.

Namiki, T., & Nagamine, K. (2012). Present situation and problems of education in Kampo medicine for undergraduate students and postgraduate doctors in Japan. *Journal of Traditional Medicines, 29*, 46–48.

Needham, J., & Gwei-Djen, L. (1962). China and the origin of qualifying examinations in medicine. In J. Needham (Ed.), *Clerks and Craftsman in China and the West: Lectures and Addresses on the History of Science and Technology* (pp. 379–395). Cambridge University Press.

Nguyen, X. T. (1993). A glimpse of the traditional medicines of animal origin. In H. B. Chau, P. D. Thuc, & H. Ngoc (Eds.), *Vietnamese Traditional Medicine* (pp. 144–156). The Gioi Publishers.

Nisbett, R. (2004). *The Geography of Thought: How Asians and Westerners Think Differently... and Why*. Simon and Schuster.

Noland, M., Robinson, S., & Wang, T. (2001). Famine in North Korea: Causes and cures. *Economic Development and Cultural Change*, *49*(4), 741–767.

Ock, S. M., Choi, J. Y., Cha, Y. S., Lee, J., Chun, M. S., Huh, C. H., ... & Lee, S. J. (2009). The use of complementary and alternative medicine in a general population in South Korea: Results from a national survey in 2006. *Journal of Korean Medical Science*, *24*(1), 1–6.

Oh, C., & Shin, D.-W. (2023). How did the clinical medicine progress during the Unified Silla Era: Installment of the medical education center 'Uihak 醫學', and its effects. *Korean Journal of Medical History*, *32*(1), 203–239.

Ohnuki-Tierney, E. (1981). *Illness and Healing among the Sakhalin Ainu: A Symbolic Interpretation*. CUP Archive.

Ohnuki-Tierney, E. (1984). *Illness and Culture in Contemporary Japan: An Anthropological View*. Cambridge University Press.

Olsen, J. W., & Miller-Antonio, S. (1992). The palaeolithic in southern China. *Asian Perspectives*, 31, 129–160.

Onishi, H. (2018). History of Japanese medical education. *Korean Journal of Medical Education*, *30*(4), 283.

O'Regan, S., Molloy, E., Watterson, L., & Nestel, D. (2016). Observer roles that optimise learning in healthcare simulation education: A systematic review. *Advances in Simulation*, *1*, 1–10.

Oyebode, O., Kandala, N. B., Chilton, P. J., & Lilford, R. J. (2016). Use of traditional medicine in middle-income countries: A WHO-SAGE study. *Health Policy and Planning*, *31*(8), 984–991.

Ozioma, E. O. J., & Chinwe, O. A. N. (2019). Herbal medicines in African traditional medicine. *Herbal Medicine*, *10*, 191–214.

Panova, E. I. (2019). The categories of health and disease in evolution of paradigms of medicine. *Sociology of Medicine*, *18*, 110–117.

Park, J. E., Kim, K. H., Kang, S., Lee, E. K., Kim, J. C., Jang, B. H., ... & Ko, S. G. (2019). Usage status and satisfaction with pharmacopuncture in Korea: A survey among Korean medicine doctors. *European Journal of Integrative Medicine*, *27*, 121–130–76.

Park, K. H., Park, J. H., Kim, S., Rhee, J., Kim, J. H., Ahn, Y. J., ... & Suh, D. J. (2015). Students' perception of the educational environment of medical schools in Korea: Findings from a nationwide survey. *Korean Journal of Medical Education*, *27*, 117–130.

Park, Y. (2012). Formation and Development of North Korean Medical Care (북한의료의 형성과 발전). In Yeo, I. et al., *History of Korean Medicine*. Yeonglim Cardinal.

Park, Y., & Park, H. (1998). A study on the medical education system in North Korea (북한의 의학교육제도 연구), 7, *Medical History* (醫史學), 7–1.

Park, Y. J., & Park, H. W. (1998). A study on medical educational system in North Korea [Korean]. *Korean Journal of Medical History*, *7*(1), 63.

Park, Y. L., Huang, C. W., Sasaki, Y. et al. (2016). Comparative study on the education system of traditional medicine in China, Japan, Korea, and Taiwan. *EXPLORE: The Journal of Science and Healing, 12*, 375–383.

Park, Y. S., Park, S. M., Jun, J. Y., & Kim, S. J. (2014). Psychiatry in former socialist countries: Implications for North Korean psychiatry. *Psychiatry Investigation, 11*, 363–370.

Park, H.-L., Lee, H.-S., Shin, B.-C., et al. (2012). Traditional medicine in China, Korea, and Japan: A brief introduction and comparison. *Evidence-Based Complementary and Alternative Medicine*, 2012, 429103.

Pyo, C. K. (1987). The significance of Dongje Medical School in medical history. *Journal of Korean Medical Classic*, *1*, 16–18.

Redvers, N., & Blondin, B. S. (2020). Traditional Indigenous medicine in North America: A scoping review. *PloS One*, *15*(8), e0237531.

Rhi, B. Y., Ha, K. S., Kim, Y. S., Sasaki, Y., Young, D., Woon, T. H., ... & Yanchun, Y. (1995). The health care seeking behavior of schizophrenic patients in 6 East Asian areas. *International Journal of Social Psychiatry*, *41*(3), 190–209.

Rodriguez, M., Parola, R., Andreola, S., Pereyra, C., & Martínez-Noël, G. (2019). TOR and SnRK1 signaling pathways in plant response to abiotic stresses: Do they always act according to the "yin-yang" model? *Plant Science*, *288*, 110220.

Rosch, E. H. (1973). On the internal structure of perceptual and semantic categories. In *Cognitive Development and Acquisition of Language* (pp. 111–144). Academic Press.

Ross, B., & Del Maestro, R. F. (2023). From Canadian surgeon to Chinese Martyr: Dr. Norman Bethune and the making of a medical folk hero. *Journal of the History of Medicine and Allied Sciences*, 79, jrad053.

Saad, B., Azaizeh, H., & Said, O. (2005). Tradition and perspectives of Arab herbal medicine: A review. *Evidence-Based Complementary and Alternative Medicine*, *2*, 475–479.

Saiki, T., Imafuku, R., Suzuki, Y., & Ban, N. (2017). The truth lies somewhere in the middle: swinging between globalization and regionalization of medical education in Japan. *Medical Teacher*, *39*(10), 1016–1022.

Schoenherr, J. R. (2017). Prestige technology in the evolution and social organization of early psychological science. *Theory & Psychology*, *27*(1), 6–33.

Schoenherr, J. R. (2019). Moral economies and codes of conduct: The social organization of Canadian experimental psychology. *Scientia Canadensis*, *41*(1), 31–54.

Schoenherr, J. R. (2021). Trust and explainability in A/IS-mediated healthcare: Operationalizing the therapeutic alliance in a distributed system. In *2021 IEEE International Symposium on Technology and Society (ISTAS)* (pp. 1–8). IEEE.

Schoenherr, J. R. (2022). Vaccination, values, and health information search behaviour in the New Folk Medicine. In *2022 IEEE International Symposium on Technology and Society (ISTAS)* (Vol. *1*, pp. 1–10). IEEE.

Schoenherr, J. R. (2027a). Innovation and implementation in health professions education and healthcare delivery. In J. R. Schoenherr (Ed.), *Fundamentals and Frontiers in Medical Education and Decision-Making: Innovation, Implementation, and Translational Research*. Routledge.

Schoenherr, J. R. (2027b). The development and dynamics of the heterarchical structure of Mayan medical education and healthcare ecosystem. In Schoenherr, J. R. (Ed.), *Fundamentals and Frontiers of Medical Education and Decision-Making: Innovation, Implementation, and Translational Research*. Routledge.

Schoenherr, J. R. (2027c). Human-centered artificial intelligence in health professions education and decision-making: A sociotechnical systems perspective. In Schoenherr, J. R. (Eds.), *Fundamentals and Frontiers of Medical Education and Decision-Making: Innovation, Implementation, and Translational Research*. Routledge.

Schoenherr, J. R., Chiou, E., & Goldshtein, M. (2023). Building trust with the ethical affordances of education technologies: A sociotechnical systems perspective. In Llinas et al. (Eds.), *Putting AI in the Critical Loop*. Elsevier.

Schoenherr, J. R., & Dopko, R. L. (2019). Heterarchical social organizations and relational models: Understanding gender biases in psychological science. *Theory & Psychology, 29*(2), 258–281.

Schoenherr, J. R., & Hamstra, S. J. (2017). Beyond fidelity: Deconstructing the seductive simplicity of fidelity in simulator-based education in the health care professions. *Simulation in Healthcare, 12*(2), 117–123.

Schoenherr, J. R., & Hamstra, S. J. (2024). Validity in health professions education: From assessment instruments to program innovation and evaluation. In Schoenherr, J. R. & McConnell, M. (Eds.), *Fundamentals and Frontiers of Medical Education and Decision-Making: Educational Theory and Psychological Practice*. Routledge.

Schoenherr, J. R., & Le Bouar, C. (2024). Communication in healthcare settings: From normal interpersonal processes to social networks during health crises. In Schoenherr, J. R. & McConnell, M. (Eds.), *Fundamentals and Frontiers of Medical Education and Decision-Making: Educational Theory and Psychological Practice*. Routledge.

Schoenherr, J. R., Mahias-Ito, I., & Li, X. (2027). Collective competence in the health professions: Learning, thinking, and deciding in groups. In J. R. Schoenherr (Ed.), *Fundamentals and Frontiers of Medical Education and Decision-Making: Innovation, Implementation, and Translational Research*. Routledge.

Schoenherr, J. R., & McConnell, M. (2024). Human-centered design in health professions education: Informing competency-based education with psychological science. In J. R. Schoenherr & M. McConnell (Eds.), *Fundamentals and Frontiers of Medical Education and Decision-Making: Educational Theory and Psychological Practice*. Routledge.

Shelton, T. V. (2020). *Herbs and Roots: A History of Chinese Doctors in the American Medical Marketplace*. Yale University Press.

Shih, C. C., Su, Y. C., Liao, C. C., & Lin, J. G. (2010). Patterns of medical pluralism among adults: Results from the 2001 National Health Interview Survey in Taiwan. *BMC Health Services Research, 10*, 1–9.

Shim, J.-M. (2016). The relationship between the use of complementary and alternative medicine and the use of biomedical services: Evidence from East Asian medical systems. *Asia-Pacific Journal of Public Health, 28*, 51–60.

Shim, J.-M., & Kim, J. (2016). Cross-national differences in the holistic use of traditional East Asian medicine in East Asia. *Health Promotion International, 33*, 1–9.

Shim, J.-M., & Kim, J. (2018). Cross-national differences in the holistic use of traditional East Asian medicine in East Asia. *Health Promotion International, 33*(3), 536–544.

Shin, D. (2008). How four different political systems have shaped the modernization of traditional Korean medicine between 1900 and 1960. *Historia Scientiarum, 17*, 225–41.

Shin, D. (2010). The difficult road to success as a medical officer. In *Kyujanggak Institute for Korean Studies, Life of a Joseon Expert*. Geuljar.

Sica, A., Invernizzi, P., & Mantovani, A. (2014). Macrophage plasticity and polarization in liver homeostasis and pathology. *Hepatology, 59*(5), 2034–2042.

Sinclair, S. (1997). *Making Doctors: An Institutional Apprenticeship*. Berg.

Soon, W. (2024). Health insurance, medicine, and society in Taiwan: Chinese authoritarianism, Taiwanese ethnicities, and global actuarial science. *East Asian Science, Technology and Society: An International Journal, 18*, 389–412.

Starr, P. (1982). *The Social Transformation of American Medicine*. Basic Books, Inc.

Stevenson, F. A., Britten, N., Barry, C. A., Bradley, C. P., & Barber, N. (2003). Self-treatment and its discussion in medical consultations: How is medical pluralism managed in practice? *Social Science & Medicine, 57*(3), 513–527.

Suh, S. (2015). *Reconstructing Bodies: Biomedicine, Health, and Nation-Building in South Korea since 1945*. Stanford University Press.

Suh, S. (2020). *Naming the Local: Medicine, Language, and Identity in Korea since the Fifteenth Century* (Vol. *404*). BRILL.

Tangkiatkumjai, M., Boardman, H., & Walker, D. M. (2020). Potential factors that influence usage of complementary and alternative medicine worldwide: A systematic review. *BMC Complementary Medicine and Therapies*, *20*, 1–15.

Taylor, K. (2004). *Chinese Medicine in Early Communist China, 1945-63: A Medicine of Revolution*. Psychology Press.

Thompson, M. C. (2001). Mission to Macau: Smallpox, vaccinia, and the Nguyen Dynasty. *Portuguese Studies Review*, *9*(1 & 2; Special Issue *The Evolution of Portuguese Asia*), 1498–1998.

Thompson, C. M. (2017). The implications of gia truyền: Family transmission texts, medical authors, and social class within the healing community in Vietnam. *South East Asia Research*, *25*(1), 34–46.

Touchie, C., & ten Cate, O. (2016). The promise, perils, problems and progress of competency-based medical education. *Medical Education*, *50*(1), 93–100.

Trambaiolo, D. (2013). Native and foreign in Tokugawa medicine. *The Journal of Japanese Studies*, *39*, 299–324.

Trejaut, J. A., Poloni, E. S., Yen, J. C., Lai, Y. H., Loo, J. H., Lee, C. L., ... & Lin, M. (2014). Taiwan Y-chromosomal DNA variation and its relationship with Island Southeast Asia. *BMC Genetics*, *15*(1), 1–23.

Tsai, P. S., Ke, T. L., Huang, C. J., Hsaio, F. H., Wang, M. Y., & Cheng, Y. H. (2006). Demographic characteristics and perceived health status of users of folk therapies in Taiwan. *Journal of Alternative & Complementary Medicine*, *12*(6), 549–554.

Tsai, P. S., Lee, P. H., & Wang, M. Y. (2008). Demographics, training, and practice patterns of practitioners of folk medicine in Taiwan: A survey of the Taipei metropolitan area. *The Journal of Alternative and Complementary Medicine*, *14*(10), 1243–1248.

Tsang, C. H. (2005). Recent discoveries at the Tapenkeng Culture Sites in Taiwan: Implications for the problem of Austronesian origins. In L. Sagart, R. Blench, & A. Sanchez-Mazas (Eds.), *The Peopling of East Asia: Putting Together Archaeology, Linguistics, and Genetics* (pp. 63–73). Routledge Curzon.

Tsurumi, E. P. (1977). *Japanese Colonial Education in Taiwan, 1895–1945*. Harvard University Press.

Venosa, A. R., Baroneza, J. E., & Fernandes, R. A. F. (2027). Medical Education in Brazil: A History of An Evolving Pluralistic Health Care System. In J. R. Schoenherr (Ed.), *Fundamentals and Frontiers of Medical Education and Decision-Making: Innovation, Implementation, and Translational Research* (pp. 310–335). Routledge.

Wade, D. T., & Halligan, P. W. (2017). The biopsychosocial model of illness: A model whose time has come. *Clinical Rehabilitation*, *31*(8), 995–1004.

Wagstaff, A. (2007). Health systems in East Asia: What can developing countries learn from Japan and the Asian Tigers? *Health Economics*, *16*, 441–456.

Wahlberg, A. (2006). Bio-politics and the promotion of traditional herbal medicine in Vietnam. *Health*, *10*, 123–147.

Wahlberg, A. (2007). A quackery with a difference—New medical pluralism and the problem of 'dangerous practitioners' in the United Kingdom. *Social Science & Medicine*, *65*(11), 2307–2316.

Wang, W. (2021). Medical education in China: Progress in the past 70 years and a vision for the future. *BMC Medical Education*, *21*(1), 453.

Welch, A. (2019). Higher education in Asia. In L. Rury & E. H. Tamura (Eds.), *The Oxford Handbook of the History of Education* (pp. 302–315).

World Bank (2014). *Vietnam Health Professionals Education and Training for Health System Reforms Project Appraisal Document.*

World Health Organization (WHO) (2002). *WHO Traditional Medicine Strategy 2002–2005.* World Health Organization, Switzerland.

World Health Organization (WHO) (2019). *WHO Global Report on Traditional and Complementary Medicine 2019.* Integrated Health Services (IHS), Traditional, Complementary and Integrative Medicine (TCI).

World Health Organization (WHO) (2022). *Global Competency and Outcomes Framework for Universal Health Coverage*. World Health Organization.

World Health Organization (WHO) (2023). *WHO Traditional Medicine Strategy 2014–2023.* World Health Organization, Switzerland.

World Health Organization. Regional Office for the Western Pacific (2015). Republic of Korea health system review. *Health Systems in Transition, 5*(4), WHO Regional Office for the Western Pacific.

Wu, A. C. C., & Hu, Y. H. (1980). Many ways to health: A study of 2,000 rural and urban Taiwan families. *The American Journal of Chinese Medicine*, *8*, 313–330.

Wu, L., Wang, Y., Peng, X., Song, M., Guo, X., Nelson, H., & Wang, W. (2014). Development of a medical academic degree system in China. *Medical Education Online*, *19*, 23141.

Xu, J., & Yang, Y. (2009). Traditional Chinese medicine in the Chinese health care system. *Health Policy*, *90*, 133–139.

Yang, E. B. (2002). A study on the classification validity and predictive validity of accreditation standards for medical schools in Korea. *Korean Journal of Medical Education*, *14*(2), 213–226.

Yeh, Y. H., Chou, Y. J., Huang, N., Pu, C., & Chou, P. (2016). The trends of utilization in traditional Chinese medicine in Taiwan from 2000 to 2010: A population-based study. *Medicine*, *95*(27).

Yim, Y. S., Sohn, I. C., Kang, Y. S., Kim, S. C., & Kim, J. H. (2009). Archeological Quest on the origin and formation of the stone needle in the Korean Peninsula. *Korean Journal of Oriental Medicine*, *15*(2), 51–61.

Yoo, H. H., Kim, M. K., Yoon, Y. S., Lee, K. M., Lee, J. H., Hong, S. J., ... & Park, W. K. (2020). Changes in the accreditation standards of medical schools by the Korean Institute of Medical Education and Evaluation from 2000 to 2019. *Journal of Educational Evaluation for Health Professions*, *17, 1–10.*

Yoon, K.-J., & Kim, D.-S. (2013). *Ways of Integrating Oriental Medicine and Western Medicine*. Korea Institute of Health and Social Affairs.

Young, J. C., & Garro, L. (1982). Variation in the choice of treatment in two Mexican communities. *Social Science & Medicine, 16*(16), 1453–1465.

Yun, K. (2019). *The Shaman's Wages: Trading in Ritual on Cheju Island.* University of Washington Press.

Zhang, X., Tan, R., Lam, W. C., Yao, L., Wang, X., Cheng, C. W., ... & Bian, Z. (2020). PRISMA (preferred reporting items for systematic reviews and meta-analyses) extension for Chinese herbal medicines 2020 (PRISMA-CHM 2020). *The American Journal of Chinese Medicine*, *48*(06), 1279–1313.

Zhu, J., Li, W., & Chen, L. (2016). Doctors in China: Improving quality through modernisation of residency education. *The Lancet*, *388*(10054), 1922–1929.

INDEX

Note: Page references in *italics* indicate figures. Page references in **bold** indicate tables. Page number followed by b and n indicates box and end notes.